Fourth Edition

HUMAN
DISEASES

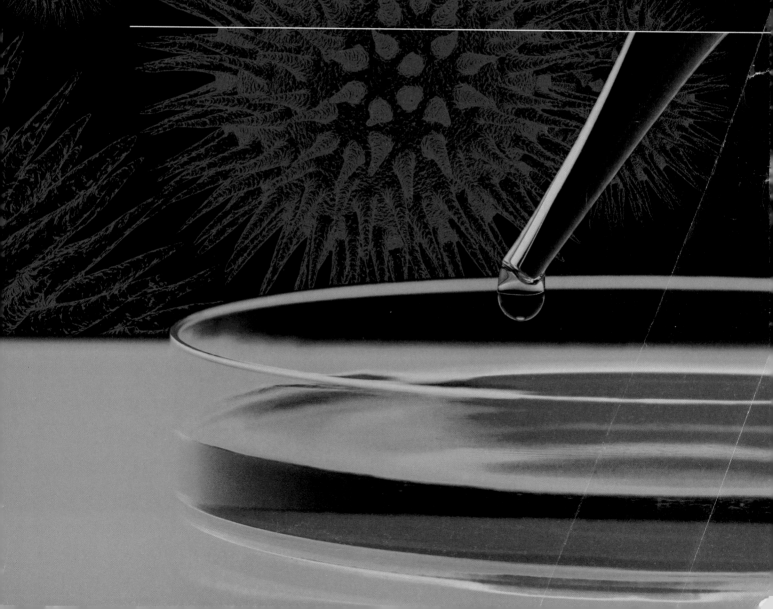

Fourth Edition

HUMAN DISEASES

Marianne Neighbors, EdD, RN

Ruth Tannehill-Jones, MS, RN

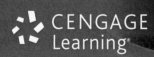

CENGAGE
Learning®

Australia • Brazil • Japan • Korea • Mexico • Singapore • Spain • United Kingdom • United States

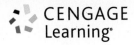

Human Diseases, Fourth Edition
Marianne Neighbors and Ruth Tannehill-Jones

Senior VP/General Manager, Skills & Product Planning: Dawn Gerrain

Product Director, Health Care Skills: Stephen Helba

Product Team Manager: Matthew Seeley

Senior Director, Development: Marah Bellegarde

Product Development Manager, Health Care Skills: Juliet Steiner

Senior Content Developer, Health Care Skills: Debra M. Myette-Flis

Product Assistant: Jennifer Wheaton

Marketing Brand Manager: Wendy Mapstone

Senior Production Director: Wendy Troeger

Production Manager: Andrew Crouth

Content Project Manager: Thomas Heffernan

Senior Art Director: Jack Pendleton

Cover image(s): iStock.com/traffic_analyzer

For product information and technology assistance, contact us at
Cengage Learning Customer & Sales Support, 1-800-354-9706
For permission to use material from this text or product,
submit all requests online at **www.cengage.com/permissions**.
Further permissions questions can be e-mailed to
permissionrequest@cengage.com

Library of Congress Control Number: 2013948334

ISBN-13: 978-1-2850-6592-2

Cengage Learning
200 First Stamford Place, 4th Floor
Stamford, CT 06902
USA

Cengage Learning is a leading provider of customized learning solutions with office locations around the globe, including Singapore, the United Kingdom, Australia, Mexico, Brazil, and Japan. Locate your local office at: **www.cengage.com/global**

Cengage Learning products are represented in Canada by Nelson Education, Ltd.

To learn more about Cengage Learning, visit **www.cengage.com**

Purchase any of our products at your local college store or at our preferred online store **www.cengagebrain.com**

Notice to the Reader

Publisher does not warrant or guarantee any of the products described herein or perform any independent analysis in connection with any of the product information contained herein. Publisher does not assume, and expressly disclaims, any obligation to obtain and include information other than that provided to it by the manufacturer. The reader is expressly warned to consider and adopt all safety precautions that might be indicated by the activities described herein and to avoid all potential hazards. By following the instructions contained herein, the reader willingly assumes all risks in connection with such instructions. The publisher makes no representations or warranties of any kind, including, but not limited to, the warranties of fitness for particular purpose or merchantability, nor are any such representations implied with respect to the material set forth herein, and the publisher takes no responsibility with respect to such material. The publisher shall not be liable for any special, consequential, or exemplary damages resulting, in whole or part, from the readers' use of, or reliance upon, this material.

Printed in the United States of America
2 3 4 5 6 7 8 18 17 16 15 14

To my husband, Larry Butler, who is my inspiration and computer guru. I love you and thank you. Marianne

To my husband, Jim, the quiet, solid, love of my life for over 40 years, and to the other man in my life, my brother Bob Tannehill, who has always loved and supported me "his younger, little sister." Ruth

Contents

List of Tables

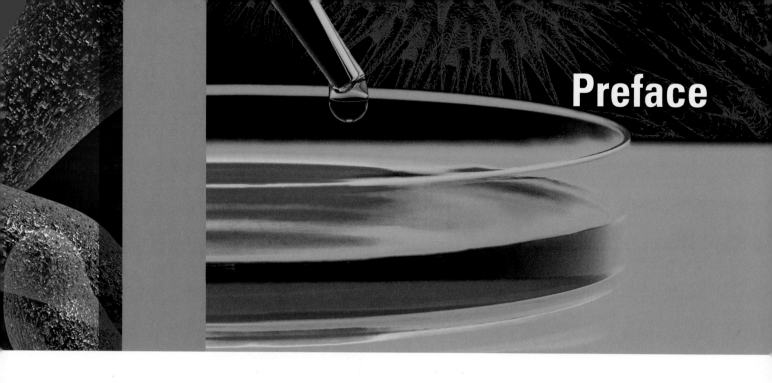

Preface

As the medical field has undergone an explosion in new techniques and therapies, there has been a matched explosion in the need for technicians, patient care providers, and general health care professionals to support this growth. These new and developing careers assist and support physicians in a variety of health care settings and include nurses, medical assistants, nursing assistants, surgical technologists, respiratory therapy assistants, physical therapy assistants, radiographic technologists, medical transcriptionists, medical office assistants, and emergency medical technicians, to name only a few.

■ APPROACH

Many pathophysiology books have been written to address the informational needs of the medical community, but few basic disease textbooks exist for the benefit of the health care professional, especially those in allied health care disciplines. This book has been designed and written specifically for this group. It is intended to meet the needs of the student in the classroom as well as serve as a valuable resource for health care professionals on the job. In addition, this text may be used as a resource on basic diseases by anyone within the medical arena or lay community. Current information for this book was based on the authors' own experiences and research sought from current literature, books, Internet resources, and physician consultations. Students will understand this text best if a basic medical terminology or anatomy

and physiology course has been completed before this course of study.

Several dilemmas immediately emerge when one considers writing a textbook for such a large and diverse audience as the health care field. Questions arise as to how much content to include, what to exclude, how detailed the content should be, and how to organize the content in the most understandable manner. Another common concern is the question of the appropriate reading level.

In an attempt to resolve these dilemmas, it was decided to organize the book in such a way that blocks of material or even entire chapters could be omitted or covered in detail, depending on the format of the class and needs of the student. At the same time, information on each disease is written in such a way that it can stand alone or be viewed as all inclusive. This concept allows the instructor, student, or individual to select and study only those specific diseases or individual disease of interest. Not all health conditions are covered in the text, so the conditions chosen to be included are those that are most common, along with the new and emerging diseases. A few rare conditions are also included. Of the conditions chosen for the text, only general information is covered. The text is designed to be a basic overview of common diseases and disorders, not an in-depth study. Thus, the diseases presented are not described on a cellular physiological level, which would be too complex for the intended audience. The intention also was to keep the reading level of the text at an easy-to-read basic level to promote understanding. We did not want to write beneath the level of the student but, at the same time, felt that a difficult reading level would only increase the complexity of the material and thus fail to promote understanding of the subject matter.

ORGANIZATION OF THE TEXT

Human Diseases, Fourth Edition, consists of 21 chapters organized into three units. Unit I, Chapters 1 through 4, lays the foundation for some basic disease concepts, including mechanisms of disease, neoplasms, inflammation, and infection. Unit II, Chapters 5 through 18, is organized by body systems, and opens with a basic Anatomy and Physiology review of the system before discussion of the Common System Diseases and Disorders. Included with this discussion, where appropriate, are Common Signs and Symptoms, Diagnostic Tests, Trauma, and Rare Diseases. In addition, a unique section toward the end of each chapter discusses the Effects of Aging to help learners understand the natural aging process of the human body. Unit III, Chapters 19 through 21, includes specialty areas covering genetics, childhood diseases, and mental health disorders. Each disease is broken down into Description, Etiology, Symptoms, Diagnosis, Treatment, and Prevention (where applicable). Although this might appear to be very title-heavy when there is only a sentence or two under each, it will assist the reader to clearly identify these components of each disease. It also maintains consistency throughout the textbook.

Several features were especially developed to promote learning and accessibility of information. Review the "How to Use" on page xxii for a detailed description and benefit of each feature.

CHANGES TO THE FOURTH EDITION

Major changes to the fourth edition include:

- All new "Glimpse of the Future" boxes that detail cutting-edge information or treatments
- All new "Complementary and Alternative Therapy" boxes that discuss herbal and other nontraditional treatments
- All new "Consider This" comments to enlighten and entertain the reader
- Some additional Healthy Highlight boxes added

- More illustrations replaced with color photographs to enhance understanding of the diseases and disorders presented in the text
- Disease statistics updated to reflect the latest statistics available
- New diagnostic tests added
- Changes in some case studies to better reflect chapter information
- Bibliographies updated to include references used in each chapter

LEARNING SUPPLEMENTS

Workbook

ISBN 978-1-2850-6593-9
The workbook offers additional practice with exercises corresponding to each chapter in the book, including multiple choice, fill-in-the-blank, true/false, short answer, and matching questions.

ONLINE RESOURCES

A student companion website is available to accompany the text that includes slide presentations created in Microsoft PowerPoint, and anatomy, physiology, and pathophysiology animations.

Accessing the student companion website:

1. Go to http://www.CengageBrain.com.
2. Register as a new user or log in as an existing user if you already have an account with Cengage Learning or CengageBrain.com.
3. Select **Go to MY Account.**
4. Open the product from the My Account page.

INSTRUCTOR COMPANION SITE

Comprehensive instructor tools are designed to assist you in teaching the content.

- The Instructor's Manual includes a sample course syllabus and outline as a guide for setting up a course. Additional materials for each chapter include detailed content outlines, learning objectives, expanded chapter summaries, discussion topics, learning activities, answers to the text review questions, answers to the workbook activities, and chapter tests with answer keys.

- Conversion Grid to help you change previously developed curriculum to this text.
- Cognero Testbank contains 1,000 questions. You can use these questions to create your own tests.
- Instructor slides created in Microsoft PowerPoint® are designed to help you plan your class presentations. Images within the presentation enhance your lectures.

ABOUT THE AUTHORS

Ruth Tannehill-Jones worked as a registered nurse for more than 30 years. She began her nursing education at the University of Arkansas, Fayetteville, with completion of an associate degree in nursing. Ms. Tannehill-Jones was not a newcomer to this campus; she had previously completed a bachelor's degree in home economics some years previous. On receiving her RN license, she worked at St. Mary-Rogers Memorial Hospital in the capacities of staff nurse, head nurse, and nursing supervisor. Her other nursing experience includes assisting orthopedic surgeons while employed by Ozark Orthopedic and Sports Medicine Clinic located in the Northwest Arkansas area. Ms. Tannehill-Jones gained experience in education by working as an instructor of surgical technology while serving as the Divisional Chair of Nursing and Allied Health Programs at Northwest Technical Institute in Springdale, Arkansas. She obtained her bachelor's degree in nursing from Missouri Southern State College in Joplin and her master's degree in health service administration at Southwest Baptist University in Bolivar, Missouri. She worked for St. Mary's—Mercy Health System for more than 20 years in a variety of nursing positions with her last position being Vice President of Patient Care Services, Chief Nurse Executive. Ms. Tannehill-Jones retired from Regency Hospital of Northwest Arkansas in 2011.

Dr. Marianne Neighbors has been in nursing practice and nursing education for more than 40 years. She received her bachelor's degree in nursing at Mankato State, a master's degree in health education at the University of Arkansas, a master's degree in nursing at the University of Oklahoma, and a doctoral degree in education with a focus on health science at the University of Arkansas. Dr. Neighbors has taught in associate degree nursing education for 18 years, focusing on medical/surgical nursing, and in baccalaureate nursing education for 23 years, focusing on health promotion and community health. She also taught advanced health promotion and nurse educator classes at the master's level. She has coauthored many research articles; four medical/surgical nursing texts, along with two medical/surgical handbooks; a health assessment handbook; and a home health handbook. Dr. Neighbors has also written chapters for other nursing authors' books. She is currently an Emeritus professor in the Eleanor Mann School of Nursing at the University of Arkansas, Fayetteville, Arkansas.

ACKNOWLEDGMENTS

A special thanks goes out to all our colleagues, friends, and family members who have supported us throughout this project.

Feedback from the User(s)

The authors would like to hear from instructors, learners, or anyone using the textbook about its strengths and/or suggestions for revisions. They are truly interested in making the textbook user friendly and comprehensive but not too detailed or too in-depth for the reader. The authors want to know how the text is being used and what features are most helpful. Please feel free to forward comments to the authors through Cengage Learning or directly by e-mail to Dr. Neighbors at neighbo@uark.edu and Ms. Tannehill-Jones at rjonesnwark@hotmail.com.

Marianne Neighbors, EdD, RN
Ruth Tannehill-Jones, MS, RN

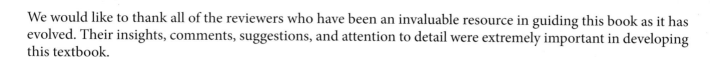

Reviewers

We would like to thank all of the reviewers who have been an invaluable resource in guiding this book as it has evolved. Their insights, comments, suggestions, and attention to detail were extremely important in developing this textbook.

Carole Berube, MA, MSN, BSN, RN
Professor Emerita in Nursing

Cheri Goretti, MA, MT(ASCP), CMA(AAMA)
Professor and Coordinator
Medical Assisting and Allied Health Programs
Quinebaug Valley Community College

Deborah Cipale, RN, MSN
Coordinator, Nursing Resource Lab/Online Adjunct Professor
Des Moines Area Community College

Jaime Nguyen, MD, MPH, MS, RMA
Director of Health Care Education
National College

Michael Volz, MS
Assistant Professor of Biology
Rock Valley College

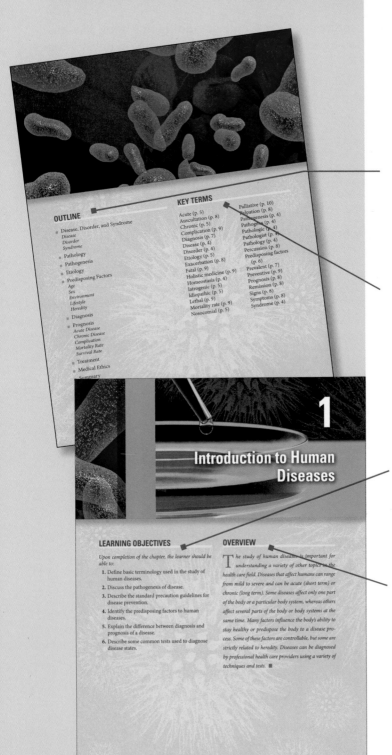

Human Diseases, Fourth Edition, helps you learn basic disease information. The following features are integrated throughout the text to assist you in learning and mastering human disease core concepts and terms.

■ OUTLINE

The content outline provides you with an overview of concepts by presenting the major topics you will learn in the chapter.

■ KEY TERMS

A list of key terms at the beginning of each chapter references the page number where each term can be found within the text. Turn to the page to understand the term used in context; turn to the glossary for the term definition. Within the text, the term is highlighted in color for easy identification.

■ LEARNING OBJECTIVES

The learning objectives alert you to concepts you should understand after reading the chapter and completing the review questions.

■ OVERVIEW

The overview provides a snapshot of the core concepts you will learn about in the chapter.

■ HEALTHY HIGHLIGHT

Healthy Highlight boxes include tips for health promotion and disease prevention. They are presented to help learners more fully understand how they, as health professionals, can help promote healthy living for themselves and their patients.

■ COMPLEMENTARY AND ALTERNATIVE THERAPY

This feature highlights information about treatments or special therapies that have research-based evidence of success. Many of these therapies are being used by consumers of health care and health care practitioners, either in combination with traditional therapy and medicines or as an alternative to traditional treatments. Some have been around for many years but might not have been used in this country, some are age-old remedies that only recently have been tested for effectiveness, and others are new discoveries. Some boxes also present material about therapies that are being promoted but might not be effective or for which there is not an evidence base for the therapy.

■ GLIMPSE OF THE FUTURE

This feature focuses on new procedures, medicines, or therapies that are presently being tested for usefulness in medical regimens or as alternative therapies. These cutting-edge treatments might soon be commonplace therapies.

■ END-OF-CHAPTER FEATURES

- The **Summary** is a succinct textual conclusion of basic chapter concepts. This differs from the overview because it consolidates the material rather than highlighting basic ideas.

- **Review Questions** reinforce material learned by testing comprehension through structured questions that directly relate to chapter content.

- The **Case Studies** present real-life scenarios that might occur in health care situations. Learners think critically about questions posed to arrive at a deeper understanding of the effects of pathological conditions. These scenarios often delve into critical ethical and legal issues. The cases could also be used for in-class discussions.

- The **Study Tools** feature directs you to additional practice activities in the Workbook, and PowerPoint® slides and animations on the Online Resources.

- The **bibliography** includes the references used in the chapter but also up-to-date articles and Internet sites for more information about content included in the chapter. It is a good resource for further reading for the instructor or students.

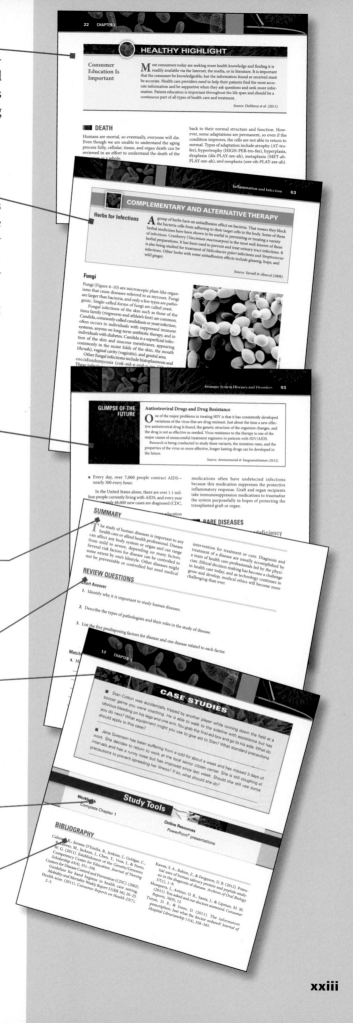

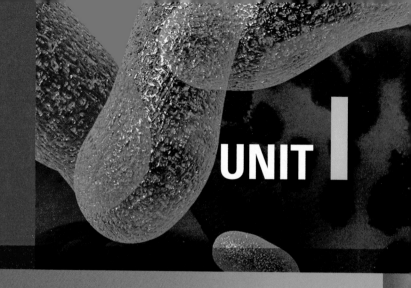

UNIT I

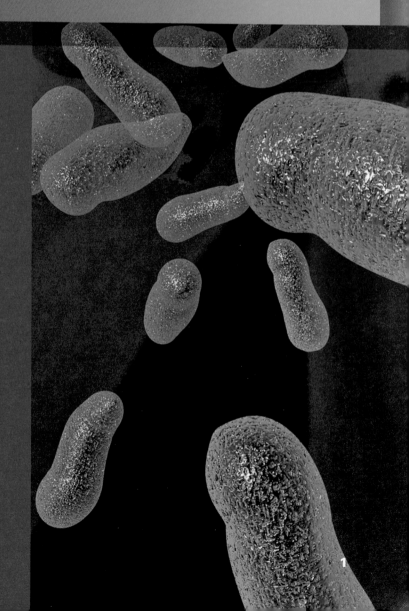

Concepts of Human Disease

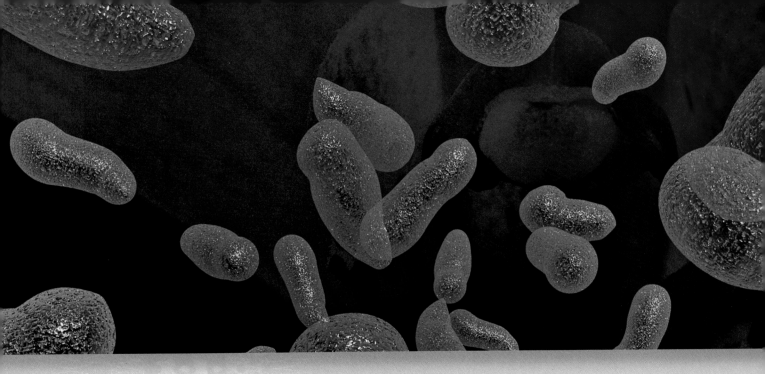

OUTLINE

KEY TERMS

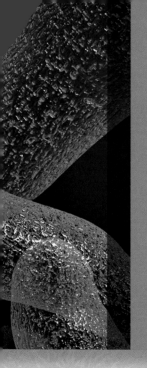

1

Introduction to Human Diseases

LEARNING OBJECTIVES

Upon completion of the chapter, the learner should be able to:

1. Define basic terminology used in the study of human diseases.

2. Discuss the pathogenesis of disease.

3. Describe the standard precaution guidelines for disease prevention.

4. Identify the predisposing factors to human diseases.

5. Explain the difference between diagnosis and prognosis of a disease.

6. Describe some common tests used to diagnose disease states.

OVERVIEW

The study of human diseases is important for understanding a variety of other topics in the health care field. Diseases that affect humans can range from mild to severe and can be acute (short term) or chronic (long term). Some diseases affect only one part of the body or a particular body system, whereas others affect several parts of the body or body systems at the same time. Many factors influence the body's ability to stay healthy or predispose the body to a disease process. Some of these factors are controllable, but some are strictly related to heredity. Diseases can be diagnosed by professional health care providers using a variety of techniques and tests. ■

DISEASE, DISORDER, AND SYNDROME

In the study of human disease, several terms may be similar and often used interchangeably but might not have identical definitions.

Disease

Disease may be defined in several ways. It may be called a change in structure or function that is considered to be abnormal within the body, or it may be defined as any change from normal. It usually refers to a condition in which symptoms occur and a pathologic state is present such as in pneumonia or leukemia. Both of these definitions have one underlying concept: the alteration of **homeostasis** (HOME-ee-oh-STAY-sis).

Homeostasis is the state of sameness or normalcy the body strives to maintain. The body is remarkable in its ability to maintain homeostasis, but when this homeostasis is no longer maintained, the body is diseased or "not at ease."

Disorder

Disorder is defined as a derangement or abnormality of function. The term *disorder* can also refer to a pathologic condition of the body or mind but more commonly is used to refer to a problem such as a vitamin deficiency (nutritional disorder). It is also used to refer to structural problems such as a malformation of a joint (bone disorder) or a condition in which the term *disease* does not seem to apply, such as dysphagia (swallowing disorder). Because *disease* and *disorder* are so closely related, they are often used synonymously.

Syndrome

Syndrome (SIN-drome) refers to a group of symptoms, which might be caused by a specific disease but might also be caused by several interrelated problems. Examples include Tourette's syndrome, Down syndrome, and acquired immunodeficiency syndrome (AIDS), which are discussed later in the text.

PATHOLOGY

Pathology (pah-THOL-oh-jee) can be broadly defined as the study of disease (patho = disease, ology = study).

TABLE 1–1 Types of Pathologists

Pathologist	Role or Subject
Experimental	Research
Academic	Teaching
Anatomic	Clinical examinations
Autopsy	Postmortem
Surgical	Biopsies
Clinical	Laboratory examinations
Hematology	Blood
Immunology	Antigen/antibodies
Microbiology	Microorganisms

© Cengage Learning®. All Rights Reserved.

A **pathologist** (pah-THOL-oh-jist) is one who studies disease. Even a student studying diseases might be considered a pathologist, using the strict definition of the word.

There are many types of pathologists because there are numerous ways to study disease. One of the more commonly known pathologists is the surgical pathologist, who inspects surgical tissue or biopsies for evidence of disease. The medical examiner or coroner can be a pathologist who studies human tissue to determine the cause of death and provide evidence of criminal involvement in a death. Other types of pathologists are outlined in Table 1–1.

The prefix *patho-* can be used in a variety of ways to describe disease processes or the disease itself. Microorganisms or agents that cause disease are called **pathogens** (PATH-oh-jens). These include some types of bacteria, viruses, fungi, protozoans, and helminths (worms). All pathogens have the ability to cause a disease or disorder. Fractures that are caused by a disease process that weakens the bone, such as osteoporosis, would be called **pathologic** (path-oh-LODGE-ick) fractures.

PATHOGENESIS

The **pathogenesis** (PATH-oh-JEN-ah-sis; patho = disease, genesis = arising) is a description of how a particular disease progresses. Many of us are familiar with the pathogenesis of the common cold.

A cold begins with an inoculation of the cold virus. This can occur following a simple handshake with someone who has a cold. Afterward, the target person might rub his or her eyes or nose, allowing entry of the virus into the body. After the inoculation

TABLE 1–2 Examples of Acute and Chronic Diseases/Disorders

Acute	Chronic
Upper respiratory infections	Arthritis
Lacerations	Hypertension
Middle ear infections	Diabetes mellitus
Gastroenteritis	Low back pain
Pneumonia	Heart disease
Fractures	Asthma

© Cengage Learning®. All Rights Reserved.

period comes incubation time. During this period, the virus multiplies, and the target person begins to have symptoms such as a runny nose and itchy eyes. The pathogenesis of the cold then moves into full-blown illness, usually followed by recovery and return to the previous state of health.

The pathogenesis of a disease can be explained in terms of time. An **acute** (a-CUTE) disease is short term and usually has a sudden onset. If the disease lasts for an extended period of time or the healing process is progressing slowly, it is classified as a **chronic** (KRON-ick) condition. See Table 1–2 for examples of acute and chronic diseases.

ETIOLOGY

The **etiology** (EE-tee-OL-oh-jee) of a disease means the study of cause. The term *etiology* is commonly used to mean simply "the cause." One might say that the cause is unknown or "of unknown etiology." The cause or etiology of pneumonia can be a virus or a bacterium. The etiology of athlete's foot is a fungus named tinea pedis.

Another term used to mean "the cause is unknown" is **idiopathic** (ID-ee-oh-PATH-ick). If an individual is diagnosed as having idiopathic gastric pain, it means the cause of the pain in the stomach is unknown.

Other terms related to cause of disease are **iatrogenic** (eye-AT-roh-JEN-ick) and **nosocomial** (NOS-oh-KOH-me-al). Iatrogenic (iatro = medicine, physician, genic = arising from) means that the problem arose from a prescribed treatment. An example of an iatrogenic problem is the development of anemia in a patient undergoing chemotherapy treatments for cancer.

Nosocomial is a closely related term; it implies that the disease was acquired from a hospital environment. An example would be a postoperative patient developing an incisional staphylococcal infection. The best way to prevent nosocomial infections is

HEALTHY HIGHLIGHT

Hand-Washing Technique

To prevent the spread of disease between oneself and others, good and frequent hand washing is the best prevention. Follow these good hand-washing steps.

- Use an antimicrobial soap when possible. Have paper towels available to dry hands and to turn off the water.
- Adjust water temperature and force. Wet hands and wrists and use a fingernail cleaner (if available) to clean under the nails gently on both hands while holding hands under the running water.
- Apply a small amount of liquid soap. Work into a lather on wrists and hands. Briskly rub hands together for 15 seconds being sure to wash areas between fingers and around each wrist.
- Rinse well from wrists to fingertips. Be careful not to touch the sides of the basin or let the water run down the arm off the elbow.
- Dry each hand from fingertips to wrist using a paper towel. When finished, turn off the water, using a paper towel as a barrier between the hands and the faucet.
- Discard soiled towels in the trash basket.

Source: Centers for Disease Control and Prevention (CDC) (2002).

HEALTHY HIGHLIGHT

Standard Precautions

Using standard precautions is recommended by the Centers for Disease Control and Prevention for the care of all patients or when administering first aid to anyone. These standards also include respiratory hygiene and cough etiquette, safe injection techniques, and wearing masks for spinal insertions.

- **Hand washing** Wash hands after touching blood, body fluids, or both, even if gloves are worn; use an antimicrobial soap.
- **Respiratory etiquette** Cover mouth, nose, or both with a tissue when coughing and dispose of used tissue immediately. Wear mask if possible. Maintain distance from others, ideally greater than 3 feet. Wash hands after contact with secretions.
- **Gloves** Wear gloves when touching blood, body fluids, and contaminated items; change gloves after patient contact or contact with contaminated items; wash hands before and after.
- **Eye wear, mask, and face shield** Wear protection for the eyes, mouth, and face when performing procedures when a risk of splashing or spraying of blood or body secretions exists. This includes insertion of catheters or injection of material into spinal or epidural spaces. A mask should also be worn if the caregiver has a respiratory infection but cannot avoid direct patient contact.
- **Gown** Wear a waterproof gown to protect the clothing from splashing or spraying blood or body fluids.
- **Equipment** Wear gloves when handling equipment contaminated with blood or body fluids; clean equipment appropriately after use; discard disposable equipment in proper containers.
- **Environment control** Follow proper procedures for cleaning and disinfecting the patient's environment after completion of a procedure.
- **Linen** Use proper procedure for disposing of linen contaminated with blood or body fluids.
- **Blood-borne pathogens** Do not recap needles; dispose of used needles and other sharp instruments in proper containers; use a mouthpiece for resuscitation; keep a mouthpiece available in areas where there is likelihood of need.

through the practice of good hand washing. A good hand-washing technique is described in the Healthy Highlight on page 5.

Media Link

Watch the video on proper hand washing on the Online Resources.

PREDISPOSING FACTORS

Predisposing factors, also known as risk factors, make a person more susceptible to disease. Predisposing factors are not the cause of the disease, and people

with predisposing factors do not always develop the disease. These factors include age, sex, environment, lifestyle, and heredity. Some risk factors are controllable, such as lifestyle behaviors, whereas others, such as age, are not.

Age

From the beginning of life until death, our risk of disease follows our age. Newborns are at risk of disease because their immune systems are not fully developed. On the other hand, older persons are at risk because their immune systems are degenerating or wearing out. Girls in their early teens and women over the age of 30 are at high risk for a difficult or problem pregnancy. The older we become, the higher the risk for

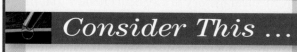

diseases such as cancer, heart disease, stroke, senile dementia, and Alzheimer's.

Sex

Some diseases are more **prevalent** (occurring more often) in one gender or the other. Men are more at risk for diseases such as lung cancer, gout, and Parkinsonism. Other disorders or diseases occur more often in women including osteoporosis, rheumatoid arthritis, and breast cancer.

Environment

Air and water pollution can lead to respiratory and gastrointestinal disease. Poor sanitation, excessive noise, and stress are also environmental risk factors. Occupational diseases such as lung disease are high among miners and persons working in areas where there are increased amounts of dust or other particles in the air.

Farmers are considered to be at higher risk for diseases because of their increased exposure to dust, pesticides, and other pollutants. Farmers are also at higher risk for trauma injuries due to safety problems around farm machinery. People living in remote, rural areas do not have health care availability comparable to those living in urban areas. This increases their risk for chronic illnesses.

Lifestyle

Lifestyle factors fall into a category over which the individual has some control. Choosing to improve health behaviors in these areas could lead to a reduction in risk and thus a possibility of avoiding the occurrence of the disease. Such factors include smoking, drinking alcohol, poor nutrition (excessive fat, salt, and sugar and not enough fruits, vegetables, and fiber), lack of exercise, and stress.

Practicing health behaviors to prevent contamination, and thus disease, is also an important lifestyle behavior. The Centers for Disease Control and Prevention recommend the use of standard precautions when caring for any individual when there is a chance of being contaminated with blood or body fluids (see Healthy Highlight box Standard Precautions on page 6). This is an important measure to prevent transmission of any disease that can be passed between humans in blood or body fluids, such as hepatitis, *Escherichia coli* infections, and AIDS.

Consider This ...

About 90% of diseases are partially caused or affected by stress.

Heredity

Although one cannot change genetic makeup, being aware of hereditary risk factors might encourage the individual to change lifestyle behaviors to reduce the risk of disease. For example, coronary heart disease has been shown to have a high familial tendency. Persons with this family inheritance are compounding their chances if they smoke, have poor nutritional intake, and do not exercise routinely.

Breast cancer and cervical cancer also have familial tendencies. Women with family members who have been diagnosed with breast cancer or cervical cancer are at a higher risk for developing these diseases. These women should be screened routinely for evidence of cancer and should complete monthly breast self-exams. With this knowledge about hereditary factors, individuals can choose to decrease their overall risk by improving their lifestyle health behaviors.

▮ DIAGNOSIS

Diagnosis (DIE-ag-KNOW-sis) is the identification or naming of a disease or condition. When an individual seeks medical attention, it is the duty of the physician to determine a diagnosis of the problem. A diagnosis is made after a methodical study by the physician, using data collected from a medical history, physical examination, and diagnostic tests (Figure 1–1).

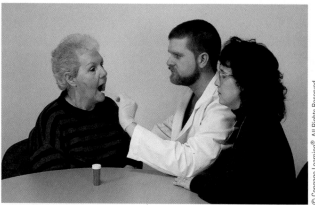

FIGURE 1–1 Physician checking a patient.

A medical history is a systems review that might include such information as previous illnesses, family illness, predisposing factors, medication allergies, current illnesses, and current **symptoms** (SIMP-tums, what patients report as their problem or problems). Examples of symptoms might include stomach pain, headache, and nausea.

The physician proceeds with a head-to-toe physical examination of the patient, looking for signs of the disease. **Signs** differ from symptoms in that signs are observable or measurable. Signs are what the physician sees or measures. Examples of signs could include vomiting, elevated blood pressure, and elevated temperature.

In some cases, a patient's concern might be considered as both a symptom and a sign. Some references call this an objective or observable symptom, whereas others state that it is also a sign. An example would be a patient complaining of a runny nose. The runny nose is the patient's symptom and, because it is observable to the physician, it is also a sign.

During the physical examination, the physician might use other skills such as **auscultation** (AWS-kul-TAY-shun, using a stethoscope to listen to body cavities), **palpation** (pal-PAY-shun, feeling lightly or pressing firmly on internal organs or structures), and **percussion** (per-KUSH-un; tapping over various body areas to produce a vibrating sound). All the results are compared to a normal standard to identify problems.

Diagnostic tests and procedures to assist in determining a diagnosis are numerous. The routine or most common include urinalysis, complete blood count (CBC), chest X-ray (CXR), and electrocardiography (EKG or ECG). See Table 1–3 for examples of common diagnostic tests and procedures.

▮ PROGNOSIS

Prognosis (prawg-KNOW-sis) is the predicted or expected outcome of the disease. For example, the prognosis of the common cold would be that the individual should feel better in 7 to 10 days.

Acute Disease

The duration of the disease can be described as acute in nature. An acute disease is one that usually has a sudden onset and lasts a short amount of time (days or weeks). Most acute diseases are related to the respiratory system. Again, the common cold would be a good example.

Chronic Disease

If the disease persists for a long time, it is considered to be chronic. Chronic diseases might begin insidiously (slowly and without symptoms) and last for the entire life of the individual. As one ages, the occurrence of chronic disease increases. One of the most common chronic diseases is hypertension, or high blood pressure.

Chronic diseases often go through periods of **remission** and **exacerbation** (ex-AS-er-BAY-shun). Remission refers to a time when symptoms are diminished or temporarily resolved. Exacerbation refers to

TABLE 1–3   Examples of Common Diagnostic Tests and Procedures

Test	Description
Complete blood count (CBC)	An examination of blood for cell counts and abnormalities
Urinalysis (UA)	An examination of urine for abnormalities
Chest X-ray (CXR)	X-ray examination of the chest cavity
Electrocardiography (ECG or EKG)	A procedure for recording the electrical activity of the heart
Blood glucose	A test of the blood to determine its glucose or sugar levels
Computerized axial tomography (CT or CAT)	A special X-ray examination showing detailed images of body structures and organs
Serum electrolytes	An examination of blood serum to determine the levels of the common electrolytes (sodium, potassium, chloride, and carbon dioxide)

a time when symptoms flare up or become worse. Leukemia is a disease that progresses through periods of remission and exacerbation. Both acute and chronic diseases can range from mild to life threatening.

Complication

The prognosis might be altered or changed at times if the individual develops a **complication**. A complication is the onset of a second disease or disorder in an individual who is already affected with a disease. An individual with a fractured arm might have a prognosis of the arm healing in 6 to 8 weeks. If the individual suffers the complication of bone infection, the prognosis might change drastically.

Mortality Rate

Mortality is defined as the quality of being mortal, that is, destined to die. Diseases commonly leading to the death of an individual have a high **mortality rate**. The mortality rate of a disease (also called death rate) is related to the number of people who die with the disease in a certain amount of time. Other terms the medical community uses to refer to a deadly disease include **fatal** and **lethal**.

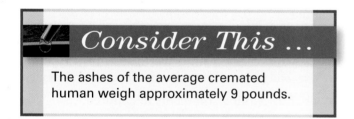

Consider This ...

The ashes of the average cremated human weigh approximately 9 pounds.

Survival Rate

A physician's prognosis can also consider survival rate. Survival rate is the percentage of people with a particular disease who live for a set period of time. For example, the 2-year survival rate of individuals with lung cancer would be the percentage of people alive 2 years after diagnosis.

▉ TREATMENT

After the diagnosis is established, the physician will work with the individual to explain or outline a plan of care. The physician might offer treatment options to the individual with expected outcomes or

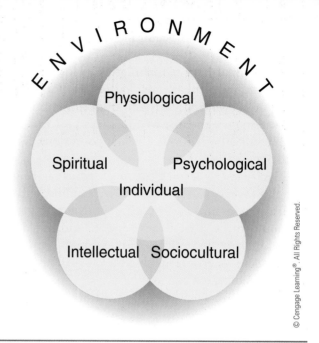

FIGURE 1–2   Holistic medicine.

prognoses. The individual's entire being should be taken into consideration. The concept of considering the whole person rather than just the physical being is called **holistic medicine**.

From a holistic viewpoint, there is interaction between the spiritual, cognitive, social, physical, and emotional being. These areas do not work independently, but have a dynamic interaction (Figure 1–2).

Treatment interventions might include (1) medications, (2) surgery, (3) exercise, (4) nutritional modifications, (5) physical therapy, and (6) education. Individuals and family members should be educated and involved in the treatment plan. Failure to involve the individual and family can decrease compliance and lead to failure of the plan.

After the treatment plan is implemented, the physician will follow up with the individual to determine effectiveness. The individual and physician should work together to modify the plan if it is found to be ineffective. Implementation of the plan usually requires an entire health care team. The team can include nurses, a physical therapist, a social worker, clergy, and other health care professionals as needed.

The best treatment option is a **preventive** plan. In preventive treatment, care is given to prevent disease. Examples of preventive care are breast mammograms to screen for breast cancer, blood pressure screening for hypertension, routine dental care to prevent dental caries, and a fecal occult blood test to screen for colon cancer.

Other treatment plans might include **palliative** (PAL-ee-ay-tiv) treatment. Palliative treatment is aimed at preventing pain and discomfort but does not seek to cure the disease. Treatment for end-term cancer and other serious chronic conditions can be palliative.

Decisions concerning treatment plans can be very difficult for the patient, the patient's family, and the health care team. This is especially true when those decisions involve palliative treatment and end-of-life issues. During these times, professionals often seek assistance in decision making by using their knowledge of medical ethics.

MEDICAL ETHICS

Webster's dictionary defines ethics as "the study of standards of conduct and moral judgment." More simply put, ethics deals with the "rightness and wrongness" or "goodness and badness" of human actions. Ethics covers many areas of conduct and judgment in our society.

Bioethics is a branch of ethics concerned with what is right or wrong in bio (life) decisions. Because bioethics is a study of life ethics, it covers or becomes entwined with medical ethics. Medical ethics includes the values and decisions in medical practice, including relationships to patients, patients' families, peer physicians, and society.

Part of the ethical challenge in this age of rapidly advancing technologies is actually determining what is right, wrong, good, or bad. New scientific discoveries are challenging familiar or usual human behaviors, leading to reconsideration of actions, thoughts, and emotions. Ethical dilemmas, once rare, are now common and often happen so quickly that society is unable to understand completely the impact these decisions will have on the future.

Bioethical decisions are often very difficult because they touch the core of humanity in dealing with issues of birth, death, sickness, health, and dignity. This generation and generations to come will be faced with ethical decisions formerly unknown to man. Many of these decisions will have great impact on medical ethics and will actually shape the future of mankind.

When challenges concerning medical ethics arise in a health care facility, an ethics committee might be called on to make a decision. This committee might involve one or more persons at each of these levels: physician, nurse, ethicist, social worker, case manager, chaplain, legal representative, and administrator, or director.

Groups or committees involved in decision making might need to consider previous works of philosophy, history, law, and religion to assist them in reaching a conclusion. Participation in ethical decision making requires members to follow some basic rules, which can include:

- Keeping the discussion focused and civil.
- Listening with an open mind to all opinions.
- Entertaining diverse ideas.
- Weighing out the pros and cons of each idea.
- Considering the impact of the decision on all persons involved.

Every individual at some time or another will encounter or be called on to make a decision that is bioethical in nature. Examples of these can include one's willingness to:

- Use a surrogate mother or father to have a biological child.
- Control the sex of children through chromosome selection.
- Use fetal stem cells to grow new organs and tissues.
- Use prescription stimulants in children.
- Legalize abortion.
- Use mood-altering drugs for older persons.
- Clone humans.
- Treat disease by replacing damaged or abnormal genes with normal genes.
- Use animal organs or tissues (xenotransplants) in humans.
- Support euthanasia.
- Allow physician-assisted suicide.

Each of the preceding issues can be overwhelming. Even so, yet another concern must be addressed, involving the economics of these choices.

Consider, for example, the economics of human cloning. How will research, technology, and intervention be funded? If costs are funded by individuals, only wealthy individuals would be able to afford clones. Is that fair or right? If costs are funded by the government, what criteria will be used for selection? Will selection be based on intelligence, physical ability, or artistic skills? Who decides?

Medical ethics includes some very complicated life issues. Bioethical decision making, or determining the rightness or wrongness of such issues, will continue to be a challenge for society well into the future.

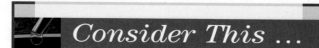

Consider This ...

A study in the Netherlands determined that smokers and obese persons benefit a socialized health care system due to earlier deaths. Health care costs for a lifetime for a healthy person will average $417,000, whereas the obese person will cost $371,000 and the smoker will cost $326,000.

SUMMARY

The study of human diseases is important to any health care or allied health professional. Disease can affect any body system or organ and can range from mild to severe, depending on many factors. Several risk factors for disease can be controlled to some extent by one's lifestyle. Other diseases might not be preventable or controlled but need medical intervention for treatment or cure. Diagnosis and treatment of a disease are usually accomplished by a team of health care professionals led by the physician. Ethical decision making has become a challenge in health care today, and as technology continues to grow and develop, medical ethics will become more challenging than ever.

REVIEW QUESTIONS

Short Answer

1. Identify why it is important to study human diseases.

2. Describe the types of pathologists and their roles in the study of disease.

3. List the five predisposing factors for disease and one disease related to each factor.

Matching

4. Match the terms in the left column with the correct definition in the right column.

_____ Pathogenesis

_____ Etiology

_____ Diagnosis

_____ Prognosis

_____ Treatment

a. The cause of a disease

b. Interventions to cure or control a disease

c. The development of a disease

d. The identification or naming of a disease

e. The predicted or expected outcome of a disease

CASE STUDIES

■ Stan Cotton was accidentally tripped by another player while running down the field at a soccer game you were coaching. He is able to walk to the sideline with assistance but has obvious bleeding on his legs and one arm. You grab the first-aid box and go to his side. What do you do next? What equipment might you use to give aid to Stan? What standard precautions should apply to this case?

■ Jane Swenson has been suffering from a cold for about a week and has missed 3 days of work. She decides to return to work at the local senior citizen center. She is still coughing at intervals and has a runny nose but has improved since last week. Should she still use some precautions to prevent spreading her illness? If so, what should she do?

Study Tools

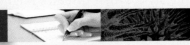

Workbook

Complete Chapter 1

Online Resources

PowerPoint® presentations

BIBLIOGRAPHY

Calzone, K., Jerome-D'Emilia, B., Jenkins, J., Goldgar, C., Rackover, M., Jackson, J., Chen, Y., Voss, J., & Feero, W. G. (2011). Establishment of the Genetic/Genomic Competency Center for Education. *Journal of Nursing Scholarship 43*(4), 351–358.

Centers for Disease Control and Prevention (CDC). (2002). Guideline for hand hygiene in health care setting. *Mobidity and Mortality Weekly Report 51*(RR 16), 20–25.

Health wire. (2011). *Consumer Reports on Health 23*(7), 2–3.

Kawas, S. A., Rahim, Z., & Ferguson, D. B. (2012). Potential uses of human salivary protein and peptide analysis in the diagnosis of disease. *Archives of Oral Biology 57*(1), 1–9.

Mosquera, J., Avitzur, O. R., Santa, J., & Lipman, M. M. (2011). You asked and our doctors answered. *Consumer Reports, 76*(9), 12.

Timm, D. F., & Jones, D. (2011). The information prescription: Just what the doctor ordered! *Journal of Hospital Librarianship 11*(4), 358–365.

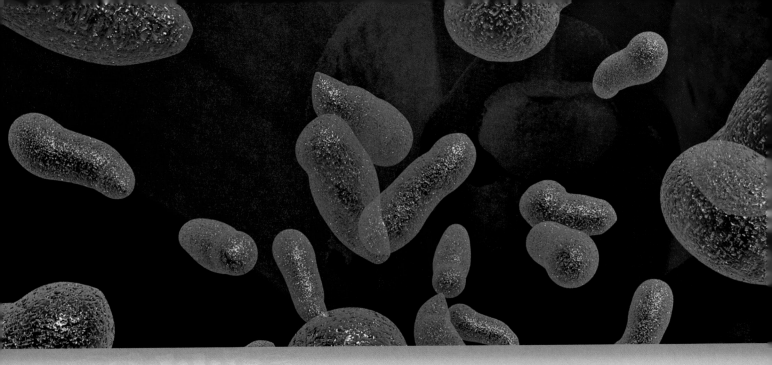

OUTLINE

KEY TERMS

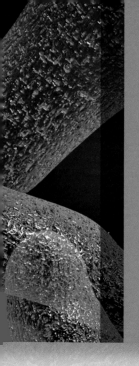

2

Mechanisms of Disease

LEARNING OBJECTIVES

Upon completion of the chapter, the learner should be able to:

1. Identify important terminology related to the mechanisms of human disease.
2. Describe the causes of disease.
3. Identify disorders in each category of the causes of disease.
4. Describe behaviors important to a healthy lifestyle.
5. Compare the various types of impaired immunity.
6. Identify the basic changes in the body occurring in the aging process.
7. Describe the process of cell and tissue injury, adaptation, and death.

OVERVIEW

The human body is a complex machine that normally runs in an efficient, balanced manner, but when changes occur in the body due to lifestyle behaviors, abnormal growths, nutritional problems, bacterial invasion, or any other factor that upsets the balance, the result might be a disease process. Human disease can be very minor or life threatening. Diseases are caused by a variety of factors; some are controllable and some are not. Even normal changes such as aging can put the individual at higher risk for developing disease. Many changes or alterations in cell and tissue structure can occur. Some of these changes are reversible, but some might cause cellular, tissue, organ, or system death. ■

▨▨ CAUSES OF DISEASE

To gain a better understanding of the different causes of diseases, it is usually helpful to classify or divide them into smaller groups. This classification can be approached in several different yet logical ways. One commonly used approach is to divide the causes of disease into the following six categories:

1. Heredity
2. Trauma
3. Inflammation and infection
4. Hyperplasias and neoplasms
5. Nutritional imbalance
6. Impaired immunity

Heredity

Hereditary diseases are caused by an abnormality in the individual's genetic or chromosomal makeup. These diseases might or might not be apparent at birth. Hereditary diseases that are present at birth, even if not apparent, are called **congenital** (kon-JEN-ih-tahl) disorders. However, not all congenital disorders are inherited. Some other causes of congenital disorders include disease during pregnancy (fetal alcohol syndrome) or difficulty with delivery (cerebral palsy), to name only a couple.

Hereditary diseases are classified in three basic ways, as (1) a single gene abnormality, (2) an abnormality of several genes (polygenic), or (3) an abnormality of a chromosome (either entire absence of a chromosome or the presence of an additional chromosome). See Table 2–1 for the classification of hereditary diseases and examples.

Chromosomal and genetic abnormalities might or might not be compatible with life. Some abnormalities might be present but cause no effect on the individual, whereas others might lead to the death and spontaneous abortion of the unborn child.

More information related to hereditary diseases can be found in Chapter 19, "Genetic and Developmental Diseases and Disorders."

Trauma

Traumatic diseases are caused by a physical injury from an external force. Trauma is the leading cause of death in children and young adults. The type of **trauma** (TRAW-mah) or traumatic disease most commonly affecting individuals varies with age, race, and residence. For example, accidents, especially falls, are a common cause of traumatic disorders in older adults, whereas gunshot wounds are the most common cause of traumatic disease and even death in young adult black males living in urban areas. However, motor vehicle accidents (**MVAs**) are the most frequent cause of serious injury overall.

The Centers for Disease Control and Prevention (CDC) lists deaths caused by trauma, in order of prevalence (or occurrence), as follows:

- MVAs
- Poison
- Firearms
- Falls
- Suicide
- Suffocation
- Homicide

Emergency management of trauma is often necessary to prevent the complications of shock, hemorrhage, and infection. On arrival at an emergency department, patients are assessed according to signs and symptoms, age, and medical history. Needs are then prioritized, and care is given in order of severity of injury. This prioritizing of care is called **triage** (tree-AUZH) and incorporates an ABC prioritizing method, with A for airway, B for breathing, and C for cardiac function. After these areas are assessed, other areas of

---

TABLE 2–1　Classification of Hereditary Disease with Examples

Single Gene	Polygenic	Chromosomal
Cystic fibrosis	Gout	Klinefelter's syndrome
Phenylketonuria	Hypertension	Turner's syndrome
Sickle cell anemia	Congenital heart anomalies	Down syndrome

trauma such as bleeding and fractures are addressed. An example of triage, in general, would be giving priority care to a patient who is not breathing before assisting a patient who has a bleeding leg wound.

Types of trauma commonly occurring in each body system are discussed in the specific system chapters.

Inflammation and Infection

Inflammation (IN-flah-MAY-shun) is a protective immune response that is triggered by any type of injury or irritant. Even the slightest trauma can initiate the inflammatory response. Signs of inflammation are redness, heat, swelling, pain, and loss of motion. An example of inflammation is sunburn. The tissue is red, warm to the touch, swollen, painful, and uncomfortable when moving. Although this area is inflamed, it is usually not infected.

Infection (in-FECT-shun) refers to the invasion of microorganisms into tissue that causes cell or tissue injury. Inflammation and infection are often used synonymously even though they are quite different. A tissue can be inflamed but not infected, as in sunburn, but usually, tissue that is infected will also be inflamed.

For tissue to be infected or for infection to occur, there has to be an invasion of microorganisms. Usually, inflammation and infection go hand in hand. For example, when the skin is cut, the tissue around the cut will undergo a mild inflammation. As skin bacteria invade the cut tissue, the area becomes infected and usually becomes even more inflamed due to the irritation to the tissue caused by the bacteria (Figure 2–1).

Diseases that are related to inflammation are identified with the suffix "itis." Examples include appendicitis (inflammation of the appendix), gastritis (inflammation of the stomach), colitis (inflammation of the colon), and encephalitis (inflammation of the brain). In many cases, the inflammation will progress to an infection due to the presence of bacteria in the region. For example, appendicitis can be caused by an obstruction of the appendix. Because the bacteria *Escherichia coli* (*E. coli*) are commonly found in the colon, the appendix becomes infected.

Hyperplasias and Neoplasms

Hyperplasias (HIGH-per-PLAY-zee-ahs; hyper = excessive, plasia = growth) and **neoplasms** (NEE-oh-plazms; neo = new, plasm = growth) are similar because, in both, an increase in cell number leads to an increase in tissue size.

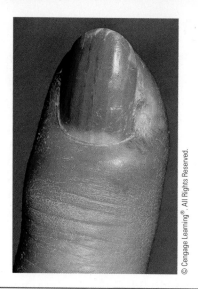

FIGURE 2–1   Inflammation of a finger.

Hyperplasias

Hyperplasias differ from neoplasms in terms of cause and growth limits. Hyperplasias are an overgrowth in response to some type of stimulus. An example of a hyperplasia would be enlargement of the thyroid gland (goiter) in response to a hormone deficiency.

Neoplasms

Neoplasms (new growths) are commonly called **tumors**. The Latin word *tumor* means "swelling" and originally was used in the description of the swelling related to inflammation. The Greek term for swelling is *onkos*, which has been used to construct the word **oncology** (ong-KOL-oh-jee; onco = tumor, logy = study of, or the study of cancer). Although all tumors are not neoplasms, as described in more detail in Chapter 3, "Neoplasms," the words are often used synonymously.

Diseases with tumor involvement usually end with the suffix *oma*. Examples include lipoma, carcinoma, melanoma, and sarcoma (Table 2–2). An exception to this is the word *hematoma*, which is a clot of blood in an area. A hematoma on the head due to a blunt blow would be an example.

Neoplasms or tumors (-omas) may be classified as **benign** (beh-NINE) or **malignant** (mah-LIG-nant). Generally speaking, benign tumors have a limited growth, are **encapsulated** (enclosed in a capsule) and thus easily removed, and are not deadly. Malignant tumors are just the opposite. These tumors grow uncontrollably; have finger-like projections into surrounding tissue, making removal very difficult; and

TABLE 2–2 Examples of Neoplasms or Tumors

Neoplasm/Tumor	Description
Adenoma	Usually benign tumor arising from glandular epithelial tissue
Carcinoma	Malignant tumor of epithelial tissue
Fibroma	Benign encapsulated tumor of connective tissue
Glioma	Malignant tumor of neurologic cells
Lipoma	Benign fatty tumor
Melanoma	Malignant tumor of the skin
Sarcoma	Malignant tumor arising from connective tissue such as muscle or bone

© Cengage Learning®. All Rights Reserved.

are usually deadly. *Malignant* means deadly or progressing to death. With these definitions, it is understandable why the terms *tumor*, *malignancy*, and *cancer* bring fear to an individual. Some -omas, or tumor diseases, are commonly called cancer. **Cancer** is defined as any malignant tumor.

The finger-like or crab-like projections that characterize malignant tumors give cancer its name, from the Greek *karkinos*, meaning "crab." This characteristic makes surgical removal of cancer quite difficult (Figure 2–2). Another characteristic of malignant neoplasms is that they **metastasize** (meh-TAS-tah-sighz), or move. **Metastatic** (MET-ah-STAT-ic) cancers move from a site of origin to a secondary site in the body. For example, lung cancer commonly metastasizes to the bone. Chapter 3 discusses more detailed information about hyperplasias and neoplasms.

Nutritional Imbalance

Good nutrition is important in maintaining good health and reducing the chance of disease. Nutritional disorders can cause problems with physical growth, mental and intellectual retardation, and even death in extreme cases. Most nutritional diseases are related to overconsumption or underconsumption of nutrients. Specific problems are malnutrition, obesity, and excessive or deficient vitamins, minerals, or both.

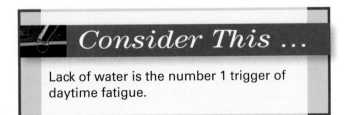

Consider This ...

Lack of water is the number 1 trigger of daytime fatigue.

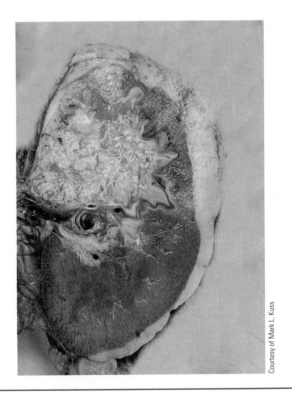

Courtesy of Mark L. Kuss

FIGURE 2–2 Crab-like appearance of cancer in a kidney.

Malnutrition

Malnutrition can be due to inadequate nutrient intake or to intake of an adequate amount with poor nutritive value. Diseases that cause a problem with absorption of nutrients can also lead to malnutrition. Children and older persons are the age groups most affected by malnutrition. Persons suffering with cancer often experience problems with malnutrition and develop cachexia. **Cachexia** (ca-KECK-see-ah) is a term that describes any individual who has an ill, thin, wasted appearance (Figure 2–3).

= skin), intramuscular (intra = within, muscular = muscle), or intravenous (intra = within, venous = vein) administration. The intravenous route is the most commonly used parenteral route. Providing the total nutrition needed by giving nutritive liquid through a venous (vein) route is called total parenteral nutrition (**TPN**).

Nutrition can also be provided through an **enteral** (small intestine) route. A nasogastric (naso = nose, gastric = stomach) tube or a tube running through the nose and into the stomach can be used for feedings if the supplement is planned short term. For longer term enteral feeding, a gastrostomy (gastro = stomach, ostomy = opening; opening into the stomach) procedure is performed to place a tube through the abdominal and stomach wall. Enteral feeding, commonly called "tube feeding," is accomplished by this method (Figure 2–4).

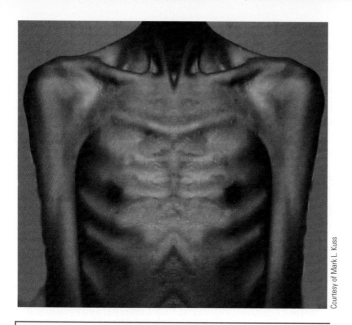

FIGURE 2–3   Cachexia.

Persons who are unable to eat enough to maintain their body weight can receive nutritional supplements in a liquid drink. Another way to supplement or provide for total nutritional intake is not through the alimentary canal or digestive system but through a **parenteral** (pah-REN-ter-al; to administer by injection) route. Parenteral routes can include subcutaneous (sub = under, cutaneous

Obesity

Although many individuals in the United States have a nutritional deficiency, the most common problem is obesity, which is primarily due to overconsumption of nutrients and lack of exercise. According to the American Heart Association, obesity is a national health concern with nearly one in three (31.7%) U.S. children ages 2 to 19 being obese and over one-third

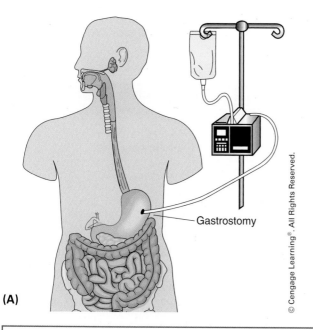

Gastrostomy

(A)

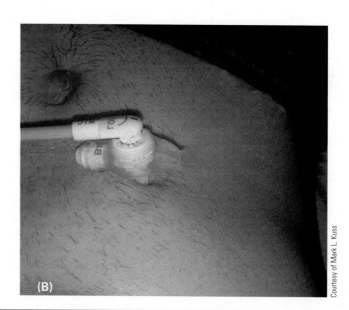

(B)

FIGURE 2–4   Gastrostomy. (A) Feeding. (B) Insertion site.

(33.7%) of adults being obese. Obesity shortens the life span of the individual by increasing the chance for arteriosclerosis, leading to cardiovascular diseases. It also affects the individual's risk for developing bone or joint problems due to the increased pressure on the skeletal system.

Obesity is simply defined as too much body fat. It is medically determined when an individual has a **body mass index (BMI)** of greater than 29.9. BMI is obtained by dividing the individual's weight in pounds by the square of his or her height, multiplied by 703. For example, a person weighing 250 pounds who is 5 feet 6 inches tall (66 inches) has a BMI of 40.3. This is calculated as 250 divided by (66 × 66) × 703. This person is considered extremely obese.

A simple BMI scale uses these figures to determine levels of obesity:

BMI

<18.5: underweight

18.5–24.9: normal

25–29: overweight

30–35: obese

36–40: moderately obese

>40: extremely obese

Bariatrics (BEAR-e-at-tricks) is a branch of medicine that deals with the prevention and treatment of obesity. First-line treatment for obesity often includes diet, exercise, antiobesity medication, and behavior modification. These treatments in the severely obese population often have poor long-term success. In these cases, bariatric or weight loss surgery may be recommended. Gastric banding and gastric bypass are two of the most common types of surgery.

Obesity is one of the most preventable causes of death. Worldwide, it is viewed as one of the most serious public health problems of the twenty-first century.

Vitamin or Mineral Excess or Deficiency

Vitamin and mineral excesses and deficiencies are usually related to diet, metabolic disorders, and some medications. Hypervitaminosis can occur in individuals who consume large amounts of vitamins for an extended period of time.

Nutritional guidelines for a healthy lifestyle are difficult to determine because they must cover a variety of ages and nutritional needs. Children, teens, and pregnant women have very specific nutritional needs. See the Healthy Highlight box General Guidelines for a Healthy Lifestyle for more information.

Impaired Immunity

The immune system of the body is a specialized group of cells, tissues, and organs that are designed to defend the body against pathogenic attacks. The body's first line of defense against pathogens is its normal structure and function, including an intact skin; mucous membranes; tears; and secretions. The immune system protects the body in two additional ways, through:

1. The inflammatory response in which leukocytes play a vital part in killing foreign invaders.
2. The specific antigen–antibody reaction in which the body responds to antigens (AN-tih-jens) by

HEALTHY HIGHLIGHT

General Guidelines for a Healthy Lifestyle

General guidelines for a healthy lifestyle include the following tips:

- Maintain proper body weight.
- Eat a variety of foods.
- Avoid excessive fat, salt, and sugar.
- Eat adequate amounts of fiber.
- Consume alcohol in moderation, no more than two drinks per day for men and one for women.
- Get enough rest and sleep, at least 7 or more hours per day.
- Always eat breakfast.
- Maintain a moderate exercise schedule.

producing antibodies. **Antigens** are substances that cause the body some type of harm, thus setting off this specific reaction. **Antibodies**, also called immune bodies, are proteins that the body produces to react to the antigen and render it harmless.

Impaired immunity occurs when some part of this system malfunctions. Following are some common ways the system malfunctions.

Allergy

The immune response is too intense or hypersensitive to an environmental substance. The **allergen** (environmental substance that causes a reaction) in an **allergy** might be such things as house dust, grass, pets, perfumes, or insect bites, to name a few. These allergens do not usually cause this type of reaction in most persons but do cause an allergic reaction in persons sensitive to them.

Autoimmunity

The immune response attacks itself. In **autoimmunity** (auto = self), the body's lymphocytes (a white blood cell that produces antibodies) cannot identify the body's own self-antigens, which are harmless. In response, the lymphocytes form antibodies that then attack the body's own cells. Examples of autoimmune diseases include rheumatoid arthritis and rheumatic fever.

Immunodeficiency

The immune response is unable to defend the body due to a decrease or absence of leukocytes, primarily lymphocytes. Persons with **immunodeficiency** are usually asymptomatic (without symptoms) except for recurrent infections. It is these recurrent infections that often lead to death. An example of an immunodeficiency disease is acquired immunodeficiency syndrome (**AIDS**). Immunodeficiency also can be caused by medications, chemotherapy, or radiation. Organ recipients are intentionally immunosuppressed or immunodeficient to save their transplanted organ. Without immunosuppressant medications, the body's immune system would recognize the organ as foreign and attack it, leading to organ death. This process is called **organ rejection**. Cancer patients often undergo chemotherapy and radiation treatments that can cause immunodeficiency. Some medications also affect the system by depressing its ability to function properly. Chapter 5, "Immune System Diseases and Disorders," discusses the immune system and related diseases in more detail.

◼ AGING

There is no definite age in years when an individual becomes aged. However, some statisticians consider the retirement age of 65 as aged. An individual's body actually begins to age at physical maturity, around age 18, in a complicated process that is not completely understood but is progressive and irreversible. Diseases related to aging are often called **degenerative** diseases. Tissue degeneration is a change in functional activity to a lower or lesser level. Examples of degenerative diseases are degenerative joint disease and degenerative disk disease.

The mechanisms of aging are complex and thought to include such factors as heredity, lifestyle, stress, diet, and environment. One might slow the process of aging to some degree by living a healthy lifestyle and controlling stress and environmental factors.

Hereditary factors can include increased life span related to an inherited ability to resist disease. Just as families have a history of disease patterns, they also appear to have a pattern of longevity. Thus, individuals who have relatives who live to be in their nineties might themselves live to that age. Individuals with a family history of members who have died of heart disease in their early years might also suffer the same problem. Although hereditary patterns cannot be controlled, longevity can be increased and disease decreased by controlling lifestyle behaviors that increase risk of chronic disease.

The body replaces and repairs itself throughout its lifetime, but with aging, this process slows. As early as age 40, there are changes in skin, endocrine function, vision, and muscle strength. Other changes in the aging process might include bone loss leading to osteoporosis, decreased melanin pigment production leading to graying of the hair, decreased immunity leading to an increase in infections and possible development of cancer, loss of brain and nerve cells that might lead to senile dementia, and decrease in intestinal motility leading to constipation and possible diverticulosis.

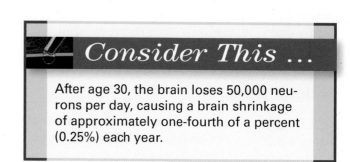

Consider This ...

After age 30, the brain loses 50,000 neurons per day, causing a brain shrinkage of approximately one-fourth of a percent (0.25%) each year.

■ DEATH

Humans are mortal, so eventually, everyone will die. Even though we are unable to understand the aging process fully, cellular, tissue, and organ death can be reviewed in an effort to understand the death of the organism as a whole.

Cellular Injury

Cellular injury and death can be due to some type of trauma, **hypoxia** (HIGH-POCK-see-ah; not enough oxygen), **anoxia** (ah-NOCK-see-ah; no oxygen), drug or bacterial toxins, or viruses. Cells can undergo near-death experiences and actually recuperate in what is considered to be reversible cell injury.

The ability of the cell to survive depends on several factors, including the amount of time the cell suffers and the type of cell injury that occurred. If the cause of the injury is short term, the cell has a greater chance of survival.

The type of cell also plays a part in its ability to recuperate. The heart, brain, and nerve cells are easily injured and often suffer death. This is particularly important because these cells do not replace themselves. Even short-term injury might readily lead to death in these cells. Other cells are not as easily damaged. Connective and epithelial cells often recuperate and even readily replace themselves by mitosis (cell division).

Cellular Adaptation

Cells that are exposed to adverse conditions often go through a process of adaptation. When the condition is changed, these cells might be able to change back to their normal structure and function. However, some adaptations are permanent, so even if the condition improves, the cells are not able to return to normal. Types of adaptation include **atrophy** (AT-tro-fee), **hypertrophy** (HIGH-PER-tro-fee), hyperplasia, **dysplasia** (dis-PLAY-zee-ah), **metaplasia** (MET-ah-PLAY-zee-ah), and **neoplasia** (nee-oh-PLAY-zee-ah).

Atrophy

Atrophy (a = without, trophy = growth) is a decrease in cell size, which leads to a decrease in the size of the tissue and organ (Figure 2–5). Atrophy is often due to the aging process itself or to disease. An example of atrophy related to aging would be the smaller size of the muscles and bones of older people. As the female ages, the breasts and female reproductive organs atrophy, especially after menopause. Examples of disease or pathologic atrophy are usually related to decreased use of the organ, especially muscles. Spinal cord injuries

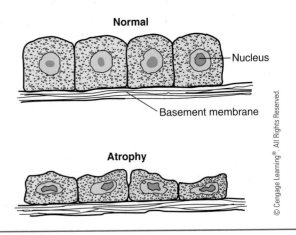

© Cengage Learning®. All Rights Reserved.

FIGURE 2–5 Normal cell versus atrophied cell.

Normal

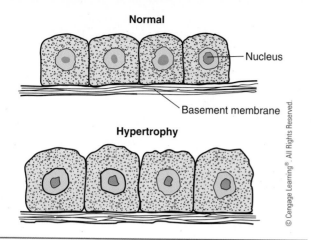

Nucleus

Basement membrane

Hypertrophy

FIGURE 2–6 Normal cell versus hypertrophied cell.

Normal

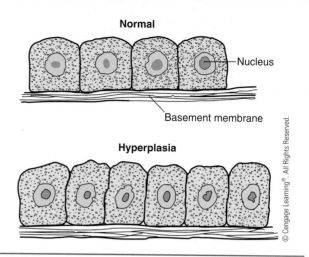

Nucleus

Basement membrane

Hyperplasia

FIGURE 2–7 Normal tissue versus hyperplasia.

lead to an inability to move muscles. Without use, muscle cells decrease in size and the muscle atrophies.

Hypertrophy

Hypertrophy (hyper = excessive, trophy = growth) is an increase in the size of the cell leading to an increase in tissue and organ size (Figure 2–6). Skeletal muscle and heart muscle cells do not increase in number by mitosis. Literally, what an individual has at birth is what the individual has throughout life. This helps explain why some athletes bulk up with exercise while others do not. The inherited number of muscle cells does not change with exercise; only the size of each cell changes. To adapt to an increased workload, muscle cells increase in size. Increased workload on the skeletal muscles causes cellular hypertrophy and an increase in muscle size. Heart muscle hypertrophy is usually seen in the left ventricle of the heart (left ventricular hypertrophy) when the left ventricle must work harder to pump blood through diseased valves and arteries. To adapt to this need, the cells increase in size and the left side of the heart enlarges.

Hyperplasia

Hyperplasia (hyper = increased, plasia = growth) is an increase in cell number that is commonly due to hormonal stimulation (Figure 2–7). Hyperplasia is discussed in more detail in Chapter 3.

Dysplasia

Dysplasia (dys = bad or difficult, plasia = growth) usually follows hyperplasia. It is an alteration in size,

shape, and organization of cells (Figure 2–8). Dysplastic cells might change back to the normal cell structure if the irritant or stimulus is removed, but usually, these cells progress to neoplasia.

Metaplasia

Metaplasia (meta = changed, plasia = growth) is a cellular adaptation in which the cell changes to another type of cell (Figure 2–9). An example is the columnar epithelial cells of the respiratory tree, which often change to stratified squamous epithelial cells when exposed to the irritants of cigarette smoking. This protective adaptation might be reversible if the individual quits smoking.

Normal

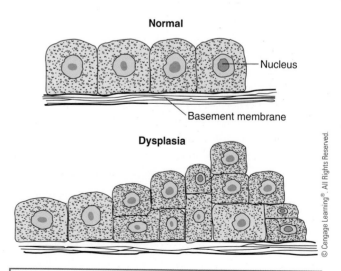

Nucleus

Basement membrane

Dysplasia

FIGURE 2–8 Normal tissue versus dysplasia.

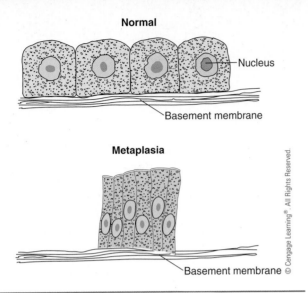

FIGURE 2–9 Normal tissue versus metaplasia.

Neoplasia

Neoplasia (neo = new, plasia = growth) is the development of a new type of cell with an uncontrolled growth pattern (Figure 2–10). Neoplasia is discussed in more detail in Chapter 3.

Cell and Tissue Death

Cell death, as previously mentioned, can be caused by trauma, hypoxia, anoxia, drug or bacterial toxins, or viruses. The most common causes of cell death are hypoxia and anoxia.

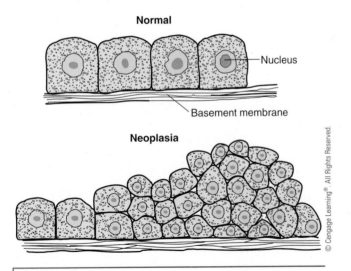

FIGURE 2–10 Normal tissue versus neoplasia.

Cell hypoxia caused by decreased blood flow is called **ischemia** (iss-KEE-me-ah; isch = hold back, emia = blood). A cell without oxygen cannot produce needed energy and eventually dies.

Cellular death, called **necrosis** (neh-CROW-sis), can involve a group of cells and, thus, tissue. When referring to dead cells or tissue, one would describe the area as necrotic. When necrosis occurs due to ischemia, the area of dead cells (ischemic necrosis) is called an **infarct** (IN-farkt). Infarcts are commonly due to obstruction of arteries. The most common infarct affects tissues of the heart, leading to a myocardial infarction, or heart attack.

Cells that are injured and not able to recover eventually die. The cause of cell death can be determined by a pathologist because the gross (visible with the eye) and microscopic appearance of the tissue differs with the type of death. There are several types of necrosis, primarily named by the microscopic appearance of the dead cells.

The most common type of necrosis is called coagulation necrosis and is due to cellular anoxia. Coagulation necrosis is the type of cell death experienced with myocardial infarction.

A common alteration in necrosis occurs when saprophytic (dead tissue–loving) bacteria become involved in the necrotic tissue. With this occurrence, the necrotic tissue is now described as gangrenous or having **gangrene** (GANG-green). The type of gangrene can be wet, dry, or gas, depending on the appearance of the necrotic tissue.

Wet gangrene usually occurs when the necrosis was caused by the sudden stoppage of blood flow, as in the trauma of burning, freezing, or embolism.

Dry gangrene occurs when blood flow has been slowed for a long period of time before necrosis occurred, as in the case of arteriosclerosis and advanced diabetes. In dry gangrene, the tissue is black, shriveled, or mummified. This type of gangrene occurs on the extremities only, primarily on the feet and toes.

Gas gangrene occurs with dirty, infected wounds. The tissue becomes infected with anaerobic (growing without oxygen) bacteria that produce a toxic gas. This is an acute, painful, and often fatal type of gangrene.

Organism Death

Human death can be related to any of the aforementioned causes of disease. The aging process leads to death due to a change in the normal structure of the individual's organs or a decrease in the ability to fight disease. Diseases that would not be lethal in our younger years, such as respiratory infections, can be the cause of death in an older individual.

According to Centers for Disease Control and Prevention (CDC), the most common cause of death in the United States is heart disease, followed by cancer and strokes (cerebrovascular accident). Although heart disease is the leading cause of death, stroke is the leading cause of serious, long-term disability in the United States. (See Chapter 8, "Cardiovascular System Diseases and Disorders," for more information.)

Many times, the human organism—like the cell—does not die but becomes disabled. Disability is called **morbidity** (state of being diseased). Often, morbidity is so extreme that the individual's quality of life is severely limited. This is often seen in cases of severe brain injury or even in some congenital disorders.

Prior to death, major organs such as the heart, lungs, and brain stop functioning. When the brain ceases to function, the individual is considered brain dead. Although death is difficult to define and difficult to determine in some cases, one guideline used is that of brain death. The criteria for determining brain death include:

- Lack of response to stimuli.
- Loss of all reflexes.
- Absence of respirations or breathing effort.
- Lack of brain activity as shown by an electroencephalogram (EEG).

This issue of defining death and when an individual is actually dead is still controversial in the medical profession.

SUMMARY

Human diseases are caused by heredity; trauma; inflammation, infection, or both; hyperplasias, neoplasms, or both; nutritional imbalances; impaired immunity; or some or all of these. Lifestyle behaviors can also be contributing factors to disease development, as can the aging process. Eventually, all organisms die, and the process of death can occur at the cellular, tissue, or whole organism level.

REVIEW QUESTIONS

Matching

1. Match the cause of diseases in the left column with the example of a disease for that category in the right column.

_____ Heredity   a. Pneumonia

_____ Trauma   b. Motor vehicle accident

_____ Inflammation/infection   c. Cancer

_____ Hyperplasias/neoplasms   d. Obesity

_____ Nutritional imbalance   e. Allergies

_____ Impaired immunity   f. Cystic fibrosis

True or False

2. T F   In autoimmunity, the body's immune system attacks itself.
3. T F   Some medications used to prevent or cure some diseases can cause immunodeficiency.
4. T F   Diseases related to the aging process are called regenerative disorders.
5. T F   All congenital disorders are easily recognized at birth.
6. T F   Heart and brain cells are easily injured by hypoxia.

7. T F   Heredity does not affect the aging process.

8. T F   Cellular death occurs only in the event of hypoxia (lack of oxygen).

Short Answer

9. List the factors that affect a cell's ability to survive after injury.

10. How do cells adapt when exposed to adverse conditions?

CASE STUDIES

■ Cann Ragland, age 29, was seriously injured in a motorcycle accident. He is comatose and on life support equipment to maintain his breathing. He has not improved in 2 weeks with aggressive medical treatment. The family is questioning whether he is alive or dead at this time. What criteria can be used to determine this? What are the issues surrounding this determination? How could you help the family through this difficult time? What resources are available to help people make decisions about end-of-life care?

■ Jessie Leher, age 69, is concerned about her aging status and loss of short-term memory at times. Her sister told her to take *Ginkgo biloba* and Co-Q10, over-the-counter herbal products. Jessie has high blood pressure and some circulatory problems. She takes several prescription medications for these disorders and for a couple of other problems, such as arthritis. Should she be cautioned about also taking the herbal remedies? How much should she actually know about her medications? Should health care providers provide more education for patients? Are consumers more interested in knowing about their health care treatments in today's world than in the past? Is that a good change?

Study Tools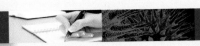

Workbook

Complete Chapter 2

Online Resources

PowerPoint® presentations

BIBLIOGRAPHY

American Heart Association. (2011). Heart disease and stroke statistics: 2011 update. *Circulation 123*(4), E18–E209.

Aschenbrenner, D. S. (2011). Drug watch. *American Journal of Nursing 11*(9), 22–23.

Begley, S. (2011). Could this be the end of cancer? *Newsweek 158*(25), 36–39.

Berrington de Gonzalez, A. (2010). Body mass index and mortality among 1.46 million white adults. *New England Journal of Medicine 363*(23), 2211–2219.

Burton, B., & Zeppetella, G. (2011). Assessing the impact of breakthrough cancer pain. *British Journal of Nursing 20*(Suppl), S14–S19.

Campbell, M. K. (2011). Cancer is a team sport. *Clinical Journal of Oncology Nursing 15*(4), 349.

Centers for Disease Control and Prevention. (2011). Deaths, injuries. In: *National Vital Statistics Report, 2007*. Atlanta, GA: Centers for Disease Control and Prevention.

Demarco, J., Nystrom, M., & Salvatore, K. (2011). The importance of patient education throughout the continuum of health care. *Journal of Consumer Health on the Internet 15*(1), 22–31.

Drug news. (2011). *Nursing 41*(4), 24.

Drug news. (2011). *Nursing 41*(6), 16.

Drug news. (2011). *Nursing 41*(8), 16.

Hamling, K. (2011). The management of nausea and vomiting in advanced cancer. *International Journal of Palliative Nursing 17*(7), 321–327.

Hanssens, S., Luyten, R., Watthy, C., Fontaine, C., Decoster, L., Baillon, C., Trullemans, F., Cortoos, A., & De Grève, J. (2011). Evaluation of a comprehensive rehabilitation program for post-treatment patients with cancer. *Oncology Nursing Forum 38*(6), E418–E424.

Lynch, E. (2011). A testing dilemma. *Nursing Standard 26*(7), 22–23.

Mellman, I., Coukos, G., & Dranoff, G. (2011). Cancer immunotherapy comes of age. *Nature 480*(7378), 480–489.

National Cancer Institute. (2012). Cancer trends progress report—2009–2010 update. *http://progressreport.cancer.gov/* (accessed January 2012).

Shepherd, H. L., Butow, P. N., & Tattersall, M. H. N. (2011). Factors which motivate cancer doctors to involve their patients in reaching treatment decisions. *Patient Education & Counseling 84*(2), 229–235.

Smart, M. (2011). Oncology update. *Oncology Nursing Forum 38*(4), 485–486.

Smart, M. (2011). Oncology update. *Oncology Nursing Forum 38*(5), 597–598.

van Mossel, C., Alford, M., & Watson, H. (2011). Challenges of patient-centered care: Practice or rhetoric. *Nursing Inquiry 18*(4), 278–228.

Watson, E. K., Rose, P. W., Neal, R. D., Hulbert-Williams, N., Donnelly, P., Hubbard, G. E., Campbell, C., Weller, D., & Wilkinson, C. (2012). Personalized cancer follow up: Risk stratification, needs assessment or both? *British Journal of Cancer 106*(1), 1–5.

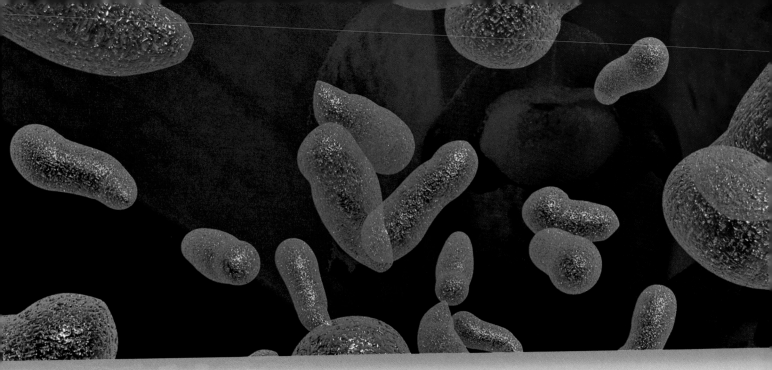

OUTLINE

KEY TERMS

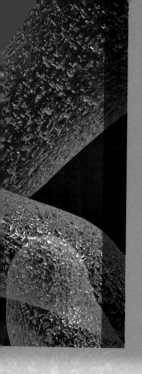
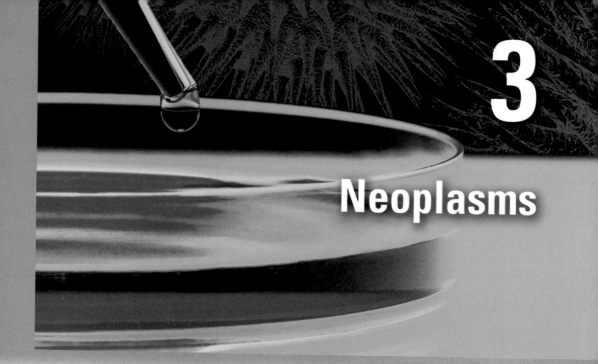

3

Neoplasms

LEARNING OBJECTIVES

Upon completion of the chapter, the learner should be able to:

1. Define basic terminology used in the study of neoplasms.
2. Explain the system used to classify neoplasms.
3. Compare hyperplasias to neoplasms.
4. Identify the progression of cancer development.
5. State the signs and symptoms of cancer.
6. Identify some common carcinogenic substances.
7. Identify high-risk behaviors for cancer development.
8. State the frequency of cancer development in the population.
9. Describe the curative, palliative, and preventive methods used in cancer treatment.

OVERVIEW

Thousands of individuals are diagnosed with neoplasms each year. The diagnostic statement, "You have a tumor," often causes instant fear, dread, and tears for the individuals and families involved; few statements in our society carry the emotional impact this one does. To most people, this diagnosis is equivalent to a pronouncement of death. But not all tumors are malignant, and not all are deadly. However, more than 1.3 million individuals are diagnosed with malignant neoplasms each year. This includes all types of cancers. Approximately 1,500 die each day, with about a half million deaths per year in the United States. However, the survival rate is about 68% now compared with only 50% just a few years ago. Prostate cancer is the most commonly diagnosed cancer among men, whereas breast cancer is the most commonly diagnosed type in women (National Cancer Institute, 2012). Cancer can be diagnosed using a variety of diagnostic tests, and treatment of cancer is most successful when the cancer has been diagnosed early. Individuals can reduce their risk of developing some types of cancer by following preventive measures recommended by the American Cancer Society. ■

TERMINOLOGY RELATED TO NEOPLASMS AND TUMORS

The term **neoplasm** (NEE-oh-plazm; neo = new, plasm = growth) means a new growth. The term **tumor** may be defined simply as a swelling or as a neoplasm. Tumor is used as a sign of inflammation and, in this instance, describes swelling. The term *tumor* as related to neoplasm means a new growth. Even though the terms *tumor* and *neoplasm* are used synonymously, not all neoplasms form tumors (Table 3–1). For instance, **leukemia** (loo-KEE-me-ah; leuk = white, emia = blood) is a malignant disease of the bone marrow that causes an increase in white blood cell production and might not form distinctive tumors. Likewise, not all tumors are neoplasms—a **hematoma** (HEM-ah-TOH-mah; hemat = blood, oma = tumor) is a large tumor or swelling filled with blood, commonly called a bruise or contusion (Figure 3–1).

CLASSIFICATION OF NEOPLASMS

Neoplasms may be classified in a variety of ways. Two of the most common ways are according to the (1) appearance and growth pattern and (2) tissue of origin, or type of body tissue from which they grow.

Appearance and Growth Pattern

Classification by appearance and growth pattern identifies neoplasms (tumors) as **benign** (beh-NINE) or **malignant** (mah-LIG-nant).

Benign Neoplasm

Neoplasms that are confined to a local area and do not spread are called benign. Benign neoplasms are more commonly called tumors. They are generally harmless unless they are growing in a confined space such as the brain.

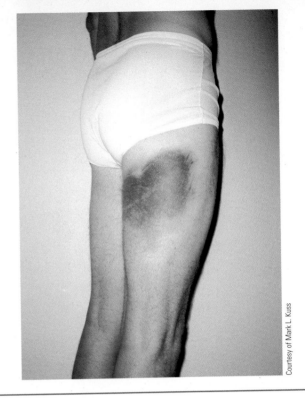

Courtesy of Mark L. Kuss

FIGURE 3–1 Hematoma.

Malignant Neoplasm

Malignant (deadly) neoplasms are so named because they exhibit characteristics of invasion and metastasis. **Invasion** refers to the spreading of the neoplasm into local or surrounding tissue. **Metastasis** (meh-TAS-tah-sis) is the spread of the neoplasm to distant sites. The general term for any malignant neoplasm is *cancer*.

Tissue of Origin

Neoplasms are classified or named according to the tissue from which they grow along with the suffix "oma" for tumor. A benign tumor will have the suffix "oma" added after the name of the tissue. An example would be lipoma, a benign tumor of fatty tissue. A malignant neoplasm will have the term **carcinoma** (KAR-sih-NO-mah) or **sarcoma** (sar-KOH-mah) added to the name of the tissue type.

Epithelial Tissue (Skin or Gland)

A benign tumor of epithelial tissue such as a gland would be adenoma; if it is a malignant neoplasm, the name becomes adenocarcinoma. *Carcinoma* denotes the largest group of malignant neoplasms

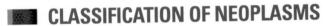

TABLE 3–1 Neoplasm vs. Nonneoplasm

| Neoplasm—new growth | Swelling: Can be called tumor
No swelling: No tumor, but is a neoplasm—e.g., leukemia |
| Nonneoplasm | Swelling: Hematoma, inflammation |

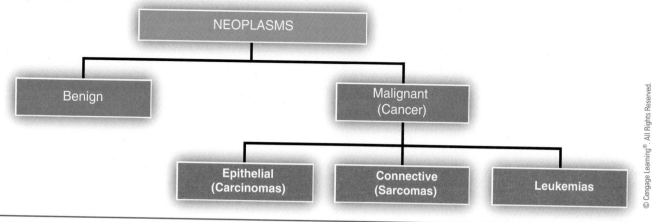

FIGURE 3–2 Classification of neoplasms.

and indicates a tumor of epithelial tissue found on external or internal body surfaces.

Connective Tissue (Bone, Muscle, or Fat)

A benign tumor of connective tissue such as bone would be an osteoma; if it is a malignant neoplasm, the name is osteosarcoma—*sarcoma* is the term used if the neoplasm is from connective tissue such as muscle, fat, and bone. Sarcomas are less common than carcinomas but spread more rapidly and are highly malignant.

Lymphatic or Blood-Forming Tissue

Lymphomas (lim-FOH-mas) and leukemias are malignant neoplasms of lymphatic and blood-forming organs and lymphatic tissues, respectively. These malignant neoplasms do not have benign counterparts. All leukemias and lymphomas are malignant, although their prognoses can vary considerably (Figure 3–2).

Other Tissues

Some tumors, of course, do not follow this pattern. For example, malignant melanoma, a malignant neoplasm of melanocytes (skin cells), is not a benign tumor, as its name would suggest. *Glioma* refers to all tumors of the glial cells of the brain, but gliomas do not fit truly the terms of this classification system. They are benign in appearance and do not metastasize, but they are malignant (deadly) because most are fatal. Examples of benign and malignant neoplasms are listed in Table 3–2.

▉ GROWTH OF BENIGN AND MALIGNANT NEOPLASMS

Normal cells grow and function for a purpose and are regulated by several factors. First, the built-in genetic program of each cell regulates its growth pattern. Second, normal cellular growth is limited by contact

TABLE 3–2 Origins and Names for Benign and Malignant Neoplasms

Cell or Tissue of Origin	Name of Benign Neoplasm	Name of Malignant Neoplasm
Glandular epithelium	Adenoma	Adenocarcinoma
Squamous epithelium	Epithelioma	Squamous cell carcinoma
Adipose (fat)	Lipoma	Liposarcoma
Cartilage	Chondroma	Chondrosarcoma
Bone	Osteoma	Osteosarcoma
Glial cell		Glioma
Blood		Leukemia

with other cells. When two normal cells come in contact with one another, they tend to stick together and transmit a signal, called contact inhibition, to each other to stop growing (Figure 3–3).

Finally, normal cellular growth is regulated by growth-promoting or growth-inhibiting substances. When the normal cells stop growing, they begin performing their specialized function. For example, epithelial cells begin functioning to cover and protect the organism, whereas bone cells function to provide structure and support. This process of individual specialization is called **differentiation** (Figure 3–4).

Benign Neoplasm Growth

Benign neoplasm or tumors might retain some normal structure and function. These cells often resemble cells of their origin, and even though they have an abnormal appearance, their appearance is uniform. Benign neoplasms also can function to some degree like normal cells. They are encapsulated, or covered with a capsule-like material, that makes removal or excision easier. These tumor cells have a limited growth potential and are slower growing than metastatic neoplasms.

Benign neoplasms are expansive (grow and enlarge in the area) but are not invasive or metastatic. This does not mean that benign tumors are harmless. The presence and growth of any tumor can obstruct passageways such as those in the digestive and respiratory systems, leading to difficulty with eating or breathing.

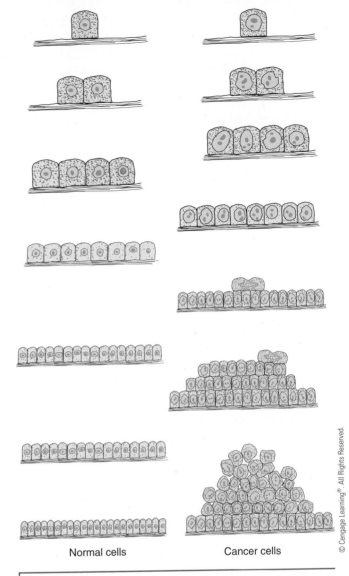

Normal cells   Cancer cells

FIGURE 3–3   Cellular growth patterns.

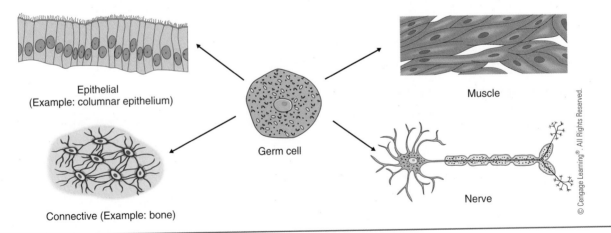

Epithelial
(Example: columnar epithelium)

Germ cell

Muscle

Nerve

Connective (Example: bone)

FIGURE 3–4   The process of cell differentiation.

Tumors also can exert pressure on nerves, causing pain and loss of sensation or movement. Benign tumors affecting a gland might cause over- or undersecretion of hormones, with resulting disorders. A benign tumor growing in an enclosed area such as the brain can place pressure on normal tissue, leading to death of the tissue and, potentially, death of the individual.

Malignant Neoplasm Growth

Malignant neoplasms are cells whose growth pattern has no purpose and is uncontrollable. Neoplastic cells grow autonomously or independent of growth factors. These cells grow excessively, without regard to normal regulatory factors such as contact inhibition.

Malignant neoplastic cells do not have the structure or function of the cells of their origin. Unlike benign tumor cells, neoplastic cells do not look alike. Their structure is not uniform but rather is haphazard and inconsistent. They are not differentiated and do not perform specialized functions. The surface area of the malignant neoplasm is not encapsulated. Rather, it is more crab-like in appearance, with multiple claw-like extensions that invade surrounding tissue. A malignant neoplasm (cancer) also metastasizes to distant areas or organs. A comparison of benign and malignant neoplasms is listed in Table 3-3.

Cancer (malignant neoplasm) cells are fast growing. The entire metabolism of the cancerous cell is aimed at rapid reproduction and growth, far outpacing the growth of the normal cell, and leads to an increase in the need for nutrients and oxygen. To meet this need, **angiogenesis** (AN-jee-oh-JEN-eh-sis; angio = vessel, genesis = growth or new growth of blood vessels) occurs to increase blood flow, providing increased nutrients to the neoplasm and allowing it to continue this rapid, uncontrolled growth. During this time, normal cells are deprived of needed nutrients, and the individual begins to lose weight and appear thin, frail, and weak, a condition called **cachexia**.

Consider This ...

Fight cancer with bright-colored fruits and vegetables—the brighter the color, the higher the antioxidant content. Blueberries, other bright-colored berries, red cabbage, and eggplant, to name a few, are good sources of antioxidants. These bright-colored foods are thought to not only stop tumor growth but also kill tumor cells.

▮ HYPERPLASIAS AND NEOPLASMS

It is important to note that there is another type of cellular growth that closely resembles a neoplasm. **Hyperplasia** (HIGH-per-PLAY-zee-ah; hyper = too much, plasia = growth) and neoplasia (neo = new, plasia = growth) are both overgrowths of cells that cause an increase in the size of the tissue.

Both commonly produce masses that, once discovered, must be identified as either hyperplasia or neoplasm because the treatment of each is drastically different. Hyperplasias and neoplasms differ in the cause and extent of their growth.

TABLE 3–3   Comparison of Benign and Malignant Neoplasms

Feature	Benign	Malignant
Growth	Slow, expansive	Fast, invasive, metastatic
Appearance	Symmetrical	Crab-like
Capsule	Yes	No
Tissue type	Resembles tissue of origin	Does not resemble tissue of origin
Cells	Differentiated	Undifferentiated
Surface	Smooth	Irregular, may ulcerate and hemorrhage

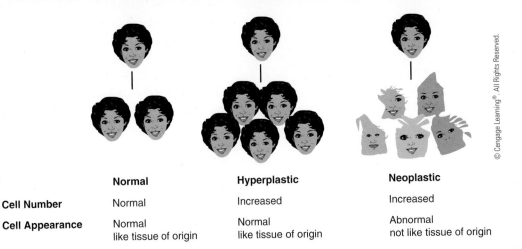

	Normal	Hyperplastic	Neoplastic
Cell Number	Normal	Increased	Increased
Cell Appearance	Normal like tissue of origin	Normal like tissue of origin	Abnormal not like tissue of origin

FIGURE 3–5 Comparison of hyperplasia and neoplasm.

Hyperplasias

Hyperplasia usually occurs in response to a stimulus, and the growth stops when the stimulus stops. Hyperplasias can be caused by a variety of stimuli. An example of a hyperplasia caused by tissue irritation is a skin callus on the foot; the stimulus is the irritation or rubbing of a shoe on that particular area. When the shoe size is corrected, the stimulus ends, the hyperplasia stops, and the callus eventually disappears.

Hyperplasias can develop due to hormone excess or deficiency such as the hormone deficiency hyperplasia causing enlargement of the thyroid gland, called goiter. Chronic inflammation can also lead to hyperplasia, as in lymph node hyperplasia or adenoid hyperplasia. Finally, hyperplasia can be caused by an unknown stimulus, as in the case of prostatic hyperplasia in older men.

Hyperplasias are an increase of cells that look like cells of their origin. To simplify this concept, one might consider the cells as daughter cells that still look like their mother (Figure 3–5).

Neoplasms

Hyperplasias and neoplasms both represent an increase in cell number, but neoplasms grow independently, excessively, and usually unceasingly.

Neoplasms are not only an increase in cell number but new (neo = new) or different in their appearance from their cell of origin, or mother, unlike hyperplasia. This difference in appearance is important to the clinical pathologist who determines or diagnoses the mass as hyperplasia or neoplasm.

DEVELOPMENT OF MALIGNANT NEOPLASMS (CANCER)

Genetic alteration is the basis for the development of malignant neoplasm, or cancer. Cells throughout the body can undergo genetic alteration or mutation, but amazingly, few develop into cancer. A cell must undergo a change or series of changes in its DNA structure to acquire the altered growth pattern of cancer. Genetic mutation or change is brought about by a virus, chemicals, **radiation** (the process of using light, short waves such as ultraviolet or X-ray), or other biologic agent called a **carcinogen** (kar-SIN-oh-jen; carcino = cancer, gen = arising), or cancer-causing agent or substance.

Continued exposure to a carcinogen or to several carcinogens can increase or promote the abnormality of the cell. Abnormal cells might revert to normal cells, appear as benign tumors, or digress to a malignant neoplasm. The body's immune system might prevent or reverse the development of cancer. Just removing or stopping the carcinogen can also reverse cancer development.

If development is not halted, abnormal cells begin to establish themselves in an effort to become cancerous and must now grow rapidly enough to establish a site. They must fight for space and nutrition, so the body and the abnormal cells are at odds with each other at this point. If the body wins, the abnormal cells might die out and disappear. If the abnormal cells attain the upper hand, they can become established and thrive.

As long as the abnormal cells are not firmly established, they are considered preneoplastic or

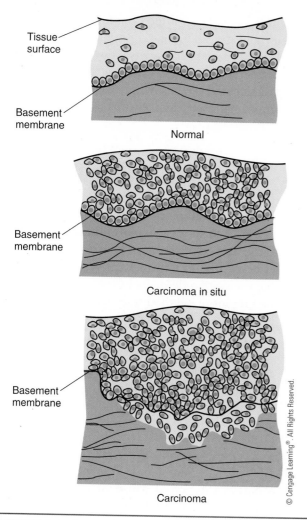

Tissue surface

Basement membrane

Normal

Basement membrane

Carcinoma in situ

Basement membrane

Carcinoma

FIGURE 3–6   Normal, carcinoma in situ, and carcinoma tissue.

precancerous. If these cells are discovered at this point, surgical removal can occur before cancer actually develops. Unfortunately, very few potential cancers are discovered at this stage. Squamous epithelial tissue often progresses through a slow series of changes, including hyperplasia, abnormal hyperplasia called **dysplasia** (DIS-PLAY-zee-ah), and, finally, a stage called **carcinoma in situ**.

In carcinoma in situ, the atypical cells are "just sitting" in the epithelial layer of the tissue and have not broken through the basement membrane and invaded the surrounding tissue. Carcinoma in situ commonly occurs in the uterine cervix, larynx, and mouth. Cancer can be avoided at this stage by surgical removal of the dysplasia, or in situ tumor.

The final stage in cancer development is the invasion by the precancerous cells into the surrounding tissue, signifying a change from precancerous to malignant neoplasm. In epithelial tissue,

this is the point at which neoplastic cells (carcinomas) break through the basement membrane that separates the epithelium from the connective tissue below (Figure 3–6). When this break occurs, the neoplastic cells can spread quickly, not only with local tissue invasion but via the lymphatic system (lymph fluid) and circulatory system (blood).

■ INVASION BY AND METASTASIS OF CANCER

Local invasion by cancer is similar to the way plants sink their roots into the soil. The finger-like projections of the neoplasms force themselves along the lines of least resistance. Pressure from the growing tumor occludes blood supply, leading to local tissue necrosis, weakening the tissue, which eases further spread of the neoplasm.

Spread of cancer from this primary location or site to secondary sites in the body is called metastasis. Cancer cells are carried, or metastasize, through the lymphatic system or through the blood. In some cases, metastasis occurs by seeding or spreading within a cavity.

Lymphatic System Metastasis

Carcinomas—epithelial tissue neoplasms—commonly spread through the lymphatics or lymphatic system. Because lymph nodes can catch or filter cancer cells, lymph nodes are commonly removed surgically and examined for the presence of cancerous cells. Lymph nodes near the tumor are generally the first to filter cancerous cells. As more and more neoplastic cells spread into the lymphatic system, the filters fill with neoplastic cells and, eventually, the nodes become full and unable to filter more cells. When this occurs, the neoplastic cells can spill over into the bloodstream.

Absence of lymph node involvement with cancer is a favorable sign and can mean that surgical cure is possible. Usually, the higher the number of lymph nodes involved, the poorer the chance of survival.

Bloodstream Metastasis

Sarcomas do not use the lymphatic system as readily as carcinomas (Table 3–4). These tumors shed neoplastic cells directly into the blood, by which they can

TABLE 3–4 Comparison of Carcinomas and Sarcomas

Feature	Carcinoma	Sarcoma
Tissue	Epithelial	Connective
Occurrence	Very common	Less common
Growth	Slow	Rapid
Metastasis	Primarily through lymph	Primarily through blood

be widely distributed throughout the body. Common sites of bloodstream metastasis are the liver, lungs, and brain. Frequently, and unfortunately, it is the secondary cancer site that is discovered first.

Cavity Metastasis

Metastasis can also occur by invasion and implantation within a serous (watery or fluid-filled) cavity. When neoplastic cells reach a serous cavity such as the pleural or peritoneal cavity, they can seed and implant freely within that cavity.

Media Link

View an animation about cancer metastasizing on the Online Resources.

GRADING AND STAGING OF CANCER

Grading and staging of malignant tumors are used to plan treatment and predict possibility of a cure. Grading determines the degree of abnormality of the neoplasm, and staging considers the degree of spread.

Grading

Grading is the microscopic examination of the tumor to determine the degree of differentiation. The more differentiated the tumor, the more it looks like the tissue of its origin. The more abnormal the tissue appears in comparison to its normal tissue, the more undifferentiated or **anaplastic** (AN-ah-PLAST-ic) it is. The higher the degree of differentiation, the better the prognosis.

Tumors that are undifferentiated or anaplastic do not resemble the tissue of origin, are highly malignant, and offer a poor prognosis. Tumors are typically placed into grades from I to IV. Grade I tumors are the less aggressive and serious, whereas grade IV tumors are the most aggressive and serious in nature.

Staging

Staging determines the extent of spread of the neoplasm. Clinical examination, X-rays, **biopsy** (BYE-op-see; removing a small piece of tissue for microscopic examination), and surgical exploration can be used to evaluate the degree of spread. Tumors can be placed in stages according to a numerical system (I to IV), much like the system described for grading.

A second, more detailed staging is the TNM system. In this system, tumors are staged according to the size and extent of the primary tumor, number of lymph nodes involved, and metastasis to other sites.

Grading and staging are two predictors of prognosis. Of the two predictors, staging is the better indicator.

CAUSES OF CANCER

Unfortunately, the actual cause of most cancer is unknown. Cancer appears to occur due to a variety of circumstances, which suggests that more than one factor is involved in its development. One thing remains constant in the development of cancer: the genetic alteration that allows the cell to grow independently and uncontrollably. It is thought that cellular mutations actually occur frequently in humans. It is further theorized that the human immune system catches and destroys these abnormal cells as soon as they occur. So, in some respects, cancer might represent some failure of the immune system in the individual. Prevention and cure of cancer will depend on finding the initiating agents that cause the genetic alteration in the cell or the event that causes an altered cell to become malignant. Currently, hundreds of carcinogenic compounds have been identified.

The process of **carcinogenesis** (KAR-sin-oh-JEN-eh-sis; cancer development) in an individual might take many years to develop, might stop and start, or might even be reversed, but usually there will be a continual progression of cellular changes from hyperplasia to dysplasia to **metaplasia** (MET-ah-PLAY-zee-ah) to neoplasia (Figure 3–7).

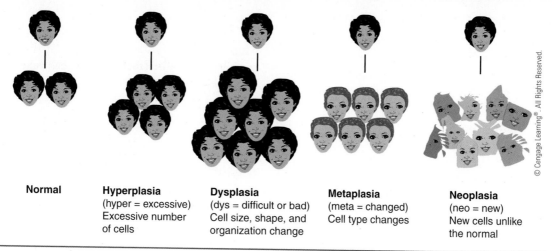

| Normal | Hyperplasia (hyper = excessive) Excessive number of cells | Dysplasia (dys = difficult or bad) Cell size, shape, and organization change | Metaplasia (meta = changed) Cell type changes | Neoplasia (neo = new) New cells unlike the normal |

FIGURE 3–7 Cellular changes progressing to neoplasm.

Chemical Carcinogens

Chemical carcinogenesis is quite complex. The frequency of exposure and the strength or potency of the chemical are important factors in the development of cancer. Chemicals that do not cause a problem by themselves might enhance cancer development when used in combination with other chemicals.

Chemical carcinogens abound in our environment, and exposure to certain chemicals used in industry can lead to cancer among workers. For instance, naphthylamine, found in certain types of dye, has been found to cause bladder cancer; asbestos, previously used in roofing and insulating materials, has been identified as a carcinogen leading to lung cancer. Miners of nickel ore have a high rate of nasal cancer, and farmers using arsenic as an insecticide often suffer from skin and lung cancers.

Currently, chemicals used as food additives, cosmetics, and certain plastics are the focus of intensive research investigating the possible relationship of these chemicals to cancer.

Hormones

Hormones can increase the incidence of cancer, yet, at times, hormones can be used as a form of cancer treatment. The action of hormones as related to cancer is not clearly understood. For example, a benign mole normally does not become malignant until sex hormones increase at puberty, but administration of diethylstilbestrol, a synthetic estrogen compound, to pregnant women during the 1940s and 1950s led to an increase in a rare vaginal adenocarcinoma in their female children and to testicular abnormalities in their male children.

Excessive production of estrogen in the female can lead to cancer of the breast and uterus. Estrogen medication used to treat menopausal symptoms in women has been shown to lead to an increase in endometrial cancer. The ovaries are sometimes removed after a female has breast cancer in an effort to decrease stimulation of other possible tumors.

Although much research has been done to correlate cancer with birth control pills, the findings are inconclusive. The most widely used combination pill, combining estrogen and progestin, a synthetic form of progesterone, might actually decrease the risk of ovarian and endometrial cancer.

Cancer of the prostate is stimulated by the male hormone testosterone but is slowed or inhibited by estrogen treatment. Males who suffer with prostatic cancer can undergo treatment with estrogen medication to counteract the effects of testosterone. Treatment to decrease testosterone production might also include an orchiectomy—removal of the testes—in an effort to decrease or slow the growth of the prostatic tumor or decrease stimulation of other possible tumors.

Radiation

Ultraviolet (UV) radiation, X-radiation, and radioactive materials are all known carcinogens. More than 2 million cases of skin cancer are diagnosed each year (National Cancer Institute, 2012). Sunbathers, farmers, fishermen, construction workers, mariners, and anyone else with an extended exposure to the UV rays of the sun or tanning lights have an increased risk of developing basal or squamous cell carcinomas. Although basal and squamous cell carcinomas tend to occur from cumulative exposure to the sun, melanoma occurs more frequently due to extreme, blistering burns at a young age. Fair-skinned people are at greatest risk for skin cancer because they lack the protective effects of melanin. UV-related skin cancer is uncommon among the black population.

X-rays have been used extensively as a diagnostic tool since discovery by Wilhelm Roentgen in 1895. Radiologists commonly developed cancers before the correlation of radiation and cancer—Roentgen himself developed skin cancer. In the late 1800s, radiation dosage was determined by taking repeated X-rays of the operator's hand, and soon after X-ray discovery, the development of the first hand cancer was reported. Presently, radiation is considered a professional risk for radiologists and those working in the field of radiology. Proper use of protective clothing and equipment minimizes the risk.

High doses of radiation might actually be used as treatment for some cancers, but this treatment does carry a risk of developing secondary tumors. These tumors usually develop after a lengthy period of time (20 to 25 years), which makes the benefits of radiation therapy far outweigh its risk.

Radioactive materials that emit alpha, beta, and gamma rays are potential carcinogens. Most of these materials are used in medicine and research and are under strict regulation. With the use of protective clothing, the risk to workers in these areas is minimal. The most devastating and dramatic link between radiation and cancer was the increase shown in leukemia and thyroid cancers in the survivors of the atomic bombs dropped on Hiroshima and Nagasaki in 1945.

Viruses

Viruses have been proven to cause cancer in laboratory animals, but the proof is not as clear-cut in humans. Some examples worth noting include the Epstein-Barr virus, which causes infectious mononucleosis and has been associated with Burkitt's lymphoma, a malignant neoplasm seen primarily in Africa. Hepatitis B virus has been closely connected to liver cancer. Individuals with cervical cancer also tend to have the herpes simplex virus.

Genetic Predisposition

There is some evidence of genetic predisposition for cancer, as demonstrated by the increased occurrence of certain types of cancers in the same family. This knowledge has led to intensive research. Discovery of certain cancer suppressor genes, and most recently a breast cancer gene, has aided research efforts, but complete understanding of the correlation of genetics and cancer has not yet been reached.

It is known that colon and breast cancer have a higher incidence in certain families. A woman whose mother or sisters have, or have had, breast cancer runs a fivefold greater chance of developing breast cancer than women who do not have this family history. Genetic testing is now available for the breast cancer gene.

Personal Risk Behaviors

Several personal behaviors common in our society—smoking cigarettes and other tobacco product use, some dietary practices, alcohol use, and certain sexual behavior—put an individual at increased risk for developing cancer.

Smoking and Tobacco Product Use

Cigarette smoking is carcinogenic. Approximately 443,000 deaths occur yearly from tobacco use (American Cancer Society [ACS], 2011). According to the ACS, smoking kills more people in the United States each year than car accidents, alcohol, acquired immunodeficiency syndrome (AIDS), murders, illegal drugs, and suicides combined. It is the major cause of lung cancer. Smokers are 10 to 20 times more likely to get lung cancer than nonsmokers.

Smoking also doubles the incidence of cancer of the bladder and pancreas. Chemicals in cigarette smoke affect all organs of the body because the chemicals are absorbed from the lungs into the blood and circulated to all organs. These chemicals are found in increased concentrations in the urine of smokers. Secondhand smoke has now also been proven to be detrimental, leading to approximately 46,000 heart disease deaths and 3,400 lung cancer deaths per year in nonsmokers. Currently, it is estimated that cigarette smoking costs the United States approximately $193 billion per year in health care costs and related losses.

The chemicals in smokeless tobacco are absorbed into the blood and, again, circulate to the entire body with detrimental effects. Oral cancer occurs more frequently in users of smokeless tobacco than in nontobacco users.

Diet

Identifying the carcinogenic nature of dietary practices is difficult because many factors are involved. Diet seems to function over a period of time to place an individual at risk for cancer. There is a consistent relationship between increased weight in women and the risk of cancer, although there is not a relationship between the two for men. Obesity and a high consumption of dietary fat in women is a consistent risk factor for endometrial, breast, and colon cancer.

Much controversy exists concerning food additives, especially saccharin and nitrates. Saccharin has been shown to cause bladder cancer in rats, but this correlation has not been clear in humans. Nitrates are used as preservatives in meat and fish and have been shown to produce stomach cancer in animals. Countries with high nitrate consumption, Japan for example, have high rates of gastric cancer.

Colon cancer rates are lower in countries that have a lower consumption of dietary fat and a higher consumption of dietary fiber than the United States. The western plains area of the United States is high in selenium and has the lowest colon cancer rates, thus supporting the concept of some correlation between selenium levels and colon cancer.

Alcohol Use

Cancer of the mouth, throat, and esophagus occurs more often in people who smoke and consume large quantities of alcohol. Alcohol has not been proven as a carcinogen per se, but recent studies have also shown a higher incidence of breast cancer in women who drink even moderate amounts (three drinks per week).

Sexual Behavior

The risk of developing cervical cancer is related to the age of first sexual intercourse and the number of sexual partners. The younger the female and the larger the number of sex partners, the greater the risk, and females who have only one sexual partner are at risk if that partner has had multiple partners. Medical studies have confirmed that human papilloma virus (HPV) is associated with most cervical cancers and that it is easily transmitted between partners.

The incidence of cervical cancer is two times greater in black women than in white and is found more commonly in women from lower socioeconomic groups. Women marrying men whose previous sexual partners had developed cervical cancer also are at greater risk of developing cervical cancer.

Pregnancy and childbirth appear to be protective mechanisms from cancer of the ovary, endometrium, and breast for women. Females who start menstrual cycles at a later age, have early menopause, bear the first child at an early age, or experience some or all these behaviors are at decreased risk for breast cancer.

CANCER PREVENTION

Cancer of the lung, breast, prostate, and colon are responsible for the majority of cancer deaths. Many of these cancers can be prevented by lifestyle changes. Smoking and tobacco use lead to approximately 30% of all cancers. Cigarette smoking is considered the single most preventable cause of lung cancer, other diseases of the lung, and heart disease.

Diet and nutrition play a significant role in the prevention of cancer. **Preventive** measures include reduction of fat intake and an increase in consumption of high-fiber food such as bran, whole grains, and fibrous vegetables and fruits. Monitor caloric intake and exercise properly.

Americans' passion for a suntan encourages people to lie in the sun and use tanning lights. The most widespread cancer—skin cancer—can be prevented by avoiding unnecessary exposure to the sun and tanning lights. If exposure to the sun is necessary, the use of a sunblock agent with 15 or higher sun protection factor (SPF) is recommended.

Consider This ...

Slip! Slop! Slap! and Wrap

The ACS's awareness campaign for skin cancer prevention promotes the slogan "Slip! Slop! Slap! and Wrap!," which is a catch phrase that reminds people of the four key ways they can protect themselves from UV radiation:

- Slip on a shirt,
- Slop on sunscreen,
- Slap on a hat, and
- Wrap on sunglasses to protect the eyes and sensitive skin around them from ultraviolet light. (ACS, 2012)

The ACS recommends the following preventive measures.

- Do not smoke. Smoking damages nearly every organ in the body, is associated with at least 15 cancers, and accounts for about one-third of all cancer deaths. This lifestyle behavior choice is the most preventable cause of early death in our society.

- Limit alcohol intake. Women should not drink more than one drink per day and men no more than two per day. Heavy drinking increases the risk of cancer of the esophagus, mouth, throat, larynx, and liver.

- Protect skin from excessive sun exposure. Use SPF 15 or greater when outdoors. Approximately 1 million cases of nonmelanoma skin cancer diagnosed yearly in the United States are thought to be sun-related.

- Refuse needless X-rays. Take special precautions to protect the unborn child if X-rays are necessary.

- Avoid heavily polluted air and long exposure to household solvent cleaners, paint thinners, and the like.

- Follow label instructions carefully when using pesticides, fungicides, and other home garden and lawn chemicals.

- Maintain a healthy body weight. Eat fewer fatty foods and more high-fiber food such as bran, whole grains, and fibrous vegetables and fruits.

- Women should perform breast self-examinations regularly.

- Exercise regularly. The recommendation is 30 minutes of moderate to vigorous activity at least 5 days a week. Those who engage in regular moderate exercise might lower their chance of developing cancer by 30%.

- Routine HPV vaccination is recommended for girls and boys to prevent HPV infection. Gardasil® and Cervarix® are both Food and Drug Administration (FDA)-approved vaccines. These vaccines should be completed before the individual becomes sexually active. Neither of the vaccines will treat an existing infection. (For more information on HPV infection, see Chapter 17.)

- Have regular checkups by physicians. For women over 50, a mammogram is recommended as part of the routine examination. Also, the **Pap test** (a test to screen for cervical cancer) should be performed at regular intervals.

- The American Cancer Society (ACS) no longer recommends monthly testicular self-exams for men because they have not been shown to affect early diagnosis. However, the ACS does recommend that men report to their health care provider changes in how the testicle feels or looks (ACS, 2012).

- A rectal examination should be part of every medical checkup for men and women, and stool samples should be examined for blood, which might be an indication of colon cancer.

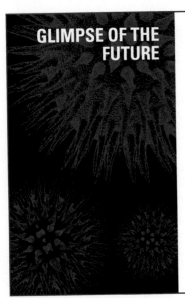

GLIMPSE OF THE FUTURE

New Cancer Research May Help Prevent the Disease

The American Cancer Society has initiated a study on "cancer prevention" to try to determine what contributes to humans developing cancer and how it can be prevented through lifestyle or environmental changes. Although researchers already know what contributes to some types of cancer (like smoking), all the factors contributing to other types of cancer are not yet known. The study will continue over many years following groups of volunteer participants who have not been diagnosed with cancer. The researchers hope to better understand the disease, its cause, and what preventive measures are important in the prevention plan. The longitudinal study should bring interesting new knowledge to the field of cancer research and prevention. Perhaps in the future, many types of cancer will be preventable by following a recommended set of lifestyle behaviors or by changing the environment.

Source: American Cancer Society (2013).

FREQUENCY OF CANCER

Cancer is a focus of major concern for our society because it strikes more than a million individuals per year. Cancer, along with heart disease, causes more than half of all deaths in the United States. One in two men and one in three women will be diagnosed with cancer during their lifespan. Since 1990, over 11 million cases of cancer have been diagnosed, with 5 million deaths occurring. One out of four deaths (1,500 per day) is due to cancer. It affects many lives, causing extreme grief, suffering, and financial loss. However, between 1990 and 2007, cancer death rates decreased 22.2% in men and 13.9% in women.

The term *cancer* covers a large number of specific types of malignant neoplasms. Each of these types might vary considerably from each other in behavior and treatment, and the prognosis for these individual types will depend on the individual cancer's metastatic rate, the extent of spread when discovered, and the effectiveness of current treatments.

In general, the survival rate of cancer is approximately 68%. Even though all malignant neoplasms might fit into a classification of carcinomas, sarcomas, leukemias, or lymphomas, there is a great difference in the way they behave. Some types, such as pancreatic carcinoma, are usually deadly, whereas skin carcinoma seldom is.

Cancer affects people of all ages and both males and females. The most common type of cancer is basal and squamous cell skin cancer. These neoplasms are seldom fatal because they are very visible, are slow

TABLE 3–5   Lifetime Risk of Being Diagnosed with Cancer—Both Sexes, All Races

Site/Type	Risk by Percent
All sites	41.21
Brain	0.61
Breast	6.37
Colon/rectum	5.08
Kidney	1.56
Leukemia	1.34
Liver	0.80
Lung	6.94
Oral cavity	1.05
Pancreas	1.45
Urinary bladder	2.41

Modified from National Cancer Institute. (2011). SEER cancer statistics review 1975–2008. Devcan Version 6.6.0, October 2011. *http://surveillance.cancer.gov/devcan/* (accessed January 2012).

TABLE 3–6   Lifetime Risk of Dying from Cancer—Both Sexes, All Races

Site/Type	Risk by Percent
All sites	21.07
Brain	0.43
Breast	1.47
Colon/rectum	2.06
Kidney	0.47
Leukemia	0.85
Liver	0.60
Lung	5.87
Oral cavity	1.05
Pancreas	1.29
Urinary bladder	0.57

Modified from National Cancer Institute. (2011). SEER cancer statistics review 1975–2008. Devcan Version 6.6.0, October 2011. *http://surveillance.cancer.gov/devcan/* (accessed January 2012).

growing, and can be completely excised. Because these tumors are generally treated in a physician's office, they are difficult to track statistically and are usually excluded in statistical data. Malignant melanoma, however, is a deadly form of skin cancer that comprises approximately only 1% of all skin malignancies but is statistically recorded as skin cancer.

The most common types of cancer, excluding skin cancers, are cancers of the lung, colon/rectum, breast, and prostate. The lifetime probability of being diagnosed with cancer and the lifetime risk of dying from cancer are presented in Tables 3–5 and 3–6.

DIAGNOSIS OF CANCER

The prognosis for the individual with a malignant neoplasm is best if the cancer is located and treated early. Routine screening can be very effective in discovery and early diagnosis of cancer. Screening measures include monthly breast self-examinations, regular Pap tests, and mammograms for females. Screening for males no longer includes a routine testicular self-examination, but any change in how the testicle feels or looks should be noticed and reported to the individual's physician. Occult stool examinations after age 40 to screen for colon cancer are important for both sexes.

Discovery of tumors can occur through routine screening or accidentally during other diagnostic procedures. For instance, X-ray examinations of the chest prior to surgery might reveal a mass, or annual physical examinations can lead to the discovery.

Recognition of cancer warning signs by an individual is important. The ACS lists several of these signs, with the initial letters forming the acronym CAUTION. They might be indicative of cancer development, so the individual with one or more of these signs should be evaluated immediately by a physician.

- Change in bowel or bladder habits
- A sore that does not heal
- Unusual bleeding or discharge
- Thickening or lump in breast or elsewhere
- Indigestion or difficulty swallowing
- Obvious change in a wart or mole
- Nagging cough or hoarseness

When discovered, more detailed radiologic exams such as computerized tomography (CT), magnetic resonance imaging (MRI), and positron emission tomography (PET) can be used to gain more information on size and location of tumor(s). (More detailed information on these exams can be found in Chapter 6, "Musculoskeletal System Diseases and Disorders," and Chapter 8, "Cardiovascular System Diseases and Disorders.")

Diagnosis of a tumor is made by microscopic examination of the cells and tissue. Examination of cells is called **cytology** (sigh-TOL-oh-jee; cyto = cell, ology = study) or a cytologic examination. Live tissue examination is a biopsy, which is the most definitive (clear-cut or without question) test used to diagnose a tumor.

A Papanicolaou, or Pap test, named after its developer, Dr. George Papanicolaou, can be used to examine the cells. Although most people think of a Pap test as a test only for cervical cytology, in reality, this simple staining test can be used to examine other body fluids such as urine, feces, sputum, prostatic fluid, or vaginal fluids. After the sample is stained, it is placed under a microscope and examined for abnormal cells.

To microscopically examine live tissue, a biopsy must be done. A biopsy can be obtained by aspiration, needle biopsy, endoscopy, or surgery. Aspiration biopsy uses a needle attached to a suction device to remove a small piece of tissue from the tumor. Needle biopsy is obtained by punching a needle through the tumor and using the tissue caught in the lumen of the needle for examination. If the size of the needle is quite small, the biopsy is called a fine needle biopsy. During endoscopy, the tissue is removed by use of the appropriate scope, for example, bronchoscope, colonoscope, or gastroscope. For surgical biopsy, the tissue is removed by cutting or incising the tissue (Figure 3–8).

Surgical biopsy can be performed with the patient's consent to excise the tumor if it is found to

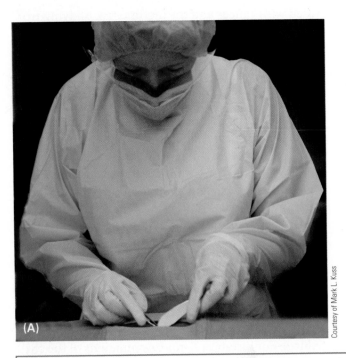
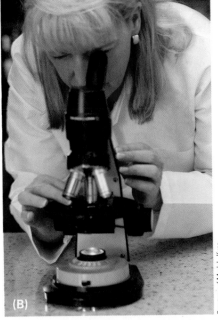

FIGURE 3–8 (A) Tissue biopsy. A small piece of tissue is surgically removed. (B) Pathologist views tissue under microscope looking for presence of disease.

be cancerous. After the biopsy is obtained, it is sent immediately to the pathologist for diagnosis. The patient often remains in the surgical suite under anesthesia while the surgeon awaits these results. A technique called a **frozen section** enables the pathologist to make a rapid determination of the tumor condition: benign or malignant.

◼◼ SIGNS AND SYMPTOMS OF CANCER

Signs and symptoms of cancer are highly variable according to the site and type of malignancy. Pain, obstruction, hemorrhage, anemia, fracture, infection, and cachexia might be manifestations of cancer. Any one of these or a combination can be present, but often, cancer is asymptomatic until late in its developmental stage, including metastasis.

Pain

Pain from cancer is usually not an early symptom. Cancer causes pain by growing to the point of causing destruction of normal tissue, obstructing the lumen of hollow organs like the intestine, placing pressure on nerve endings, causing inflammation leading to discomfort, or any of these.

Obstruction

Obstruction of a hollow organ can occur from a tumor growing inside the organ or from tumor growth outside the organ that compresses or pushes into the organ. Examples of obstruction could include the bronchus of the lung and any area of the intestine.

Hemorrhage

Hemorrhage can be caused by the cancerous tissue ulcerating and bleeding. This might lead to acute or chronic blood loss and often results in anemia. Hidden blood in the feces can be detected by an occult blood stool test.

Anemia

Anemia is very common in individuals with malignant neoplasm and might be the result of tumor hemorrhage or a decrease in red blood cell production as a result of cancer treatments.

Fractures

Pathologic fractures might occur if a tumor has invaded the bone and caused weakness at that site. A fracture occurring from a minimal injury might be indicative of a cancer but, in an older person, might also be due to osteoporosis. The bone tumor might be primary or secondary with cancer of the lung, breast, or prostate readily metastasizing to the bone.

Infection

Infection is common and can lead to the demise of the individual. Tumor ulceration can allow entry of microorganisms that cause infection, or the individual might have impaired immunity due to **chemotherapy** (chemo = chemical, therapy = treatment) and radiation treatments, affecting the bone marrow and causing a decrease in production of white blood cells.

Individuals with cancer often have a loss of appetite, leading to a poor nutritional state and an increase in the chance of infection. Immune deficiency often leads to infection of the individual by a host of organisms such as fungi, viruses, protozoa, and bacteria that are not usually pathogenic.

Cachexia

Cachexia is a condition of general ill health and malnutrition often seen in the terminally ill patient. (Refer to Figure 2–3 in Chapter 2, "Mechanisms of Disease.") This condition is evidence of the demands on the body by the rapidly growing tumor and treatment modalities, coupled with poor nutritional intake.

◼◼ CANCER TREATMENT

New technological advances lead to ever-changing treatment of malignant neoplasms. Treatment might be aimed at cure (**curative**), at relief of symptoms (**palliative**; PAL-ee-AY-tiv), or at prevention (preventive). Major types of treatment include surgery, chemotherapy, and radiation, and hormone treatment might be the treatment of choice in some instances. The oncologist might recommend one of these treatments or a combination of them, depending on the type of cancer and treatment plan.

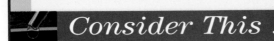

Consider This ...

A recent study revealed that cancer patients who keep their sense of humor are 70% more likely to survive than those with little or no sense of humor.

Surgery

Surgery for cancer can be curative, palliative, or preventive.

Curative surgery is aimed at complete removal of the tumor. Cancer of the lung, stomach, skin, breast, intestine, and female reproductive organs responds well to this type of surgery.

Palliative surgery is usually indicated when cure is not possible but when surgery will alleviate pain and discomfort. The intestine is an area commonly undergoing this type of surgery for obstruction, bleeding, or perforation. Surgery also might be performed to sever nerves in an effort to reduce pain.

Preventive surgery might be performed to prevent development of cancer. Polyps in the colon can be removed if they are thought to be precancerous, and a woman might choose to undergo prophylactic mastectomy if she has been identified as being at high risk for breast cancer.

Chemotherapy

Chemotherapy can be the medication of choice or used in combination with surgery and radiation therapy. Generally, chemotherapy is effective to treat rapidly growing metastatic neoplasms. It is aimed at rapidly growing neoplastic cells with the idea that it will kill or inhibit the growth of these cells while having minimal effect on normal cells.

In some instances, the growth rate of normal cells and neoplastic cells is not varied enough, and normal body cells suffer from the effects of the treatment. Rapidly growing normal cells such as those found in the epithelium, hair, and bone marrow suffer the most, leading to nausea, vomiting, loss of appetite, hair loss, anemia, and impaired immunity.

Radiation

Radiation is generally used in treatment of residual neoplasm postoperatively and to treat tumors that are not surgically accessible or operable. Palliative radiation treatments can shrink the tumor and relieve discomfort. Radiation treatment can be external with direct radiation or internal using radioisotope beads, seeds, or ribbons that are implanted inside the body. Both methods are aimed at disrupting DNA and interfering with cell growth and replication.

The goal is to destroy as much of the tumor as possible without affecting the normal tissue surrounding it. Adverse effects generally occur in the skin, mucous membranes, and bone marrow, leading to nausea, vomiting, loss of appetite, hair loss, and impaired immunity.

Hormone Therapy

Hormone therapy can cause regression in tumors of the breast and prostate. Administration of antagonistic hormones or excision of hormone-producing organs such as the ovaries and testes can be effective in prolonging life. Hormone therapy is generally used as a palliative treatment for metastatic tumors.

COMPLEMENTARY AND ALTERNATIVE THERAPY

Does Fennel Seed Extract Have Anticancer Potential?

Alternative medicines and therapies are being studied for their anticancer potential. In one study, researchers tested fennel seed methanolic extract (FSME) for its antioxidant, cytotoxic, and antitumor potential. The study showed that FSME may have some anticancer potential for breast cancer and liver cancer. It is also a safe and easily accessible source of antioxidants. Antioxidants have been shown in some studies to prevent disease and improve health.

Source: Ragaa et al. (2011).

SUMMARY

Neoplasms are new growths, either benign or malignant, that can arise from cells almost anywhere in the body. *Tumor* is the term commonly used to describe a neoplasm, but not all neoplasms form tumors. Hyperplasias are similar to neoplasms because they are an overgrowth of cells, but they resemble their cell of origin, whereas neoplasms do not. Neoplasms that are malignant are usually called cancers and are usually named for the type of tissue from which they developed. Metastatic cancers are those that spread to other parts of the body.

The cause of most cancer is unknown, but research has identified high-risk behaviors as well as some carcinogens in the environment that might contribute to cancer development. The ACS has recommended preventive measures and lists seven warning signs of cancer. Although the mortality rate for cancer in general is still very high in the United States, early diagnosis and treatment can yield a good prognosis for many types of cancer.

REVIEW QUESTIONS

Short Answer

1. What is the difference between a neoplasm and a tumor?

2. How are neoplasms classified?

3. What is the largest group of malignant neoplasms?

4. When a malignant neoplasm moves to various parts or organs of the body, it is said to be a _____ tumor.

5. What is the difference between hyperplasias and neoplasms?

True or False

6. T   F   Grading is the microscopic examination of the tumor to determine the degree of differentiation.
7. T   F   Tumors that are undifferentiated or anaplastic do not resemble the tissue of origin, are highly malignant, and have a poor prognosis.
8. T   F   Radioactive materials that emit alpha, beta, and gamma rays are not considered to be potential carcinogens.
9. T   F   There is no known genetic predisposition for cancer.
10. T   F   There are several personal risk behaviors common in our society that put an individual at increased risk for developing cancer.

Matching

11. Match the term in the left column with the phrase that best describes it from the column on the right.

_____ Metastatic neoplasm

_____ Cancer of the lung, breast, prostate, and colon

_____ CAUTION

_____ Basal and squamous skin cancer

_____ Biopsy

_____ Liver, lungs, and brain

_____ Ultraviolet (UV) radiation, X-ray, and radioactive materials

_____ Routine screening

_____ Surgery, chemotherapy, and radiation

_____ Palliative

a. Known carcinogens

b. An acronym for the seven warning signs of cancer

c. Microscopic examination of live tissue

d. Responsible for the majority of cancer deaths

e. Cells whose growth pattern has no purpose and is uncontrollable

f. Common sites of bloodstream metastasis

g. The most common type of cancer

h. Major types of cancer treatment

i. Treatment aimed at relieving symptoms

j. Very effective in the discovery and early diagnosis of cancer

CASE STUDIES

■ Mr. Holloway, age 65, who has made an appointment for a routine checkup. He has not complained of any unusual symptoms but feels he should have a yearly examination because of his age. What are some routine screening tests that should be performed on Mr. Holloway because of his age and gender? What important cancer prevention strategies should you discuss with Mr. Holloway during his visit?

■ Mrs. Holloway, age 55, is also visiting her physician for routine screening. She is concerned because her sister, who is age 47, was recently diagnosed with breast cancer. What types of cancer are most commonly diagnosed in patients like Mrs. Holloway, based on her age and gender? Should she be concerned about developing breast cancer? If she has never performed breast self-exams, what would you tell her about this screening procedure? How could you help her understand the correct procedure for completing a breast self-exam?

Study Tools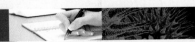

Workbook

Complete Chapter 3

Online Resources

PowerPoint® presentations

Animation

BIBLIOGRAPHY

American Cancer Society. (2011). Cancer facts and figures 2011. *www.cancer.org* (accessed January 2012).

American Cancer Society. (2012). Detailed guide: Testicular cancer. *www.cancer.org* (accessed July 2012).

American Cancer Society. (2012). American Cancer Society skin cancer prevention activities. *www.cancer.org* (accessed June 2012).

American Cancer Society. (2013). Cancer Prevention Study-3. *www.cancer.org* (accessed August 2013).

Aschenbrenner, D. S. (2011). Drug Watch. *American Journal of Nursing 11*(9), 22–23.

Begley, S. (2011). Could this be the end of cancer? *Newsweek 158*(25), 36–39.

Burton, B., & Zeppetella, G. (2011). Assessing the impact of breakthrough cancer pain. *British Journal of Nursing 20*(Suppl), S14–S19.

Campbell, M. K. (2011). Cancer is a team sport. *Clinical Journal of Oncology Nursing 15*(4), 349.

Centers for Disease Control and Prevention. (2008). Smoking-attributable mortality, years of potential life lost, and productivity losses—United States, 2000–2004. *Morbidity and Mortality Weekly Report 57*(45), 1226–1228.

Centers for Disease Control and Prevention. (2010). FDA licensure of bivalent human papillomavirus vaccine (HPV2, Cervarix) for use in females and updated HPV vaccination recommendations from the Advisory Committee on Immunization Practices (ACIP). *Morbidity and Mortality Weekly Report 59*(20), 626–629.

Centers for Disease Control and Prevention. (2010). Vital signs: Nonsmokers' exposure to secondhand smoke—United States, 1999–2008. *Morbidity and Mortality Weekly Report 59*(35), 1141–1146.

Centers for Disease Control and Prevention. (2011). Recommendations on the use of quadrivalent human papillomavirus vaccine in males—Advisory Committee on Immunization Practices (ACIP), 2011. *Morbidity and Mortality Weekly Report 60*(50), 1705–1708.

Drug news. (2011). *Nursing 41*(4), 24.

Drug news. (2011). *Nursing 41*(6), 16.

Drug news. (2011). *Nursing 41*(8), 16.

Hamling, K. (2011). The management of nausea and vomiting in advanced cancer. *International Journal of Palliative Nursing 17*(7), 321–327.

Hanssens, S., Luyten, R., Watthy, C., Fontaine, C., Decoster, L., Baillon, C., Trullemans, F., Cortoos, A., & De Grève, J. (2011). Evaluation of a comprehensive rehabilitation program for post-treatment patients with cancer. *Oncology Nursing Forum 38*(6), E418–E424.

Lynch, E. (2011). A testing dilemma. *Nursing Standard 26*(7), 22–23.

Mellman, I., Coukos, G., & Dranoff, G. (2011). Cancer immunotherapy comes of age. *Nature 480*(7378), 480–489.

National Cancer Institute. (2011). SEER cancer statistics review 1975–2008. Devcan Version 6.6.0, October 2011. *http://surveillance.cancer.gov/devcan/* (accessed January 2012).

National Cancer Institute. (2012). Cancer trends progress report—2009–2010 update. *www.progressreport.cancer* (accessed January 2012).

Ragaa, H., Amal, M., Mohamad, G., Assmaa, M., Hussain, A., Sabry, M., & Mahmuod, M. (2011). Antioxidant and anticarcinogenic effects of methanolic extract and volatile oil of fennel seeds (*Foeniculum vulgare*). *Journal of Medicinal Food 14*(9), 986–1001.

Shepherd, H. L., Butow, P. N., & Tattersall, M. H. N. (2011). Factors which motivate cancer doctors to involve their patients in reaching treatment decisions. *Patient Education & Counseling 84*(2), 229–235.

Siegel, R., Ward, E., Brawley, O., & Jemal, A. (2011). Cancer statistics, 2011. *CA: A Cancer Journal for Clinicians 61*(4), 212–236.

Smart, M. (2011). Oncology update. *Oncology Nursing Forum 38*(4), 485–486.

Smart, M. (2011). Oncology update. *Oncology Nursing Forum 38*(5), 597–598.

Van Mossel, C., Alford, M., & Watson, H. (2011). Challenges of patient-centered care: Practice or rhetoric. *Nursing Inquiry 18*(4), 278–280.

Watson, E. K., Rose, P. W., Neal, R. D., Hulbert-Williams, N., Donnelly, P., Hubbard, G. E., Campbell, C., Weller, D., & Wilkinson, C. (2012). Personalized cancer follow-up: Risk stratification, needs assessment or both? *British Journal of Cancer 106*(1), 1–5.

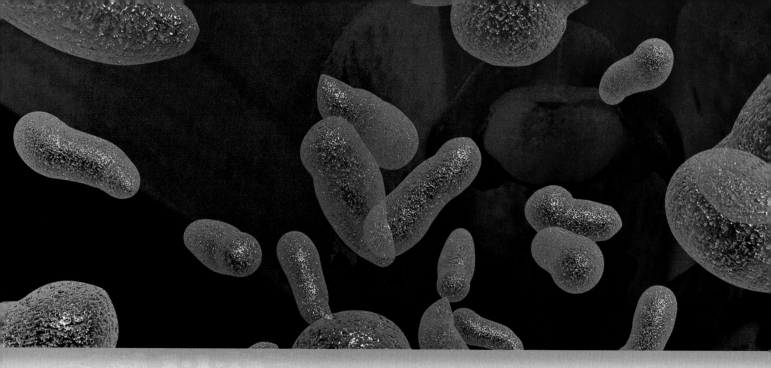

OUTLINE

KEY TERMS

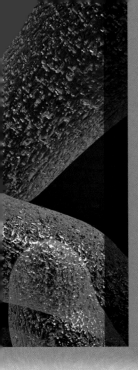
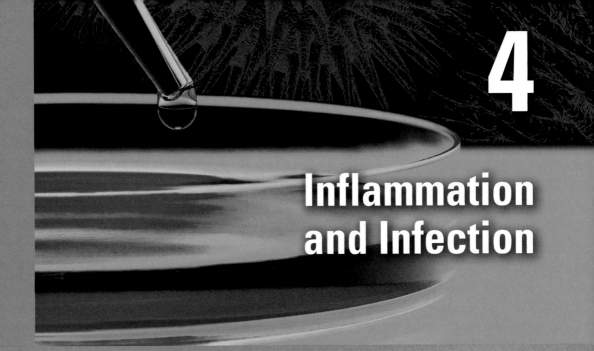

4

Inflammation and Infection

LEARNING OBJECTIVES

Upon completion of the chapter, the learner should be able to:

1. Identify important terminology related to the defense mechanisms.
2. Describe the basic defense mechanisms in the body.
3. Explain the steps in the inflammatory process.
4. Describe the process of tissue repair and healing.
5. Identify complications of wound healing.
6. Describe the process of infection development.
7. Identify the common infectious microorganisms and the resulting diseases.
8. Identify the common laboratory test conducted to identify pathogenic organisms.

OVERVIEW

The human body is in a constant state of activity, part of which is to prevent trauma and maintain homeostasis against foreign invaders and pathogens. It maintains defense mechanisms—inflammation is a natural one—for this protection, but when these protective mechanisms fail, the usual result is an infection. Infections are diagnosed and treated in a variety of ways. ■

DEFENSE MECHANISMS

The immune system has the difficult job of protecting the body against foreign invasion. Defense can be nonspecific, protecting the body against any and all invaders; or it can be specific, identifying the invader prior to killing it. This system uses three basic lines of defense to accomplish its protective goals.

Physical or Surface Barriers (Nonspecific)

An intact skin is the body's first line of defense. The skin is a physical barrier and an acidic, antimicrobial surface that is an effective barrier against infection most of the time. The skin has more than 650,000 microorganisms per square inch on its surface, adding up to more than 100 trillion microorganisms per person. The normal bacterial flora of the skin acts as a placeholder, preventing habitation by other **bacteria** (microscopic, one-celled organisms). Sebaceous (oil secreting) and odoriferous (perspiration secreting) glands secrete antibacterial acids and enzymes. Mucous membranes serve to trap invaders.

Inflammation (Nonspecific)

If physical barriers are broken and the foreign invader penetrates the cells and tissues, it triggers the second line of defense, the inflammatory response. This response begins a stereotypic vascular response within seconds of an unwanted invasion. In other words, the process unfolds or follows the same pattern regardless of the type of invader. The primary goals of the inflammatory response are to isolate the invader, destroy it, and clean up the debris, thereby promoting healing.

Immune Response (Specific)

The last line of defense reacts to invasion much slower than inflammation but with specific killing ability. All cells, even human body cells, have protein or saccharide markers called **antigens** (AN-tih-jenz) on their surfaces that identify the cell. During the immune response, the body actually identifies the invader by the antigen. Once the antigen is identified, lymphocytes produce **antibodies**. These antibodies link with the cell antigen, thus killing the cell or disabling it. This immunologic defense has the unique ability to

remember the invader and produce more antibodies if the invader returns (Figure 4–1).

INFLAMMATION

Inflammation is a nonspecific cellular and vascular reaction to any tissue **trauma** (TRAW-mah; injury). One limiting factor of inflammation, however, is that it cannot occur in tissue that does not have a blood supply.

If tissue is destroyed by injury, the inflammatory process will occur only along borders of the injury where blood supply is maintained. In gangrenous tissue, for example, inflammation cannot occur in the dead or necrotic tissue, but there is an observable reaction along its borders.

The fact that inflammation occurs only in vascularized (supplied with blood) tissue is important in forensic medicine. Evidence of inflammation in tissue confirms that an injury occurred while the individual was alive. If no evidence of inflammation exists, the pathologist can be assured that the person was dead when the injury was inflicted.

Inflammation is designed to be a beneficial, protective defense mechanism. In some instances, the reaction can become so intense that it becomes harmful to tissues. Such an acute hypersensitive reaction can lead not only to local tissue damage but also to anaphylactic shock and death of the individual. If the process goes awry, producing an autoimmune reaction, the body basically begins to destroy itself, and anti-inflammatory medications might be needed to stop the reaction if it becomes injurious.

The Inflammatory Process

When any tissue undergoes trauma, regardless of the cause—physical injury, invasion of microorganisms, ischemia (decreased oxygen in cells), freezing, burning, electrocution, radiation, or chemical irritation, for instance—inflammation will occur.

Mast cells, also called tissue histiocytes, exist in all tissues of the body and play a major role in the inflammatory process. When injured or irritated, these cells release **histamine**. Histamine causes local arterioles, venules, and capillaries to dilate, resulting in an increase in blood flow to the area. This increase in blood flow, called **hyperemia** (HIGH-per-EE-me-ah; hyper = increased, emia = blood), causes increased redness and heat in the area.

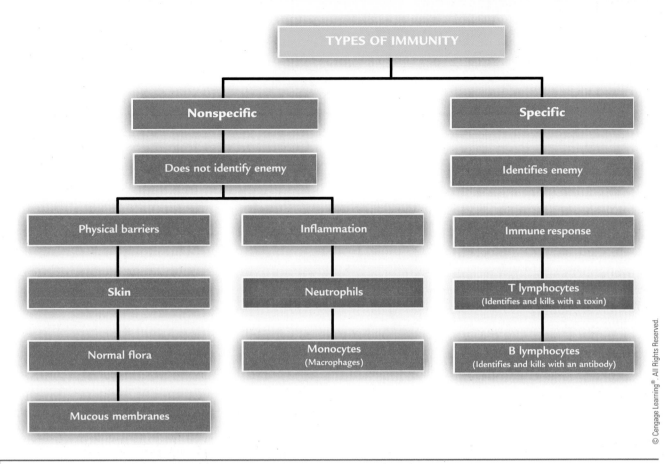

FIGURE 4–1   Immunity—lines of defense.

Hyperemia also brings increased numbers of leukocytes (white blood cells) to the area. The white cells that move into this area first and in the greatest numbers are neutrophils, also called polymorphonuclear cells (PMNs) (poly = many, morphic = shaped nucleus). These white cells line the endothelium of the vessels, awaiting the opportunity to move into the tissue.

As the capillaries dilate under the influence of histamine, vascular permeability occurs. In other words, the capillary becomes permeable, or leaky, as the endothelial cells are stretched apart. This permeability allows blood fluid called **exudate** (ECKS-you-dayt) to leak into the tissue. This leakage of fluid is the cause of the swelling or edema observed with inflammation.

As edema increases, more pressure is exerted on nerve endings, leading to increased pain. With increased pain and tenderness, the individual tends to guard the area and may experience loss of function. These vascular and cellular responses produce the five cardinal signs of inflammation: heat, redness, swelling, pain, and loss of function (Figure 4–2).

Vascular permeability also allows the waiting neutrophils to escape into the tissue. The neutrophils extend part of their bodies between the epithelial cells and squeeze through the capillary wall by a process called **diapedesis** (DYE-ah-pe-DEE-sis) (see Figure 4–2). The process of diapedesis is very effective, delivering millions of neutrophils to the area within a few hours.

Neutrophils can be considered the foot soldiers of the inflammatory process. They arrive first, they arrive in great numbers, and they readily move into action in the tissue, drawn or directed to the injured area by a process called **chemotaxis**. One might think of this process as a chemical taxi cab. Chemicals, detected through chemoreceptors on the neutrophil's outer membrane, are released by a variety of elements such as bacteria, injured tissue, and plasma proteins. These chemoreceptors also draw the neutrophil in the direction of the highest chemical concentration (see Figure 4–2).

When the neutrophil arrives at the scene of the trauma, it begins the job of phagocytosis, or cell eating. The neutrophil eats and destroys microorganisms,

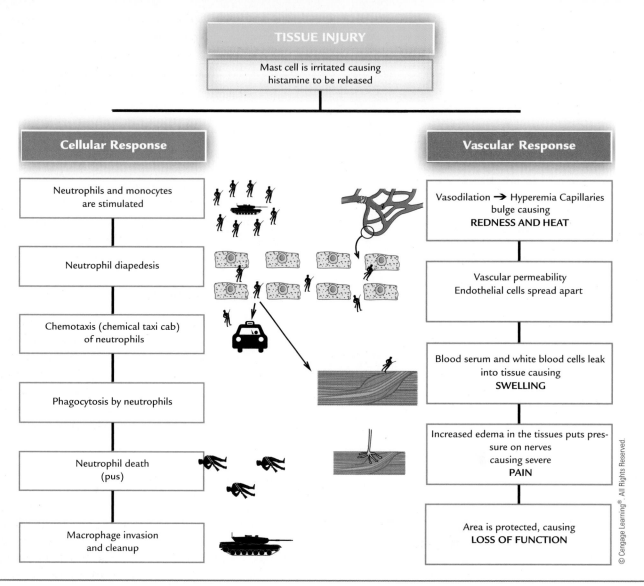

FIGURE 4–2 Acute inflammation—cellular and vascular response.

foreign materials, and dead cells. However, the life of the neutrophil is short. The death of numerous neutrophils mixed with exudate or blood fluid make up, in part, the white fluid identified as **pus**.

Approximately 3 to 4 days after the inflammatory process begins, large numbers of another type of white cell, the large, slow-moving monocyte, begin to arrive at the scene. As the monocyte leaves the bloodstream and moves into the tissue, it too becomes phagocytic and is called a **macrophage** (macro = large, phage = eat). As the name suggests, a macrophage is a large eater of microorganisms, foreign material, and dead cells. This cell might be considered the tank of the war because it is slower moving but has more killing power than the neutrophil. Another job of the macrophage is to act as

the cleanup crew, removing the dead neutrophils and tissue debris in the inflamed area.

Until this point, the **inflammation** is considered an acute (short-lived) situation. If the inflammation persists for a longer period of time, it is considered a chronic problem. This time period is difficult to establish because some chronic inflammations will exhibit periods of exacerbation (flare up), eliciting a new outpouring of neutrophils. Likewise, some acute inflammations will trigger the response of an unusually high number of macrophages.

After approximately 7 to 10 days, if the inflammatory process has not overcome the invader, the nuclear warheads of the defense system—the lymphocytes—are called on to respond. Lymphocytes are slow but powerful, specific killers, part of the body's third line of defense: the immune response. They identify the enemy, make an antibody to kill it, and then remember the enemy and the killing process (see Figure 4–1). Refer to Chapter 5, "Immune System Diseases and Disorders," for more detailed information on the immune system.

Chronic Inflammation

Generally speaking, a chronic inflammation can be considered one that lasts 2 weeks or longer. If the acute attack by neutrophils and macrophages is unsuccessful, the battle can become chronic. Microscopic examination of chronic inflammation will reveal a large number of macrophages and fewer neutrophils.

If macrophages are unable to overcome the invader and protect the host, the body might try to isolate the area by forming a granuloma. A granuloma is formed by macrophages and fibrous deposits of collagen and may be hardened by calcium deposits. This granuloma protects the surrounding tissue and allows healing to begin. A classic cause of granuloma formation is tuberculosis. These granulomas may become quite large, form a fibrous rim, and eventually calcify. Another cause of granuloma is foreign body involvement such as a wood splinter, gravel, suture, glass sliver, or metal fragments embedded in the tissue. The body walls off the material to protect the adjacent tissue. This granuloma may become hardened with fibrous tissue and remain for the life of the individual.

Inflammatory Exudates

The duration and extent of an inflammatory **lesion** (LEE-zhun; any discontinuity of tissue) may be determined by direct visualization of the site. External inflammatory lesions are observed easily, whereas internal inflammatory lesions in organs and cavities might require surgical or endoscopic examination. The appearance and amount of exudate or blood fluid can assist in identifying an acute or a chronic condition.

Serous Exudate

Serous exudate is a clear, serum-like fluid containing small amounts of protein. It implies a lesser degree of damage and occurs in the acute stage of inflammation. Examples of serous exudate include the fluid in skin blisters, cold sores, and injured joints, for example. Serous exudate is easily reabsorbed after the inflammatory response is halted and healing begins.

Fibrinous Exudate

Fibrinous exudate is composed of fluid and large amounts of fibrinogen. In comparison to serous exudate, the leakage of fibrinogen indicates a larger injury with more severe inflammation. Fibrinous exudate can be observed in strep throat or bacterial pneumonia, forming a mesh-like lesion. A superficial skin wound might be covered with dried fibrinous exudate commonly called a scab.

Purulent Exudate

Purulent (PURR-you-lent) exudate is loaded with dead and dying PMNs or neutrophils, tissue debris, and **pyogenic** (PYE-oh-JEN-ick; pyo = pus, genic = arising), or pus-forming, bacteria. Purulent exudate is commonly called pus. A localized collection of pus is called an **abscess**; an accumulation of pus in a body cavity is called **empyema** (EM-pye-EE-mah). For example, pus accumulated in the chest or thoracic cavity would be called thoracic empyema.

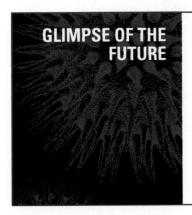

GLIMPSE OF THE FUTURE

Smoking and Inflammation

Inflammation is a component of normal tissue healing and is important in the body's defense mechanisms. Researchers are trying to understand the effects of smoking on inflammation by looking at the mechanisms that occur in the immune-inflammatory response. It has been reported that smoking causes an immunosuppressant state in the body, which is also what happens in some immune diseases (see Chapter 5). The relationship between smoking and inflammation continues to be studied.

Source: Gonçalves et al. (2011).

Inflammatory Lesions

Any discontinuity or abnormality of tissue is called a lesion, a broad term that includes wounds, ulcers, wheals, blisters, vesicles, pustules, or tumors, to name a few. Lesions are due to physical or pathologic injury. Inflammatory lesions include abscesses, ulcers, and **cellulitis** (SELL-you-LYE-tis; inflammation of connective tissue).

Abscesses

Abscesses are typically caused by streptococcal and staphylococcal (pyogenic) bacteria. During the inflammatory response, the body attempts to contain or stop the spread of the bacteria into adjacent tissue by forming a wall around the area. When this wall forms around a purulent exudate, an abscess is formed. Boils, furuncles, and pimples are examples of abscesses.

Typically, a small abscess shows signs of acute inflammation: redness, heat, swelling, and pain. When the central portion of the abscess softens or develops a head, puncturing the head will cause an outpouring of pus, relief of pain, and onset of healing. Puncturing the abscess before the area is walled off and the head is soft, however, can lead to a spread of the infecting organism.

A small abscess might rupture and heal spontaneously, but a large abscess might need to be surgically incised and drained. Draining an abscess speeds healing; without drainage, the body must continue to battle the invading organisms. If the body is successful, it will eventually win the battle, reabsorb the exudate, and replace the area with fibrous tissue. A large abscess, such as in appendicitis, can spread and become fatal if not contained. If a large abscess ruptures, it tends to form a tract, or opening to the surface of the skin called a **sinus**. If this tract connects two organs or cavities to each other or to the surface of the skin, it is called a **fistula** (FIST-you-lah) (Figure 4–3).

Ulcer

An **ulcer** is a crater-like lesion in the skin or mucous membrane. It is the result of an injury and the subsequent inflammatory response. The tissue in this area becomes necrotic (dead) and sloughs off, leaving a crater or excavated area. Ulcers are commonly seen in the stomach and duodenum as a result of injury by bacteria and stomach acid. Pressure ulcers, commonly called bedsores or decubitus ulcers, are caused by excessive pressure on tissue. Pressure ulcers primarily appear over bony prominences of the body, especially those affected in the reclining position, such as the heel, sacrum, hip, elbow, and scapula (Figure 4–4).

Cellulitis

Cellulitis is a diffuse, or widespread, acute inflammatory process. It is commonly seen in the skin and subcutaneous tissues. Cellulitis is characterized by general edema and redness. Cellulitis of the face primarily involves the cheeks and periorbital (peri = around, orbital = eye) areas. This type of cellulitis must receive special attention because it can spread to the sinuses of the brain. Cellulitis is often caused by *Streptococcus* or *Staphylococcus* bacteria and is due to the body's inability to confine or wall off the causative organism. Cellulitis is potentially dangerous but usually can be treated effectively with antibiotics.

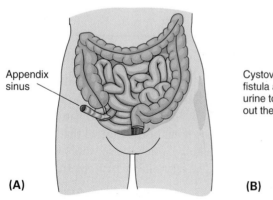

Appendix sinus

(A)

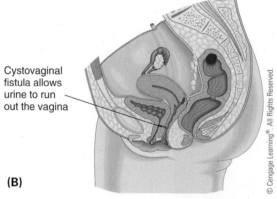

Cystovaginal fistula allows urine to run out the vagina

(B)

FIGURE 4–3   (A) Sinus. (B) Fistula.

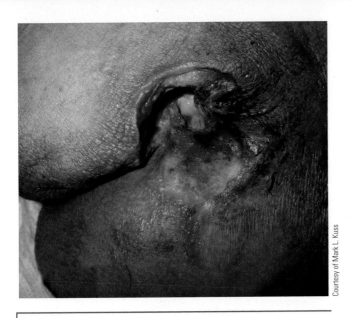

Courtesy of Mark L. Kuss

| **FIGURE 4–4**   Pressure ulcer.

■ TISSUE REPAIR AND HEALING

Proper tissue repair and healing is an ongoing process much like any other body process and occurs in most instances, but this process can be influenced by many other factors. Healing can be impaired or slowed when secondary diseases are present, the body is malnourished, or the immune system is compromised.

Tissue Repair

During the final phase of the inflammatory process, macrophages are responsible for cleaning up the area and producing growth factors that aid the repair process. Repair of tissue also depends on cellular regeneration and the type of cells that make up the tissue. Some cells divide quite readily, but others do not. Cellular proliferation, or division, can be grouped into three general categories.

1. **Mitotic cells** continuously divide throughout life. They exist in the skin and mucosa of internal organs and readily replace damaged tissue.

2. **Facultative mitotic cells** do not divide regularly but can be stimulated to divide when necessary. They exist in such organs as the liver and kidney. Some part of these organs must remain intact for these cells to be available to divide and replace the lost tissue.

3. **Nondividing cells** do not divide under any condition. Cells of this type include central nerves,

brain cells, and heart muscle cells. Repair of these tissues is by fibrous scarring.

The body's two basic methods of repair involve healing by regeneration and by fibrous connective tissue repair, or **scar** formation. Regeneration is the best type of repair because it usually leads to restoration of normal function, whereas fibrous connective tissue repair does not.

Regeneration

Regeneration involves mitotic cell division. During regeneration, the damaged tissue is replaced by cellular division of healthy tissue. For example, skin tissue is replaced by epithelial cell division, and bone tissue is replaced by osteocyte division. Regeneration can usually occur in internal organs if the major framework of the organ has not been destroyed. Complex structures such as lung tissue and glomeruli (in the kidney), however, do not regenerate. Regeneration is particularly important when there is damage to a large amount of tissue; for instance, epithelial regeneration is very beneficial with massive burns. Bone cells, osteocytes, and blood-forming bone cells have a remarkable ability to regenerate from a few remaining cells and can be transplanted from another individual by bone marrow transplant.

Fibrous Connective Tissue Repair (Scar Formation)

Fibrous connective tissue repair, or scar formation, can occur in any tissue and produces the same result, no matter the location—a tough, fibrous tissue called a scar. A scar provides a bridge between the normal tissue and the wound, but it does not restore function. Wound repair of nerves, brain tissue, and heart muscle is by fibrous connective tissue repair (Figure 4–5).

Tissue Healing

Tissue healing can be separated into categories of healing by primary union or secondary union. Categorization is determined by whether the wound edges are approximated (pulled together) or left separated during the healing process.

Primary Union (First Intention)

Primary union, also called healing by first intention, involves approximating the edges of the wound. A classic example of healing by primary union is the

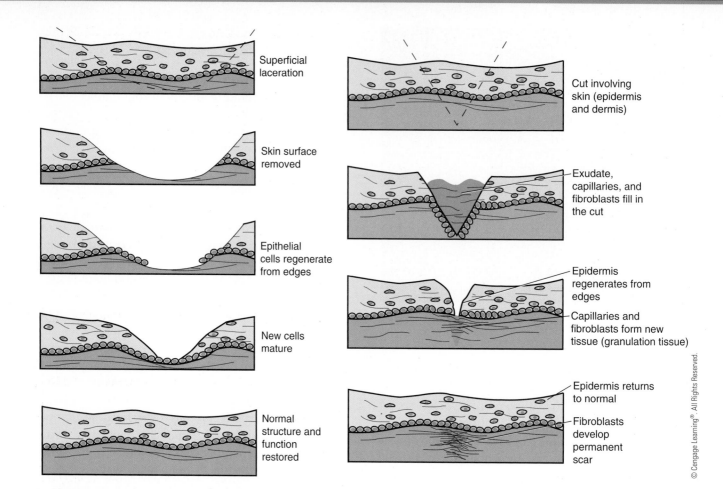

Superficial laceration

Skin surface removed

Epithelial cells regenerate from edges

New cells mature

Normal structure and function restored

Cut involving skin (epidermis and dermis)

Exudate, capillaries, and fibroblasts fill in the cut

Epidermis regenerates from edges

Capillaries and fibroblasts form new tissue (granulation tissue)

Epidermis returns to normal

Fibroblasts develop permanent scar

FIGURE 4–5 Tissue repair—complete regeneration and fibrous connective tissue repair.

healing process following a clean surgical incision. The wound edges are clean, there is minimal tissue damage, and the edges are approximated with sutures, staples, or tape.

Primary healing occurs in an orderly fashion. The steps of primary healing include the following:

1. The incisional line quickly fills with serum, forming a scab.

2. Within 1 to 2 days, new capillaries begin to bridge the gap between the wound edges.

3. In the next few days, fibroblasts grow across the deeper wound layers and begin to deposit collagen in this fibrous network. This tissue is called granulation tissue.

4. The collagen begins to contract, pulling the wound edges together and forming a scar.

After a few weeks, the incision might appear healed, but the deeper layers of tissue might not be healed for a month or more. Usually, an incisional scar will pale in color and shrink in size over a period of months or years.

Secondary Union (Secondary Intention)

Large wounds and those infected by dirt, debris, and bacteria cannot be pulled together to heal by primary intention. The process of healing by **secondary union** is the same process as that of primary union but involves a larger degree of tissue damage and more inflammation to resolve (Figure 4–6). To fill the wound, large numbers of capillaries, fibroblasts, and collagen must be produced. After a week or so, the new, soft, red tissue is called granulation tissue, which is eventually replaced as more collagen is deposited in the area. The collagen contracts, pulling the wound edges together and beginning the formation of a scar. Healing time varies depending on the size of the wound; large wounds can take a long time to heal by secondary union because additional time will

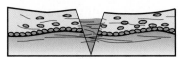
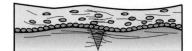
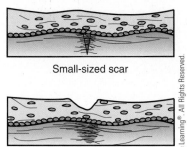

Small amount of exudate	Small amount of granulation tissue	Small-sized scar
	Primary union	

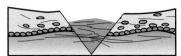
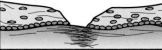

Large amount of exudate	Large amount of granulation tissue	Large-sized scar
	Secondary union	

FIGURE 4–6 Tissue healing—primary and secondary union.

be needed for the scar to develop the strength of the surrounding tissue. If the wound is too large, the epithelium might not be able to bridge the gap, and a skin graft might be needed.

Media Link

View an animation on tissue repair and healing on the Online Resources.

Delayed Wound Healing

One of the greatest impediments to wound healing is the amount of dead tissue and debris—dirt, bacteria, dead leukocytes, or a variety of other contaminates—in the wound. It might take the body's leukocytes weeks or months to phagocytize (eat up) all the debris. In the meantime, bacteria might be producing dead cells and necrotic tissue as fast as the cleanup effort can advance. To speed healing, dirty wounds must be cleaned and débrided. **Débridement** (day-breed-MON), commonly pronounced (day-breed-MENT), is a process of washing or cutting away necrotic tissue and foreign material.

Consider This ...

Maggot treatment, also called biotherapy, is often more effective than modern antibiotics for treating open wounds. Maggots will gently eat away the decaying tissue, will leave the healthy tissue intact, and will not cause any side effects.

Other factors affecting healing time include the following:

1. **Age** Younger people heal more rapidly than older people.
2. **Size** Smaller wounds heal faster than larger ones.
3. **Location** Epithelial tissue heals rapidly, compared to other tissue types.
4. **Nutrition** Good nutritional status promotes wound healing. Protein and vitamin C are essential to healing.
5. **Immobility** Wound tissue heals more rapidly if it is kept immobile.
6. **Circulation** Tissue with good blood supply heals more rapidly. Epithelial tissue heals more readily than cartilage. Individuals with diabetes have small-blood-vessel disease (diabetic microangiopathy), leading to ischemia of the tissue and poor wound healing.
7. **Organism virulence** Wounds infected with **virulent** (VIR-you-lent; poisonous) microorganisms are slower to heal than those that are not infected.
8. **Steroids** Steroid therapy inhibits the inflammatory response, giving the invading offender the upper hand.

Complications of Wound Healing

Prolonged wound healing can occur as a result of any one or a combination of the factors previously discussed. Other complications of wound healing involve poor or excessive scar formation. A scar that does not have adequate strength can lead to wound **dehiscence** (dee-HISS-ens), or separation of tissue margins. Excessive collagen formation often results in a hard, raised

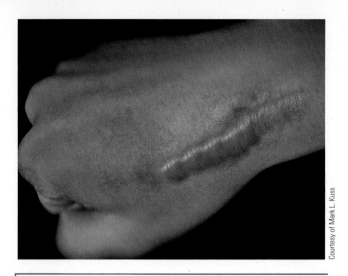

Courtesy of Mark L. Kuss

| **FIGURE 4–7**   Keloid.

scar called a **keloid** (KEE-loid) (Figure 4–7). Keloid scars are often unsightly but harmless and occur more often in the African-American population. Surgical removal can result in the formation of another keloid.

Adhesions (ad-HE-zhuns) from scar tissue can be a complication of surgery, especially abdominal surgery. As normal fibrous scar tissue develops in the operative organ, part of this tissue can cling to the surface of the adjoining organs, forming a fibrous band called an **adhesion**. Adhesions are often asymptomatic and cause no difficulties, but in some cases, they can become painful and lead to obstruction of the adjacent organ. The intestine frequently is obstructed by adhesions following abdominal surgery. Further surgery to release painful or obstructive adhesions may be needed.

▒ INFECTION

In Chapter 2, "Mechanisms of Disease," the fact that inflammation and infection are different responses or reactions was introduced. Inflammation is a protective immune response and can occur without bacterial invasion. **Infection**, however, refers to the invasion of microorganisms in the tissue, causing cell or tissue injury and leading to the inflammatory response.

Humans live with disease-causing microorganisms all around them. Some bacteria even live on the skin surface, in the respiratory tract, and in the intestine without causing illness, and some are actually beneficial. These bacteria are called *normal flora*.

Microorganisms that produce disease are called pathogenic. Normal flora can become pathogenic

under certain conditions. When this occurs, the normal flora bacteria become **opportunistic** because they take the opportunity to cause infection in the host.

Certain conditions must be present for a microorganism to cause an infection in the host. Pathogens must have an area to enter, be resistant enough and enter in great enough numbers to survive, and overcome the defenses of the individual.

First, the microorganism must successfully gain access into the body through a portal of entry; any break in the skin offers this. Common openings such as the nose, mouth, eyes, and ears are also portals of entry. The most common port of entry is the respiratory system. Other portals include the digestive system, urinary tract, and reproductive tract.

Second, the pathogen must be resistant to the defenses of the host. The ability of a microorganism to overcome the defense of the host is its virulence. A virulent microorganism has an aggressive or invasive nature and can produce a toxin, or poison, that injures tissues. The degree of virulence of a microorganism varies. Generally speaking, organisms that come from an infected host are more virulent than those grown in laboratory conditions.

Third, the number of invading pathogens can determine the risk for infection—even weak pathogenic organisms can cause infection if they invade in large enough numbers to overcome the body's defense system. Generally speaking, the higher the number of invading pathogens, the greater the risk of infection.

Finally, the condition of the individual or the host is a determinant of infection risk. An individual who is in good physical and emotional health, has good nutrition, practices risk-reducing habits, and is relatively young has a good chance of avoiding infection.

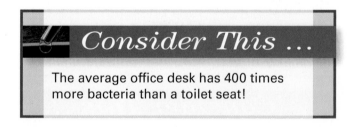

Consider This ...

The average office desk has 400 times more bacteria than a toilet seat!

Frequency and Types of Infection

Infectious diseases are the leading cause of death in the world, so a country's ability to track and identify infectious diseases is an important weapon in the control of disease. In the United States, the Centers

TABLE 4–1   Some Common Infections Caused by Microorganisms in Humans

Bacteria	Virus	Fungus
Staphylococcus	Common cold	Ringworm (tinea)
Streptococcus	Herpes simplex	Athlete's foot
Escherichia coli	Mononucleosis	Candidiasis
Klebsiella	HIV	Thrush
Pseudomonas	Measles	Vaginitis
Shigella	Mumps	Histoplasmosis
Salmonella	Rubella	Coccidioidomycosis
	Influenza (flu)	

Rickettsial	Protozoan	Helminths
Rocky Mountain spotted fever	Malaria	Roundworms
	Giardiasis	Flatworms
		Pinworms
		Tapeworms

for Disease Control and Prevention (CDC), based in Atlanta, provide these services.

Respiratory infections, including upper respiratory infections, influenza-like infections, pneumonia, and bronchitis, account for more than 80% of all infections. Childhood infections, wound infections, viral infections, and other types of infection account for the remaining number of infections diagnosed.

Microorganisms that produce infection in humans include bacteria, **viruses, fungi, rickettsiae** (ric-KET-see-ah), **protozoa,** and **helminths** (Table 4–1). These organisms can produce infections in the host that range from very mild to life threatening.

Bacteria

Bacterial infections (Figure 4–8) can occur as a primary or secondary disease. Primary bacterial infections occur when a person is exposed to a pathogen. Secondary infection occurs after the onset of another disease process or condition. Secondary infections are very common. The most common cause for them is obstruction of a body passageway. For example, nasal obstruction can lead to sinusitis, and obstruction of the eustachian tubes can lead to otitis media, or middle-ear infection.

Normal flora bacteria live on or in the skin, mouth, nose, genital tract, and intestines of humans. These bacteria often become pathogenic when they gain access into the body or when the body's resistance is less robust than normal. *Staphylococcus* is a bacterium of the skin that often enters the body and can infect any organ. *Staphylococcus aureus* is an important member of the *Staphylococcus* family because it can develop strains, such as methicillin-resistant

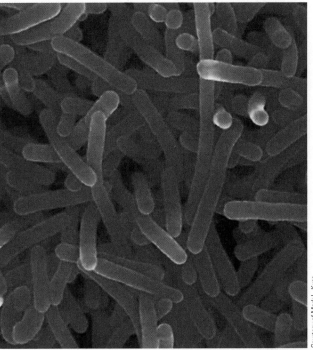

FIGURE 4–8   Bacteria.

Staphylococcus aureus (MRSA), that are resistant to penicillin and other antibiotics. These antibiotic-resistant strains are particularly dangerous because they are difficult to control and eliminate. For instance, a form of MRSA called community-acquired MRSA (CA-MRSA) is the most dangerous form of MRSA. It has become epidemic in the United States in the past few years with an estimated 2.3 million people carrying the infection without symptoms. It is second only to human immunodeficiency virus (HIV) as the major public health threat. CA-MRSA starts out as a skin infection but soon becomes a serious systemic infection. It can rapidly cause severe respiratory distress leading to respiratory failure.

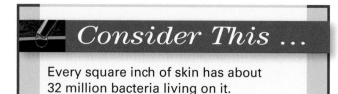

Consider This ...

Every square inch of skin has about 32 million bacteria living on it.

Streptococcus bacteria normally live on the skin and in the throat. Common infections caused by *Streptococcus* bacteria include strep throat, scarlet fever, pneumonia, and meningitis. In a select group of individuals, strep throat can lead to rheumatic fever and glomerulonephritis.

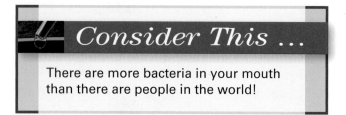

Consider This ...

There are more bacteria in your mouth than there are people in the world!

Enteric bacteria are those living in the intestinal tract, and common forms include *Escherichia coli* (*E. coli*), *Klebsiella*, *Pseudomonas*, *Shigella*, and *Salmonella*. *E. coli* causes enteritis in infants and adults and can be the cause of travelers' diarrhea. *E. coli* and *Klebsiella* are common causes of urinary tract infections. *Pseudomonas* commonly infects wounds and is associated with a foul odor and green pus production. *Shigella* and *Salmonella* infections cause diarrhea; *Salmonella* is the causative organism of food poisoning.

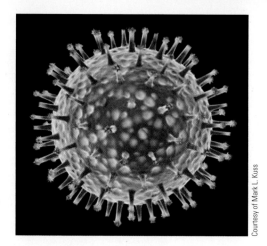

Courtesy of Mark L. Kuss

FIGURE 4–9 Virus.

Viruses

Viruses (Figure 4–9) are the smallest infective organisms and must be visualized by an electron microscope. They cannot reproduce or live outside the cell and must invade the cell and use it to reproduce their genetic information. Lymphocytes of the immune system are the body's primary defense against viruses. Some viruses can mutate or change, so the body must develop more than one kind of antibody to kill that type of virus.

Viral infections cannot be treated easily. Some antiviral agents can be given to individuals who have reduced resistance to infections to try to prevent such infection. Antibiotic therapy does not kill a virus. Usually, supportive care is given by treating the symptoms the virus causes, such as fever, sore throat, runny nose, headache, and chest congestion. Antibiotics will help in treatment of a secondary bacterial infection occurring with the viral infection.

Viral infections of the upper respiratory system, including the common cold, far outnumber other viral diseases. Cold sores, also known as herpes simplex, are very common and affect many individuals. Infectious mononucleosis frequently affects adolescents and young adults. HIV causes acquired immunodeficiency syndrome (AIDS) and has become the most noted virus due to its fatal outcome.

Immunizations are effective in preventing many viral diseases such as measles, mumps, rubella, and small pox. Influenza virus (flu) mutates and requires new vaccines with each mutation. Some viruses are latent types, meaning they live inside the cell, causing no harm until the body becomes stressed or impaired. Latent viruses, such as those in the herpes family, replicate and cause symptoms during stressful periods.

COMPLEMENTARY AND ALTERNATIVE THERAPY

Herbs for Infections

A group of herbs have an antiadhesion effect on bacteria. That means they block the bacteria cells from adhering to their target cells in the body. Some of these herbal medicines have been shown to be useful in preventing or treating a variety of infections. Cranberry (*Vaccinium macrocarpon*) is the most well-known of these herbal preparations. It has been used to prevent and treat urinary tract infections. It is also being studied for treatment of *Helicobacter pylori* infections and *Streptococcus* infections. Other herbs with some antiadhesion effects include ginseng, hops, and wild ginger.

Source: Yarnell & Abascal (2008).

Fungi

Fungi (Figure 4–10) are microscopic plant-like organisms that cause diseases referred to as mycoses. Fungi are larger than bacteria, and only a few types are pathogenic. Single-celled forms of fungi are called yeast.

Fungal infections of the skin such as those of the tinea family (ringworm and athlete's foot) are common. Candida, commonly called candidiasis or yeast infection, often occurs in individuals with suppressed immune systems, anyone on long-term antibiotic therapy, and in individuals with diabetes. Candida is a superficial infection of the skin and mucous membranes, appearing commonly in the moist folds of the skin, the mouth (thrush), vaginal cavity (vaginitis), and genital area.

Other fungal infections include histoplasmosis and coccidioidomycosis (cok-sid-e-oyd-o-my-CO-sis). These infections are common to certain geographical

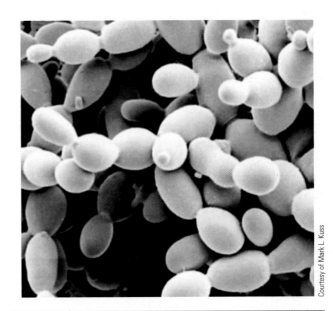

Courtesy of Mark L. Kuss

FIGURE 4–10   Fungi.

HEALTHY HIGHLIGHT

Medication Precautions

WARNING! Anyone taking a prescribed antibiotic medication should always take ALL of the medication even if the symptoms stop. Antibiotics should not be saved for the next illness. Failure to complete antibiotic therapy can lead to the development of antibiotic-resistant strains of bacteria because the first doses of medication might kill weaker bacteria and stun the stronger ones, but if therapy is halted prematurely, the stronger bacteria might survive and reproduce strains that can resist the antibiotic. When this occurs, stronger and usually more expensive medications must be used to treat the same infection at a later date. Mismanagement of antibiotic therapy has led to development of strains of bacteria that now must be treated with stronger oral antibiotics or intravenous (IV) antibiotics.

HEALTHY HIGHLIGHT

Prevention for the Common Cold

The common cold virus has more than 100 strains, and the body must identify and kill each virus as the body becomes infected. An individual will not suffer with the same cold virus twice, which explains why young children have more colds than adults. As we age, we have become ill with many cold viruses and have developed immunity to this greater number. Cold viruses are very contagious, entering the body primarily through the respiratory tract. Good hand washing is the best preventive measure for the common cold, and using antibacterial hand gels and sanitizers is also recommended.

locations but are not common in the general population. Fungal infections can be treated with antifungal and antibiotic medications but often are difficult to cure and might require long-term therapy.

Rickettsiae

Rickettsiae (Figure 4–11) are microscopic organisms that are intermediate between bacteria and viruses. They must live in the host cell like a virus. Rickettsiae are spread by fleas, ticks, mites, and lice and can cause fatal infections in humans, the most common of which is Rocky Mountain spotted fever.

Protozoa

Protozoa (Figure 4–12) are single-celled microscopic members of the animal kingdom. They are found in

the soil and live on dead or decaying material. Infection is by ingestion of spores or by infected insect bites.

Malaria, which is spread by mosquitoes, is the most prevalent protozoan infection worldwide but is uncommon in the United States. The protozoa causing malaria live in and destroy the red blood cell of the host. Giardiasis (gee-ar-DIE-a-sis) is an intestinal infection caused by drinking water infected with the *Giardia lamblia* protozoan; it is treated with antibiotic therapy.

Helminths

Helminths (Figure 4–13) are any of the roundworms or flatworms. Helminth infestation is common worldwide

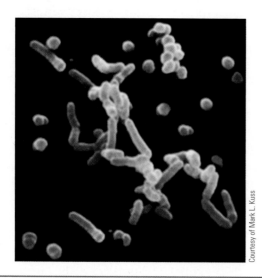

FIGURE 4–11 Rickettsiae.

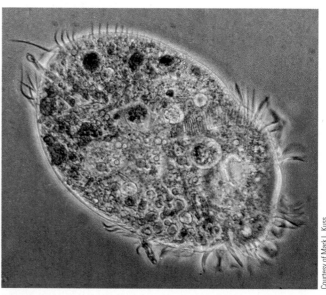

FIGURE 4–12 Protozoa.

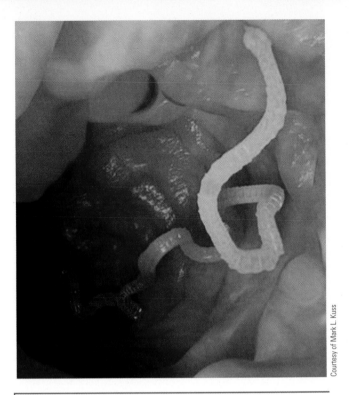

Courtesy of Mark L. Kuss

FIGURE 4–13   Helminth.

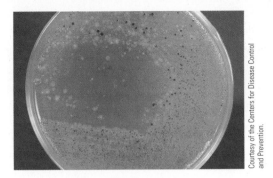

Courtesy of the Centers for Disease Control and Prevention.

FIGURE 4–14   Bacterial culture.

but not as common in the United States. Pinworms and tapeworms are the most common helminths. Pinworms cause anal itching but do not cause serious illness. Tapeworms, acquired by eating uncooked or inadequately cooked meat, can cause intestinal disease in humans.

Testing for Infection

Symptoms of infection in an individual can include fever, **tachycardia** (TACH-ee-KAR-dee-ah; tachy = rapid, cardia = heart rate), and **malaise** (general ill feeling). Often, blood studies will reveal **leukocytosis** (leuko = white, cyto = cell, osis = condition), or an increase in the white cell count, and blood from an individual with **septicemia** (SEP-tih-SEE-me-ah) will reveal the presence of the pathogen in the blood. Infection in the meninges, or meningitis, can show presence of pathogens in the individual's spinal fluid.

A culture is the process of growing pathogenic cells on or in a gelatin-like substance called media that pathogenic organisms use for food (Figure 4–14). Media can be made of different nutrient agars of which a common one is sheep's blood agar. Laboratory studies of how the microorganism uses this food assist in the determination of the type of pathogen.

A culture is the most definitive test for organisms in a lesion or wound. Cultures are most commonly used for bacteria identification, but can also identify viral and fungal infections. Most specimens are obtained from the throat, urine, sputum, purulent wound lesions, feces, blood, and spinal fluid.

After identification of the pathogen, a sensitivity test is used to identify the type of treatment needed. The combined test for these is called a **culture and sensitivity** test. During a sensitivity test, the microorganisms are grown on the entire surface of the agar plate. An antibiotic-permeated disk or strip is placed on the agar plate to determine if the antibiotic will kill the organism. The larger the kill zone, the more effective that antibiotic is at killing the organism. Use of the antibiotic-permeated strip, known as the epsilometer test (Etest®), not only shows the kill zone, but also uses graduated markings to indicate the concentration of antibiotic needed to kill the organism (Figure 4–15).

Specific antigen–antibody reactive tests can be used to determine the presence of pathogens. For example, a rapid diagnosis of strep throat can be made by testing for the presence of an antigen in a throat specimen. The *Streptococcus* antigen will clot or clump when mixed with a laboratory *Streptococcus* antibody.

Bacterial, rickettsial, and some other pathogenic infections can be determined by serologic testing, which uses the individual's blood serum to test for antibodies against the pathogen.

Skin testing also uses antibody presence to determine exposure to pathogens. Tuberculosis (TB) skin testing (also called the Mantoux test) is one of the most common skin tests and involves the intradermal (under the skin) injection of tuberculin bacteria particles (antigen) (Figure 4–16). If an

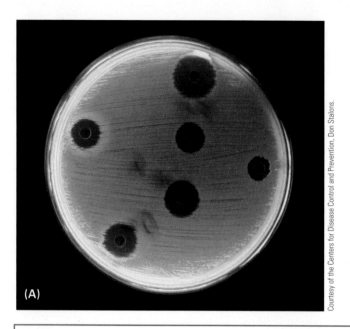

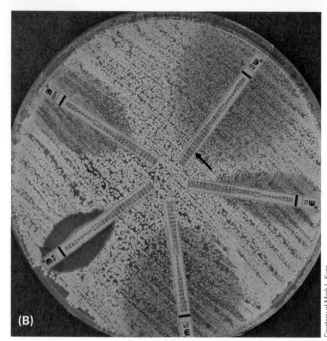

FIGURE 4–15   Sensitivity test. (A) Disk method. (B) Etest®.

individual has been exposed to TB and has developed the TB antibody, this antibody will attack the antigen and cause an **induration** (IN-dur-RAY-shun; hardened tissue), displaying a positive skin test (Figure 4–17).

Testing for MRSA includes culture and sensitivity of infected body tissues or nasal secretions. Treatment is often delayed since completion of this test takes a minimum of 48 hours. The Xpert MRSA® uses DNA-type technology to test for the drug-resistant strain.

This test can determine the presence of MRSA within an hour, but the cost is often prohibitive, especially for smaller health care facilities.

A positive skin test and serology testing might not indicate current infection or the degree of infection. These tests are only a few of the many laboratory tests used in diagnosing pathogenic infections and indicate only that the individual has been exposed to the pathogen and has developed antibodies.

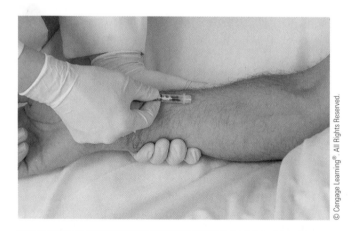

FIGURE 4–16   Tuberculosis (TB) skin test.

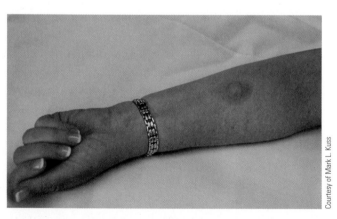

FIGURE 4–17   Positive skin test.

SUMMARY

The body responds to the invasions of pathogens by using its defense mechanisms. Inflammation is a natural protective mechanism that occurs when physical barriers are broken and the invader penetrates the tissues. The inflammatory process consists of a series of events that eventually, if functioning properly, destroy the invading pathogen.

When this system of protection fails, infection can occur. Infections are caused by a variety of organisms, most commonly by bacteria and viruses. They are diagnosed and treated in a variety of ways. Several kinds of laboratory tests can be used to identify the organism and determine the appropriate therapy.

REVIEW QUESTIONS

Short Answer

1. What are the three defense mechanisms of the body? (Describe them.)

2. What are the steps in the inflammatory process?

3. How do inflammatory exudates and inflammatory lesions differ?

4. What are the five cardinal signs of inflammation?

5. What is the difference between a keloid and an adhesion?

6. Compare and contrast some microorganisms that produce infection in humans.

7. What type of testing is used to identify the organism causing an infection?

Fill in the Blanks

8. Cellular proliferation can be grouped into the three categories of _____, _____, and _____.

9. The body's two main methods of repair involve _____ and _____.

10. Primary union is also called _____.

11. The process of secondary union involves a larger degree of _____ and more _____ to resolve it than primary union requires.

12. The greatest impediments to wound healing are _____ and _____.

CASE STUDIES

■ Ms. Jannicet is an 85-year-old resident in a local long-term care facility. She is very thin and frail and, except for meals, stays in bed most of the day. This puts her at risk for developing pressure ulcers. On what areas of her body would she most likely develop pressure ulcers? How can they be prevented? How would you describe a pressure ulcer? Describe the healing process of a pressure ulcer.

■ Mr. Jordan has a sore throat and frequent cough, so he made an appointment with his physician for an evaluation. He was diagnosed with an upper respiratory infection. The physician prescribed an antibiotic to be taken four times a day for 10 days. What are some important points about taking the medication that Mr. Jordan should know? Although he already has an infection, is good hand washing still important? If so, why?

Study Tools

Workbook

Complete Chapter 4

Online Resources

PowerPoint® presentations

Animation

BIBLIOGRAPHY

Baron, E. (2011). Acinetobacter spreads its wings. *Infectious Disease Alert* (Suppl), 23–24.

Benbow, M. (2011). Wound care: Ensuring a holistic and collaborative assessment. *British Journal of Community Nursing 16*(Suppl), S6–S16.

Cadogan, J., Baldwin, D., Carpenter, S., Davey, J., Harris, H., Purser, K., & Wicks, G. (2011). Identification, diagnosis and treatment of wound infection. *Nursing Standard, 26*(11), 44–48.

Cowman, S., Gethin, G., Clarke, E., Moore, Z., Craig, G., Jordan-O'Brien, J., & Strapp, H. (2012). An international eDelphi study identifying the research and education priorities in wound management and tissue repair. *Journal of Clinical Nursing, 21*(3/4), 344–353.

Gethin, G. (2011). The role of antiseptics in pressure ulcer management. *Nursing Standard, 26*(7), 53–60.

Gonçalves, R. B., Coletta, R. D., Silvério, K. G., Benevides, L. L., Casati, M. Z., da Silva, J. S., & Nociti Jr., F. H. (2011). Impact of smoking on inflammation: Overview of molecular mechanisms. *Inflammation Research, 60*(5), 409–424.

Imran, I., Hussain, L., Zia-Ul-Haq, M. M., Janbaz, K., Gilani, A. H., & De Feo, V. (2011). Gastrointestial and respiratory activities of *Acacia leucophloea. Journal of Ethnopharmacology, 138*(3), 676–682.

Matsui, Y., Furue, M., Sanada, H., Tachibana, T., Nakayama, T., Sugama, J., & Miyachi, Y. (2011). Development of the DESIGN-R with an observational study: An absolute evaluation tool for monitoring pressure ulcer wound healing. *Wound Repair & Regeneration, 19*(3), 309–315.

McKeeney, L. (2011). Evaluating the effectiveness of wound management products. *Nursing Standard, 26*(7), 72–76.

McVeigh, H. (2011). Topical silver for preventing wound infection. *International Journal of Evidence-Based Healthcare, 9*(4), 454–455.

Powell, G. (2011). Wound care for injecting drug users: Part 1. *Nursing Standard, 25*(46), 51–60.

Vítor, J. B., & Vale, F. F. (2011). Alternative therapies for *Helicobacter pylori*: Probiotics and phytomedicine. *FEMS Immunology & Medical Microbiology, 63*(2), 153–164.

Yarnell, E., & Abascal, K. (2008). Antiadhesion herbs. *Alternative & Complementary Therapies, 14*(3), 139–144.

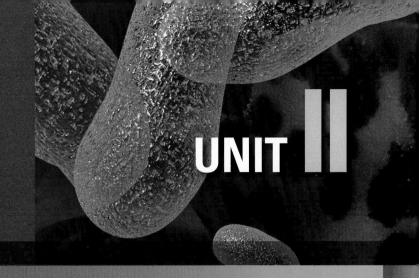

UNIT II

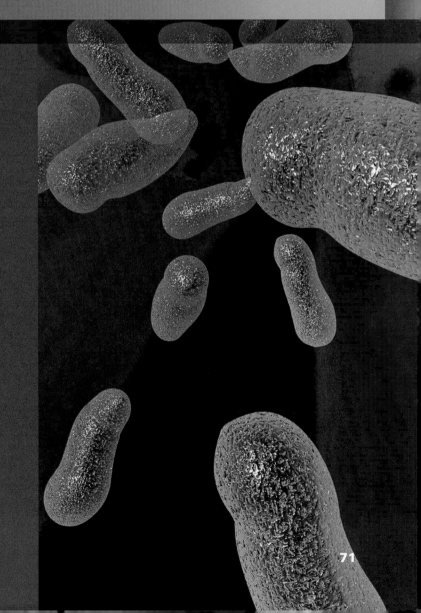

Common Diseases and Disorders of Body Systems

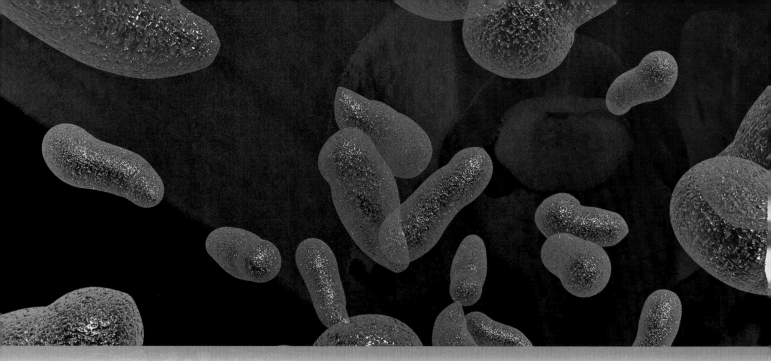

OUTLINE

KEY TERMS

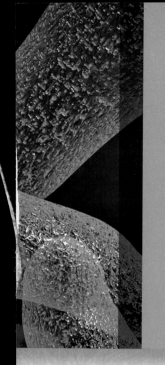

Immune System Diseases and Disorders

5

LEARNING OBJECTIVES

Upon completion of the chapter, the learner should be able to:

1. Define the terminology common to the immune system and the disorders of the system.
2. Discuss the basic anatomy and physiology of the immune system.
3. Identify the important signs and symptoms associated with common immune system disorders.
4. Describe the common diagnostics used to determine type, cause, or both of an immune system disorder.
5. Identify disorders of the immune system.
6. Describe the typical course and management of common immune system disorders.
7. Describe the effects of aging on the immune system and the common disorders of the system associated with aging.

OVERVIEW

The immune system protects the body through the processes of defense, attack, and removal of pathogens. The immune system also helps the body by removing aged or dead cells and other debris. Diseases or disorders of the immune system can range from mild to severe and can affect individuals of any age, race, or gender. Many of the disorders of the system are extremely debilitating and require long-term therapy. If the immune system is not functioning properly due to disease or other influencing factors, the result may be a secondary disease of the body resulting from the compromised immune system. ∎

ANATOMY AND PHYSIOLOGY

The immune system is made up of a complex group of cells and organs found throughout the body. The system includes primary organs, such as the thymus gland and the bone marrow, and secondary organs such as the lymph nodes, spleen, liver, and tonsils (Figure 5–1). Lymphocytes, the major cells of the immune system, arise and develop in the primary organs. The secondary organs are responsible for filtering foreign substances and providing the space for antigen reactions.

The cells of the immune system include four types of leukocytes: polymorphonuclear leukocytes, monocytes, macrophages, and lymphocytes. The polymorphonuclear leukocytes (PMNs), also known as granulocytes, are active in the inflammatory process. Some leukocytes react when infection threatens the body; others respond to prevent damage to cells and tissues from an allergic reaction. The monocytes and macrophages become phagocytic in the presence of pathogens and foreign substances. The lymphocytes are the major players in the immune response (Table 5–1).

Lymphocytes are formed in the bone marrow. Those remaining and maturing in the bone marrow become B lymphocytes. Others migrate and mature in the thymus and become T lymphocytes. When mature, both B and T lymphocytes enter the blood and circulate and colonize the lymphatic organs, predominately the spleen and lymph nodes.

T lymphocytes, or T cells, are responsible for the cell-mediated response. These cells destroy microorganisms

TABLE 5–1 Types and Functions of Leukocytes

Type	Function
Polymorphonuclear leukocytes	
Neutrophils	Phagocytosis
Eosinophils	Allergic response
Basophils	Histamine release
Monocytes	Become macrophages (phagocytosis)
Macrophages	Phagocytosis
Lymphocytes	
T lymphocytes	Cell-mediated immunity
B lymphocytes	Humoral immunity
Plasma cells	Antibody production

that invade the body. These reactions do not require antibodies produced by the B lymphocytes or B cells because the T cells have been previously sensitized by circulating antigens. Several types of T cells function to stimulate B cells to produce antibodies, destroy foreign cells in the body, stop the immune response, and remember previous exposure to antigens.

B lymphocytes are responsible for humoral immunity. Humoral immunity is associated with circulating antibodies in contrast to cell-mediated immunity. The B lymphocytes enlarge and divide to become mature plasma cells. The plasma cells secrete antibodies into the blood and lymph to protect the body against infections and toxins produced by microorganisms.

There are two types of immune responses in the body: specific and nonspecific. Specific immune response is associated with antigens and the antibody reaction. It is the body's watch-guard system for foreign invaders. The antibody response occurs after exposure to an antigen. Antibodies may neutralize, kill, or cause clumping of the foreign microorganism. Antibodies may be assisted by the complement system. This system is a group of proteins that are formed in the liver and circulate in the serum. The complement system works with and enhances the work of the antibodies to destroy the invader.

The nonspecific immune response includes inflammation, phagocytosis, physical barriers (the skin and mucous membranes), and chemical barriers (acids and other secretions). These immune response defenses are the body's first line of protection against foreign invaders.

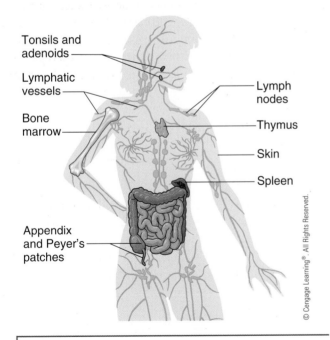

Tonsils and adenoids
Lymphatic vessels
Bone marrow
Appendix and Peyer's patches
Lymph nodes
Thymus
Skin
Spleen

FIGURE 5–1 Organs of the immune system.

TABLE 5–2 Types of Immunity

Type of Immunity	Example
Active natural immunity	Having the disease (such as mumps)
Active artificial immunity	Receiving a vaccination (such as MMR)
Passive natural immunity	Antibodies produced by the body itself or received from maternal–fetus transmission
Passive artificial immunity	Injection of antibodies

© Cengage Learning®. All Rights Reserved.

There are several ways to classify types of immunity, but the most common method is to divide immunity into passive and active then further divide these types into natural and artificial. Table 5–2 outlines the types of immunity and gives examples of each. In addition, some classification systems use the term *natural resistance* when describing immunity. Natural resistance is the inherited immunity the individual may possess due to race, species, or ethnic background. Some races, species, or particular groups of populations are naturally resistant to certain diseases, just as some are more susceptible to certain diseases.

COMMON SIGNS AND SYMPTOMS

In some cases, a patient's concern can be considered as both a symptom and a sign. Some references call this an objective or observable symptom, whereas others state that it is also a sign. An example would be a patient complaining of a runny nose. The runny nose is the patient's symptom, and because it is observable to the physician, it is also a sign.

The common signs and symptoms related to the various immune system diseases are quite varied, depending on the organ or organ system affected. Symptoms common to allergic reactions include local or systemic inflammatory responses (redness, heat, swelling, and itching) and respiratory symptoms (runny nose, coughing, sneezing, and nasal congestion).

The classic clinical problem with immune deficiency disorders is the development of unusual and severe infections such as pneumonia, meningitis, or septicemia, to name just a few. Also, the development of infections by microorganisms that are not usually pathogenic (opportunistic infections) might be indicative of an **immunodeficiency** (lack of immunity) disorder. The common signs and symptoms related to the various **autoimmune** (immunity against self) and **isoimmune** (immunity against other humans) disorders are also varied, depending on the organ or organ system affected and the invading pathogen. For this reason, signs and symptoms of these diseases are identified in the discussion of the specific disease.

DIAGNOSTIC TESTS

Determining the cause of an allergic reaction might be quite difficult. There are hundreds of possible **antigens (allergens)** that cause allergic reactions. Some of the more common allergens are house dust, pet hair, chocolate, ragweed, cigarette smoke, pollen, seafood, nickel, plants, paints, dyes, and chemical cleaners.

The most important test for diagnosing allergies is the skin test. A skin test may be performed by intradermal injection involving injection of a small amount of the suspected antigen under the skin. A skin patch test utilizes placement of a small antigen-soaked patch placed against the individual's skin. Another skin test is a scratch test in which a small amount of suspected antigen is placed in a small scratch. All three types of tests are used to identify an allergen.

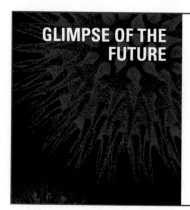

GLIMPSE OF THE FUTURE

Vaccines to Stimulate T-Cell Production

Research has shown that T cells play an important role in protecting the body from infectious diseases. Recent vaccine development has moved to creating products that stimulate T-cell production. These vaccines have been successful in inducing T-cell development for diseases such as HIV/AIDS and malaria. Continued research is needed to find similar vaccines for other infectious and parasitic diseases. In the future, researchers may also find a T-cell–inducing vaccine that is effective for some types of cancer.

Source: Gilbert (2012).

Allergy to the antigen is positive if an inflammatory response or wheal occurs at the injection site. The size of the wheal is usually indicative of the individual's sensitivity to the allergen. There are hundreds of allergic antigens that may be used in skin testing.

After an antigen has been identified, a desensitization treatment may be attempted. Desensitization requires the injection of an increasing amount of allergen over a long period of time with the goal of desensitizing the body to the allergen. Other treatments include antihistamine medications and avoiding exposure to the allergen.

Hypersensitivity reactions to transfused blood cells are usually identified by a blood count indicating low levels of red cells, white cells, and platelets. Antibodies can form against all these blood elements, leading to anemia, leukopenia, and thrombocytopenia, respectively.

A Coombs test will indicate the formation of antibodies on the red blood cell. This test can be used to determine blood type and diagnose certain **hemolytic** (HE-moh-LIT-ick; hemo = blood, lytic = destroying) anemias. A Coombs test can also indicate the presence of maternal antibodies against the fetal blood type, as occurs in erythroblastosis fetalis.

Autoimmune disorders can be diagnosed using blood tests that measure for specific diseases. For example, individuals with systemic lupus erythematosus will have a positive antinuclear antibody (ANA) test. Rheumatoid factor (RF) in the blood is often indicative of rheumatoid arthritis. Another test for rheumatoid arthritis is the presence of anti-cyclic citrullinated peptide (CCP) antibodies. This test is also used to predict those who will have more severe effects of the disease.

Immunodeficiency disorders are usually diagnosed by blood testing that reveals low white cell counts, specifically B and T lymphocytes. Presence of an antibody in the blood against a causative pathogen can also be used. Finding an antibody against the human immunodeficiency virus (HIV) is indicative of exposure to acquired immunodeficiency syndrome (AIDS).

■ COMMON DISEASES OF THE IMMUNE SYSTEM

Diseases of the immune system can be divided into two main groups: hypersensitivity disorders and immune deficiency disorders. Several specific diseases are within each grouping. Each of these has some unique problems associated with the disease, but some of the signs and symptoms may be quite similar.

PHARMACOLOGY HIGHLIGHT

Common Drugs for Immune Disorders

CATEGORY	EXAMPLES OF MEDICATIONS
Antihistamines Drugs used to reduce the symptoms from allergies	carbinoxamine or levocabastine (prescription drugs) fexofenadine, cetirizine, or loratadine (over-the-counter drugs)
Anti-inflammatories Drugs used to reduce inflammation	hydrocortisone, beclomethasone, or amcinonide (steroids) acetaminophen, aspirin, or ibuprofen (nonsteroidal)
Antipyretics/Analgesics Drugs used to reduce fever and pain	acetaminophen, aspirin, ibuprofen, or naproxen
Antivirals Drugs used to stop the action of the virus	acyclovir, imiquimod, or cidofovir
Bronchodilators Drugs used to improve breathing	albuterol, aminophylline, epinephrine, theophylline, or salmeterol

Consider This ...

Stress hormones, cortisol and epinephrine, which suppress the body's immune system, will actually decrease after a good dose of laughter.

Hypersensitivity Disorders

Hypersensitivity disorders are the result of an overreaction of the immune system to an antigen or allergen. Hypersensitivity disorders can be further classified as those related to allergy, autoimmunity, and isoimmunity (Figure 5–2).

ALLERGIES

■ *DESCRIPTION.* Allergies are among the most prevalent types of hypersensitivity problems. Millions of people suffer from some type of allergy. Hay fever, asthma (AZ-ma), **urticaria** (UR-tih-KAR-ree-ah;

a reaction characterized by intense wheals and itching), and contact dermatitis are common allergic reactions. These reactions are usually just bothersome, but they can be a serious health threat. Severe asthma, for example, may be life threatening. Food allergies are also common in some populations but may be difficult to diagnose.

■ *ETIOLOGY.* Allergy is an acquired hypersensitivity. The individual with an allergy must first be exposed or sensitized to the antigen. Subsequent or repeated exposure leads to a reaction, identified as an allergy or an allergic reaction, by the immune system. Allergens can cause an immediate response like those identified with hay fever, asthma, or food allergy. Delayed-response allergies are slower to react and are usually less harmful. An example of delayed response allergy would be contact dermatitis, caused by exposure to poison ivy.

■ *SYMPTOMS.* Most allergens are airborne. Respiratory symptoms can include runny nose, coughing, sneezing, wheezing, and nasal congestion. Other allergies can lead to redness, heat, swelling, and itching of the involved tissue.

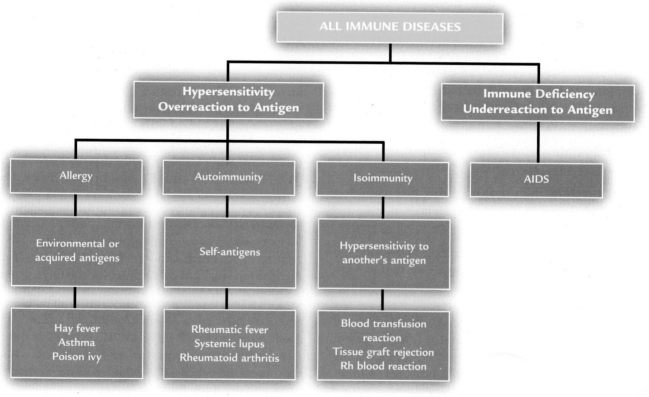

FIGURE 5–2 Classification of hypersensitivity disorders.

■ **DIAGNOSIS.** Diagnosis of allergies is often made on the basis of history and physical exam along with testing. Positive skin sensitivity testing and blood testing, including an elevated blood eosinophil (a white blood cell that responds in allergic conditions) level, are indicative of allergies.

■ **TREATMENT.** Treatments include avoidance of the allergen, allergy desensitization injections, and antihistamine and steroid medications.

■ **PREVENTION.** Prevention of all hypersensitivity disorders is total avoidance of the allergen or, in the case of autoimmune diseases, minimizing the hyperimmune symptoms.

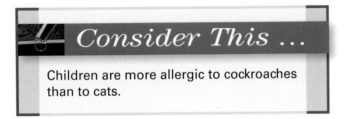

Consider This ...

Children are more allergic to cockroaches than to cats.

HAY FEVER

■ **DESCRIPTION.** Hay fever is a reaction in the mucous membranes of the nose and upper respiratory tract to an allergen.

■ **ETIOLOGY.** The allergen is usually airborne and can be seasonal. Tree pollen, grasses, agricultural crops, and ragweed pollen can cause an increase in symptoms during the different seasons of the year. Nonseasonal hay fever can be the result of house dust, pet dander, or food allergies.

■ **SYMPTOMS.** Symptoms include sneezing, watery eyes, runny nose, and itching.

■ **DIAGNOSIS.** Skin testing is the most common method of allergy testing for hay fever.

■ **TREATMENT.** Treatment of hay fever includes removal of the allergen or separation of the allergen and the hay fever sufferer. Individuals who suffer from hay fever can choose to move permanently to a different climate or to vacation in a different area when the pollen count is high in their area. An air-conditioned environment is beneficial because it filters much of the allergen. Antihistamines and other drugs can be given orally—and in nose drops and sprays—in an effort to control symptoms. Allergy desensitization might be of benefit.

ASTHMA

■ **DESCRIPTION.** This chronic allergic condition is also known as bronchial asthma. It affects 5–10% of children, making it the leading cause of chronic illness in childhood. Male children have asthma twice as often as girls prior to puberty. After puberty, the ratio is more equal.

■ **ETIOLOGY.** When exposed to an allergen, the hypersensitive individual has episodes of wheezing due to **bronchospasm** (BRONG-ko-SPA-zm) or muscular constriction of the bronchi of the respiratory tract. The individual appears perfectly normal between episodes.

Asthma can be caused by allergens in the environment, such as pollen, dust, pet dander, smoke, or various fumes. Other causes of asthma are nonallergic and include events that produce stress. Triggers for nonallergic asthma include respiratory infections such as the common cold, changes in temperature and humidity, exercise, and emotional stress.

■ **SYMPTOMS.** Symptoms of an attack are extreme shortness of breath, difficulty breathing, wheezing, and anxiety. Attacks vary in severity from mild to almost suffocating. Coughing during the attack usually begins with a mild, dry cough, but progresses to production of large amounts of mucus as the attack continues. Skin might be pale and moist in mild attacks, with cyanosis of the nail beds and lips occurring in more severe attacks. During an attack, asthmatics often assume a sitting position, leaning forward with hands resting on the knees. This position helps the individual breathe by using all the respiratory muscles (Figure 5–3). A severe attack that does not respond to treatment with bronchodilators and/or lasts for several days is called **status asthmaticus** (AZ-MAH-ti-kus) and is a life-threatening medical emergency.

■ **DIAGNOSIS.** Diagnosis is made after a complete history and physical exam along with lung function testing. A trial medication might be ordered. If the medication works, the diagnosis is probably asthma.

■ **TREATMENT.** Treatment includes avoidance of causative allergens, desensitization, education, and medications to treat symptoms. Deep breathing exercises, maintenance of proper posture, and relaxation techniques are beneficial. A regimen of medications to relax and open the bronchi (bronchodilators) and to thin the excessive mucus (mucolytics) is important.

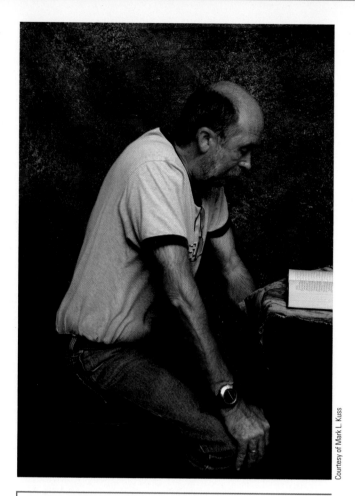

FIGURE 5–3   Positioning in an asthma attack.

There is no cure for asthma, but it can be controlled by a combination of therapies including strict compliance to a medication regimen, relaxation techniques, exercise, and avoidance of allergens.

Media Link

View an animation about asthma on the Online Resources.

URTICARIA

■ **DESCRIPTION.** Commonly called hives or nettle rash, urticaria is a vascular reaction of the skin.

■ **ETIOLOGY.** This condition is caused by contact with an external irritant such as insect bites, pollen, drugs, food, or plants.

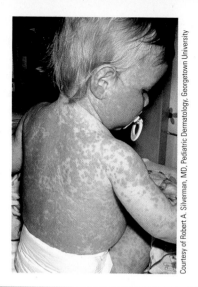

FIGURE 5–4   Urticaria.

■ **SYMPTOMS.** The condition is characterized by slightly elevated lesions that are redder or paler than the surrounding skin and is associated with severe itching. The elevated areas are called wheals or hives. Scratching or rubbing the hypersensitive area can lead to formation of larger or additional wheals (Figure 5–4).

■ **DIAGNOSIS.** A physical examination will help diagnose this skin reaction. A history of recent exposure to plants, insect bites, pets, new foods, or medications might assist in identifying the allergen.

■ **TREATMENT.** Treatment includes antihistamines and avoidance of the allergen.

ANAPHYLAXIS

■ **DESCRIPTION.** This is a severe allergic response to an allergen, often leading to anaphylactic shock.

■ **ETIOLOGY.** Anaphylaxis (AN-ah-fih-LACK-sis), also known as an anaphylactic reaction, is caused by absorption of the antigen into the blood directly or through the mucous membranes. Food allergy is believed to be the leading cause of anaphylaxis outside the hospital (Food Allergy and Anaphylaxis Network, 2008). Other common causes of anaphylaxis include medications, insect stings, and latex.

■ **SYMPTOMS.** A local anaphylactic reaction might be mild and produce generalized itching, swelling, and urticaria. This reaction should be closely monitored because it might rapidly progress to systemic anaphylaxis. Systemic anaphylaxis is a true medical emergency involving the release of histamine throughout body tissues. Within minutes, the individual feels itching of the throat, tongue, and scalp. Edema or swelling of the face and airways leads to difficulty breathing. The individual suffers a huge drop in blood pressure (shock) and body temperature. Unconsciousness usually occurs with the drop in blood pressure. If these symptoms are not reversed with medical attention, death from respiratory and cardiac arrest can occur within 15 to 20 minutes.

■ **DIAGNOSIS.** Symptoms of anaphylaxis generally initiate within minutes and last less than 24 hours. A diagnosis is made rapidly, based on the presenting symptoms.

■ **TREATMENT.** Treatment during an attack might include performance of an emergency tracheostomy (TRAY-kee-OS-toh-me; trache = trachea, ostomy = new opening) or endotracheal (endo = within, trachea = windpipe) intubation with mechanical ventilation. Immediate administration of epinephrine medication is necessary. Epinephrine (adrenalin) is a vasoconstrictor and a smooth-muscle relaxant. Effects of epinephrine will raise the blood pressure, dilate the bronchi, and decrease laryngeal spasms. Antihistamines and **corticosteroids** (KORT-ti-ko-STEHR-oyds; powerful anti-inflammatory hormones) are given to limit histamine production, thus slowing the allergic reaction.

Follow-up treatment should include identifying the allergen. The individual is taught to identify and avoid the allergen and recognize the onset of a reaction. These individuals should wear an allergy identification necklace or bracelet. Individuals who experience this severe reaction should always carry an allergy kit containing Benadryl (an antihistamine), syringes, and vials of epinephrine, or an epinephrine auto-injector (EpiPen® or Auvi-Q®). The individual and family members should understand and practice the appropriate steps in treatment of a reaction.

FOOD ALLERGIES

■ **DESCRIPTION.** Gastrointestinal food allergies are often difficult to diagnose. The process involves elimination of certain foods and then adding these to the diet one at a time.

■ **ETIOLOGY.** Chocolate and shellfish are common food allergies. Often, the allergy is not to a specific food but to additives or preservatives in the food. Allergy to milk might not be a true allergy but rather an intolerance to the lactose in the milk. Lactose intolerance can be treated by taking lactose enzyme (lactase) before consumption of dairy products.

■ **SYMPTOMS.** Symptoms of food allergies may include skin rash, abdominal cramping, diarrhea, and vomiting.

■ **DIAGNOSIS.** A thorough history from the patient and the patient's documented food diary aids in diagnosis. Testing, including skin tests, blood test, and food challenges, is also helpful.

■ **TREATMENT.** If the allergic reaction is mild, treatment with antihistamines might be sufficient. In a severe reaction, the first priority is to maintain the airway. Activation of the emergency medical system might be needed.

CONTACT DERMATITIS

■ **DESCRIPTION.** Contact dermatitis is an acute or chronic allergic reaction affecting the skin.

■ **ETIOLOGY.** Often the allergen is some type of cosmetic, laundry product, plant, jewelry, paint, drug, plastic, or a variety of other agents (Figure 5–5). Often, it is difficult to determine the causative agent, and once found, complete avoidance might not be possible.

■ **SYMPTOMS.** Allergic lesions can range from small, red, localized lesions to vesicular lesions that cover the entire body. A common example of contact dermatitis is poison ivy.

■ **DIAGNOSIS.** Skin patch testing helps determine the diagnosis of the allergen (Figure 5–6).

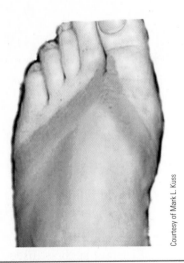

Courtesy of Mark L. Kuss

FIGURE 5–5 Contact dermatitis.

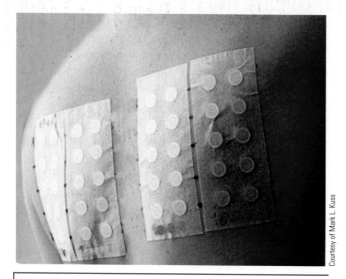

FIGURE 5–6   Skin patch testing.

■ TREATMENT. Treatment is not available until the allergen is diagnosed. Avoiding the allergen is the most effective treatment.

Autoimmune Disorders

Autoimmune disorders are hypersensitivities in which the body fails to recognize its own antigens or **self-antigen**. An individual's body cells have specific antigen on the cell surfaces. Failure to recognize this antigen as a self-antigen leads to the body attacking and destroying its own tissues. Several theories exist as to the cause of this type of disorder, but currently, the cause for autoimmune disorders is unknown. Autoimmune disorders include rheumatic fever, rheumatoid arthritis, myasthenia gravis, type 1 diabetes, lupus erythematosus, and scleroderma.

RHEUMATIC FEVER

■ DESCRIPTION. Rheumatic (ROO-MAT-ik) fever is an inflammatory disease that can affect the heart, joints, and skin.

■ ETIOLOGY. In a small number of individuals, rheumatic fever occurs following a group A **streptococcal** (STREHP-toh-KAHK-al) infection, usually strep throat. In this select number of individuals, the proteins in their hearts and other connective tissues are similar to the protein of the strep bacteria. For this reason, rheumatic fever tends to run in families. Exposure to strep bacteria causes the immune system to make antibodies to fight the bacteria.

These antibodies also attack the tissues of the heart and joints because they cannot distinguish the differences in the proteins. Rheumatic fever is characterized by myocarditis (myo = muscle, cardi = heart, itis = inflammation) and arthritis.

■ SYMPTOMS. Rheumatic fever usually occurs 1 to 4 weeks after a streptococcal infection. Children and adolescents are most commonly affected. Onset of the disease can be sudden or gradual and includes symptoms of fever, malaise, and joint pain. The first occurrence of rheumatic fever might be mild and resolve without any permanent damage. Further episodes are usually more severe and might lead to permanent scarring and deformity of the heart valves (Figure 5–7). Deformity of the mitral and aortic valve can eventually lead to heart failure.

■ DIAGNOSIS. There is no definitive test for diagnosing rheumatic fever. Blood testing along with electrocardiogram to determine heart muscle damage are part of the diagnostic workup, and a positive throat culture for *Streptococcus* bacteria is also indicative of the diagnosis.

■ TREATMENT. Culturing for strep infections and prolonged treatment (at least 10 days) with antibiotics are most effective. **Prophylactic** (pro-fil-LACK-tic; works to prevent) antibiotics can be given to susceptible individuals. Surgical replacement of the heart valves might be necessary for individuals with severe valve deformity.

■ PREVENTION. Prompt and accurate diagnosis and treatment of group A streptococcal infections are the best preventive measures against rheumatic fever.

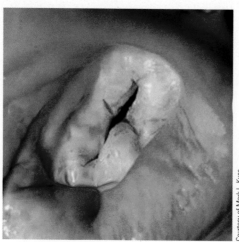

FIGURE 5–7   Rheumatic fever: damaged heart valve.

RHEUMATOID ARTHRITIS

■ **DESCRIPTION.** Rheumatoid arthritis is an auto-immune disease that causes chronic inflammation of connective tissue. Joint tissue is primarily affected, but any connective tissue of the body might be involved.

■ **ETIOLOGY.** The exact cause of rheumatoid arthritis is unknown, but it is associated with the production of an abnormal antibody that attacks or attaches to the body's own cells and tissues. Presence of the antibody called *rheumatoid factor (RF)* in the affected individual's blood is indicative of the disease.

■ **SYMPTOMS.** Commonly, metacarpal-phalangeal joints of the hands are initially affected with rheumatoid arthritis. This leads to a classic sign of rheumatoid arthritis called ulnar deviation of the fingers (Figure 5–8). As the disease progresses, involvement of other synovial joints can occur. Joints affected can include those of the fingers, wrists, elbows, feet, ankles, and knees. Symptoms of rheumatoid arthritis can vary in severity from mild to severe and might go through periods of remission and exacerbation.

Rheumatoid arthritis begins with inflammation of the synovial lining of the joint, leading to pain, stiffness, and joint deformity. Eventually, the cartilage of the joint is destroyed and replaced with a granulation tissue called pannus (PAN-nus). As the disease progresses, the entire joint surface is destroyed and replaced with fibrous tissue, making the joint less movable. Fusion or total loss of joint function is called ankylosis (ANG-kih-LOH-sis) (Figure 5–9).

In addition to joint changes, the individual might also have lesions in the collagen of the lungs, blood vessels, heart, and eyes, leading to pleuritis (PLOO-RIGH-tis; pleura = pleura or lining of the lung, itis = inflammation), anemia, valvulitis (VAL-view-LYE-tis; valvul = valve, itis = inflammation), and glaucoma (glaw-KOH-mah), respectively. Rheumatoid nodules characteristically appear in the subcutaneous tissue around the fingers, toes, and elbows (Figure 5–10). Individuals with rheumatoid arthritis often appear frail and chronically ill. Anemia and infection are common secondary problems.

This chronic disease affects both sexes and all ages, but onset is most common in women between the ages of 20 and 40. Women are affected three times more often than men. Rheumatoid arthritis in children usually affects infants to children aged 16, can be very severe, and is called juvenile rheumatoid arthritis or Still's disease.

■ **DIAGNOSIS.** Diagnosis is based on physical examination, characteristic symptoms, and blood tests

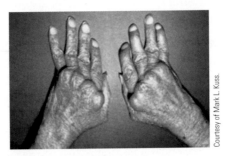

FIGURE 5–8 Ulnar deviation from rheumatoid arthritis.

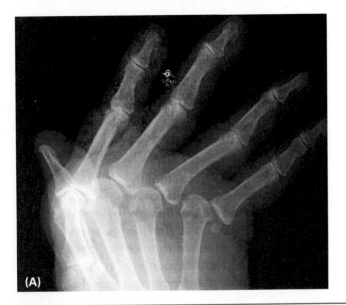

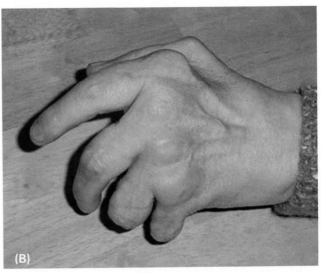

FIGURE 5–9 Joint changes from rheumatoid arthritis. (A) X-ray view. (B) Ankylosis.

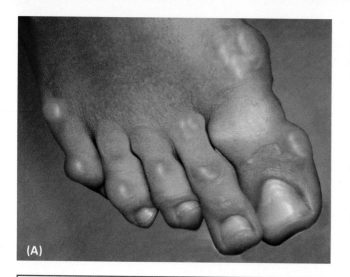
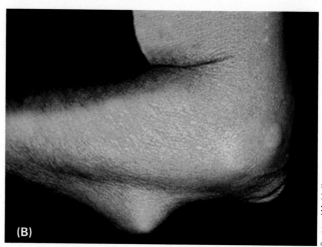

Courtesy of Mark L. Kuss

FIGURE 5–10   Rheumatoid nodules. (A) Foot. (B) Elbow.

including positive rheumatoid factor, anti-CCP antibodies, and elevated erythrocyte sedimentation rate (ESR).

■ **TREATMENT.** Rheumatoid arthritis, like other auto-immune disorders, cannot be cured. Treatment includes use of anti-inflammatory medications and analgesics. Disease-modifying antirheumatic drugs (DMARDs) and biologic drugs act on the immune system and are showing favorable progress in slowing the progression of rheumatoid arthritis. DMARDs include Imutrex® (methotrexate), Plaquenil® (hydroxychloroquine), and Azulfidine® (sulfasalazine). Biologic medications are the newest and include Humira® (adalimumab), Enbrel® (etanercept), and Actemra® (tocilizumab). Other medications used in the treatment of rheuma-toid arthritis include Minocin® (minocycline), Neoral® (cyclosporin), and Imuran® (azathioprine).

Corticosteroids can be prescribed short term dur-ing periods of exacerbation. An exercise and rest rou-tine is essential to maintain joint function. Surgical joint replacement might also be beneficial.

■ **PREVENTION.** There is no known way to prevent rheumatoid arthritis.

MYASTHENIA GRAVIS

■ **DESCRIPTION.** Myasthenia gravis (MY-uh-STHEE-nee-uh GRAV-iss) is characterized by severe muscle fatigue.

■ **ETIOLOGY.** This disease affects the transmission of nerve signals to muscle at the neuromuscular junc-tion, but there is no muscle or nerve tissue disease. Nerve impulses are carried to the muscle by the neu-rotransmitter acetylcholine (ah-SEE-til-KOH-leen).

COMPLEMENTARY AND ALTERNATIVE THERAPY

Alternative Medicines for Rheumatoid Arthritis

Alternative medicines and therapies for rheumatoid arthritis may vary from oral preparations to topical creams. Studies have been done on the effectiveness of these treatments. The review of these studies has shown that there was no "consistent evidence" to show that the alternative treatments were beneficial. However, in some studies, borage seed oil (*Borago officinalis*) and thunder god vine (*Tripterygium wilfordii*) have been shown to be helpful, so research on these two therapies should be continued to see if they really are effective in treating rheumatoid arthritis. (See Complementary and Alternative Therapy box Complications from Using Borage Oil: Seizures on page 84.)

Source: Macfarlane et al. (2011).

COMPLEMENTARY AND ALTERNATIVE THERAPY

Complications from Using Borage Oil: Seizures

Research has shown borage oil might be effective for treating rheumatoid arthritis, but it may also cause serious side effects. Borage oil comes from the seed of the borage plant (*Borago officinalis*) and has been sold as an alternative treatment for arthritis, dermatitis, nerve pain, and other ailments. Seizures were reported in people after just a short time of ingesting borage oil. Caution should be taken if using this product. (See Complementary and Alternative Therapy box Alternative Medicines for Rheumatoid Arthritis on page 83.)

Source: Al-Khamees et al. (2011).

These impulses are sent by the nerve but are not properly received by the muscle. This error in transmission is due to antibodies attacking the muscle receptors, which blocks the transmission by acetylcholine (Figure 5–11). This poor transmission of information to the muscle leads to weak muscle contractions and fatigue.

Myasthenia gravis is one of the less common autoimmune disorders, with an estimated 20 cases per 100,000 people (Myasthenia Gravis Foundation of America, 2010). Myasthenia can be categorized as an autoimmune, musculoskeletal, or neurologic disease because it has characteristics of problems in each of these systems.

■ **SYMPTOMS.** Onset of the disease is usually slow, and diagnosis might be difficult because it can affect any muscle of the body. Commonly, facial muscles are the ones initially affected, leading to diplopia (dip-PLOHP-ee-ah; double vision), ptosis (TOE-sis; drooping eyelids) (Figure 5–12), dysphagia (dys-FAY-jee-ah; difficulty swallowing), dysphonia (dys-FOH-nee-ah; difficulty talking), and difficulty with facial expressions, which can leave the individual with an expressionless facial appearance. Other symptoms relate to fatigue of all voluntary muscles and include difficulty rising from a sitting position, lifting the arms, standing, and walking.

The degree of weakness varies with the time of day and activities. Generally, these individuals feel stronger in the morning due to a buildup of acetylcholine and become weaker as the day progresses because acetylcholine stores diminish. Short rest periods are necessary to help restore muscle function.

Periods of exacerbation and remission do occur. During exacerbation, complete bed rest might be necessary.

■ **DIAGNOSIS.** Myasthenia is difficult to diagnose because symptoms can be hard to distinguish from

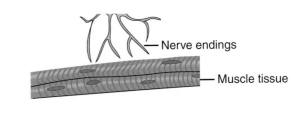

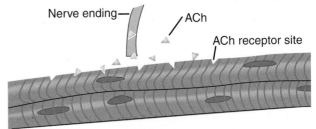

Normal (Magnified)

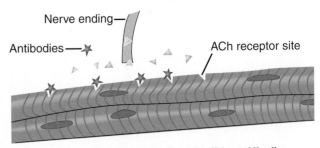

Myasthenia Gravis (Magnified)

Nerves do not touch muscle tissue to stimulate movement. Nerve endings secrete a neurotransmitter, acetylcholine (ACh), that sticks to muscle tissue receptor sites causing muscle contraction.

Antibodies produced with myasthenia gravis block these receptor sites thus blocking muscle stimulus and movement.

FIGURE 5–11   Blocking of receptor sites in myasthenia gravis.

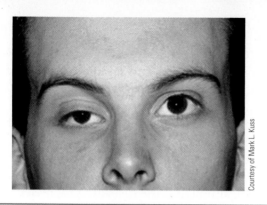

Courtesy of Mark L. Kuss

FIGURE 5–12   Myesthenia gravis: ptosis.

other neurologic disorders. A thorough physical exam might reveal fatigue of the muscles; blood testing for antibodies against the acetylcholine receptor is also suggestive of myasthenia. Other tests include electromyography to test muscle fatigue and respiratory spirometry to assess respiratory function.

■ **TREATMENT.** Treatment can include cholinergic medications that do not allow the normal breakdown of the neurotransmitter acetylcholine, allowing a buildup of the neurotransmitter, thus improving neuromuscular transmission. Plasma exchange to remove the circulating antibodies provides some improvement in the condition. Recent advances in care and treatment have reduced the mortality rate to 3–4%. Death is usually due to muscle weakness leading to respiratory failure.

■ **PREVENTION.** Myasthenia gravis cannot be prevented, but avoiding stress, extremes in temperature, fever, illness, and overexertion can help prevent exacerbations.

TYPE 1 DIABETES MELLITUS (INSULIN-DEPENDENT DIABETES MELLITUS)

■ **DESCRIPTION.** Type 1 diabetes mellitus, formerly known as insulin-dependent diabetes mellitus (IDDM), is a disease that alters the body's carbohydrate or sugar metabolism.

■ **ETIOLOGY.** Type 1 diabetes mellitus is believed to be caused by an autoimmune disorder triggered by a viral infection. The most common viral infections that might lead to diabetes include rubella, mumps, and influenza. The infecting virus inflames insulin-producing beta cells of the pancreas, and the inflammatory process, for reasons that remain unclear, seems to stimulate the beta cells to produce

an abnormal cell antigen. Lymphocytes recognize the abnormal antigen as nonself and destroy it along with the beta cells. Without insulin-producing beta cells, the individual becomes dependent on insulin injections to manage carbohydrate usage.

The normal antigens in the cells of the pancreas are human leukocyte antigens (HLAs). Individuals genetically inherit the HLAs of the pancreas. The tendency to develop an autoimmune response, and thus diabetes mellitus, is considered hereditary in nature.

There are other types of diabetes that are not caused by autoimmunity. Because all types of diabetes affect the endocrine system, they will be discussed and compared in detail in Chapter 14, "Endocrine System Diseases and Disorders."

LUPUS ERYTHEMATOSUS

■ **DESCRIPTION.** The term *lupus* originally referred to any chronic, destructive type of skin lesion. The Latin word *lupus* means *wolf*, and erythematosus refers to redness. The term *lupus erythematosus* has been used since the thirteenth century because physicians of that time thought the shape and color of the skin lesions resembled a wolf bite. The word *lupus* is often used to refer to lupus erythematosus, although used alone, this term truly has no meaning. There are several forms of lupus, including lupus pernio, lupus vulgarus, drug-induced lupus, and lupus erythematosus.

There are two types of lupus erythematosus: cutaneous (discoid) and systemic (diffuse). Cutaneous or discoid lupus erythematosus (DLE) is limited to skin or cutaneous involvement. DLE does not affect multiple systems, as does systemic lupus erythematosus (SLE). DLE can be thought of as a type of systemic lupus because cause, testing, and treatment are similar for cutaneous involvement. DLE is the less serious type of lupus erythematosus.

SLE affects approximately 1 in 2,400 people. It primarily affects women, occurring 10 times more frequently in women than in men. Onset is usually between ages 30 and 40, but it can appear at any age. The disease is most severe among individuals of African-American descent.

■ **ETIOLOGY.** SLE is an autoimmune disorder in which B lymphocytes produce autoantibodies that attack body cells. Individuals with SLE have a high number of antinuclear antibodies (ANAs). These antibodies attack the body's own cell nuclei, destroying the RNA and DNA of the cell. Detection of ANA by microscopic immunofluorescence supports the diagnosis of SLE.

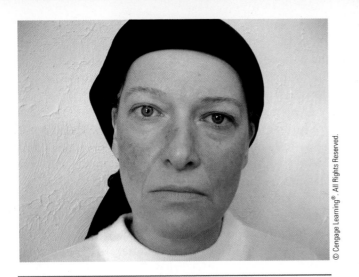

FIGURE 5-13 Butterfly rash of systemic lupus erythematosus (SLE).

■ **SYMPTOMS.** SLE often affects the skin and a number of other organs or systems. A classic sign is the presence of a persistent, red, facial butterfly-shaped rash across the bridge of the nose and cheeks (Figure 5–13). Symptomatic individuals often complain of fever, joint pain, weight loss, and facial rash. Joint, kidney, and muscle involvement can lead to complaints of arthritis, glomerulonephritis (inflammation of the glomerulus, or filtering unit of the kidney), and atrophy, respectively. Heart valve deformities and abnormal blood composition are not unusual findings.

■ **DIAGNOSIS.** Diagnosis is often very difficult, but tests including electrolytes, renal function, liver enzymes, complete blood count, and ANA are helpful. The most definitive testing is a positive result on an ANA test.

■ **TREATMENT.** SLE is a chronic disease that goes through periods of exacerbation and remission. Complete remission is very rare. Treatment is symptomatic. Nonsteroidal anti-inflammatory, antipyretic, and analgesic medications can be used to treat symptoms. Life-threatening exacerbations are often treated with corticosteroids. Prognosis depends on which organs are affected and the severity of the infection. Survival in patients with SLE in the United States, Canada, Europe, and China is approximately 95% at 5 years, 90% at 10 years, and 78% at 20 years (Longo et al., 2012). Renal insufficiency, bacterial endocarditis, cardiac failure, sepsis, and pneumonia commonly lead to death.

■ **PREVENTION.** SLE cannot be prevented or cured.

SCLERODERMA

■ **DESCRIPTION.** Scleroderma (skle-ro-DER-mah; sclero = hardening, derma = skin) is a chronic autoimmune disorder characterized by hardening, thickening, and shrinking of the connective tissues of the body, including the skin. Like many other chronic diseases, scleroderma might exhibit periods of remission and exacerbation. The generally slow progression of the disease allows the individual a reasonably long life, although if the disorder progresses rapidly, affecting vital organs, early death can result. Death is usually related to kidney failure.

■ **ETIOLOGY.** It is thought that this autoimmune reaction begins with the skin and connective tissues, attracting lymph cells. These lymph cells stimulate the production of collagen, leading to the disorder.

Milder forms of scleroderma commonly affect women 30–50 years of age and include those limited to the skin, face, and extremities. The more severe forms, called systemic or diffuse, usually affect men and older persons. This type not only affects the skin but also internal organs, including the heart, lungs, and kidney. These tissues become hardened, thickened, and often limited in function.

■ **SYMPTOMS.** Characteristically, individuals with scleroderma have thick, leather-like, shiny, taut skin and joint contractures. The first symptom is usually Raynaud's phenomenon, an episodic vasoconstriction affecting the hands. The mouth area often becomes wrinkled with a tight, purse-lipped appearance, leading to difficulty eating (Figure 5–14). Diagnosis can be confirmed by clinical examination and tissue biopsy.

■ **DIAGNOSIS.** Diagnosis is difficult because this disease initially mimics other disorders such as bursitis and arthritis.

Physical symptoms indicative of scleroderma include:

- Tight skin around the hands, face, and mouth
- Changes in the capillaries at the base of the fingernails
- Calcium deposits under the skin

These physical symptoms, coupled with special blood testing for the presence of anticentromere antibodies, often yields a positive diagnosis.

■ **TREATMENT.** Currently, there is no treatment or cure to stop the progression of scleroderma.

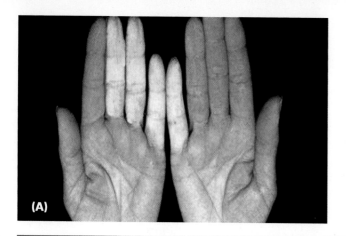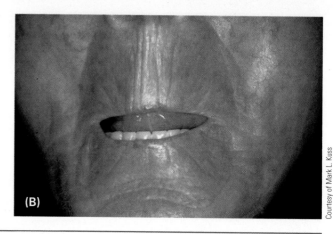

Courtesy of Mark L. Kuss

FIGURE 5–14   Scleraderma. (A) Raynaud's phenomenon. (B) Mouth tightening.

Treatment with anti-inflammatory medications, immunosuppressives, and antibiotics might be beneficial. Muscle stretching and strengthening exercises might also be beneficial to maintain muscle strength and joint mobility.

■ **PREVENTION.** No one really knows what causes scleroderma, so at this time, there are no preventive methods identified.

Isoimmune Disorders

Isoimmunity refers to a hypersensitivity of one individual to another individual's tissues. Examples include blood type reactions, tissue rejections, and maternal–fetal reactions.

BLOOD TRANSFUSION REACTION

■ **DESCRIPTION.** As previously stated, all body cells have a specific antigen that identifies them. Red blood cells (RBCs) have surface antigens. Transfusion of blood from one individual to another is, in a sense, a type of tissue transplant. RBCs have to be typed and cross-matched to identify antigens properly and prevent rejection.

The blood types are identified by antigens and can be divided into four groups: A, B, AB, and O. Types O and A are the most common. Each RBC has an antigen and a corresponding antibody. Blood type A has an A antigen and anti-B antibody. B type has a B antigen and anti-A antibody. O has no antigen and both anti-A and anti-B antibodies. AB has an A and a B antigen and no antibody. These antigen–antibody patterns make type O the universal blood donor and type AB the universal blood recipient (Figure 5–15).

■ **ETIOLOGY.** If a blood type with an antigen is given to a type that has antibodies against that antigen, the antibodies will attack the antigen and break down the donor RBCs. For example, if type A (with antigen A and anti-B antibody) is given to type B (with antigen B and anti-A antibody), the anti-A antibody in the B type recipient's blood will attack the A antigen and break down the type A donor blood (see Figure 5–15).

As antibodies react with the antigen, they also cause clumping of the blood, leading to microthrombi (microscopic-sized blood clots). These microthrombi can lead to multiple organ emboli and have fatal consequences.

■ **SYMPTOMS.** Symptoms of transfusion reaction include chills, shivering, and fever.

■ **TREATMENT.** Reactions should be treated immediately by discontinuing the transfusion and contacting the director of the blood bank, medical physician, and nephrologist. Anticipation of complications such as hypotension, renal failure, disseminated intravascular coagulation (DIC), and possibly death should be expected and treated preventively or as symptoms arise.

■ **DIAGNOSIS.** Most transfusion reactions are diagnosed by watching for any significant change in a patient's condition during transfusion. Diagnosis depends on recognition of a significant change in vital signs along with development of the signs and symptoms of a reaction.

■ **PREVENTION.** Prevention is aimed at ensuring that the blood transfused is compatible by typing, cross-matching, and checking for antibody reaction.

Type	Percent of Population with Type	Antigen	Antibody	Color Jar Example	Donate Blood To:	Receive Blood From:
A	41	A	B	RED	A and AB	A and O
B	12	B	A	BLUE	B and AB	B and O
O	44	None	A and B	CLEAR	A, B, AB, O	O
AB	3	A and B	None	PURPLE	AB	A, B, AB, O

To understand the concept of transfusion reaction with antigen and antibodies, consider this example. The particular blood type can give blood to any type that does not change the color in the jar and receive blood from any type that does not change the color in the jar. For example, A can give blood to AB because adding red to purple will not change the purple color. However, A cannot give to B because giving red to blue will change the color. Since O is in the clear jar, it can give to all types but could not receive from anything but O or the clear color would change.

FIGURE 5–15   Blood types for donors and recipients.

ERYTHROBLASTOSIS FETALIS

■ **DESCRIPTION.** Erythroblastosis fetalis (eh-RITH-roh-blas-TOH-sis feh-TAH-lis) is an isoimmune condition in which antibodies in a mother's blood attack and destroy the antigen on the baby's RBCs, ultimately killing the unborn fetus. This condition is also known as hemolytic (hemo = blood, lytic = breaking or crushing) disease of the newborn.

Antigens on the RBCs give each type of cell a special identity. In addition to antigens that determine blood type, 85% of Americans have another antigen called the Rh factor. This group is collectively called Rh positive (Rh+) because they have the factor or antigen. Those who do not have the factor—approximately 15% of the population—are Rh negative (Rh−). Crossmatching for transfusions must match the appropriate type and Rh factor. The common rule of Rh factor is, "those who don't have it don't want it; those who have it don't care." In other words, Rh− individuals cannot receive Rh+ blood. On the other hand, Rh+ individuals "don't care," so they can receive Rh+ or Rh− blood. Blood type and factor are genetically determined or received from an individual's mother or father.

Because blood type and factor are determined by one's mother or father, it is possible for a mother to be pregnant with a baby of different blood type and factor (received from the father) (Figure 5–16).

Mothers pregnant with babies of different blood types do not have a problem because RBCs do not cross the placenta. Oxygen and nutrients simply diffuse across placental membranes to nourish the baby. RBCs do not normally exchange between the mother and the infant. Mothers who are Rh− and "don't want" Rh+ factor might have difficulty with Rh+ babies.

■ **ETIOLOGY.** Rh− mothers pregnant with Rh+ babies usually do not have a problem with the first baby. During the first pregnancy, the mother's blood has not had the opportunity to identify the antigen because there has been no exchange of blood cells or antigens. However, there may be some slight mixing of blood during the birthing process. As this blood intermingles, the Rh+ antigen is picked up by the mother's blood. The mother's immune system recognizes this antigen as a foreign invader and builds antibodies to destroy it. Subsequent Rh+ babies are not as fortunate as the first Rh+ baby.

■ **SYMPTOMS.** If this Rh− mother becomes pregnant with another Rh+ baby, antibodies against the Rh factor that she has built up in her blood do cross the placental membranes. These antibodies attack the blood of the unborn child, breaking down the RBCs and leading to anemia and possible death of the baby.

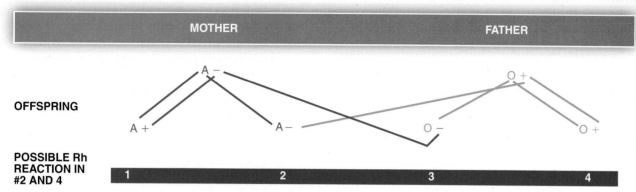

The offspring of this mother and father have the possibility of four different blood types. Since this is an Rh− mother, there is a possibility of an Rh reaction with the two Rh+ children. If the father was also Rh−, all offspring would be Rh− and no reaction would occur in any of the children. If the mother were Rh+ no Rh reaction could occur in any of the offspring since Rh+ mothers are not sensitive to the Rh antigen.

FIGURE 5–16   Blood type in inheritance patterns and identification of possible Rh reactions.

This condition affects only Rh+ babies carried by Rh− mothers. Rh+ mothers "don't care" about the factor. Rh+ mothers have the antigen, so they do not build up antibodies against it.

■ **DIAGNOSIS.** Prenatal diagnosis of erythroblastosis fetalis is accomplished by ultrasound. An abnormal or increased fluid accumulation might be noted in the abdomen, lungs, heart, skin, or all of these in the baby. There is also an increase in the amount of amniotic fluid along with thickening of the placenta.

■ **TREATMENT.** Treatment for erythroblastosis fetalis is exchange transfusion of the baby's blood with Rh+ blood at birth. This treatment stops the destruction of the baby's RBCs. Over a period of time, the transfused Rh+ blood is replaced by the baby's own blood. If erythroblastosis fetalis is a possibility in an Rh− mother, the baby's condition can be monitored by amniocentesis. Babies who are mildly affected might be carried to full term. Severe cases, however, might indicate the need to induce labor and premature delivery of the baby to begin lifesaving treatment.

Historically, an Rh factor marital mismatch might have been the reason queens or wives of royalty were beheaded when unable to produce living heirs to the throne. If the king was Rh+ and the queen Rh−, every child after the first would have been at successively higher risk of fetal death. Erythroblastosis fetalis rarely occurs in the modern world. The development of RhoGAM®, a special immune globulin, has halted this condition.

■ **PREVENTION.** RhoGAM® is an injectable medication given to Rh− females to prevent the development of antibodies against Rh+ factor. It is given prophylactically after the delivery of the first and any subsequent Rh+ fetuses to prevent development of Rh antibodies.

ORGAN REJECTION

■ **DESCRIPTION.** Organs such as the liver, kidney, heart, and lungs could be easily transplanted if not for the human immune system.

■ **ETIOLOGY.** The immune system recognizes transplanted tissue as foreign and attacks it. This attack by lymphocytes brings about donor tissue destruction recognized as tissue or organ rejection.

■ **SYMPTOMS.** Transplant rejection might be hyperacute in nature and actually occur during the surgical procedure. Acute rejection occurs within the first few weeks, whereas chronic rejection occurs over a period of time, usually months to years. Chronic rejection occurs slowly and is due to vessel damage that decreases blood flow to the donor tissue. Decreased blood flow causes chronic ischemia and, ultimately, death of the donor organ.

■ **DIAGNOSIS.** Diagnosis is made by physical examination and testing of the function of the newly transplanted organ. A biopsy of the organ can confirm rejection.

■ **TREATMENT.** Donated organs are matched to possible recipients. The closer the donor antigen matches that of the recipient, the less chance the organ will be rejected. Administration of immunosuppression medications also decreases the possibility of rejection.

■ **PREVENTION.** Immunosuppression medications must be taken prior to transplantation surgery and for the remainder of the organ recipient's life. This medication suppresses or decreases the body's ability to wage war against the donor tissue and thus prevents organ rejection.

Immune Deficiency Disorders

The last classification of immune disorders is immunodeficiency. These disorders represent an inability of the immune system to protect the individual against disease. This deficiency might be congenital due to a genetic disorder, or it might be acquired during the individual's lifetime. Acquired disorders are the most common type and can be due to disease therapies, such as chemotherapy and radiation treatments, by suppressing bone marrow, thus decreasing leukocyte production. Medications given to organ transplant recipients purposefully suppress the immune system. The most common immunodeficiency disorder is AIDS.

The classic clinical problem with immunodeficiency disorders is the development of unusual and severe infections such as pneumonia, meningitis, or septicemia, to name a few. Also, the development of infections by microorganisms that are not usually pathogenic (opportunistic infections) can be indicative of an immunodeficiency disorder. Other signs and symptoms are numerous and varied, depending on the organs or organ systems affected and the invading pathogen. Specific signs and symptoms will be included in the discussion of the disorder.

ACQUIRED IMMUNODEFICIENCY SYNDROME (AIDS)

■ **DESCRIPTION.** The name of this disease briefly describes its pathology. It is an acquired disease that causes the immune system to be deficient in protecting the body, leading to a syndrome of symptoms or secondary diseases.

AIDS was first diagnosed in the United States in the early 1980s. The first diagnosed cases were found in a group of homosexual men who became ill with a series of opportunistic diseases and eventually died. These individuals had surprisingly suppressed immune systems. Further research led to the discovery of the virus and mode of transmission.

■ **ETIOLOGY.** The cause of AIDS is a virus called human immunodeficiency virus (HIV). The wicked characteristic of HIV is its battle plan to wipe out the individual's lymphocytes, thus leaving the body defenseless against attack by all pathogenic organisms. The primary target is the T lymphocyte, but macrophages are affected as well. HIV is **cytotoxic** (cyto = cell, toxic = killing). Ultimately, the HIV-infected individual will have a low T lymphocyte cell count, indicative of a positive diagnosis of AIDS.

HIV is transmitted from one individual to another through intimate contact and sharing of body fluids. The virus must enter the body and bloodstream to infect the individual. HIV is fragile and easily killed by temperature changes. Many misconceptions and fears about the transmission of AIDS are still prevalent in society today. An individual cannot get HIV infection from toilet seats, doorknobs, furniture, water fountains, and other objects. An individual cannot get HIV from social kissing, coughing, sneezing, or even sharing eating utensils. HIV is not transmitted through air, food, urine, feces, or water. HIV is primarily transmitted in three ways:

1. **Sexual intercourse** Semen and vaginal secretions carry HIV. Transmission rate is higher from male to female because females might have microscopic vaginal tears during intercourse. Transmission rate is very high with anal intercourse because the internal lining of the rectum is very thin. Approximately 75% of infected individuals in the United States contract AIDS through sexual intercourse.

2. **Sharing of hypodermic needles** HIV-infected blood is injected into the body by sharing needles. This type of transmission accounts for 18–25% of infected individuals in the United States.

3. **In utero from infected mother to unborn child** HIV passes across the placenta to infect the baby. This accounts for 1–3% of AIDS cases.

Transmission of HIV through blood transfusions has been virtually eliminated by effective screening methods. Health professionals following appropriate precautions are at very little risk of contracting HIV.

■ **SYMPTOMS.** HIV was first staged in 1990. Staging is helpful in diagnosis, evaluation, and management of HIV/AIDS. Several health organizations have developed staging processes often based on T-cell counts.

One of the most current staging processes has been developed by AIDS.gov, a resource provided by the U.S. Department of Health and Human Services. The AIDS.gov system (2012) includes a five-stage progression.

Acute Infection

- Occurs within 2 to 4 weeks after infection with HIV.
- Symptoms are similar to a bad flu.
- Large amounts of virus are produced in the body, attacking CD4 T cells.

Clinical Latency

- No symptoms—asymptomatic.
- If testing is done, the person would test positive for HIV.
- Lymphadenopathy—larger-than-normal lymph nodes.
- May persist for a period of 8 years or longer.

Early-Stage AIDS

- Development of mild bacterial, viral, and fungal infections.
- Mild symptoms such as skin rashes, fatigue, night sweats, slight weight loss, fungal skin and nail infections, headache, and fatigue may appear.

Middle-Stage AIDS

- Characterized by an increase in severity of infections.
- Persistent fungal infections of the mouth or vagina called thrush.
- Herpes infection of the mouth and genitals (cold sores).
- Diarrhea.
- More dramatic weight loss and persistent fevers.

Late-Stage AIDS

- Infected person is severely sick.
- T-cell count drops below 200.
- Infections include *Mycobacterium avium* complex disease (caused by a fungus).
- *Pneumocystis carinii* pneumonia (caused by a bacteria).
- Cytomegalovirus (caused by a virus).

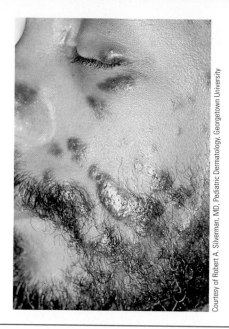

Courtesy of Robert A. Silverman, MD, Pediatric Dermatology, Georgetown University

FIGURE 5–17 Kaposi's sarcoma.

- Chronic severe diarrhea, intense night sweats, memory loss, depression and other disorders of the brain, severe weight loss. Two diseases that are primarily identified with late-stage HIV/AIDS are:

1. *Pneumocystis carinii* (NEW-moh-SIS-tis kah-RYE-nee-eye) **pneumonia,** an infection of the lungs with a protozoan. This organism has never been documented as a cause of pneumonia in persons with normal immune systems.
2. **Kaposi's sarcoma** (KAP-oh-seez sar-KOH-mah), a blood vessel cancer that causes reddish-purple skin lesions (Figure 5–17).

■ *DIAGNOSIS.* AIDS is diagnosed when the T-cell count drops below 200 cells per microliter.

■ *TREATMENT.* AIDS was 100% fatal from the time of discovery until treatment became available. Historically, there have been three eras of treatment: 1980–1995, before effective HIV treatment became available; 1996–1999, the beginning of effective treatment; and 2000–2003, when contemporary HIV treatment became readily available. A U.S. scientific study (*AIDS*, 2007) reported with excitement that mortality rates for people living with HIV had plummeted since the introduction of highly active antiretroviral therapy (HAART) in 1996.

The study also revealed that the mortality rate of HIV went from 488 per 1,000 persons in 1995 to 101 per 1,000 persons in 2002. Since that time, with early diagnosis and proper treatment with antiretroviral therapy (ART), life expectancy can be very near the normal range.

If AIDS is diagnosed while the T-cell count is over 400 cells per microliter and ART is successfully utilized, it is estimated that the median age of death (life expectancy) for those with AIDS will be an approximately 75.0 years of age. This is roughly 7 years short of the general population life expectancy (Nakagawa et al., 2012).

The main challenges in improving survival rates with AIDS include early detection and treatment costs. It is estimated that one in five infected individuals are unaware of their condition until they become symptomatic.

The lifetime cost of treatment for one individual with AIDS is projected to be over $379,000 (Centers for Disease Control and Prevention [CDC], 2012). Approximately 33% of HIV patients are unable to afford their treatment because they have no health insurance coverage. Late detection combined with inadequate treatment increases mortality rate. With over 17,000 deaths per year, AIDS still ranks as the sixth leading cause of death in persons 25 to 44 years of age (U.S. National Library of Medicine [NLM], 2012).

Those persons who do not survive usually have a variety of symptoms and diseases as the individual's immune system crumbles and becomes incapacitated (Figure 5–18). Ultimately, superinfections and massive diarrhea may be the cause of death.

■ **PREVENTION.** AIDS continues to be a worldwide epidemic or pandemic. Since the beginning of AIDS, approximately 60 million people have been diagnosed and over 30 million have died.

Worldwide statistics (American Foundation for AIDS Research, 2012) for the year 2011 include:

- An estimated 34 million have AIDS.
- Over 2.5 million were newly infected.

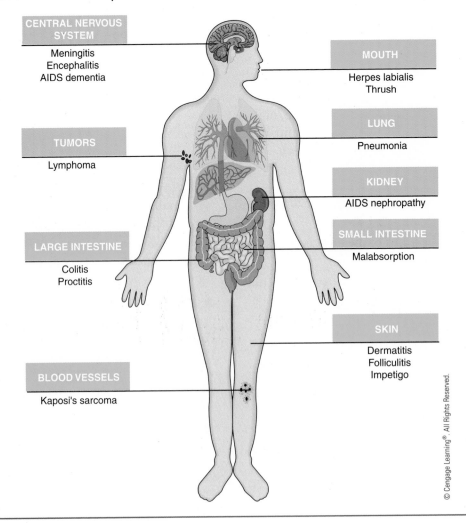

FIGURE 5–18 Pathologies associated with AIDS.

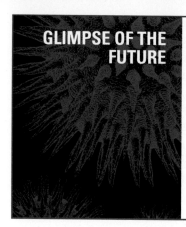

GLIMPSE OF THE FUTURE

Antiretroviral Drugs and Drug Resistance

One of the major problems in treating HIV is that it has consistently developed variations of the virus that are drug resistant. Just about the time a new effective antiretroviral drug is found, the genetic structure of the organism changes, and the drug is not as effective as needed. Virus resistance to the therapy is one of the major causes of unsuccessful treatment regimens in patients with HIV/AIDS.

Research is being conducted to study these variants, the mutation rates, and the properties of the virus so more effective, longer-lasting drugs can be developed in the future.

Source: Ammaranond & Sanguansittianan (2012).

- Every day, over 7,000 people contract AIDS—nearly 300 every hour.

In the United States alone, there are over 1.1 million people currently living with AIDS, and every year approximately 48,000 new cases are diagnosed (CDC, 2010).

AIDS can be stopped with preventive education and action. The only known method of prevention is avoiding exposure to the virus.

TRAUMA

Trauma to the immune system is generally limited to treatments or medications, such as chemotherapy and radiation treatments, that often lead to immunosuppression. Individuals on corticosteroid medications often have undetected infections because this medication suppresses the protective inflammatory response. Graft and organ recipients take immunosuppression medications to traumatize the system purposefully in hopes of protecting the transplanted graft or organ.

RARE DISEASES

Severe Combined Immunodeficiency Disease (SCID)

SCID is a group of inherited disorders in which there is partial or complete dysfunction of the immune system or complete deficiency. Untreated children usually die at a young age. Treatment can include a

HEALTHY HIGHLIGHT

Preventive Strategies for HIV and AIDS

Preventive Strategies for HIV and AIDS

- Abstain from sexual intercourse or develop a monogamous relationship with a partner who is not infected and is not an intravenous drug user.
- Do not abuse alcohol or drugs in a manner that prevents you from being in control of your behavior.
- Do not use intravenous drugs. If you are an intravenous drug user, always use a sterile needle or one soaked in bleach, and do not share your needles.

Other Behaviors That Will Help Prevent the Spread of HIV

- Refrain from multiple sex partners or sex with intravenous drug users.
- Refrain from unprotected sex with homosexuals or bisexual men.
- Always use a latex condom with a spermicide and virucide if you are uncertain about your partner's sexual history.

bone marrow transplant from a matched sibling and has restored complete immune function in some children. Protective isolation is necessary to prevent lethal infections. This protected environment has led to these children being called "bubble babies."

EFFECTS OF AGING ON THE IMMUNE SYSTEM

Presently, not all age-related changes in the immune system are well understood. It is known that the thymus gland degenerates with age. The thymus reaches its maximum size in early childhood and then slowly decreases in size after puberty. As the gland decreases in size, so does the number of T cells because they originate in the cortex of the thymus. The remaining T cells do not function as well, increasing the chance of developing invasive diseases, such as cancer. Some defects in lymph cells also occur in the aging process.

The B-cell levels remain stable throughout life, but the antibodies in older persons might not function as well as in younger years. Thus, infections are common in the older population. The antibodies are more likely to attack the body's own tissue (autoantibodies) as a result of loss of tolerance to self-antigens. General resistance to disease seems to decrease with age, but this might be due to many other factors such as general nutrition, exercise, medications, and psychosocial influences rather than to changes in the immune system.

Consider This ...

Laughing lowers stress hormones and strengthens the immune system. A 6-year-old laughs an average of 300 times a day, while the average adult only laughs 15–100 times a day.

SUMMARY

The immune system consists of organs such as the thymus gland, bone marrow, lymph nodes, spleen, liver, and tonsils, and major cells such as the lymphocytes. The immune system is an important defense system for the body because a malfunctioning or compromised immune system weakens the body's defenses against invading microorganisms. Many secondary disorders such as infections are due to a compromised immune response. Primary diseases or disorders of the immune system are categorized as hypersensitivity disorders or immune deficiency disorders. Hypersensitivity disorders include allergies, autoimmune disorders, and isoimmune disorders. The immune deficiency disease, AIDS, is one of the most common and debilitating conditions of the immune system. Diagnostic testing for immune disorders includes skin testing, complete blood cell counts, and some specific antibody studies. Treatment for immune disorders varies with the specific problem. Some immune disorders are quite mild, whereas others are severe and require long-term therapy.

REVIEW QUESTIONS

Short Answer

1. What are the functions of the immune system?

2. Which signs and symptoms are associated with common immune system disorders?

3. Which diagnostic tests are most commonly used to determine the type, cause, or both of an immune system disorder?

Matching

4. Match the disorders listed in the left column with the correct category of immune system diseases in the right column. (Right-hand column categories may be used more than once.)

_____ Hay fever

_____ AIDS

_____ Anaphylaxis

_____ Rheumatic fever

_____ Erythroblastosis fetalis

_____ Organ rejection

a. Allergies

b. Autoimmune disorders

c. Isoimmune disorders

d. Immune deficiency disorders

Multiple Choice

5. Which of the following behaviors might contribute to increased risk for HIV transmission?

a. Donating blood

b. Sharing intravenous needles

c. Failure to wash hands after toileting

d. Unprotected sex

e. Sharing eating utensils

f. Direct contact with body fluids

g. Frequent use of laxatives and enemas

True or False

6. T F   The immune system is the body's only defense system against invading organisms.

7. T F   Signs and symptoms of hypersensitivity disorders might include rash, redness, heat, swelling, nasal congestion, coughing, and sneezing.

8. T F   The Coombs test is used to detect certain antibodies in the blood.

9. T F   Autoimmune disorders are hyposensitivities in which the body fails to recognize its own antigens.

10. T F   The effects of aging put the older adult at an increased risk for immune system problems.

CASE STUDIES

■ Terry Stephens is a 26-year-old male who has been diagnosed as HIV positive. He has told you that he and his girlfriend have unprotected sex. You have been close friends for many years. What are some strategies you could use to inform Terry about the danger of this behavior? Should you also talk to his girlfriend? When Terry was hospitalized, you noticed his caregivers wore gloves when starting his IV and drawing blood. Was this because he is HIV positive? Would this be a routine precaution?

■ Your friend, Janet, is suffering from rheumatoid arthritis. She asks you if she should take an over-the-counter preparation containing borage oil. She read an advertisement about the benefits of this product for arthritis sufferers. How would you answer her question? Can you safely say it is a good idea to try this treatment? Would it help relieve her symptoms? What does the research say about the side effects?

Study Tools

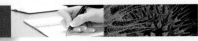

Workbook

    Complete Chapter 5

Online Resources

    PowerPoint® presentations

    Animation

BIBLIOGRAPHY

AIDS.gov. (2012). AIDS basics. *http://www.aids.gov/hiv-aids-basics* (accessed June 2012).

AIDS Healthcare Foundation. (2012). *http://www.aidshealth.org/* (accessed January 2012).

Alderuccio, F. (2011). Stem cell based therapy for autoimmunity. *Current Stem Cell Research & Therapy 6*(1), 1–2.

Al-Khamees, W. A., Schwartz, M. D., Alrashdi, S., Algren, A. D., & Morgan, B. W. (2011). Status epilepticus associated with borage oil ingestion. *Journal of Medical Toxicology 7*(2), 154–157.

American Foundation for AIDS Research. (2012). *http://www.amfar.org/* (accessed January 2012).

Ammaranond, P., & Sanguansittianan, S. (2012). Mechanism of HIV antiretroviral drugs progress toward drug resistance. *Fundamental & Clinical Pharmacology 26*(1), 146–161.

ART for autoimmune illness. (2011). *Australian Nursing Journal 19*(5), 24.

Arthritis Foundation. (2012). *http://www.arthritis.org/* (accessed January 2012).

Asselah, T., & Marcellin, P. (2012). Direct acting antivirals for the treatment of chronic hepatitis C: One pill a day for tomorrow. *Liver International 32*(S), 88–102.

Better meds pummel HIV mortality. (2007). *AIDS*, October 3 edition. http://www.poz.com/articles/aids_mortality_rate_1_13154.shtml (Accessed June 2013).

Brodkey, M., Ben-Zacharia, A., & Reardon, J. (2011). Living well with multiple sclerosis. *American Journal of Nursing 111*(7), 40–50.

Centers for Disease Control (CDC). (2012). HIV cost effectiveness. *http://www.cdc.gov/hiv/prefention/ongoing* (accessed August 2013).

Cranwell-Bruce, L. A. (2011). Biological disease modifying anti-rheumatic drugs. *Medsurg Nursing 20*(3), 147–150.

Firth, J., & Critchley, S. (2011). Treating to target in rheumatoid arthritis: Biologic therapies. *British Journal of Nursing 20*(20), 1284–1291.

Food Allergy and Anaphylaxis Network. (2008). Frequently asked questions. *www.foodallergy.org* (accessed May 2008).

Fuschiotti, P. (2011). Role of IL-13 in systemic sclerosis. *Cytokine 56*(3), 544–549.

Gilbert, S. C. (2012). T-cell-inducing vaccines: What's the future. *Immunology 135*(1), 19–26.

Lee, S., & Margolin, K. (2011). Cytokines in cancer immunotherapy. *Cancers 3*(4), 3856–3896.

Leyshon, J. (2011). Improving inhaler technique in patients with asthma. *Nursing Standard 26*(9), 49–56.

Longo, D., Fauci, A., Kasper, D., Hauser, S., Jameson, J., & Loscalzo, J. *Harrison's Principles of Internal Medicine*, 18th ed. New York: McGraw Hill, 2012.

Lupus Foundation of America, Inc. (2012). *www.lupus.org/* (accessed January 2012).

Macfarlane, G. J., El-Metwally, A., De Silva, V., Ernst, E., Dowds, G. L., & Moots, R. J. (2011). Evidence for the efficacy of complementary and alternative medicines in the management of rheumatoid arthritis: A systematic review. *Rheumatology 50*(9), 1672–1683.

Myasthenia Gravis Foundation of America. (2010). What is myasthenia gravis? *www.myasthenia.org* (accessed September 2012).

Nakagawa, F., Lodwick, R. K., Smith, C. J., Smith, R., Cambiano, V., Lundgren, J. D., Delpech, V., & Phillips, A. N. (2012). Projected life expectancy of people with HIV according to timing of diagnosis. *AIDS 26*(3), 335–343.

Neimark, J. (2012). Altered immune cells block HIV. *Discover 33*(1), 18.

Scleroderma Foundation. (2012). *www.scleroderma.org/* (accessed January 2012).

Seidman, J. C., Richard, S. A., Viboud, C., & Miller, M. A. (2012). Quantitative review of antibody response to inactivated seasonal influenza vaccines. *Influenza & Other Respiratory Viruses 6*(1), 52–62.

Shah, P., & Schaffer, D. (2011). Antiviral RNAi: Translating science towards therapeutic success. *Pharmaceutical Research 28*(12), 2966–2982.

Simmons, S. (2011). Recognizing and managing rheumatoid arthritis. *Nursing 41*(7), 34–40.

Tobias, C. R., Downes, A., Eddens, S., & Ruiz, J. (2012). Building blocks for peer success: Lessons learned from a train-the-trainer program. *AIDS Patient Care & STDs 26*(1), 53–59.

Torre, D., & Pugliese, A. (2008). Platelets and HIV-1 infection: Old and new aspects. *Current HIV Research 6*(5), 411–418.

U.S. National Library of Medicine (NLM). (2012). Aids. *www.ncbi.nlm.nih.gov* (accessed August 2013).

van Sighem, A., Gras, L., Reiss, P., Brinkman, K., & de Wolf, F. (2010). Life expectancy of recently diagnosed asymptomatic HIV-infected patients approaches that of uninfected individuals. *AIDS 24*(10), 1527–1535.

Volberding, P. A., & Deeks, S. G. (2010). Antiretroviral therapy and management of HIV infection. *The Lancet 376*(9734), 49–62.

Wheeler, T. (2010). Systemic lupus erythematosus: The basics of nursing care. *British Journal of Nursing 19*(4), 249–253.

World Health Organization. (2007). WHO case definitions of HIV for surveillance and revised clinical staging and immunological classification of HIV-related disease in adults and children. *http://www.who.int/hiv/pub/guidelines/HIVstaging150307.pdf* (accessed June 2013).

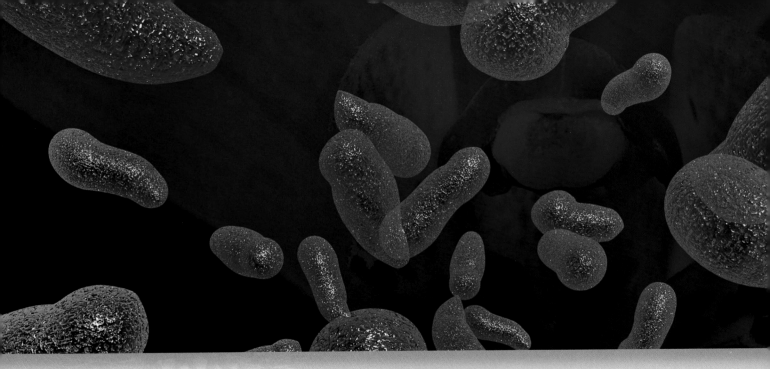

OUTLINE

- Anatomy and Physiology
- Common Signs and Symptoms
- Diagnostic Tests
- Common Diseases of the Musculoskeletal System
  Diseases of the Bone
  Diseases of the Joints
  Diseases of the Muscles and Connective Tissue
  Neoplasms
- Trauma
  Fracture
  Strains and Sprains
  Dislocations and Subluxations
  Low Back Pain (LBP)
  Herniated Nucleus Pulposus (HNP)
  Bursitis
  Tendonitis
  Carpal Tunnel Syndrome
  Plantar Fasciitis
  Torn Rotator Cuff
  Torn Meniscus
  Cruciate Ligament Tears
  Shin Splints
- Rare Diseases
  de Quervain's Disease
  Tuberculosis of the Bone
  Paget's Disease
  Myasthenia Gravis
- Effects of Aging on the System
- Summary
- Review Questions
- Case Studies
- Bibliography

KEY TERMS

Anaerobic (p. 113)
Bone mass density (BMD) (p. 102)
Calcaneal (p. 123)
Computerized axial tomography (CAT or CT) (p. 102)
Densitometry (p. 102)
Diskectomy (p. 121)
Dowager's hump (p. 106)
Dual energy X-ray absorptiometry (DEXA) (p. 102)
Electromyography (p. 102)
Fascia (p. 123)
Interphalangeal (p. 109)
Laminectomy (p. 121)
Magnetic resonance imaging (MRI) (p. 102)
Meniscus (p. 124)
Metacarpophalangeal (p. 109)
Metatarsophalangeal (p. 111)
Mineralization (p. 108)
Myelogram (p. 120)
ORIF (p. 115)
Osteomyelitis (p. 107)
Radiologic (p. 102)
RICE (p. 118)
Sciatica (p. 120)
Spasms (p. 119)

Tetany (p. 113)
Tophi (p. 111)

Types of Fractures
Articular (p. 109)
Avulsion (p. 115)
Closed (p. 115)
Colles' (p. 115)
Comminuted (p. 115)
Complete (p. 115)
Compound (p. 115)
Compression (p. 106)
Displaced (p. 115)
Extracapsular (p. 115)
Femoral neck (p. 115)
Greenstick (p. 115)
Impacted (p. 115)
Incomplete (p. 115)
Intertrochanteric (p. 115)
Intracapsular (p. 115)
Longitudinal (p. 115)
Nondisplaced (p. 102)
Oblique (p. 115)
Open (p. 115)
Pathologic (p. 114)
Pott's (p. 115)
Simple (p. 115)
Spiral (p. 115)
Stellate (p. 115)
Stress (p. 114)
Subcapital (p. 115)
Transverse (p. 115)

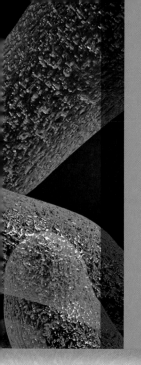

6

Musculoskeletal System Diseases and Disorders

LEARNING OBJECTIVES

Upon completion of the chapter, the learner should be able to:

1. Define the terminology common to the musculoskeletal system and the disorders of the system.

2. Discuss the basic anatomy and physiology of the musculoskeletal system.

3. Identify the important signs and symptoms associated with common musculoskeletal system disorders.

4. Describe the common diagnostics used to determine type, cause, or both of a musculoskeletal system disorder.

5. Identify the common disorders of the musculoskeletal system.

6. Describe the typical course and management of the common musculoskeletal system disorders.

7. Describe the effects of aging on the musculoskeletal system and the common disorders associated with aging of the system.

OVERVIEW

The musculoskeletal system provides the structure and movement function for the individual. Because the muscles and bones run throughout the body, disorders of the system can affect any other system, and disorders of other systems frequently affect the musculoskeletal system. This includes bones, joints, ligaments, muscles, and tendons; each of these has a unique function but also interacts with the other components of the system to support the person and provide for mobility. Problems with the musculoskeletal system frequently affect the individual's independence and, thus, the quality of life. ■

ANATOMY AND PHYSIOLOGY

The skeletal component of the musculoskeletal system is made up of bones and joints. The bones provide the framework to support the body. They also produce blood cells, store fat and minerals, protect soft tissues (such as the brain), and help create body motion. Bones are very vascular; blood circulates through them, picking up or storing body minerals such as calcium, phosphorus, magnesium, and sodium. Bones also contain osteoblasts, active bone-building cells; osteoclasts, cells that reabsorb bone; and osteocytes, mature bone cells.

Bones are often classified by shape and composition. For example, the skeletal system is composed of long bones such as the femur in the leg, short bones such as the carpal bones in the wrist and the tarsal bones in the ankles, flat bones such as the sternum or skull, irregular bones such as the vertebrae or pelvic bones, and sesamoid bones such as the knee-cap (Figure 6–1). The composition of bone is either cortical or cancellous. Cortical bone is dense, smooth, and compact, whereas cancellous bone is spongy, with many open spaces throughout. The ligaments are fibrous connective tissues that connect bones to other bones and joints.

Bone can be damaged and repair itself. The steps of bone repair include (1) bleeding at the site of injury with clot and granulation tissue formation; (2) proliferation of cells at the site, forming a callus (soft bony deposit) over the injury or fracture; (3) cells becoming bone (osteoblasts) or cartilage at the site; (4) the bone calcifying (hardened) by the deposit of inorganic salts at the site; and (5) the remodeling of the bone to the shape necessary to complete its designated function. Bone repair is dependent on many factors such as the general health status of the individual, his or her age, the degree of injury, circulation to the site, and the presence of other diseases or infection.

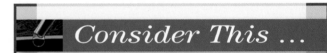

Consider This ...

Due to fusion of bones as we age, a baby has approximately 350 bones, while the adult only has 206!

The joints are where two or more bones meet. They are usually classified based on the amount of movement of the joint, as described in Table 6–1, but they also can be classified by their structure. Classification of joints by structure includes fibrous (such as the joints of the skull), cartilaginous (such as the joints of the vertebrae), and synovial (such as the joints of the knee). The synovial joints are those separated by a fluid-filled cavity.

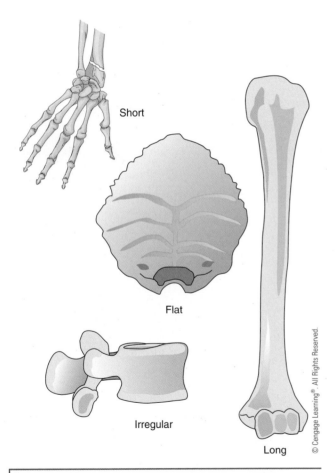

Short

Flat

Irregular

Long

© Cengage Learning®. All Rights Reserved.

FIGURE 6–1 Examples of types of bones.

TABLE 6–1 Classification of Joints by Movement

Classification	Amount of Movement	Example of Joint
Synarthrosis	No movement	Suture of the skull
Amphiarthrosis	Some movement but very limited	Pelvis
Diarthrosis	Complete movement	Knee, hip, elbow

© Cengage Learning®. All Rights Reserved.

The major movements of joints are flexion (bending), extension (reaching out or spreading out), abduction (away from the body), adduction (toward the body), rotation (turning on an axis), circumduction (circular movement), and elevation (lifting).

Cartilage is collagen tissue that supports articulating (adjoining) bones. It provides protection and a cushion to prevent friction between bones and acts like a shock absorber to reduce stress on the bone surface.

The functions of the muscles of the body are to provide structure and movement and to produce heat (Figure 6–2). The muscles of the musculoskeletal system are called striated because they look striped or banded under a microscope. They are also called voluntary muscles because most are moved by conscious control as opposed to other muscles, such as cardiac, that move involuntarily. Skeletal muscles move in response to signals from the central nervous system. Connective tissue holds the muscle fibers together, and tendons, long, fibrous, nonelastic connective tissues, attach muscle to bone.

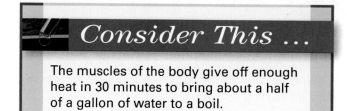

Consider This ...

The muscles of the body give off enough heat in 30 minutes to bring about a half of a gallon of water to a boil.

Each muscle fiber in the body contains myofibrils, which are composed of sarcomeres that are the contracting and relaxing component of the muscle. This contracting and relaxing characteristic provides the smooth, elastic movement of the muscle.

Consider This ...

When you take a step, you use approximately 200 muscles.

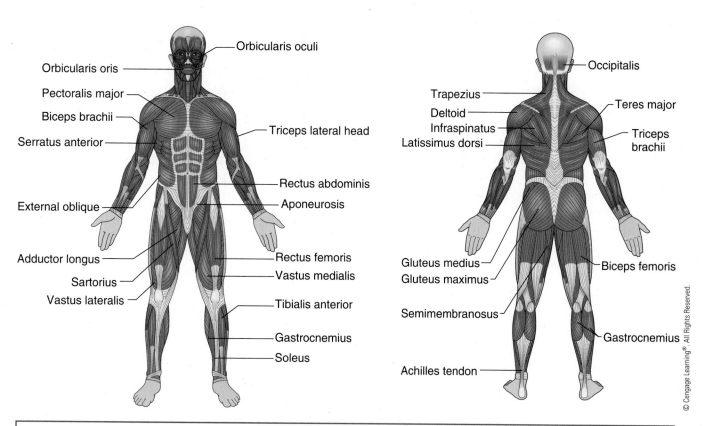

FIGURE 6–2   The skeletal muscles.

The source of energy for the movement of muscles is the metabolism of adenosine triphosphate (ATP) in the cell. ATP is produced from available glucose and glycogen (stored glucose) in the cells. Adequate amounts of oxygen and glucose are necessary for parts of this process.

COMMON SIGNS AND SYMPTOMS

The most common signs and symptoms of bone and joint disease are pain, swelling, decreased mobility, and deformity. Most fractures are associated with pain due to a disruption of the periosteum and related sensory nerves. Many fractures are easy to recognize due to the obvious displacement and related deformity. **Nondisplaced** (not out of place or position) fractures are not as easy to recognize but can cause pain just the same.

Weakness is the most common sign or symptom of muscle disorders and can be related to a primary disease of the muscle or be secondary to a neurologic disorder. Muscle tissue will atrophy if weakness persists for an extended length of time. On the other hand, just the reverse can also occur, with muscle atrophy leading to muscle weakness.

DIAGNOSTIC TESTS

Radiologic examinations (X-rays) are the primary tool in diagnosing bone and joint disorders, but **computerized axial tomography (CAT or CT)** or **magnetic resonance imaging (MRI)** might be needed for more detailed studies.

CAT involves taking specialized X-rays of the affected individual in a special tube-like scanner. The individual must be able to lie still for approximately 30 minutes. The results are detailed X-ray pictures that appear to cut the area of consideration into slices, thus the name tomogram (tomo = cutting, gram = picture) (Figure 6–3).

MRI is another detailed X-ray type of examination; it uses a large magnet to make electromagnetic images. Here also, individuals must be able to lie still and must not wear any type of metal during the test. MRI is more expensive to perform but takes more detailed images of soft tissue than a CT scanner does.

Bone mass density (BMD) screening is used to confirm low bone mass and the diagnosis of osteoporosis. Bone **densitometry** testing techniques are simple radiology scans. The newest type, **dual energy X-ray absorptiometry (DEXA scan)**, takes measurements at the spine, hip, and wrist. A score above −1 is normal; a score between −1 and −2.5 reflects osteopenia (low bone mass); and a score below −2.5 is defined as osteoporosis.

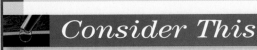

Consider This ...

By weight, bone is five times stronger than steel.

Blood studies, including calcium, phosphorus, and an enzyme (alkaline phosphatase), also can prove helpful with metabolic disorders. Infectious disorders can be cultured. Often, the specimen for culture is obtained during surgical procedures such as débridement.

Muscle disorders are often evaluated by **electromyography** (EMG), accomplished by inserting a small needle into muscle tissue and recording the electrical activity. Electromyography can assist in determining whether the disorder is muscular or neurologic in nature. Muscle tissue biopsy can be performed on difficult cases. Biopsy is the most definitive means of determining cause of muscle disorder. Biopsy is also the most reliable test for tumors of the musculoskeletal system.

COMMON DISEASES OF THE MUSCULOSKELETAL SYSTEM

Diseases of the Bone

Diseases of the bone can range from mild to severe, with the most serious causing extreme deformity or disability. Many of the disorders are more common in the older adult because changes in the system can lead to increased risk for skeletal problems. Individuals with bone disease frequently need assistive devices such as crutches, walkers, or canes to maintain mobility. Internal devices such as artificial joints, pins, and braces also might be necessary.

SPINAL DEFORMITIES

■ ***DESCRIPTION.*** Deformities might be very obvious at onset, as with congenital defects, but more

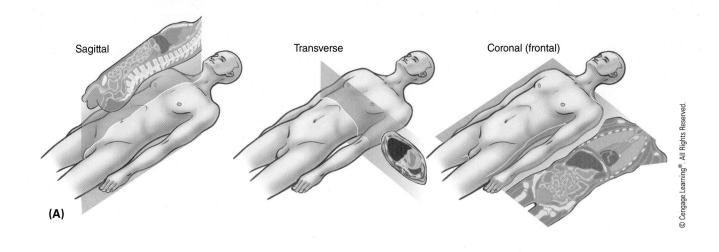

Sagittal   Transverse   Coronal (frontal)

(A)

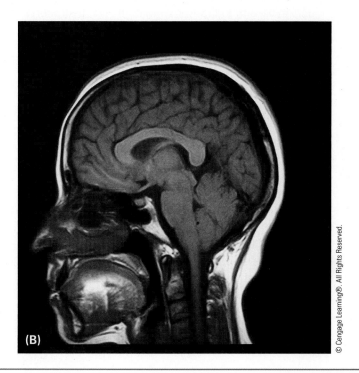

(B)

FIGURE 6–3 Computed tomography (CT scan) provides cross-sectional views of different body planes. (A) CT of chest and abdomen. (B) MRI of head.

commonly, they progress slowly and are unnoticed until symptoms arise.

■ ***ETIOLOGY.*** Deformities can be caused by a variety of factors, including congenital defects, poor posture, bone disease, and growth disorders.

■ ***SYMPTOMS.*** Symptoms commonly include back pain and fatigue. Diagnosis is generally confirmed by X-ray and clinical examination.

■ ***DIAGNOSIS.*** Spinal deformities are diagnosed by thorough physical examination and a series of X-rays of the spine. A pulmonary function test might be needed if breathing is affected. MRI scans can assist in identifying tumor or infection.

■ ***TREATMENT.*** Treatment includes eliminating or treating causative factors, bracing, and spinal surgery. Untreated spinal deformities can progress to life-threatening conditions when cardiac and respiratory function are compromised.

PHARMACOLOGY HIGHLIGHT

Common Drugs for Musculoskeletal Disorders

CATEGORY	EXAMPLES OF MEDICATIONS
Antihistamines Drugs used to reduce the symptoms from allergies	carbinoxamine or levocabastine (prescription drugs) fexofenadine, cetirizine, or loratadine (over-the-counter drugs)
Antibiotics Drugs used to prevent or stop bacterial infections	ampicillin, amoxicillin, ciprofloxacin, doxycycline, erythromycin, penicillin, or tetracycline
Anti-inflammatories Drugs used to reduce inflammation	hydrocortisone, beclomethasone, or amcinonide (steroids) acetaminophen, aspirin, or ibuprofen (nonsteroidal)
Antipyretics/Analgesics Drugs used to reduce fever and pain	acetaminophen, aspirin, ibuprofen, naproxen, or some narcotic analgesics if necessary such as oxycodone
Antirheumatics Drugs to prevent some rheumatic conditions and symptoms	adalimumab, celecoxib, glucosamine, ibuprofen, indomethacin, or tocilizumab
Bone Resorption Inhibitors Drugs used to prevent bone loss	alendronate, raloxifene, or risedronate
Vitamins/Minerals Supplements used to support or replace low levels	calcium and vitamin D (especially D_3); these may be prescribed individually or in combination with other vitamins and minerals.
Muscle Relaxants Drugs used to alleviate pain and stiffness	cyclobenzaprine or carisoprodol

■ **PREVENTION.** There is no known prevention for spinal deformities.

KYPHOSIS

Kyphosis (kie-FOE-sis) is a humped curvature of the thoracic spine, commonly called humpback or hunchback. Kyphosis often appears in postmenopausal, osteoporitic females.

LORDOSIS

Lordosis (lor-DOE-sis) is an exaggerated anterior or inward curve of the lumbar spine, also called swayback. It normally occurs with pregnancy as the individual compensates for the increased size of the abdomen. When compared to the normal spine, lordosis results in a protruding abdomen and buttocks and a swayed lower back. Obesity is a common cause of lordosis.

SCOLIOSIS

■ **DESCRIPTION.** Scoliosis (SKOLE-lee-OH-sis) is a lateral curvature of the spine. It affects both sexes, but girls usually have more severe curvatures and account for approximately 90% of the cases. Scoliosis can occur at any age but is usually noticed during the early teen years, when growth rate is accelerated.

■ **ETIOLOGY.** The cause of scoliosis, in most cases, is unknown.

■ **SYMPTOMS.** Symptoms include (1) back pain due to muscles trying to conform to the spinal curving, (2) a rib or shoulder blade hump, and (3) uneven shoulders and hips. Scoliosis is often noticed when dresses hang lower on one side or the other, and the brassiere straps need to be adjusted to different lengths.

■ **DIAGNOSIS.** Scoliosis screening in school-aged children was initiated in the 1960s and is now mandated by law in some states. Screening involves observation of the spine as the individual bends forward. Scoliosis is suspected if the spine curves to the side and the scapula shifts upward (Figure 6–4).

■ **TREATMENT.** Treatment is aimed at preventing a worsening of the condition and often includes bracing. Compliance with brace-wearing for female adolescents is often poor, leading to the need for further treatment. Most cases of scoliosis can be corrected if detected early and treated properly and promptly.

■ **PREVENTION.** Scoliosis cannot be prevented.

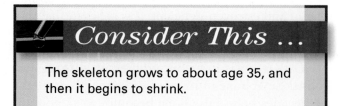

Consider This ...

The skeleton grows to about age 35, and then it begins to shrink.

OTHER DISEASES OF THE BONE

OSTEOPOROSIS

■ **DESCRIPTION.** Osteoporosis (OS-tee-oh-por-OH-sis) is a metabolic bone disease that causes a porosity or Swiss-cheese appearance of the bone, leading to a decrease in bone mass. It is the most prevalent bone disease worldwide. It is estimated to cause major orthopedic problems in approximately one-third of the women in the United States.

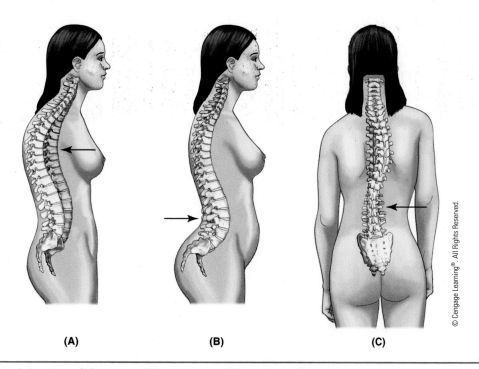

(A)　　　　(B)　　　　(C)

FIGURE 6–4 Spinal deformities: (A) kyposis, (B) lordosis, and (C) scoliosis (S curvature). Note that the normal curvature is shown in shadow.

■ *ETIOLOGY.* Many causative factors play a part in osteoporosis. Age-related osteoporosis affects both men and women equally and is due to normal age-related bone loss. Osteoporosis occurs secondary to diseases that affect mobility. For example, quadriplegia can lead to a loss of 30–40% of bone mass after 6 months of immobility. The most common type of osteoporosis is seen in women who are postmenopausal and estrogen-deficient. It is believed that this osteoporosis is due to a combination of factors, including a decrease in estrogen, calcium, and exercise.

Osteoporosis is a slow, progressive disease that robs skeletal bone of its mass and strength. It might be decades before the bone becomes weak enough to fracture. Most fractures in women over age 50 are related to osteoporosis.

■ *SYMPTOMS.* Early signs of osteoporosis include **compression** (bone mashed down on itself, common in vertebra) fractures of the spine and pathologic wrist fractures. Compression fractures of the spine lead to a decrease in height and pain in the thoracic and lumbar spine. Over a period of time, the individual might lose 4–5 inches of height, decreasing the thoracic and abdominal cavity size. This decrease in chest cavity size leads to decreased activity tolerance due to shortness of breath. A decrease in the abdominal cavity size leads to feelings of fullness after eating only small amounts of food and to a constant bloated feeling. Other symptoms are kyphosis and the appearance of a **Dowager's hump** (abnormal curvature in the upper thoracic spine; see Figure 6–5). Wrist fractures, especially of the distal radius, commonly occur in osteoporitic individuals with only a slight fall. As the disease progresses, the individual has an increased risk for fracturing a hip. More than one million hip fractures occur annually in the United States. Hip fractures in frail, older women often lead to complications that result in mortality (Figure 6–6).

■ *DIAGNOSIS.* Diagnosis can be confirmed by clinical examination, X-rays, CT scans, and bone densitometry (measurement of bone thickness).

■ *TREATMENT.* Currently, there is no treatment to reverse osteoporosis, although the progression of osteoporosis can be slowed and bone mass levels maintained by a combination of therapies. Administration of the medications Fosamax® (alendronate), Actonel® (risedronate), Boniva® (ibandronate), and Reclast® (zoledronate) appears to be helpful in preventing fractures. Reduction of risk factors includes decreasing alcohol and caffeine consumption and not smoking (Table 6–2). Other therapies include increasing

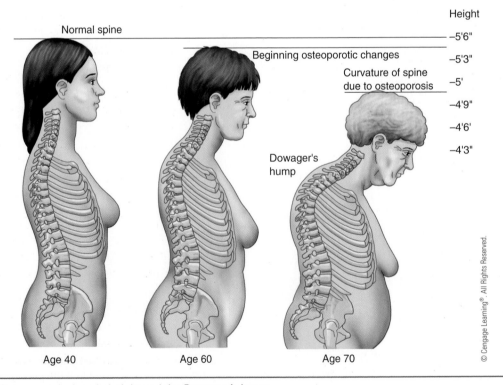

Normal spine

Beginning osteoporotic changes

Curvature of spine due to osteoporosis

Dowager's hump

Height
–5'6"
–5'3"
–5'
–4'9"
–4'6'
–4'3"

Age 40   Age 60   Age 70

FIGURE 6–5 Osteoporosis: loss in height and the Dowager's hump.

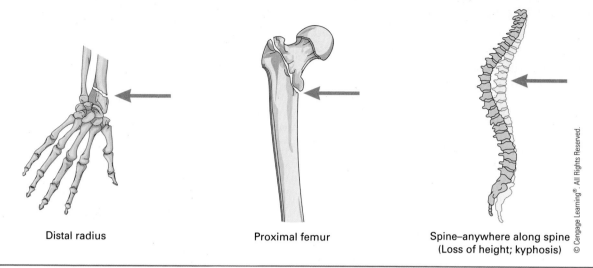

Distal radius   Proximal femur   Spine—anywhere along spine
                                                                (Loss of height; kyphosis)

© Cengage Learning®. All Rights Reserved.

FIGURE 6–6   Fracture sites related to osteoporosis.

TABLE 6–2 | **Risk Factors for Osteoporosis**

The following are considered factors that increase the risk of developing osteoporosis:
■ Family history of osteoporosis
■ Increased risk from aging
■ Medications—tetracycline, corticosteroids, aluminum antacids, some diuretics, some anticonvulsants
■ Female, white or Asian
■ Lack of exercise
■ Lack of calcium in diet or supplements
■ Increased risk from postsurgery oophorectomy (removal of ovaries)
■ Alcohol consumption
■ Caffeine consumption
■ Smoking

© Cengage Learning®. All Rights Reserved.

estrogen, increasing calcium and vitamin D intake, and a daily exercise routine that includes weight-bearing exercise. Much controversy exists concerning the use of estrogen replacement therapy because it is associated with an increase in breast and gynecologic malignancies. An increase in calcium levels also might lead to the formation of kidney stones. These treatments must be considered on an individual basis. The one treatment that is agreed on by most practitioners is the need for daily exercise. Regular exercise has been shown to reduce the rate of hip fractures by 50%.

■ **PREVENTION.** Preventive measures for osteoporosis need to begin early because bone mass is built prior to age 30. Young women should be encouraged to exercise daily, eat a balanced diet, quit smoking, and limit caffeine and alcohol consumption. Entering menopausal years with good bone mass and maintaining as much of the bone as possible is the best weapon against osteoporosis.

OSTEOMYELITIS

■ **DESCRIPTION.** Osteomyelitis (OS-tee-oh-My-ull-LIE-tis; osteo = bone, myel = marrow, itis = inflammation) is an inflammation of the bone commonly caused by infection.

■ **ETIOLOGY.** *Staphylococcus aureus* is the responsible organism in approximately 90% of cases. This bacterium can enter the bone through a wound, spread from an infection nearby, or come from a skin or throat infection. Osteomyelitis usually affects the long bones of the arms and legs. It most often occurs in children and adolescents as a result of a throat infection. In severe cases, it can affect the growth plate of the bones, leading to shortening of the limb.

■ **SYMPTOMS.** Symptoms of osteomyelitis can include sudden onset of high fever, chills, tenderness over the affected bone, leukocytosis (leuko = white, cyto = cell, osis = condition of increase), and bacteremia (bacteria = microscopic organism, emia = blood, bacteria in the blood). In adults, osteomyelitis often occurs following a traumatic accident involving the bone or following bone surgery, especially when implants such as screws, plates, or other hardware are needed.

■ **DIAGNOSIS.** Physical examination revealing pain in a bone along with an elevated white blood cell count can suggest osteomyelitis. An indicative test is an elevated erythrocyte sedimentation rate (ESR), and an X-ray exam, an MRI scan, or a CT scan can also reveal abnormality. Diagnosis can be confirmed by taking samples of bone, pus, blood, or joint fluid to identify infective organisms.

■ **TREATMENT.** Treatment for osteomyelitis is aggressive intravenous antibiotic therapy. Affected bone is often débrided surgically to speed the healing process. Surgical hardware is often removed for this same reason. Acute osteomyelitis, if not treated effectively, can become chronic and lead to a lifetime of problems for the affected individual. Chronic osteomyelitis can lead to large, gaping scar tissue and chronic wound drainage (Figure 6–7).

■ **PREVENTION.** Cleansing and properly treating wounds, especially deep wounds, aids in the prevention of osteomyelitis. Blood-borne bacteria must also be promptly diagnosed and treated. Individuals with artificial joints or metal components should take preventive antibiotics prior to any surgery or dental procedure.

OSTEOMALACIA

■ **DESCRIPTION.** Osteomalacia (OS-tee-oh-muh-LAY-shuh; osteo = bone, malacia = softening) is the general term for softening of the bones due to defective **mineralization** and the general term for softening of the bones in adults; in children, it is called rickets.

■ **ETIOLOGY.** Osteomalacia is caused by a deficiency of vitamin D, which aids in the bone mineralization that causes their characteristic hardness. Without this process, the bone becomes soft and weak. To mineralize, bones need calcium, phosphorus, and vitamin D.

Vitamin D deficiency in adults can be due to inadequate nutritional intake, inadequate exposure to sunlight (skin exposed to sunlight synthesizes vitamin D), or a malabsorption problem.

■ **SYMPTOMS.** Symptoms and signs of osteomalacia include bone pain, loss of height, bending, and deformity in weight-bearing bones such as the spine, pelvis, and legs.

■ **DIAGNOSIS.** A thorough history of diet and amount of time in the sun is helpful in diagnosis, followed by blood testing to measure vitamin D levels and X-rays to look for cracks in the bone. A bone biopsy is quite definitive but often not needed for diagnosis.

■ **TREATMENT.** Correction of the deficiency potentially cures the problem. Administration of 200,000 IU weekly of vitamin D for 4 to 6 weeks, followed by an oral dose of 1,600 IU daily, is usually an adequate treatment. However, bones that have bowed, shortened, or flattened might not regain normal appearance and function.

■ **PREVENTION.** Vitamin D deficiency can usually be avoided by:

- Exposing arms and legs to sunlight for 5 to 10 minutes a day.
- Eating foods high in vitamin D such as oily fish (salmon, sardines, mackerel) and egg yolks.
- Taking vitamin supplements if needed.

Diseases of the Joints

Most of the diseases of the joints occur as a slow, degenerative process, so they tend to be more common with age. As with diseases of the bones, diseases of the joints often result in the individual requiring assistive devices or artificial parts to maintain

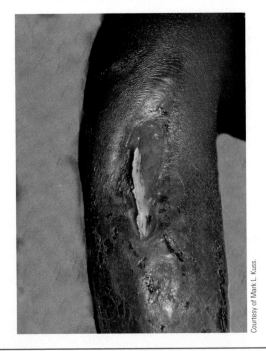

Courtesy of Mark L. Kuss.

FIGURE 6–7 Chronic osteomyelitis scar of the lower leg.

mobility. Frequently, damage to joints occurring during youth is not apparent until middle or older adulthood.

ARTHRITIS

Arthritis (arthro = joint, itis = inflammation) and *rheumatism* are terms commonly used to describe a variety of conditions that cause pain and stiffness in the musculoskeletal system. Both are terms that cover a broad group of conditions, but arthritis is a condition of inflammation in a joint, whereas rheumatism is a condition of stiffness. Arthritis is any inflammation of a joint. Everyone at some time or another has had arthritis; for example, a sprained ankle or jammed fingers are arthritic conditions. Arthritis can be divided into two main groups: osteoarthritis and rheumatoid arthritis. Osteoarthritis is the most common form of arthritis, but rheumatoid arthritis is the more serious and debilitating type.

OSTEOARTHRITIS OR DEGENERATIVE JOINT DISEASE

■ **DESCRIPTION.** Osteoarthritis, a complex, degenerative process, or wearing out of a joint, is the leading cause of disability in the United States (American College of Rheumatology, 2012). It can begin in the early 20s with 90% of all adults showing some radiologic changes.

■ **ETIOLOGY.** The exact cause of osteoarthritis is unknown. The amount or degree of wear is associated with several factors (Table 6–3). Sports injuries speed the wear and tear on the joints, leading to osteoarthritis at a younger age.

■ **SYMPTOMS.** Older adults are usually symptomatic with this type of arthritis. It often affects frequently used joints, such as those in the hands,

and joints that are weight-bearing such as those of the spine, hip, and knee. Affected joints of the hands often swell and become painful. The distal and proximal **interphalangeal** (inter = between, phalangeal = finger bones) joints are often affected and can acquire a crooked deformity of the fingers. The **metacarpophalangeal** (meta = beyond, carpo = wrist, phalangeal = finger bones) joints are usually not affected (Figure 6–8).

Osteoarthritis that affects weight-bearing joints often affects the spine, hips, and knees. As the joints of the spinal column are affected with arthritis, individuals can become symptomatic with back pain. Osteoarthritis affects the hips and knees by wearing away the **articular** (are-TICK-you-lar) cartilage at the end of the long bones where bones articulate, or meet. Eventually, the entire surface of the cartilage might be worn away, exposing areas of raw bone. When this occurs, new bone forms in and around the joint, causing the bone ends to thicken. Fragments of this new bone are called bone spurs and often lead to a decrease in joint motion. X-ray examination might reveal the spurs and only small patches of cartilage on the bone ends. This is called a bone-on-bone condition, and at this point, individuals are often candidates for total hip or knee replacement surgery. Osteoarthritis peaks in the fifth to sixth decade of life, with approximately 80% of individuals showing symptoms by age 70.

■ **TREATMENT.** Treatment for osteoarthritis includes rest, non–weight-bearing exercise such as swimming and biking, application of heat, and use of analgesics and anti-inflammatory medications. Severe osteoarthritis can be treated by steroid injections into the joint capsule to relieve pain. Total surgical joint replacement might be recommended.

■ **DIAGNOSIS.** The diagnosis is usually made based on history and physical exam because X-rays do not always correlate with symptoms.

■ **PREVENTION.** Maintaining a healthy body weight is the single best prevention. Excess weight strains joints, especially those of the knees and hips. It is estimated that every one pound of body weight places approximately three pounds of stress on the joints of the knees and even more on the hips.

RHEUMATOID ARTHRITIS

■ **DESCRIPTION.** Rheumatoid arthritis was discussed in Chapter 5, "Immune System Diseases and Disorders," as an autoimmune disorder that not only

TABLE 6–3 Risk Factors for Osteoarthritis
The following are considered factors that increase the risk of developing osteoarthritis:
■ Family history of osteoarthritis
■ Excessive wear and tear or injury to joints
■ Obesity
■ Increased risk with age
■ Female

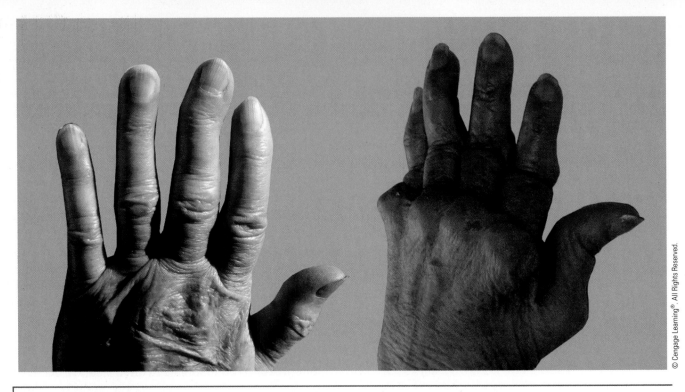

FIGURE 6–8 Comparison of (left) osteoarthritis and (right) rheumatoid arthritis: hands and joints.

affects the joints but also the connective tissues of the entire body. Rheumatoid arthritis often affects the lungs, heart, and blood vessels, causing the individual to appear chronically ill. This type of arthritis often affects people in the prime of life and affects women more often than men. It is a debilitating, chronic disease that destroys the joints.

■ *SYMPTOMS.* A noticeable difference in the way osteoarthritis and rheumatoid arthritis affect the joints can be observed in joints of the hand. Osteoarthritis affects the working joints of the hand (primarily the distal and proximal interphalangeal joints), causing swelling and pain. All joints of the

HEALTHY HIGHLIGHT

Knuckle-Cracking

"Will knuckle-cracking cause arthritis in my joints?" This is a commonly asked question by those who have developed the habit of knuckle-cracking, the sound made by the rush of synovial fluid from one area of the joint to another as the joint is forcefully pulled apart. Research supports the fact that this action does not cause an increase in osteoarthritis, but it also supports the fact that individuals who crack their knuckles eventually have decreased grip and hand function. Research does not rule out the idea of knuckle-cracking causing joint damage. Knuckle-crackers might not have to worry about an increase in osteo-arthritic pain due to chronic knuckle-cracking, but they might still develop long-term pain from chronic ligament inflammation. Some researchers feel that chronic joint pain, whether related to arthritis or not, is still chronic joint pain and thus recommend that knuckle-crackers stop this behavior. Interestingly, related research found that knuckle-crackers are also more likely to bite their fingernails, smoke, and drink alcohol.

hand can be affected in rheumatoid individuals, often with noticeable deformity and destruction in the metacarpophalangeal joints (see Figure 6–8). Also, refer to Chapter 5 for more information on rheumatoid arthritis.

GOUT

■ **DESCRIPTION.** Gout is often called gouty arthritis because this condition leads to inflammation of the affected joints.

■ **ETIOLOGY.** Gout is caused by a metabolic alteration in the breakdown of certain protein foods. Individuals with gout deposit uric acid crystals in joints of the body.

■ **SYMPTOMS.** The primary joint affected is the **metatarsophalangeal** (meta = between, tarso = foot, phalangeal = toe bones) joint of the big toe. These uric acid crystals have razor sharp edges that irritate the joint, causing an acute inflammatory response. Symptoms are redness, heat, swelling, and pain in the joint.

Approximately 95% of gout patients are male, with onset usually after age 30. Chronic gout can be characterized by uric acid deposited in subcutaneous tissue as well as in the joint. These deposits appear as small, whitish nodules called **tophi** and are commonly seen around a joint and in the soft tissue of the ear (Figure 6–9). Kidney dysfunction and an increase in the occurrence of kidney stones are also common with chronic gout.

■ **DIAGNOSIS.** Diagnosis is based on finding uric acid crystals in joint, body fluids, tissues, or all of these. Uric acid blood testing is also helpful in diagnosing gout.

■ **TREATMENT.** Treatment can include anti-gout medication (probenecid and allopurinol [Zyloprim®]) and dietary adjustments to decrease the amount of protein consumed. Weight loss in obese patients also can be beneficial.

■ **PREVENTION.** Avoiding foods high in purine such as meat, poultry, fish, and other seafood is helpful in preventing gouty attacks. Preventing dehydration by drinking plenty of fluids while avoiding diuretic drinks such as tea and alcohol is also helpful.

JOINT DEFORMITIES

HALLUX VALGUS

■ **DESCRIPTION.** Hallux (big toe) valgus (bent outward) is a deformity affecting the metatarsophalangeal joint of the big toe. It is more commonly called a bunion. This condition occurs more frequently in women and tends to run in families.

■ **ETIOLOGY.** The cause of bunions is controversial. Many experts think the cause is an inherited faulty foot formation that progresses over time and is irritated by poor or improper footwear. Others think the footwear actually causes the condition. Whatever the cause, all agree that wearing pointed-toe shoes, especially with high heels, aggravates the condition. This type of shoe forces the great toe into a valgus position and increases the pressure on the metatarsophalangeal

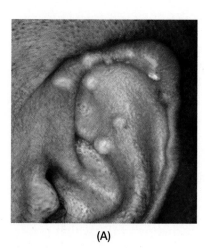 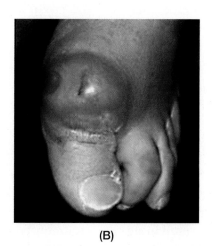 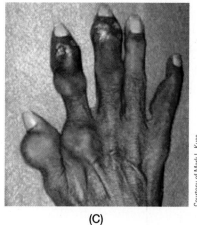

(A) (B) (C)

FIGURE 6–9 Common sites of tophi.

Courtesy of Mark L. Kuss

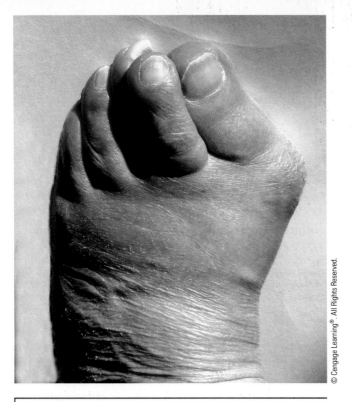

FIGURE 6–10 Hallux valgus (bunion).

joint. Over a period of time, this chronic irritation leads to a buildup of soft tissue and bone in the joint area (Figure 6–10).

■ **SYMPTOMS.** Symptoms and signs include redness, pain, and swelling in the area and, often, the inability to wear pointed-toe or high-heeled shoes.

■ **DIAGNOSIS.** Bunions are very visible and easily diagnosed by X-rays.

■ **TREATMENT.** Mild cases can be resolved by changing to a properly fitting, low-heeled shoe. Analgesic and anti-inflammatory medications can be beneficial in relieving pain. More severe cases might need surgical intervention with bunionectomy.

■ **PREVENTION.** Wearing proper footwear can prevent or at least slow the progression of bunion.

TEMPOROMANDIBULAR JOINT SYNDROME (TMJ)

■ **DESCRIPTION.** TMJ is an inflammation of the temporomandibular joint, the joint that connects the lower jaw to the skull. This disorder can result in significant pain and impairment.

■ **ETIOLOGY.** TMJ might be due to joint tissue lesions, overbite, malocclusion, or improperly fitted dentures or dental work.

■ **SYMPTOMS.** Severe headaches and pain in the jaw joint might be indicative of TMJ. This pain can be made worse by chewing. Classic signs include marked decrease in the ability to open the mouth and a clicking sound made during chewing motion.

■ **DIAGNOSIS.** Examination of the mouth along with dental X-rays, CT scan, or MRI scan aids in diagnosis of TMJ.

■ **TREATMENT.** Treatment includes correction of the causative factors, often leading to surgical intervention.

■ **PREVENTION.** Controlling or eliminating causative factors aids in prevention of TMJ.

Diseases of the Muscles and Connective Tissue

Diseases of the muscles and connective tissue, unlike many of the bone disorders, are quite common in very young or young adult individuals. Some of these disorders, such as the muscular dystrophies, are chronic, progressive, and devastating to families because they usually result in early death. Other disorders of the muscles and connective tissue are considered to be rather minor and can be treated medically or surgically.

Consider This ...

The tongue is the only muscle in the body that is attached at only one end and is, for its size, the strongest muscle in the body.

MUSCULAR DYSTROPHY (MD)

■ **DESCRIPTION.** Muscular dystrophy is an inherited genetic disorder that affects skeletal muscle. There are many types of dystrophies, but the most common type is Duchenne's MD, which primarily affects male children.

■ **SYMPTOMS.** Duchenne's MD is characterized by a wasting away of shoulder and pelvic girdle muscles. Survival beyond age 20 is rare. This disorder is discussed in detail in Chapter 19, "Genetic and Developmental Diseases and Disorders."

GANGLION CYST

■ **DESCRIPTION.** A ganglion cyst is a fluid-filled benign tumor that usually develops on a tendon sheath near the wrist area.

■ **ETIOLOGY.** The cause of these cysts is unknown, although some feel that they might be associated with a repetitive injury.

■ **SYMPTOMS.** A cyst is commonly a single, smooth, round lump just under the skin (Figure 6–11). It can be quite small or grow to the size of a dime or quarter. Usually, these are painless but unsightly. Cysts can disappear gradually over a period of months.

■ **DIAGNOSIS.** A physical exam is often all that is needed to diagnosis this condition.

■ **TREATMENT.** If they are painful or unsightly, the physician might choose to rupture the cyst or drain it. Ganglionectomy, or surgical removal, also can be performed.

■ **PREVENTION.** There are no preventive measures for ganglion cysts.

TETANUS

■ **DESCRIPTION.** Tetanus, also called lockjaw, is an acute, infectious, life-threatening disease characterized by painful, uncontrolled contractions of skeletal muscle.

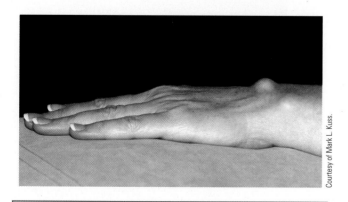

FIGURE 6–11 Ganglion cyst.

Courtesy of Mark L. Kuss.

■ **ETIOLOGY.** A toxin produced by the bacillus bacterium, *Clostridium tetani*, causes tetanus. This bacterium is commonly found in animal feces and, when excreted, lives as spores in the soil. The number of these spores is especially high in barnyards, pastures, or garden areas fertilized with animal manure. When this infectious bacterium enters the body in an **anaerobic** (ana = without, erobic = air) wound such as a puncture, it grows and produces a dangerous toxin. This toxin travels in the blood and attaches to motor or muscle neurons. The toxin irritates the nerve, producing the stimulus for skeletal muscle contraction. Because of the neurologic involvement, tetanus also may be categorized as a nervous system disorder.

■ **SYMPTOMS.** The bacterial toxin affects the nervous system rather slowly. The farther the distance between the wound and the spinal cord, the slower the progression. One to three weeks might pass before the onset of symptoms. The jaw muscles are often the first muscles affected with **tetany** (TET-ah-nee), or rigid muscle contraction, preventing the individual from opening the mouth, hence the term *lockjaw*. Eventually, muscles of the esophagus, neck, back, arms, and legs are affected. Other symptoms are a high fever, tachycardia (rapid pulse rate), dysphagia (difficulty swallowing), and intense pain.

■ **DIAGNOSIS.** Diagnosis is confirmed by a spatula test, which involves touching the posterior pharyngeal wall (the very back of the throat) with a soft-tipped instrument. A positive result is an involuntary contraction of the muscles causing the patient to bite down on the instrument.

■ **TREATMENT.** Treatment is a prompt and immediate cleansing of wounds with special consideration given to puncture-type wounds. Immunization might be needed, depending on the individual's immunization history. If the individual has not received a tetanus toxoid injection in the past 5 years, an antitoxin might be given to bind and inactivate the tetanus toxin. Initially, tetanus toxoid should be administered to children as part of basic diphtheria, pertussis, and tetanus (DPT) immunization.

Tetanus antibodies must be boosted approximately every 7 to 10 years throughout life. Individuals with low tetanus antibody levels are susceptible to tetanus. An antitoxin can be given to prevent tetanus following an injury because the body does not have time to build up its own antibodies.

Following this episode, it is usually recommended that the individual follow up with the proper tetanus toxoid booster.

Care of an individual with tetanus includes symptomatic treatment, often including respiratory, nutritional, and hydration support. Antibiotics and muscle relaxants also can be administered. Even with the best of care, tetanus is usually fatal due to respiratory failure. If the individual survives, the disease process usually lasts 6 to 8 weeks. Surprisingly, the disease usually does not leave any permanent disability, but it also does not confer any lasting immunity to tetanus.

■ **PREVENTION.** Tetanus can be prevented by vaccination. It is recommended that adults receive a booster vaccine every 10 years. Standard care practice in many places is to give the booster to any patient with a puncture wound who is uncertain of when he or she was last vaccinated or if he or she has had fewer than three lifetime doses of the vaccine.

SYSTEMIC LUPUS ERYTHEMATOSUS

■ **DESCRIPTION.** Systemic lupus erythematosus is an autoimmune disorder that affects the connective tissue throughout the body. One of the main characteristics is a butterfly-patterned rash across the nose and face. For more details, see Chapter 5.

Neoplasms

Primary neoplasms of the musculoskeletal system are uncommon. Typically, neoplasms of this system are secondary, metastasizing from the lungs, breast, and prostate. The most common primary tumor of bone is osteosarcoma, which affects the tibia, humerus, or femur. Ewing's sarcoma is also primarily a bone tumor, affecting long bones in children and teens. It is highly malignant and quickly metastasizes to nearly every organ of the body. Myeloma is the most common marrow tumor, commonly affecting the pelvis, vertebrae, and long bones of adults. Kaposi's sarcoma affects soft tissue of primarily immunosuppressed individuals. Rhabdomyosarcoma is a very rare but highly malignant tumor of skeletal muscle.

Symptoms of musculoskeletal tumors can include pathologic fracture and bone pain. Clinical examination followed by radiologic studies, CT scan, blood studies, and biopsy often confirm the diagnosis. Treatment of malignant tumors of the musculoskeletal system can include radiation, chemotherapy, and surgery.

Surgical procedures often involve excision and amputation. Even with aggressive therapy, prognosis for these malignant neoplasms is often very poor.

■ TRAUMA

Trauma is the main cause of problems in the musculoskeletal system. Fractures are by far the most common and frequent injury to bone. Tennis elbow is the most frequent ailment of the upper body. Treatment for sprains and strains is among the top 10 reasons that patients seek medical attention for acute disease. Low back pain is in the top 10 for chronic disease.

Fracture

A fracture (Figure 6–12) is any discontinuity of a bone. A fracture and a break are synonymous, although a **stress** (related to too much weight-bearing or pressure) fracture or incomplete fracture might not break the bone in two. Fractures can be caused by trauma (injury) or can be **pathologic** (caused by weakness from a disease).

Types of Fractures

Fractures may be classified in a number of ways. One method of classification is based on the condition of the overlying skin. If the bone has protruded through

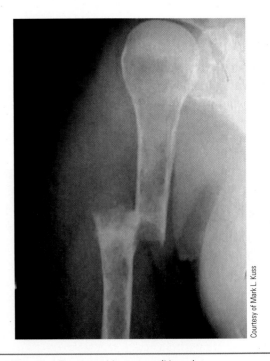

Courtesy of Mark L. Kuss

FIGURE 6–12   Fractured humerus (X-ray).

the skin or an object has punctured the skin, making an opening through the skin to the fracture site, it is an **open** fracture. Open fractures are also called **compound** fractures because the fracture, plus the open skin, is compounding the problem. An open fracture is always an emergency due to the high risk of bone infection. Patients with open fractures are taken to surgery for cleaning and débridement. If there is no opening in the skin, it is called a **closed,** or **simple, fracture.**

Another method of classification considers the condition of the bone. If the fracture goes completely through the bone, it is a **complete fracture.** If the bone is fractured but not in two, it is an **incomplete fracture.** A common incomplete fracture that occurs in children is called a **greenstick** fracture because it appears to have broken partially, like a sap-filled green stick.

Fractures also may be described by the number of fragments or the position of the fragments. A **displaced** fracture is one in which fragments are out of position, whereas nondisplaced means the fragments are still in correct position. If there are more than two ends or fragments, the break is a **comminuted** fracture. Bone appearing to be mashed down is a compression fracture. A common site of a compression fracture is in the vertebrae. An **impacted** fracture is one characterized as a bone end forced over the other end. **Avulsion** fracture describes a separation of a small bone fragment from the bone where a tendon or ligament is attached.

The position of the fracture line as compared to bone position might also describe the fracture. A **longitudinal** fracture runs the length of the bone; a **transverse** fracture runs across or at a 90-degree angle. **Oblique** fractures run in a transverse pattern, and **spiral** fractures twist around the bone. **Stellate** fractures form a star-like pattern.

Location may be used to describe the fracture. An articular fracture involves a joint surface. **Intracapsular** and **extracapsular** describe fractures inside or outside the joint capsule, respectively. **Intertrochanteric** describes fractures in the trochanter of the femur, and **femoral neck** and **subcapital** fractures describe fractures located on the femur. Finally, fractures may be named by the physician who first described them; for example, **Colles'** (Figure 6–13) and **Pott's** fractures are fractures of the wrist and ankle, respectively.

To be very specific, a fracture may be more clearly defined by using several descriptive names.

For example, a diagnosis of a closed fracture is a broad diagnosis covering many kinds of fractures. A more descriptive diagnosis would be a closed, comminuted, fracture. An even clearer diagnosis would be a closed, comminuted, femoral neck fracture.

Sites and causes of fractures vary by age and gender. Children commonly fracture their arms during falls. Teen males commonly have long bone fractures related to motor vehicle accidents (MVAs) or sports injuries. Older females suffer with hip fractures generally related to falls and osteoporosis.

Media Link

View an animation about the types of fractures on CourseMate.

Treatment of Fractures

Treatment of fractures often involves first aid at the site of the accident. First aid includes splinting the fracture site by immobilizing the area to decrease movement and prevent further injury. A splint should be applied in an as-is position. No attempt should be made to reduce the fracture or place the bone back in normal position at this time.

After medical assistance has been obtained, proper treatment might require reduction of the fracture. If this can be accomplished without a surgical incision, it is called a closed reduction, common in fractures of the extremities. Radiography can confirm proper position of the bones. If the fracture cannot be reduced without internal manipulation, the area is surgically opened, or incised, and an open reduction is performed. Open reductions commonly require some type of internal fixation or holding device such as pins, plates, screws, or rods in a procedure called an open reduction, internal fixation (**ORIF**). Open fractures require surgical intervention to clean and débride the involved tissue, usually by cleansing with copious (excessive) amounts of fluid to prevent infection and osteomyelitis.

Closed and open reductions can require the application of a splint or cast to immobilize the area during the healing process. Most fractures heal in 4 to 8 weeks, depending on the site of fracture, the type of fracture, and the age and nutritional status of the involved individual.

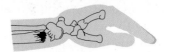

Colles'
Fracture named for physician

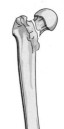

Femoral neck
Fracture based on location

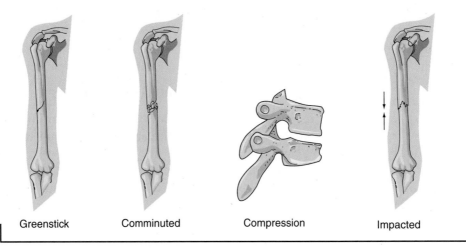

Pathologic	Open (compound)	Closed (simple)
Caused by weakness from disease		

Classification based on skin condition

Greenstick   Comminuted   Compression   Impacted

Classification based on bone condition

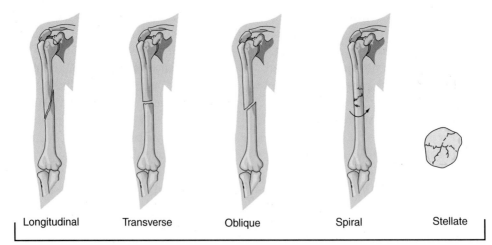

Longitudinal   Transverse   Oblique   Spiral   Stellate

Classification based on position of fracture line

FIGURE 6–13 Types of fractures.

The application of traction might be beneficial to relieve muscle spasms, to hold a fracture in correct position, or to stretch the muscles, allowing bone fragment ends to separate, thus reducing pain and further tissue damage. Traction involves the application of a device to maintain alignment and apply a pulling force.

Traction may be classified by the type of application device, two basic types of which are skeletal and skin. Skeletal traction is used for long-term traction or when large muscle groups are involved such as for a femur fracture with resultant quadriceps spasm. Skeletal traction involves placement of a pin through the bone distal to the fracture, and then ropes, pulley devices, and weights apply traction or pull to the fracture site (Figure 6–14). Skin traction is used for short-term traction or when small muscle groups are involved. The traction device is applied to the skin with the use of adhesive or elastic wrapping. The same ropes, pulleys, and weights might be used for skin traction, but the amount of weight applied is usually less than with skeletal traction.

Complications of Fractures

Complications of fractures include mal-union, nonunion, avascular necrosis, and infection. Mal-union is healing of the fracture in an abnormal or nonfunctional position; nonunion is the failure of the bone to heal. The complication of avascular necrosis occurs when the blood supply to the bone is not adequate to maintain bone health and the bone tissue dies. Infection of the bone was discussed in detail under the section titled "Osteomyelitis" (see page 107).

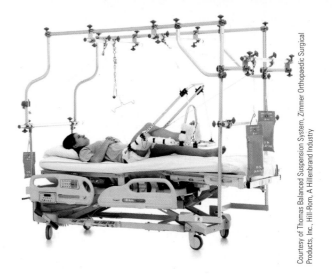

Courtesy of Thomas Balanced Suspension System, Zimmer Orthopaedic Surgical Products, Inc., Hill-Rom, A Hillenbrand Industry

FIGURE 6–14 Skeletal traction.

Media Link

View animations on injuries, resulting from a twisting force and a direct force, on the Online Resources.

Strains and Sprains

STRAIN

■ **DESCRIPTION.** A strain is a very common overstretching injury of a muscle.

HEALTHY HIGHLIGHT

Sports Injuries: When to See a Doctor

Participation in sports often results in numerous lumps, bumps, and bruises. Often, these injuries heal without medical treatment, but some injuries, left unattended, can lead to long-term difficulties. Often, individuals ask, "When should I see a doctor?"

The following may be used as general guidelines for seeking medical attention:

■ Any injury in or near a joint
■ Pain that does not subside after 10 days
■ Any time there is obvious bone deformity
■ Injury that has not improved in 5 to 7 days
■ Any sign of infection: temperature of 101°F or greater, presence of pus, red streaks in the tissue, or swollen lymph glands

■ **ETIOLOGY.** Individuals commonly have lumbar strains from lifting too much weight, lifting improperly, or lifting repetitively. Strained backs are common after a weekend of activity by an individual not in adequate physical condition.

■ **SYMPTOMS.** Symptoms include soreness, pain, and tenderness.

■ **DIAGNOSIS.** Strains, in most cases, are diagnosed based on a history and physical exam. Examination might reveal swelling and tenderness in the affected area.

■ **TREATMENT.** Treatment includes rest, moist heat, and the use of analgesics and anti-inflammatory medications. As pain subsides, physical therapy might be initiated to restore strength and flexibility. A strain is less serious than a sprain.

■ **PREVENTION.** Avoiding extreme fatigue and warming up before exercise can help prevent strains.

SPRAIN

■ **DESCRIPTION.** A sprain is a traumatic injury to a joint with partial or complete tearing of ligaments.

■ **ETIOLOGY.** Sports activities commonly lead to sprains. The ankle joint is commonly affected and can become so painful that the joint cannot be used. The degree of ligament tearing, plus involvement of associated tendons, muscles, and blood vessels, determines the degree of injury. Severe sprains can exhibit complete tearing of the ligaments.

■ **SYMPTOMS.** Symptoms include varying degrees of swelling, pain, heat, and redness to purple or dark

blue discoloration from blood vessel hemorrhage (Figure 6–15).

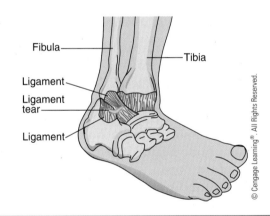

Media Link

Watch an animation about an ankle sprain on CourseMate.

■ **DIAGNOSIS.** Physical examination is often all that is needed for diagnosis, although X-rays might be taken to rule out fracture. In extreme cases, MRI and arthroscopy can be used.

■ **TREATMENT.** Treatment depends on the severity of the sprain. Mild sprains are treated by implementing the concept of **RICE**: rest, ice, compression (wrapping with an elastic bandage), and elevation. As the sprain heals and pain resolves, light exercise and gradual walking are recommended.

Fibula — Tibia
Ligament —
Ligament tear —
Ligament —

© Cengage Learning®. All Rights Reserved.

FIGURE 6–15 Sprained ankle.

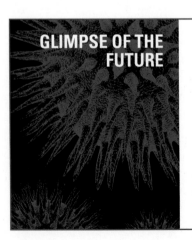

GLIMPSE OF THE FUTURE

Best Treatment for Ankle Sprains

A systematic review of the literature on treatment for acute ankle sprains found that ankle braces as well as wraps or tape were most frequently used as the treatment of choice. These treatments were reviewed to decide the best practice to use. A few studies reported that the use of an ankle brace after injury produced positive outcomes and was a cost-effective method of treatment. However, further research is needed to really determine the best treatment for the patient and the most cost-saving method. The treatment for ankle sprains may change in the future based on the continued research.

Source: Kemmler et al. (2011).

■ *PREVENTION.* Regular exercise, stretching, and strengthening to maintain good physical condition are the best preventions for sprains.

Dislocations and Subluxations

■ *DESCRIPTION.* Dislocation is the complete separation of a bone from its normal position in a joint. A subluxation is a partial separation (Figure 6–16).

■ *ETIOLOGY.* Dislocations occur with major traumatic injuries such as MVAs, contact sports, or falls and can cause a fracture as well. Dislocations can also be related to joint abnormalities or disease. In the case of disease, the dislocation might occur frequently and without cause.

■ *SYMPTOMS.* Dislocation causes acute pain and obvious joint deformity. In ball-and-socket joints, the ball can be totally anterior or posterior to the socket. The joint tissue rapidly swells, making reduction difficult.

■ *DIAGNOSIS.* A history and physical exam by a physician is adequate for a diagnosis. An X-ray can be helpful in determining the extent of the injury.

■ *TREATMENT.* Because of the swelling, a dislocated joint should be reduced or repositioned by a physician immediately. Even with emergency treatment, general anesthesia might be needed for the reduction procedure.

Individuals who suffer with recurrent dislocations and subluxations can be taught how to reduce the joint. If the joint ligaments become weakened with repeated dislocations, surgery might be necessary to tighten the ligaments, thus strengthening the joint.

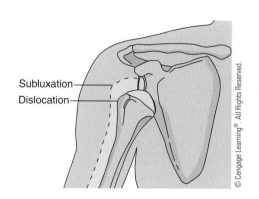

Subluxation
Dislocation

© Cengage Learning®. All Rights Reserved.

FIGURE 6–16   Dislocation and subluxation.

■ *PREVENTION.* Maintaining muscle strength around the joint will help prevent these conditions. Individual bandage wraps, braces, and special padding can also help.

Low Back Pain (LBP)

■ *DESCRIPTION.* The low back or lumbar area of the spine is very susceptible to stress or strain.

■ *ETIOLOGY.* This stress can be increased by such factors as obesity, poor posture, weak abdominal muscles, and constant or improper lifting. These factors are more likely to cause LBP in individuals who have spinal deformities or diseases affecting the spine.

Some disorders that affect the spine and often lead to LBP include spinal deformities, osteoarthritis, rheumatoid arthritis, osteoporosis, and bone cancer, to name just a few. X-ray examinations are usually helpful in determining the cause of LBP, but further detailed study with a CT scan or MRI might be needed.

■ *SYMPTOMS.* LBP is a very common disorder of the musculoskeletal system. It might be acute and resolve in a few days, or it might be a chronic discomfort that lasts a lifetime.

■ *DIAGNOSIS.* X-rays, CT, and MRI assist in the diagnosis of LBP.

■ *TREATMENT.* Treatment of acute LBP is usually rest, warm moist heat, analgesics, and anti-inflammatory medications. Lumbar **spasms** (uncontrolled muscle contractions) are common and very painful. These spasms often twist the back out of normal position. Muscle relaxants might be prescribed for acute attacks, but rest and application of heat are usually adequate to control spasms. After the acute attack subsides, a daily exercise program including aerobic walking is very beneficial in building muscle tone and decreasing the risk of further attacks. One of the most common causes of LBP is a herniated intervertebral disk or herniated nucleus pulposus.

■ *PREVENTION.* Developing and maintaining a regular walking and exercise program are the best preventive measures for back pain prevention. Lifting properly is also an important preventive measure.

COMPLEMENTARY AND ALTERNATIVE THERAPY

Complementary and Alternative Therapy for Low Back Pain

There are various complementary and alternative therapies used for low back pain. Spinal manipulation is a frequently prescribed modality. In this treatment, a practitioner places a device or hands on the back to forcefully manipulate and move a spinal joint. Another alternative treatment is massage therapy. It is used to reduce back pain and improve balance. Acupuncture is an alternative treatment that is gaining in popularity. It involves using needles placed in specific spots to resolve the low back pain.

Source: Simmons (2011).

Herniated Nucleus Pulposus (HNP)

■ **DESCRIPTION.** HNP is commonly called herniated disk (or disc), ruptured disk, slipped disk, or bulging disk. All these terms are similar.

■ **ETIOLOGY.** HNP is the protrusion of the soft center (nucleus pulposus) of a disk in the spinal cord or spinal nerve (Figure 6–17).

■ **SYMPTOMS.** Pressure on the spinal nerve can cause pain in the sciatic nerve, called **sciatica**, which radiates down the back side of the leg.

■ **DIAGNOSIS.** Diagnosis involves physical examination, often confirmed by a CT scan, MRI, or **myelogram**. A myelogram involves injecting dye into the spinal canal and taking pictures to reveal compression on the spinal cord or spinal nerves.

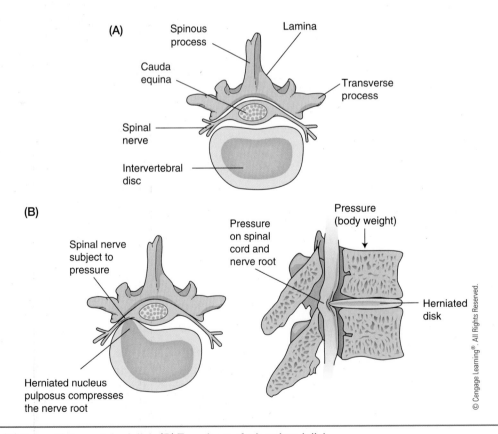

© Cengage Learning®. All Rights Reserved.

FIGURE 6–17   (A) Normal intervertebral disk. (B) Two views of a herniated disk.

■ **TREATMENT.** Treatment of HNP is often the same as for LBP. Extensive exercise therapy can reduce the size of the protrusion and relieve the associated LBP. If pain persists after therapy, or if the disk is found to be causing severe spinal cord or spinal nerve compression, surgery for disk removal might be needed. Surgery to remove the disk or to cut away vertebra to open the area around the nerve is called a **diskectomy** or **laminectomy**, respectively. A relatively new procedure to relieve the pain from osteoporotic compression fractures can also be performed. In this treatment, a large-bore needle is inserted with X-ray guidance into the compressed vertebra. A balloon is inserted into the bone through the needle and inflated, restoring the height of the vertebra. Sometimes, bone cement is injected into the bone to make sure it does not collapse again.

■ **PREVENTION.** Proper lifting, weight control, and maintaining a good exercise and walking program are all preventive measures.

Bursitis

■ **DESCRIPTION.** Bursitis (ber-SIE-tis) is the inflammation of a bursa or small, fluid-filled sac near joints. Bursae help reduce friction during movement.

■ **ETIOLOGY.** Repetitive motions often lead to irritation of the bursa, resulting in bursitis. Any joint can be affected, but bursitis of the shoulder is the most common type. Bursitis that occurs in the elbow is commonly called tennis elbow.

■ **SYMPTOMS.** Symptoms include severe pain that limits motion in the joint.

■ **DIAGNOSIS.** Bursitis is identified by location of pain or swelling and by pain with motion of the tissues in the affected area. X-ray testing can also help.

■ **TREATMENT.** Rest, application of moist heat, and use of analgesics and anti-inflammatory medications will usually resolve the condition. If bursitis persists, further treatment of the bursa includes injection with corticosteroids, draining, and surgical excision. Active range-of-motion exercises are needed after pain subsides to regain and maintain joint motion.

■ **PREVENTION.** Identifying and modifying activities that cause or aggravate the problem is the best prevention. Taking frequent breaks, especially from repetitive activities, is also helpful. Exercising and stretching to strengthen the muscle, ligaments, and tendons in the area of injury are important.

HEALTHY HIGHLIGHT

RICE

RICE, an acronym for Rest, Ice, Compression, and Elevation, can be used effectively for almost all types of injuries from a sprained ankle to a broken bone. When an injury occurs, RICE should be followed for the first 24 hours.

- **REST** Immediate, non–weight-bearing rest will prevent further damage. Rest includes use of splints, slings, and crutches.
- **ICE** Application of ice slows bleeding and swelling by causing vasoconstriction. The more blood that collects in an area, the longer the healing time. Ice should not be applied directly to the skin; rather, wrap the ice pack in a towel before application. Alternating ice treatment—30 minutes on and 15 minutes off—is a general rule. Apply heat after 24 hours to improve vascular flow and carry away tissue debris.
- **COMPRESSION** Application of a compression stocking or ace wrap will provide support and limit swelling, thereby speeding healing time. Compression devices should be snug but not so tight they cut off circulation, which could lead to increased pain and numbness.
- **ELEVATION** Place the injured area at a height above the heart to allow gravity to assist venous flow to further reduce swelling.

TENNIS ELBOW

TENNIS ELBOW

■ **DESCRIPTION.** Tennis elbow is a type of bursitis that affects the elbow area.

■ **ETIOLOGY.** This bursitis is not always caused by playing tennis, as its name suggests. Tennis elbow is a repetitive-motion injury.

■ **SYMPTOMS.** The most common symptom is a severe, burning pain on the outside of the elbow. Pain can be made worse by pressing on the outside surface of the elbow or by lifting or gripping objects. Lifting even the smallest object, such as a coffee cup, can lead to extreme pain.

■ **DIAGNOSIS.** Diagnosis can be confirmed by eliciting increased pain when the middle finger is pushed backward or extended against resistance.

■ **TREATMENT.** Treatment is the same as with bursitis. Application of a wide strap just below the elbow will change and support muscle movement in the forearm, thus reducing some of the pain.

■ **PREVENTION.** Stretching and strengthening the arm muscles so they are flexible and strong enough to support activities is the best prevention.

Tendonitis

■ **DESCRIPTION.** Tendonitis is inflammation of a tendon or connective tissue that attaches muscle to bone. Tendonitis can occur in any tendon, but most often, it affects the shoulder.

■ **ETIOLOGY.** Tendonitis is commonly a repetitive-motion injury but also can be caused by calcium deposits. Athletes in baseball, basketball, swimming, and tennis are often affected. Tendonitis also can occur in association with bursitis.

■ **SYMPTOMS.** Pain, gradual or sudden and severe, is the main symptom.

■ **DIAGNOSIS.** A physical examination revealing tenderness along the involved tendon along with pain when the muscle to which the tendon is attached is moved or worked against resistance will support the diagnosis.

■ **TREATMENT.** Treatment is rest, application of ice (which might irritate bursitis), and use of analgesics and anti-inflammatory medications. Active range-of-motion exercises can be initiated, after the pain subsides, to restore motion. If joint adhesions have developed, surgical intervention might be necessary to free the joint and restore mobility.

■ **PREVENTION.** Strengthening exercises, avoiding repetitive activities, and avoiding overuse of the arm or leg are preventive measures.

Carpal Tunnel Syndrome

■ **DESCRIPTION.** Carpal tunnel syndrome is a repetitive-motion injury affecting the hands and commonly seen in individuals who perform computer data entry, work at manufacturing jobs, or do any task that requires continuous, repetitive finger and wrist motions.

■ **ETIOLOGY.** The blood vessels, tendons, and nerves that feed or innervate the hands pass through a tunnel in the wrist area formed by the carpal tunnel ligament (Figure 6–18). The repetitive motion causes inflammation of the tendons, resulting in pressure on the medial nerve.

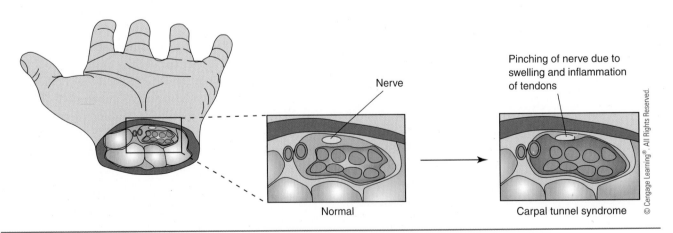

Nerve

Pinching of nerve due to swelling and inflammation of tendons

Normal

Carpal tunnel syndrome

FIGURE 6–18 Carpal tunnel syndrome.

■ *SYMPTOMS.* Symptoms of carpal tunnel syndrome often include numbness, pain, swelling, coolness, and discoloration in the affected hand and fingers.

■ *DIAGNOSIS.* Diagnosis is confirmed by history, physical examination, and testing. Positive results of a Phalen's maneuver, performed by flexing the wrist as far as possible and watching for symptoms, are sufficient for diagnosis. A positive test is one that results in numbness in the median nerve area within 60 seconds of the maneuver.

■ *TREATMENT.* Treatment consists of stopping the repetitive motion, resting the hand, splinting, administration of anti-inflammatory medications, and physical therapy. Carpal tunnel syndrome not relieved by these measures might require surgery to split the carpal ligament, enlarging the tunnel and relieving pressure on the median nerve.

■ *PREVENTION.* Prevention of carpal tunnel syndrome is the best plan and can be accomplished by ergonomic principles and job rotation to improve hand positions and provide adequate rest periods, respectively.

Plantar Fasciitis

■ *DESCRIPTION.* Plantar fasciitis (FAS-ee-EYE-tis) is also called calcaneal spur or heel spur. The plantar **fascia** is a thick, fibrous, connective tissue that runs the length of the bottom or plantar surface of the foot. The plantar fascia attaches to the heel, or **calcaneal** area of the foot, and helps develop the arch of the foot (Figure 6–19).

■ *ETIOLOGY.* Plantar fasciitis is often seen in runners due to the repeated pressure placed on the

fascia during running. This constant pressure causes inflammation and pain at the point of attachment to the calcaneus. It is not uncommon for individuals to have a small heel spur at this point of attachment, but it becomes more noticeable and more painful with this condition. Heel spurs do not cause the problem; they are the result of the problem.

■ *SYMPTOMS.* The common symptom of plantar fasciitis is an intermittent pain in the heel that is worse when taking the first few steps after sitting or standing for some time, when getting out of bed, or at the beginning of an exercise routine. Plantar fasciitis develops more often in individuals who have a sudden increase in activity or weight. Other sufferers include individuals who are flat-footed, toe runners, or overweight and have high arches and poor shoe support.

■ *DIAGNOSIS.* History and physical exam is usually sufficient for diagnosis. The classic history is a complaint of pain in the foot during the first steps after getting out of bed or after sitting for a long period of time.

■ *TREATMENT.* Treatment includes rest, application of ice, use of analgesics and anti-inflammatory medication, and use of a heel pad or orthotic that relieves pressure on the heel. After pain subsides, exercises to strengthen the foot might help prevent reinjury. Surgery to remove the heel spur and release the plantar fascia has proven ineffective in most instances.

■ *PREVENTION.* Steps to prevent plantar fasciitis include wearing shoes with good arch support, exercising to stretch the Achilles tendon, maintaining proper body weight, and avoiding going barefoot.

Torn Rotator Cuff

■ *DESCRIPTION.* The rotator cuff comprises a group of muscles that hold the head of the humerus in the shoulder socket area.

■ *ETIOLOGY.* Tears are commonly caused by traumatic injuries of baseball, basketball, and tennis.

■ *SYMPTOMS.* Tears in the tendons that hold these muscles to the bone produce a snapping sound, followed by acute pain and the inability of the individual to abduct (move away from midline) or raise the arm.

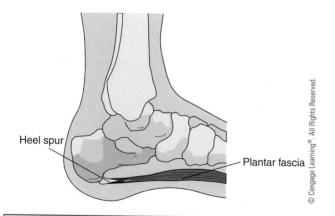

Heel spur

Plantar fascia

© Cengage Learning®. All Rights Reserved.

FIGURE 6–19 Plantar fasciitis.

■ *DIAGNOSIS.* Diagnosis is made by physical examination and can be confirmed with a CT scan or arthroscopy.

■ *TREATMENT.* Acute rotator cuff tears are surgically repaired to restore motion of the shoulder. Postoperatively, the individual is placed in a shoulder immobilizer for 3 to 4 weeks. Analgesics and anti-inflammatory medications can be administered for acute pain. Active rehabilitation exercise is needed postoperatively to restore shoulder function.

■ *PREVENTION.* Daily exercise to maintain muscle strength and flexibility in the shoulder is the best preventive measure.

Torn Meniscus

■ *DESCRIPTION.* There are two semilunar cartilages in each knee joint, forming a lateral and medial meniscus. The **meniscus** (meh-NIS-cuss) is attached to the top of the tibia and provides cushioning for the distal femur.

■ *ETIOLOGY.* Athletes participating in football, baseball, soccer, and tennis commonly suffer with this injury. The tear usually results from a sudden twisting of the leg while the knee is flexed (Figure 6–20).

■ *SYMPTOMS.* Symptoms include acute pain with weight bearing on the affected knee. The individual might feel that the knee is locking or giving. Full flexion or extension of the knee might not be possible due to increased pain.

■ *DIAGNOSIS.* Physical examination of the knee, along with X-ray or MRI, confirms the diagnosis.

■ *TREATMENT.* Treatment is immobilization, elevation, and application of ice to decrease inflammation and pain. Analgesics and anti-inflammatory medications also can be needed. If surgical treatment is needed, it is commonly done arthroscopically or with the use of a scope to look into the knee. An extensive exercise rehabilitation program is begun postoperatively.

■ *PREVENTION.* Regular exercise, including strength training, aids in prevention of tears.

Cruciate Ligament Tears

■ *DESCRIPTION.* Cruciate (shaped like a cross) ligaments are located inside the knee joint (Figure 6–20A). They work as a pair (the anterior cruciate ligament and the posterior cruciate ligament) and form a cross, giving the knee front-to-back and rotary stability.

■ *ETIOLOGY.* These ligaments are often injured when the leg is twisted or hit from the front or back while in a planted or weight-bearing position (Figure 6–20B).

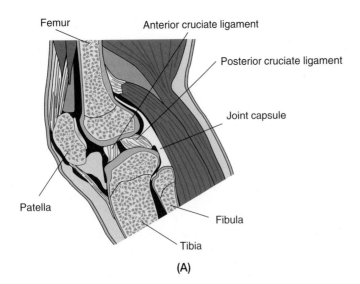

Femur
Anterior cruciate ligament
Posterior cruciate ligament
Joint capsule
Patella
Fibula
Tibia

(A)

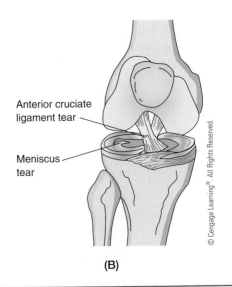

Anterior cruciate ligament tear
Meniscus tear

(B)

FIGURE 6–20 (A) Cruciate ligaments. (B) Meniscus and anterior cruciate ligament tear.

■ **SYMPTOMS.** A *popping* sound is commonly heard at the time of injury, followed by pain and swelling of the knee. Knee instability, front to back, is a primary sign of a cruciate ligament tear.

■ **DIAGNOSIS.** Diagnosis involves clinical examination, joint stability testing, and possible CT scanning.

■ **TREATMENT.** Treatment depends on the degree of injury and can vary from immobilization to surgical intervention.

■ **PREVENTION.** Maintaining excellent strength, flexibility, and endurance of the hamstrings and quadriceps muscles can prevent some anterior cruciate ligament (ACL) tears.

Shin Splints

■ **DESCRIPTION.** Shin splint is a term used to describe an overuse injury to the periosteum and extensor muscles of the lower leg.

■ **ETIOLOGY.** Shin splints occur routinely with a sudden increase in activity or a new exercise routine, commonly occurring in runners, joggers, and high-impact aerobics enthusiasts. Running on hard surfaces can also cause the problem.

■ **SYMPTOMS.** Pain and tenderness along the inner aspect of the tibia, worsening with exercise and disappearing with rest, are common symptoms.

■ **DIAGNOSIS.** Diagnosis is usually based on clinical examination, but X-ray examination can rule out a stress fracture.

■ **TREATMENT.** Rest, analgesics, anti-inflammatory medications, and alternating ice and heat treatments are usually beneficial.

■ **PREVENTION.** Proper conditioning, stretching exercises, and padded exercise shoes assist in preventing this disorder.

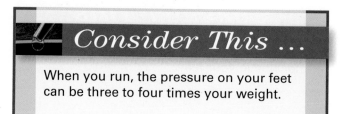

Consider This ...

When you run, the pressure on your feet can be three to four times your weight.

■ RARE DISEASES

de Quervain's Disease

de Quervain's disease is a repetitive-use tendonitis affecting the thumb. Pain can radiate up the forearm several inches and down into the thumb and increase if the individual attempts to pull the thumb and little finger together while the fingers are pointing upward. Physical examination and testing confirm the diagnosis.

Tuberculosis of the Bone

The bacterium *Mycobacterium tuberculosis* primarily affects the lungs, but it can also enter the bloodstream and travel to other organs of the body. Tuberculosis (TB) of the bone generally affects the arms and legs, and the knee is a common site for infection. Just as it does in the lungs, TB causes the development of cavities in the tissue, leading to bone weakness and pain. Antibiotic treatment is generally effective. A special form of TB in the vertebra or back of children is called Pott's disease.

Paget's Disease

Paget's (PAJ-ets) disease, also known as osteitis deformans, is a chronic metabolic bone disease that affects bone formation. Normally, bone is broken down and replaced at a consistent rate. Paget's is characterized by an overgrowth of new bone that outpaces the breakdown of old bone. The new bone is thicker than the old but much weaker, increasing the possibility of fracture. Radiologic examination reveals a mosaic bone pattern that is easily recognized as Paget's.

Paget's disease often affects the pelvis and long bones of the legs in individuals over age 40 and becomes more common with advancing age. Paget's can be asymptomatic, in which case, no treatment is necessary or beneficial. When symptomatic, individuals might complain of bone pain that becomes worse at night. Bones may fracture easily or become deformed, leading to bowed legs and curvature of the spine.

If the disease affects bones of the ear, hearing might become impaired. A secondary problem or complication of Paget's is the development of osteosarcoma, or bone cancer. The cause of Paget's is idiopathic. Treatment is primarily symptomatic, although a high-protein diet with calcium and vitamin D supplements can be beneficial.

Myasthenia Gravis

Myasthenia gravis (MY-us-THEE-nee-uh GRAV-iss) is an autoimmune disorder characterized by muscle weakness and fatigue that is somewhat relieved with rest. The problem is related to blocking of the acetylcholine neurotransmitter by antibodies in the neuromuscular junction. For more details about myasthenia gravis, see Chapter 5.

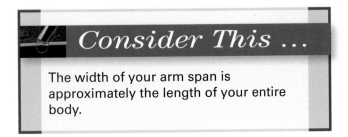

Consider This …

The width of your arm span is approximately the length of your entire body.

■ EFFECTS OF AGING ON THE SYSTEM

Normal changes that occur in bones, joints, and muscles cause a variety of problems in the older adult. Bone density decreases with age as calcium is reabsorbed from the bone. This causes greater brittleness of the bone with increased risks for fractures.

Osteoporosis is a common problem in the older adult, especially in older females, because of its association with decreasing estrogen levels in the blood.

As the individual ages, muscles decrease in strength and mass. Some muscle cells atrophy and decrease in total number. Arm and leg muscles lose tone and become somewhat flaccid and flabby in appearance.

Changes in height and curvature of the spine occur from changes in the vertebral disks and compression of the vertebrae. As muscles waste and joints stiffen, some loss of flexibility and agility is also common, along with an overall decreased mobility. Research has demonstrated the benefits of weight training and exercise classes for the older adult to prevent some of the muscle wasting, decreases in bone density, and loss of flexibility.

Musculoskeletal diseases, especially the debilitating ones such as arthritis, are extremely difficult for the older adult. Healing, such as after a fracture, is slower and often impaired by other chronic disorders common to the older adult. Pain associated with these disorders and changes in the system tend to decrease the individual's mobility and independence even more. Safety issues are of utmost importance when musculoskeletal system disorders are present because falls are one of the most common causes of injury in the older adult.

SUMMARY

The musculoskeletal system consists of bones, joints, muscles, ligaments, and tendons. It is the body's main framework and is responsible for all movements, which are the result of contraction and relaxation of the muscle fibers. The muscles are stimulated by responses from the nervous system. Most muscle movements are voluntary movements. The most common symptoms of musculoskeletal system disorders are pain, immobility, and disability. Diagnosis of a musculoskeletal system problem is usually made by assessment and X-ray or magnetic resonance imaging. However, other specific tests such as bone scans or endoscopy also can be used. Although fractures are a major group of musculoskeletal system disorders, many other diseases are common to

the system. Some of these are short term, but many are long-term, debilitating disorders. Individuals with musculoskeletal system diseases frequently need assistive devices such as crutches or walkers to maintain mobility. Changes in the musculoskeletal system in the older adult often lead to increased risk for fractures and disability.

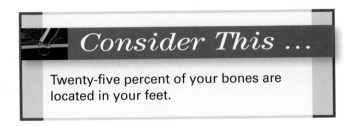

Consider This …

Twenty-five percent of your bones are located in your feet.

REVIEW QUESTIONS

Short Answer

1. What are the major functions of the musculoskeletal system?

2. What are the common signs and symptoms associated with musculoskeletal system disorders?

3. What are the most common tests used to diagnose musculoskeletal system disorders?

Fill in the Blank

4. The musculoskeletal system is composed of _____, _____, _____, _____, and _____.

5. _____ attach muscle to bone.

6. _____ joints are ones that have full movement.

7. The most common disorder of the system is _____.

8. _____ _____ is the most serious form of arthritis, but _____ is the most common type of arthritis.

Matching

9. Match the fracture-related term in the left column with the appropriate description in the right column.

_____ comminuted

_____ nondisplaced

_____ transverse

_____ greenstick

_____ stress

_____ impacted

_____ compound

a. Bone fragments are in correct position

b. One bone end is forced over another

c. More than two ends or fragments are present

d. Bone has protruded through the skin

e. An incomplete fracture common in children

f. Fracture runs across or at a 90-degree angle

g. Caused by too much weight-bearing or pressure

CASE STUDIES

■ Estella Gore is a 77-year-old resident of a local nursing home. She fell 4 weeks ago and fractured her left hip and is now in rehabilitation therapy and walking with the assistance of a physical therapy aide and a rolling walker. She states she is very frightened to walk and would rather use her wheelchair for mobility. What should you tell Ms. Gore about the importance of continuing to walk, even if she needs the assistance of a walker or personnel? Why is it important for her to be as mobile as possible? What are the overall effects of immobility? How does immobility affect other body systems?

■ Jeremy Dale is a 30-year-old recreational sports enthusiast and likes to play soccer and baseball on his days off from work. He mentions to you, his coworker, that he thinks he might have sprained his ankle over the weekend while playing soccer with some friends. He says it is swollen and very painful today and asks whether you think he should see a doctor or just wait for it to get better. What might be some good recommendations for you to give Jeremy about his sports injury? What could you tell him in general about minor sports injuries? How could he determine whether this is a sprain or a strain? Should he apply ice and elevate or compress the injured ankle? Is it too late for that treatment to be helpful?

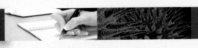

Study Tools

Workbook

Complete Chapter 6

Online Resources

PowerPoint® presentations

Animation

BIBLIOGRAPHY

American College of Rheumatology. (2012). Osteoarthritis. *www.rheumatology.org* (accessed July 2012).

Bilotti, E., Faiman, B. M., Richards, T. A., Tariman, J. D., Miceli, T. S., & Rome, S. I. (2011). Survivorship care guidelines for patients living with multiple myeloma. *Clinical Journal of Oncology Nursing 15*(S), 5–8.

Clinical Digest. (2010). Drug for osteoporosis does not increase risk of cancer. *Nursing Standard 25*(4), 16–17.

Faiman, B. M., Mangan, P., Spong, J., Tariman, J. D., & The International Myeloma Foundation Nurse Leadership Board. (2011). Renal complications in multiple myeloma and related disorders. *Clinical Journal of Oncology Nursing 15*(S), 66–76.

Granda-Cameron, C., Hanlon, A. L., Lynch, M., & Houldin, A. (2011). Experience of newly diagnosed patients with sarcoma receiving chemotherapy. *Oncology Nursing Forum 38*(2), 160–169.

Handley, A. (2011). Life and limb: Philippa Bridgeman. *Nursing Standard 26*(8), 22–23.

Hui, C., Salmon, L. J., Kok, A., Maeno, S., Linklater, J., & Pinczewski, L. A. (2011). Fifteen-year outcome of endoscopic anterior cruciate ligament reconstruction with patellar tendon autograft for "isolated" anterior cruciate ligament tear. *American Journal of Sports Medicine 39*(1), 89–98.

Hung, W. W., & Morrison, R. S. (2011). Hip fracture: A complex illness among complex patients. *Annals of Internal Medicine 155*(4), 267–268.

Kammerlander, C., Gosch, M., Kammerlander-Knauer, U., Luger, T., Blauth, M., & Roth, T. (2011). Long-term functional outcome in geriatric hip fracture patients. *Archives of Orthopaedic & Trauma Surgery 131*(10), 1435–1444.

Kemler, E., van de Port, I., Backx, F., & van Dijk, C. (2011). A systematic review on the treatment of acute ankle sprain. *Sports Medicine 41*(3), 185–197.

Kessenich, C. R. (2011). Reasoning in radiology: Do ankle injuries always require an X-ray? *Nurse Practitioner 36*(12), 17–18.

Lips, P., Bouillon, R., van Schoor, N. M., Vanderschueren, D., Verschueren, S., Kuchuk, N., & Boonen, S. (2010). Reducing fracture risk with calcium and vitamin D. *Clinical Endocrinology 73*(3), 277–285.

Messinger-Rapport, B. J., Morley, J. E., Thomas, D. R., & Gammack, J. K. (2011). Clinical update on nursing home medicine: 2011. *Journal of the American Medical Directors Association 12*(9), 615–626.

Miceli, T. S., Colson, K., Faiman, B. M., Miller, K., & Tariman, J. D. (2011). Maintaining bone health in patients with multiple myeloma. *Clinical Journal of Oncology Nursing 15*(S), 9–23.

O'Malley, N., Blauth, M., Suhm, N., & Kates, S. (2011). Hip fracture management, before and beyond surgery and medication: A synthesis of the evidence. *Archives of Orthopaedic & Trauma Surgery 131*(11), 1519–1527.

Premaor, M. O., & Compston, J. E. (2011). Testing for secondary causes of osteoporosis. *British Medical Journal 342*(7792), 330–331.

Roush, K. (2011). Prevention and treatment of osteoporosis in postmenopausal women: A review. *American Journal of Nursing 111*(8), 26–34.

Simmons, S. (2011). Controlling pain: Complementary and alternative therapies for low-back pain. *Nursing 41*(5), 54–55.

Stauber, M. A. (2011). Not all spinal cord injuries involve a fracture. *Advanced Emergency Nursing Journal 33*(3), 226–231.

Stubenrauch, J. M. (2011). Spinal manipulation therapy for low-back pain: It's no better-or worse-than other treatments. *American Journal of Nursing 111*(5), 18.

Walker, J. A. (2010). Management of patients with carpal tunnel syndrome. *Nursing Standard 24*(19), 44–48.

Wood, S. (2011). Sprains and strains. *Practice Nurse 41*(19), 33–36.

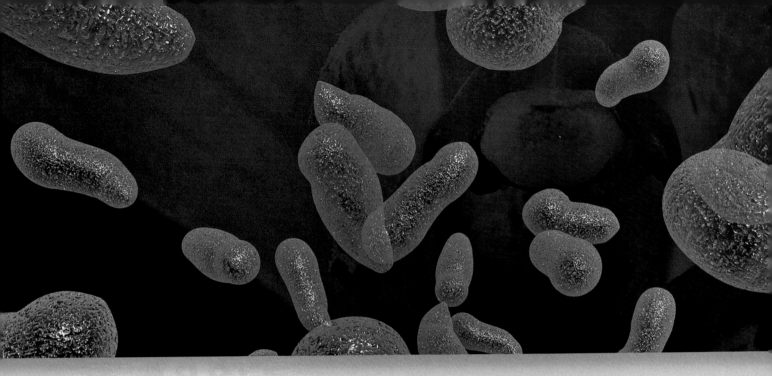

OUTLINE

- Anatomy and Physiology
- Common Signs and Symptoms
- Diagnostic Tests
- Common Diseases of the Blood and Blood-Forming Organs
  Disorders of Red Blood Cells
  Disorders of White Blood Cells
  Disorders of Platelets
- Trauma
- Rare Diseases
  Thalassemia
  Von Willebrand's Disease
  Lymphosarcoma
- Effects of Aging on the System
- Summary
- Review Questions
- Case Studies
- Bibliography

KEY TERMS

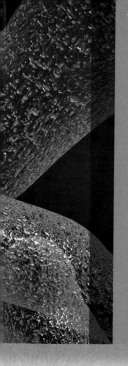

7

Blood and Blood-Forming Organs Diseases and Disorders

LEARNING OBJECTIVES

Upon completion of the chapter, the learner should be able to:

1. Define the terminology common to the blood and blood-forming organs and the disorders of the blood and blood-forming organs.

2. Discuss the basic anatomy and physiology of the blood and blood-forming organs.

3. Identify the important signs and symptoms associated with common blood and blood-forming organ disorders.

4. Describe the common diagnostics used to determine the type and cause of blood and blood-forming organ disorders.

5. Identify the common disorders of the blood and blood-forming organs.

6. Describe the typical course and management of the common blood and blood-forming organ disorders.

7. Describe the effects of aging on the blood and blood-forming organs and the common disorders associated with aging of the system.

OVERVIEW

The blood and the blood-forming organs make up the individual's hematologic system. Blood is the body's life fluid, responsible for transporting nutrients to cells and removing wastes. The blood-forming organs are the lymph nodes, bone marrow, spleen, and liver. Disorders of the system can have severe effects on other systems because of the pervasive responsibilities of the blood and blood-forming organs. Altered nutrition, medications, and diseases of other systems, in turn, can greatly affect the functioning of the hematologic system. ■

■ ANATOMY AND PHYSIOLOGY

The blood and blood-forming organs are also called the hematologic system. The major function of the blood is to transport necessary nutrients to the cells and to aid in the removal of wastes. The blood also transports hormones secreted by the endocrine system. In addition, the white blood cells (leukocytes) are important in infection prevention. The blood is composed of a variety of substances of which plasma, a straw-colored liquid, makes up about 55% of the total. The formed elements constitute the other 45%. They include the erythrocytes (red blood cells, or RBCs), leukocytes (white blood cells, or WBCs), and platelets (clotting fragments) (Figure 7–1).

Descriptive properties of the blood include its color, volume, viscosity, and pH. Blood is bright red in the arteries due to its oxygen content; blood in the veins is a dark red (often depicted as blue) due to the absence of oxygen. The average adult has about 75 ml/kg of body weight of circulating blood (5–6 liters or approximately 1.5 gallons). The viscosity or density of blood is about three or more times greater than water. Blood is slightly alkaline (pH 7.35–7.45).

The erythrocytes transport oxygen from the lungs to the tissues. The normal erythrocyte count is 4.2 to 6.3 million. Erythrocytes formed in the bone marrow do not reproduce. Erythrocyte production increases when oxygen needs increase. During their life span, which is only about 120 days, red cells become worn and often ragged from bumping and bouncing into the vessel walls of the circulatory system. The worn RBCs are filtered out of circulation by the spleen and liver. These organs are responsible for breaking down the RBCs and saving the iron component for reuse in the development of new RBCs.

Consider This ...

The average-sized human creates and kills approximately 15 million blood cells per second.

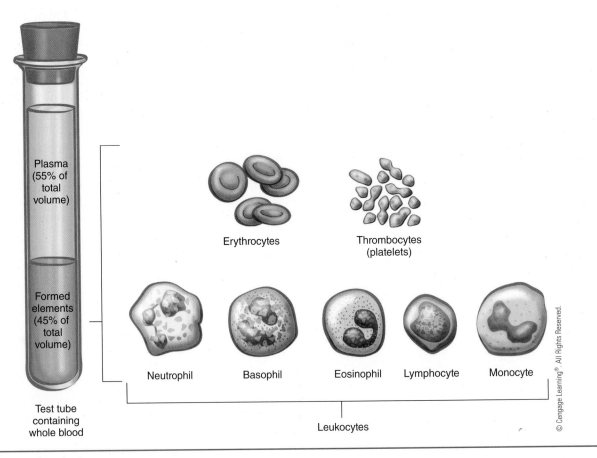

FIGURE 7–1 Blood components.

Hemoglobin, a component of the RBC, is important in the transport of oxygen. A low level of hemoglobin in the blood reduces the level of circulating oxygen. The normal level of hemoglobin for an adult male is 13.5–18 g/100 ml, and 12–16 g/100 ml for an adult female.

Leukocytes protect the individual from infections. The average white blood cell count for an adult is 4,500–11,000/mm^3. A count higher than 11,000 usually indicates the presence of an infection. See Chapter 4, "Inflammation and Infection," and Chapter 5, "Immune System Diseases and Disorders," for more information about leukocytes.

Platelets, also called thrombocytes, produce the thrombokinase used in the clotting process. The average number of platelets in adults is 150,000–350,000/mm^3 of blood.

The plasma portion of blood is composed of 91% water and 9% plasma proteins. The plasma proteins include (1) albumin, responsible for maintaining osmotic pressure; (2) globulin, responsible for infection fighting; (3) fibrinogen, responsible for part of the clotting process; and (4) prothrombin, also responsible for part of the clotting process.

Blood coagulation (clotting) occurs in phases. In the first phase, the platelets, in association with several plasma proteins, agglutinate (clump) at the site of injury or blood loss, and thromboplastin is formed. In the second phase, prothrombin is converted to thrombin in the presence of calcium. In the third phase, thrombin and fibrinogen form fibrin. With the presence of calcium, a fibrin clot is formed. In the fourth phase, the clot is removed through the process of fibrinolysis.

Blood is classified by the antigens in the RBCs and the antibodies in the plasma. The antigens are A and B, and the antibodies are anti-A and anti-B. In addition, a factor called Rh is used in the classification system. (See Chapter 5 under "Erythroblastosis Fetalis" and "Blood Transfusion Reaction" for more information.) Blood is typed as A, B, AB, and O. Type A blood has A antigens and anti-B antibodies, type B blood has B antigens and anti-A antibodies, type AB blood has A and B antigens and does not have anti-A or anti-B antibodies, and type O blood has neither A nor B antigens but has both anti-A and anti-B antibodies. The Rh designation is based on 12 distinct antigens. Rh-positive blood contains this antigen, but Rh-negative blood does not. Because of these designations and blood properties, blood transfusion recipients must have a type and cross-match of blood to be certain a reaction will not occur (Table 7–1).

TABLE 7–1 RBC Blood Donor and Recipient Chart

RBC Donor (Giver)	RBC Recipient (Receiver)			
	O	A	B	AB
O	YES	YES	YES	YES
A	NO	YES	NO	YES
B	NO	NO	YES	YES
AB	NO	NO	NO	YES

YES = This type can receive the donated RBCs.
NO = This type cannot receive the donated RBCs.

© Cengage Learning®. All Rights Reserved.

The blood-forming organs include the lymph nodes, bone marrow, spleen, and liver. The lymph nodes are found throughout the body along the lymphatic vessels. The lymph nodes filter the lymph and produce the lymphocytes and antibodies important for protection from pathogens.

Bone marrow is found in the center part of long bones and in the spongy part of other bones. It is the major blood cell–producing organ in the body.

The spleen is found in the upper left quadrant of the abdomen. It produces lymphocytes, plasma cells, and antibodies and filters microorganisms from the blood. It also removes old blood cells from the body.

The liver is a large organ found in the right upper quadrant of the abdomen. It has multiple responsibilities for many body systems. The liver functions as a blood-forming organ in intrauterine life and is active the rest of the individual's life as a producer of prothrombin and fibrinogen for blood clotting.

Media Link

View an animation on the blood on the Online Resources.

COMMON SIGNS AND SYMPTOMS

Signs and symptoms of this system include those related to increases and decreases in the number of blood cells. Diseases affecting the blood-forming organs (primarily spleen, bone marrow, and lymph nodes) can lead to decreased or increased production of cells. Diseases that hemolyze, destroy, or use up the cells lead to a decrease in cell number and volume.

Erythrocytopenia (erythro = red, cyte = cell, penia = decrease) leads to **anemia** (an = without, emia = blood). Anemia does not mean without any blood; it means low or decreased RBC volume. Signs and symptoms of anemia can be minor or major, asymptomatic to life-threatening, depending on cause. Common signs and symptoms include a low erythrocyte count, headache, fatigue, pallor, and shortness of breath.

Erythrocytosis (erythrocyte = red cell, osis = condition) is a condition of increased RBCs. Common signs and symptoms include a high RBC count, reddened skin tones, bloodshot eyes, increased blood volume and pressure, and an increase in the workload of the heart.

Leukocytopenia (leuko = white, cyte = cell, penia = decrease) is a decrease in white cell count. Leukocytopenia weakens the immune system because these cells are primary players in the defense system. **Neutropenia** (neutrophil decrease) and **lymphopenia** (lymphocyte decrease) can be associated with chronic infection because the numbers are used up during a long-term battle. Signs and symptoms are related to the particular type of infection.

Leukocytosis (leukocyto = white cell, osis = condition) is an increase in white cell count. This condition is a normal response to acute infection. If leukocytosis is related to a tumor, these numbers can be extreme, as in the case of leukemia (leuk = white, emia = blood).

Thrombocytopenia (THROM-boh-SIGH-toh-PEE-nee-ah; thrombocyte = platelet, penia = decrease) is a decrease in platelets, leading to a coagulation problem. Signs and symptoms include small hemorrhages in the skin called **petechiae** (pee-TEE-kee-eye), large areas of bruising or hemorrhage called **ecchymoses** (ECH-ih-MOH-ses), and **epistaxis** (EP-ih-STACK-sis; nosebleeds). Bleeding lesions in the mouth, gums, and mucous membranes are also common.

Thrombocytosis (THROM-boh-sigh-TOE-sis; thrombocyte = platelet, osis = condition of) is an increase in platelets. This condition is uncommon and usually has no serious side effects (Table 7–2).

■ DIAGNOSTIC TESTS

Diagnostic tests for blood and blood-forming organ disorders include complete blood count with differential and indices. Biopsy of the blood-forming organs also can be helpful in diagnosing disorders of the spleen, lymph nodes, and bone marrow.

TABLE 7–2	Blood Cell Abnormalities and Associated Symptoms	
	Condition	**Symptoms**
Red Blood Cells		
Increased	Erythrocytosis	Reddened skin, increased blood pressure, increased workload on the heart
Decreased	Erythrocytopenia	Anemia
White Blood Cells		
Increased	Leukocytosis	Usually asymptomatic
Decreased	Leukocytopenia	Weakened immune system
Thrombocytes		
Increased	Thrombocytosis	Increased clotting
Decreased	Thrombocytopenia	Increased bleeding

© Cengage Learning®. All Rights Reserved.

A **complete blood count** (CBC) identifies the number of RBCs, WBCs, and platelets per cubic millimeter (Table 7–3) and can be used in the determination of most blood diseases. RBC count and indices can assist in the determination of the different anemias, polycythemia, and erythrocytosis. A **differential** is a more detailed count, identifying the number of each type of leukocyte. A WBC count and differential can assist in determination of inflammation and infection or tumors of white cells. **Hematocrit** (Hct) reflects the amount of red cell mass as a proportion of whole blood. **Hemoglobin** (Hgb) reflects the amount of hemoglobin or oxygen-carrying potential available in the blood. Special measurements of red cells are called indices and include:

- **MCV** Mean corpuscular volume; reflects average size of the red cell
- **MCH** Mean corpuscular hemoglobin, or average hemoglobin content
- **MCHC** Mean corpuscular hemoglobin concentration, or average hemoglobin concentration

The morphology of each of the cells and platelets can be observed by performing a blood smear.

TABLE 7–3 **CBC Normal Values**

Cells	Values
Erythrocytes	**Males**
	4.6–6.3 million/mm^3
	Females
	4.2–5.4 million/mm^3
Hematocrit	**Males**
	40–54%
	Females
	38–47%
Hemoglobin	**Males**
	13–18 g/dl
	Females
	12–16 g/dl
RBC indices	
MCV	80–96 mm^3
MCH	27–31 pg
MCHC	32–36%
Leukocytes	4,300–11,000 mm^3
Differential	
Myelocytes	0/mm^3
Band neutrophils	1,500–3,000/mm^3
Segmented neutrophils	300–500/mm^3
Lymphocytes	50–250/mm^3
Monocytes	15–50/mm^3
Eosinophils	15–50/mm^3
Basophils	15–50/mm^3
Platelets	150,000–350,000/mm^3
Reticulocytes	25,000–75,000/mm^3

Key: g/dl = grams per deciliter; MCH = mean corpuscular hemoglobin; MCHC = mean corpuscular hemoglobin concentration; MCV = mean corpuscular volume; mm^3 = cubic millimeter; pg = picograms.

© Cengage Learning®. All Rights Reserved.

A blood smear is performed by placing a drop of blood on a glass slide, smearing it to spread the cells to a thin layer, and staining and examining it microscopically for abnormal cell morphology or shape. Adding a staining solution to the slide helps in the identification of granular and agranular WBCs. A blood smear can be helpful in determining the cause of anemia, especially sickle cell disease.

A **bleeding time** is used to measure the time it takes the blood to clot. It can assist in determining blood disorders such as hemophilia, thrombocytopenia, or disseminated intravascular coagulation, and liver disease, Vitamin K deficiency, or defective clotting factors. Prothrombin time (PT) and partial thromboplastin time (PTT) are often used in conjunction to evaluate both the clotting time and the function of the coagulation factors. The international normalized ratio (INR) is also used to measure bleeding time. It is most often used to monitor the effectiveness of anticlotting medications such as warfarin. It measures the time it takes for blood to clot and compares it to an average.

Biopsy of blood-forming organs can be helpful in diagnosing diseases and disorders. For instance, bone marrow biopsy is performed by boring a needle into the bone of the iliac crest of the hip to obtain tissue that is prepared and microscopically examined. Lymph node biopsy can be performed to determine functioning of the marrow, detect anemias, and diagnose neoplasms.

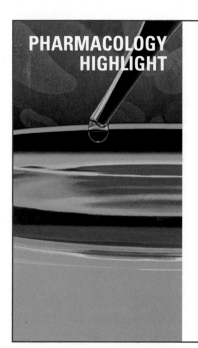

PHARMACOLOGY HIGHLIGHT

Common Drugs for Blood and Blood-Forming Disorders

CATEGORY	EXAMPLES OF MEDICATIONS
Anticoagulants	
Drugs used to prevent clotting	warfarin, heparin, or dabigatran
Antineoplastics	
Drugs used to treat cancer	
Alkylating agents	chlorambucil, cyclophosphamide, or lomustine
Antimetabolites	5-flourauracil, mercaptopurine, or methotrexate
Antitumor antibiotics	mitomycin or streptozocin
Hormones/antihormones	estrogens, androgens, flutamide, or tamoxifen
Other substances	vincristine, L-asparaginase, paclitaxel, carboplatin, cisplatin, or etoposide
Vitamins/Minerals	
Supplements used to support or replace low levels	calcium, chromium, folate, iodine, iron, magnesium, selenium, vitamins A, B$_6$, B$_{12}$, C, D, E, K, or zinc; these may be prescribed individually or in combinations.

COMMON DISEASES OF THE BLOOD AND BLOOD-FORMING ORGANS

The most common problem related to this system is anemia, a decrease in RBC mass that can be caused by a number of different disease processes. Anemia is generally a sign of a disease but is commonly used as a diagnosis until the cause is discovered. Anemia can be serious if the cause is not determined or cannot be corrected.

Disorders of WBCs are usually secondary to other diseases rather than as a primary disease. Infections demand an increased need for WBCs because they are used up while fighting the invader. This can lead to leukocytopenia, a decrease in WBC number.

Any disorders of the blood-forming organs (spleen, bone marrow, and lymph nodes) can lead to secondary disorders of this system. Leukemias, lymphomas, and myelomas are the primary tumors affecting the system.

Disorders of Red Blood Cells

Any increase or decrease in number or size of RBCs will affect the mass or volume. Red cell mass is important because it directly affects the amount of hemoglobin available (oxygen-carrying potential). Commonly, the problem is not enough red cell mass, leading to anemia. Too much red cell mass is called erythrocytosis, the most common type of which is a condition called polycythemia.

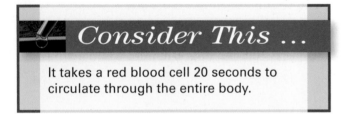

Consider This ...

It takes a red blood cell 20 seconds to circulate through the entire body.

ANEMIA

■ **DESCRIPTION.** Any decrease in oxygen-carrying ability of the RBC is anemia. There are more than 400 types of anemia affecting nearly 3.5 million women and children (Centers for Disease Control and Prevention, 2012), but the three most common types are related to deficiency of iron, folic acid, and vitamin B_{12}.

■ **ETIOLOGY.** Anemia is commonly due to a low number of RBCs or a decrease in hemoglobin in RBCs. Acute hemorrhage or chronic bleeding can lead to a low number of circulating RBCs and, thus, anemia.

Any disease of the liver, spleen, or bone marrow can also lead to anemia. For instance, if the cells are broken down (**hemolyzed**) too soon, this can lead to a decrease in cell number; if cells are not formed quickly enough to replace the worn cells, the number of circulating cells will be low. If cells are formed abnormally, their ability to carry oxygen can be impaired because although the number of cells might be adequate, their oxygen-carrying ability is not. Dietary deficiencies often lead to an inadequate supply of nutrients to make RBCs.

■ **SYMPTOMS.** Despite the cause, the symptoms of anemia are fairly common. The individual suffering from anemia commonly is pale or has a condition of **pallor**. Facial paleness can be difficult to determine, but further examination of the mucous membranes of the mouth and conjunctiva of the eyes will reveal definite paleness. The nail beds also might be noticeably pale in color.

Anemic individuals are weak and suffer from fatigue due to poor oxygenation of muscle tissue. Shortness of breath, **dyspnea** (DISP-nee-ah; dys = difficult, pnea = breathing), **tachycardia** (TACH-ee-KAR-dee-ah; tachy = fast, cardia = heart), and **tachypnea** (TACK-ip-NEE-ah; tachy = fast, pnea = breathing) are common as the heart and lungs attempt to meet the body's oxygen need. Headache, irritability, and **syncope** (SIN-koh-pee; fainting) can also be symptoms.

■ **DIAGNOSIS.** Anemia can be very simple or related to a complicated or chronic disease. For simple cases, a history and physical examination along with blood tests measuring the level of hemoglobin, hematocrit, iron, folic acid, and vitamin B_{12} assist in diagnosis. Microscopic examination of the size and shape of the red cells also provides further clues to the type of anemia.

More complicated anemias, or those caused by chronic disease, might need further testing, including urine analysis, stool sampling, endoscopy, colonoscopy, and bone marrow biopsy.

■ **TREATMENT.** Determining the cause of anemia is very important because treatment is directed at the cause. Therefore, treatment for anemia varies, depending on cause or type of anemia. Some anemias can be cured, whereas others, such as sickle cell anemia, are not curable.

■ **PREVENTION.** Eating a healthy diet including foods high in iron and B complex vitamins will prevent deficiency anemias. More complicated types might not be preventable or treatable.

IRON DEFICIENCY ANEMIA

■ **DESCRIPTION.** Iron deficiency anemia arises when there is insufficient iron for the body to produce the oxygen-carrying component, hemoglobin, within RBCs.

■ **ETIOLOGY.** Iron deficiency anemia can be due to a loss of iron, such as from chronic blood loss, or to an inadequate intake of iron such as from low dietary intake of iron. Chronic blood loss can be due to bleeding hemorrhoids, gastrointestinal bleeding, and heavy or prolonged menstrual flow. Iron deficiency anemia is commonly seen in females during times of increased iron demand as occur during pregnancy and breastfeeding. During their menstrual years, females often have iron loss due to a combination of menstruation and inadequate dietary intake of iron.

■ **SYMPTOMS.** Those symptoms previously described in the anemia section pertain here as well, but, briefly, include pallor, weakness, fatigue, and dyspnea.

■ **DIAGNOSIS.** History and physical examination along with blood tests indicating low levels of hemoglobin, iron, or both assist in diagnosis of an iron deficiency. For cases caused by bleeding, further tests include looking for the presence of blood in urine and stool samples. Gastroscopy and colonoscopy also can help determine the origin of the bleeding.

■ **TREATMENT.** Treatment is aimed at the cause and can include resolving a bleeding problem or increasing dietary intake of iron. Foods high in iron include fruits, green vegetables, lean meat, and whole-grain breads. Iron supplements like *ferrous sulfate* may also be prescribed. With treatment, iron levels are usually restored to normal within 2 months.

■ **PREVENTION.** Deficiency anemia can be prevented by eating a healthy diet high in iron. Anemia related to blood loss can be prevented by seeking medical help at the first sign of excessive bleeding.

FOLIC ACID DEFICIENCY ANEMIA

■ **DESCRIPTION.** Folic acid is a B complex vitamin necessary for the maturation of RBCs. A deficiency in folic acid leads to this type of anemia.

■ **ETIOLOGY.** Deficiency of folic acid can be related to poor diet, overcooking vegetables, or alcoholism. Deficiency can also occur during times of high folic acid need such as those associated with infancy and pregnancy.

■ **SYMPTOMS.** Symptoms can include fatigue, weight loss, abdominal pain, black or bloody stools, and chest pain.

■ **DIAGNOSIS.** Blood testing aids in the diagnosis. CBC will show anemia and abnormally large RBCs. The blood folate level will also be low. Bone marrow biopsy is seldom needed but also will show abnormally large red cell size.

■ **TREATMENT.** Treatment is aimed at increasing dietary intake of foods high in folic acid such as green leafy vegetables, mushrooms, lima beans, and kidney beans. Folic acid supplements may also be prescribed. If there are no complications to treatment, folic acid levels are usually restored to normal within 2 months.

■ **PREVENTION.** Consumption of a diet high in folic acid aids in prevention.

VITAMIN B_{12} DEFICIENCY ANEMIA

■ **DESCRIPTION.** Vitamin B_{12} anemia results from dietary deficiency in B_{12} or inability of the digestive tract to absorb it. Vitamin B_{12} is essential for the body to produce RBCs as well as to maintain a healthy nervous system.

■ **ETIOLOGY.** Inability to absorb B_{12} can be due to several factors, including (1) removal of the small intestine, where B_{12} is absorbed, (2) having a disease that affects the small intestine, such as Crohn's disease, which interferes with absorption, (3) consumption of a diet deficient in B_{12}, or (4) loss or lack of intrinsic factor. This last cause of deficiency is the most common and is also called pernicious anemia.

PERNICIOUS ANEMIA

Pernicious anemia usually affects older individuals and has an unusual cause. The mucosa, or lining, of the stomach normally secretes a protein called intrinsic factor. This factor is necessary for vitamin B_{12} absorption in the small intestine. Those affected have had an autoimmune disorder (a disorder caused by the person's own immune system) that blocks production or destroys the cells that produce this intrinsic factor.

■ **SYMPTOMS.** Common symptoms include pallor, fatigue, weakness, confusion, depression, and numbness in the hands and feet.

■ **DIAGNOSIS.** Vitamin B_{12} deficiencies are diagnosed by a thorough history and physical, CBC, and blood testing for vitamin B_{12}. A history of small-intestine surgery or chronic disease of the small intestine can be recognized easily and diagnosed. Dietary deficiency and pernicious anemia can be more difficult to diagnose and might need further testing, including a gastroscopy (looking through a scope into the stomach) to view the cells that produce intrinsic factor.

■ **TREATMENT.** Treatment depends on the cause of the deficiency. Absorption and dietary deficiency anemia can be treated with oral vitamin tablets, injectable vitamin B_{12}, or consumption of a diet high in vitamin B_{12}. Meat, fish, poultry, and milk are all sources of B_{12}. Pernicious anemia cannot be treated with a change in diet because without intrinsic factor, no amount of B_{12} can be absorbed. Treatment is a monthly injection of vitamin B_{12} for the life of the individual.

■ **PREVENTION.** Anemias related to poor diet can be prevented by eating a diet high in vitamin B_{12}. Pernicious anemia, at this time, is not preventable.

HEMOLYTIC ANEMIA

■ **DESCRIPTION.** Hemolytic anemia is characterized by increased destruction of RBCs.

■ **ETIOLOGY.** This type of anemia can be related to an antigen–antibody reaction as with Rh factor in blood transfusion reaction or erythroblastosis fetalis. (See Chapter 5 for detailed information.) Hemolytic anemia also can occur due to a disorder of the immune system leading to destruction of one's own erythrocytes. This type of anemia can be severe and lead to death of the individual. Hemolytic anemia can be brought on by exposure to chemicals such as benzene; medications, including aspirin and penicillin; and bacterial toxins.

■ **SYMPTOMS.** Symptoms include pallor, weakness, fatigue, and tachycardia, the last of which can lead to heart failure.

■ **DIAGNOSIS.** A thorough history and physical along with blood testing will aid in diagnosis. CBC will reveal anemia. A blood smear will reveal an increased number of immature and fragmented red cells.

■ **TREATMENT.** Treatment can include prompt exchange transfusion (removal of the individual's blood and replacement by donor blood). Steroid medication along with splenectomy can also help. Folic acid and iron supplements may also be prescribed.

■ **PREVENTION.** Hemolytic anemia due to genetic inheritance is not preventable. Acquired hemolytic anemias such as transfusion reactions can be prevented with proper screening.

SICKLE CELL ANEMIA

■ **DESCRIPTION.** Sickle cell anemia is a hereditary anemia, found in the African-American race that causes an abnormal sickle shape of the erythrocyte. Interestingly, sickle cell disease is thought to have developed as a defense mechanism against malaria. The parasite that causes malaria does not grow in cells that sickle, giving these individuals a health advantage in countries where malaria is prevalent.

■ **ETIOLOGY.** The sickle cell has abnormal hemoglobin that causes it to elongate or sickle when deoxygenated (as it loses the oxygen load). The cell regains its normal shape after it is reoxygenated (picks up an oxygen load) (Figure 7–2). The sickle shape causes a problem because it does not allow the cell to travel smoothly through small blood vessels. Sickle cells tend to stick and clump together in small vessels, leading to occlusion of the vessel, ischemia, and infarction. This occlusion can occur in any vessel, causing multiple thrombi (clots) and emboli (traveling clots) formations that can lead to infarctions throughout the body, including the vital organs.

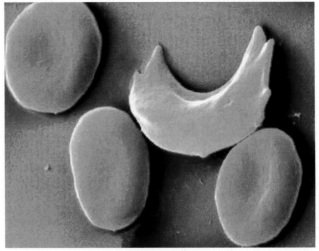

FIGURE 7–2   Sickled erythrocytes.

■ SYMPTOMS. Symptoms of the disease can vary from mild to severe. Pain in the back, legs, and abdomen is the most common symptom. Other symptoms include fatigue, irritability, swollen joints, leg sores, and gum disease. A classic mark of sickle cell anemia is a group of symptoms called sickle cell crisis, marked by episodes of pain in two or more locations. The pain is often compared in severity to cancer pain. This crisis generally occurs any time the body has an increased need for oxygen, so increased activity, physical stress, and illness can lead to a crisis. The crisis itself increases the body's need for oxygen and often sets off a vicious cycle of oxygen demand and sickling of more cells. Individuals suffering severe symptoms often die in infancy or childhood. Few severely affected individuals live beyond age 20, and even mildly affected individuals usually die before age 50.

■ DIAGNOSIS. Diagnosis is made after history and blood testing. Two blood tests determine sickle cell disease. The first is hemoglobin electrophoresis, which measures the amount of normal and abnormal hemoglobin in the blood. The second is the Sickledex® test, which measures the percentage of red sickle cells after mixing a small drop of blood with a deoxygenating agent. A positive test is one in which 25% or more of cells sickle.

■ TREATMENT. There is no cure for sickle cell disease, and treatment is symptomatic. Therapy with hydroxyurea, a drug that increases levels of hemoglobin, and planned blood transfusions have markedly improved the life expectancy of individuals with sickle cell anemia. An increase in fluid intake to twice the normal amount can also help by increasing blood volume and improving sickle cell movement.

■ PREVENTION. Because sickle cell anemia is a hereditary disorder, the only prevention is through genetic counseling and decision by potential carriers to avoid childbearing.

HEMORRHAGIC ANEMIA

■ DESCRIPTION. This anemia is caused by the loss of whole blood and can also be called blood loss anemia. A common complication of losing large amounts of blood is hypovolemic shock.

■ ETIOLOGY. Acute loss of large amounts of blood, which can be caused by such activities as surgery and any trauma or accident involving blood loss, leads to hemorrhagic anemia. Accidents such as motor vehicle accidents and accidental amputations of arms or legs can easily lead to hemorrhagic anemia.

■ SYMPTOMS. Symptoms include pallor, cool clammy skin, tachypnea, and tachycardia. If large amounts of blood have been lost, other symptoms can arise, including dizziness, fainting, and an extreme thirst as a result of dehydration.

■ DIAGNOSIS. Hemorrhagic anemia is easily diagnosed when the blood loss is external. Internal bleeding also leads to hemorrhagic anemia but is often more difficult to diagnose. A history and physical are necessary, and a CBC showing low cell mass, hemoglobin, and hematocrit is indicative of hemorrhagic anemia.

■ TREATMENT. Treatment depends on the severity of the condition. In an acute blood loss, controlling or stopping the bleeding is the primary concern. Applying oxygen immediately to increase the oxygen-carrying capacity of the remaining blood supply is also important. Intravenous fluids and liquids taken by mouth help restore fluid volume. In severe cases of blood loss, a blood transfusion might be needed.

In chronic or slower blood loss anemia, finding the cause and stopping the bleeding are again the primary focus. If the blood loss is not severe, blood fluid will be replaced within a few hours. The decreased number of circulating erythrocytes will stimulate the bone marrow to step up production of them. Bone marrow can replace large numbers of blood cells, thus correcting this type of anemia. Consuming a healthy diet especially high in protein and iron will help restore the body's blood reserves and return it to a healthy state.

■ PREVENTION. Accident prevention and controlling chronic bleeding are helpful in preventing hemorrhagic anemia.

APLASTIC ANEMIA

■ DESCRIPTION. Aplastic anemia is characterized by failure of the bone marrow to produce blood components. A severe decrease or total absence of erythrocytes, leukocytes, and thrombocytes, called **pancytopenia** (pan = all, cyto = cell, penia = decrease), is common.

■ ETIOLOGY. This anemia is due to injury or destruction of the blood-forming area of the bone marrow. Causes include chemotherapy, radiation, viruses, and chemical toxins.

■ **SYMPTOMS.** This decrease in blood cells leads to anemia, infection, and hemorrhage, respectively.

■ **DIAGNOSIS.** Aplastic anemia is diagnosed by using a history and physical examination with blood testing. A CBC will show a low hemoglobin and hematocrit, indicative of anemia. Blood can also be tested for iron and folic acid levels to rule out these types of anemia.

A reticulocyte count test measures reticulocytes, or immature RBCs, and helps determine whether the bone marrow is producing RBCs as it should. In aplastic anemia, the reticulocytes numbers will be low.

Because blood cells are formed inside bone, a bone marrow aspiration or biopsy can also be used. In both of these tests, a large-bore needle or surgical instrument removes small pieces of marrow and bone, respectively. The cells are then examined under a microscope to look for abnormal cells. In aplastic anemia, the red cell production and numbers are low.

Other tests that can be helpful in diagnosis include X-ray, computed tomography (CT) scan, and ultrasound. These tests help rule out cancer, infection, and other types of anemia.

■ **TREATMENT.** Severe cases of aplastic anemia have a poor prognosis, with 50% fatality. Treatment includes discontinuing or avoiding the causative agent. Other treatment might include bone marrow transplantation and blood transfusions.

■ **PREVENTION.** Avoiding causative agents is helpful in prevention, but too often, the causative agent is unknown or unavoidable, making prevention impossible.

POLYCYTHEMIAS

POLYCYTHEMIA (PRIMARY OR VERA)

■ **DESCRIPTION.** Polycythemia is also called primary polycythemia or polycythemia vera. It is a condition of too many blood cells.

■ **ETIOLOGY.** Primary polycythemia is caused by hyperplasia (hyper = excessive, plasia = growth) of the cell-forming tissues of the bone marrow, leading to an increase in the production of erythrocytes, leukocytes, and thrombocytes. This disease has an unknown etiology.

■ **SYMPTOMS.** The increase in erythrocytes leads to an increase in blood volume, which raises blood pressure and causes an increase in the workload on the heart. The spleen, an organ of blood cell storage, is enlarged. The mucous membranes are reddened in color, and the

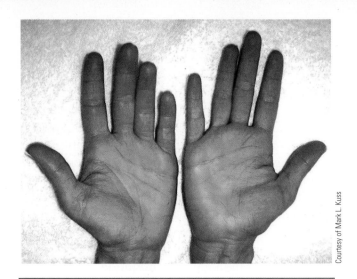

FIGURE 7–3 Polycythemia—reddened palms.

eyes often appear bloodshot. The palms of the hands are noticeably a deeper red color (Figure 7–3).

■ **DIAGNOSIS.** Polycythemia can be accidentally discovered through routine blood testing before a person has any symptoms. Hemoglobin (the protein that carries oxygen in RBCs) will be abnormally high, as will the hematocrit (the percentage of RBCs in the total blood volume). Platelets and WBCs might also be increased.

■ **TREATMENT.** Treatment is to reduce the red cell count and, thus, blood volume. Phlebotomy or removal of blood, such as with blood donation, at regular intervals will reduce the volume and is a common treatment.

■ **PREVENTION.** Polycythemia cannot be prevented. With treatment, symptoms and complications can be prevented or delayed.

SECONDARY POLYCYTHEMIA (ERYTHROCYTOSIS)

■ **DESCRIPTION.** Secondary polycythemia, or erythrocytosis (erythrocyte = red cell, osis = condition of), differs from primary polycythemia in that only red cell numbers are increased.

■ **ETIOLOGY.** Erythrocytosis is a protective mechanism of the body to meet the need for extra oxygen, a normal compensatory mechanism for people who are not getting enough oxygen. It is seen as a positive change in people in high altitudes where oxygen content of air is low. Also, highly trained athletes can have erythrocytosis to meet the high oxygen demands of the body's muscle tissue. Certain respiratory conditions and circulatory conditions cause a decrease in oxygen supply to the tissues and thus stimulate erythrocytosis also. When the conditions calling for extra oxygen are returned to normal, the erythrocytosis disappears. For example, if people living in high altitudes move to a lower altitude, the red cell count will return to a normal level. Smoking, which impairs RBCs' ability to deliver oxygen to body tissues, can cause secondary polycythemia.

■ *SYMPTOMS.* Headaches, weakness, and fatigue are often the first symptoms of secondary polycythemia; lightheadedness and shortness of breath are also common. If the polycythemia is due to disease of the lungs, the face might be reddened and become blue during exercise or other exertion.

■ *DIAGNOSIS.* Following a history and physical exam, diagnosis of secondary polycythemia is assisted by blood testing. Arterial blood gases (ABGs) testing shows the concentration of oxygen in an artery, and low oxygen levels in this test can be indicative of secondary polycythemia. Blood levels of erythropoietin, a hormone that stimulates the bone marrow to produce RBCs, can also be measured. Normal or low erythropoietin levels can indicate secondary polycythemia. X-ray and CT imaging studies also can rule out liver, kidney, or spleen disorders or tumors.

■ *TREATMENT.* Secondary polycythemia is treated by addressing the cause of the disorder. For example, lung disorders such as those caused by cigarette smoking can cause secondary polycythemia; not smoking helps treat the lung condition and improve the secondary polycythemia.

■ *PREVENTION.* In some cases, secondary polycythemia can be prevented by stopping the causative factor or by not doing the things that deprive the body of needed oxygen. Living in high altitudes and smoking, for example, can be avoided or stopped.

Disorders of White Blood Cells

Disorders of WBCs are common problems of the hematologic system. The common symptom of WBC disorders is a compromised immune response, leaving the individual susceptible to infections. Unfortunately, the etiology of most of these diseases is unknown.

MONONUCLEOSIS

Infectious mononucleosis, commonly called kissing disease, is caused by the Epstein–Barr virus. This virus affects lymphocytes, the WBC involved in providing immunity. Symptoms include sore throat, fever, malaise, fatigue, and enlarged lymph nodes. This condition is discussed in detail in Chapter 20, "Childhood Diseases and Disorders."

LEUKEMIA

■ *DESCRIPTION.* Leukemia is a malignant neoplasm of the blood-forming organs (bone marrow, lymph nodes, and spleen). It is characterized by an abnormally high production of immature leukocytes that function abnormally and cause a decrease in the production of erythrocytes and platelets.

Leukemia may be classified as acute or chronic. Acute forms commonly affect children, progress rapidly, and can be fatal. Chronic forms occur more commonly in older adults, are often asymptomatic, and might not be the cause of death. Leukemia is also classified as myelogenous (affecting the bone marrow) and lymphocytic (affecting the lymph nodes).

■ *ETIOLOGY.* The cause of leukemia is unknown.

■ *SYMPTOMS.* Symptoms of leukemia include fatigue, headache, sore throat, dyspnea, bleeding of the mucous membranes of the mouth and gastrointestinal system, bone and joint pain, and enlargement of lymph nodes, liver, and spleen. Infections are common because white cells are not functioning properly. Bleeding disorders and anemia are due to erythrocytopenia and thrombocytopenia, respectively.

■ *DIAGNOSIS.* Leukemia is usually diagnosed by clinical history and blood studies. A bone marrow biopsy is the most definitive test for confirming the diagnosis.

■ *TREATMENT.* Treatment includes aggressive chemotherapy using several neoplastic agents. When the illness is in remission, a bone marrow transplant to replace the neoplastic tissue with normal tissue can be performed. Pain from enlargement of lymph nodes, spleen, and liver can be treated with analgesics. Complete remission occurs approximately 50% of the time, depending on the type of leukemia and the individual's tolerance of the treatment.

■ *PREVENTION.* There is no known way to prevent leukemia, although avoiding toxic chemicals, cigarette smoking, and radiation might prevent some types of leukemia.

COMPLEMENTARY AND ALTERNATIVE THERAPY

Complementary Therapy for Leukemia

The fruit of *Alpinia oxyphylla*, a member of the ginger family, has long been used in Chinese herbal medicine for treatment of nausea and vomiting and overactive bladder. It has also been used for treatment of cancers such as leukemias and inflammatory conditions because it has antiangiogenic properties (inhibits the growth of new blood vessels). A study tested for the antiangiogenic properties of *A. oxyphylla* and found it did have antiangiogenic potential. However, for it to be an effective complementary treatment for leukemia or other cancers, more research needs to be completed.

Source: He et al. (2010).

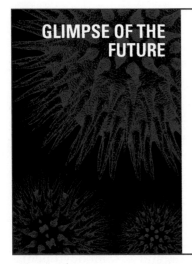

GLIMPSE OF THE FUTURE

New Drugs for Leukemia and Other Cancers

There are many new drugs on the market now for cancer chemotherapy, and many more are being tested and may be available soon. Historically, the therapy did not have much success, but drugs today target specific parts of cancer cells and are improving the survival rates. Successful treatment of some types of leukemia, specifically chronic myelogenous leukemia by imatinib, has increased hope for many other cancer victims. These target-specific drugs are showing promise for treatment regimens for a variety of cancers. However, the high cost of the new cancer drugs may cause intense debate in the health care arena. The cost versus the need for many other health care interventions for a variety of health issues could lead to fewer new drugs being available for leukemia and other cancers in the future.

Source: Peterson (2011).

LYMPHOMAS

Lymphoma refers to several types of neoplasms that affect lymphoid tissue (lymph nodes, tonsils, spleen, and lymph fluid). There are many types of lymphoma, but all affect normal lymphocyte production, leading to impaired immunity. Lymphoma is the most common type of blood cancer in the United States.

HODGKIN'S DISEASE

■ **DESCRIPTION.** Hodgkin's disease is the most common lymphoma. It is characterized clinically by the orderly spread of disease from one lymph node group to another.

■ **ETIOLOGY.** The cause is thought to be viral in nature.

■ **SYMPTOMS.** Lymphoma is characterized by painless enlargement of the lymph nodes in the neck, weight loss, and fever. Hodgkin's primarily affects young adults with an average age of 35 years. Men are affected with Hodgkin's at a slightly higher rate than women.

■ **DIAGNOSIS.** Diagnosis is made when a large connective tissue cell called the **Reed–Sternberg cell** is present in lymphatic tissue (Figure 7–4). The diagnosis can be confirmed by lymph node and bone marrow biopsy.

■ **TREATMENT.** Treatment with radiation and chemotherapy is usually effective in bringing about remission. If the disease is kept in remission for 5 years or longer, complete cure might be possible. The cure rate is about 93%, making it one of the most curable forms of cancer—if it is detected in the early stages. Mortality rate is approximately 20%.

■ **PREVENTION.** Since the cause of Hodgkin's is unknown, there are no known preventive measures.

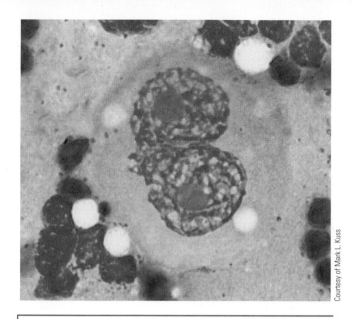

FIGURE 7–4   Reed–Sternberg cell.

NON-HODGKIN'S LYMPHOMA

■ **DESCRIPTION.** Non-Hodgkin's lymphoma (NHL) is a group of lymphomas not containing the Reed–Sternberg cell characteristic of Hodgkin's and more widespread than Hodgkin's. NHL affects older adults more often than Hodgkin's disease, with the average age of 50 years. Men are affected one and a half times more often than women.

■ **ETIOLOGY.** The cause of NHL is unknown, but individuals receiving, or who have received, immunosuppressive medications have more than a 100-times greater chance of developing NHL.

■ **SYMPTOMS.** Usually, there is painless enlargement of lymph nodes in the neck, axilla, and inguinal areas. Other symptoms include fever, night sweats, and weight loss.

■ **DIAGNOSIS.** Diagnosis is made when there is the absence of the Reed–Sternberg cell in lymphatic tissue. The diagnosis is confirmed by lymph node and bone marrow biopsy.

■ **TREATMENT.** Treatment and prognosis depend on the type of NHL, but some combination of radiation and chemotherapy is usually beneficial.

■ **PREVENTION.** Although the cause of NHL is unknown, those at increased risk include those exposed to pesticides, solvents, and fertilizers. Avoiding these risk factors might assist in prevention of the disease.

MULTIPLE MYELOMA

■ **DESCRIPTION.** Multiple myeloma is a malignant neoplasm of plasma cells, or B-lymphocytes, in which the plasma cells multiply abnormally in the bone marrow, causing weakness in the bone and leading to pathologic fractures and bone pain (Figure 7–5).

■ **ETIOLOGY.** The cause of multiple myeloma is unknown. It occurs increasingly with age, peaking in the 70s, and is more common in men. It is one of the most common neoplasms affecting the bone.

■ **SYMPTOMS.** Overgrowth of plasma cells leads to a decrease in other blood components, causing anemia, leukocytopenia, and thrombocytopenia. The breakdown of bone leads to hypercalcemia (hyper = excessive, calc = calcium, emia = blood), excessive blood calcium levels. Antibodies secreted by the plasma cells attach to kidney tubules, causing tissue damage leading to kidney failure.

■ **DIAGNOSIS.** Diagnosis is confirmed by:

■ X-ray exhibiting a honeycombed bone pattern due to tumor involvement.

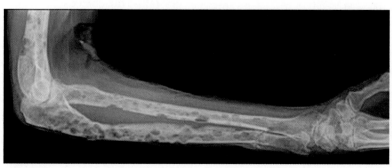

FIGURE 7–5   Multiple myeloma (X-ray)—extensive bone destruction caused by disease.

- Hypercalcemia due to the tumor breaking down bone.
- Evidence of **Bence Jones protein** (a special protein) in the blood and urine.
- A bone marrow biopsy confirming the presence of an excessive number of plasma cells.

■ **TREATMENT.** Prognosis is poor for multiple myeloma. Chemotherapy and radiation are not very effective, and death is usually within 2 to 3 years as the result of infection and kidney failure.

■ **PREVENTION.** Risk factors have been identified as herbicides, petroleum products, heavy metals, and radiation. Avoidance of these risk factors might aid in prevention of this disease.

Disorders of Platelets

Platelet and clotting disorders are varied in terms of cause, severity, treatment, and prognosis. However, they all share the common symptom of bleeding, which might be mild or severe, depending on the particular condition. Many of these disorders of platelets are inherited diseases.

HEMOPHILIA

■ **DESCRIPTION.** Hemophilia refers to a group of bleeding disorders characterized by abnormally slow clotting and long bleeding times. These characteristics make hemophiliacs "love blood" or, more realistically, need transfusions. There are several types of hemophilia, but the most common is type A.

■ **ETIOLOGY.** Hemophilia (hemo = blood, philia = lover) is an X-linked hereditary bleeding disorder. Hemophilia commonly occurs in male children and is passed on to these children, often, by their mother, who is usually asymptomatic and unaffected. Hemophiliacs lack a blood protein that plays a part in clot formation.

■ **SYMPTOMS.** Symptoms of frequent epistaxis (nosebleeds), bruising, and prolonged bleeding in a male child might be indicative of hemophilia. This condition can vary from mild to severe—a hemophiliac might experience severe and prolonged bleeding with a minor injury. Severe hemophilia often leads to **hemarthrosis** (hem = blood, arthro = joint, osis = condition) or bleeding into joints, which is extremely painful, and recurrent episodes often lead to joint deformity.

■ **DIAGNOSIS.** Diagnosis is confirmed by obtaining a detailed medical history, physical examination, and blood testing. Blood tests include measurement of clotting time and the presence of clotting proteins. An extended or lengthy clotting time and low levels or absence of clotting proteins can be indicative of hemophilia.

■ **TREATMENT.** There is no cure for hemophilia. Treatment is aimed at prevention of injury and treatment of symptoms. Whole blood transfusions can be needed along with a concentrated form of the necessary clotting protein.

■ **PREVENTION.** Because hemophilia is an inherited genetic disease, the only way it can be prevented is by genetic testing of possible carriers with the decision not to have children.

THROMBOCYTOPENIA

■ **DESCRIPTION.** Thrombocytopenia, also known as thrombocytopenia purpura, is a decrease in platelets that leads to an inability to clot blood normally.

■ **ETIOLOGY.** Thrombocytopenia can be due to inadequate or abnormal platelet production or destruction. In the case of abnormal destruction, platelet life might be reduced to hours instead of days. The cause of this disorder is frequently unknown. In these cases, the condition may be called idiopathic thrombocytopenia purpura.

■ **SYMPTOMS.** This condition is characterized by abnormal bleeding in the skin, mucous membranes, and internal organs. The skin might exhibit small hemorrhagic spots called petechiae or larger purplish hemorrhagic spots called ecchymoses. This purple coloring of the skin leads to another descriptive term, **purpura** (PER-pew-rah; purplish color of the skin caused by hemorrhaging). Symptoms of thrombocytopenia include gastrointestinal hemorrhages, frequent epistaxis (nosebleeds), and **hematuria** (HEM-ah-TOO-ree-ah; hema = blood, uria = urine, blood in the urine).

■ **DIAGNOSIS.** Diagnosis is made from individual clinical history along with platelet count and bleeding time. A low platelet count and an extended or longer than normal bleeding time can be indicative of the disease.

■ **TREATMENT.** Treatment includes avoiding tissue trauma to reduce the potential for bleeding, administration of vitamin K to improve clotting, and transfusion of platelets. If the disorder persists, a splenectomy might alleviate symptoms because the spleen is the main site of platelet destruction. Splenectomy is usually the last treatment of choice but is very effective.

■ **PREVENTION.** Certain cases of thrombocytopenia might be preventable, but most are not. Two steps that can be taken to prevent complications include:

- Avoiding medications that decrease platelet aggregation or stickiness, thus making them less likely to clot. This includes but is not limited to aspirin and ibuprofen.

- Avoiding heavy drinking because alcohol slows platelet production.

DISSEMINATED INTRAVASCULAR COAGULATION (DIC)

■ **DESCRIPTION.** DIC is a condition of abnormal clotting followed by abnormal bleeding. It is a disease process by which blood starts to coagulate or clot throughout the entire body. This overall clotting depletes platelets and clotting factors, allowing the body then to bleed freely. These two activities set up a potentially catastrophic situation in which the body can have clotting (thrombosis) and massive bleeding (hemorrhage) at the same time.

■ **ETIOLOGY.** DIC usually follows some major trauma such as blood transfusion reaction, surgery, septicemia, complicated childbirth, trauma involving massive tissue destruction, shock, malignancy, or snakebite.

■ **SYMPTOMS.** The individual with DIC might initially have microthrombi in the fingers and toes, turning these extremities blue to black in color, or larger thrombus formation, often leading to life-threatening pulmonary embolism. Lodging of clots in the small and large blood vessels and in body organs slows blood supply, often resulting in organ damage. As platelets and clotting factors are used, other symptoms appear, including oozing of blood, resulting in petechiae; ecchymosis; hematoma and hematuria; gastrointestinal bleeding that causes **hematemesis** (HEM-ah-TEM-eh-sis; hema = blood, emesis = vomiting); blood in the stool; and symptoms associated with anemia.

■ **DIAGNOSIS.** Diagnosis is made on the basis of history of trauma and blood studies. Important blood studies include CBC showing platelet levels, bleeding time, and fibrinogen level (a clotting factor). A positive test for DIC will reveal a decreased number of platelets, increased or long bleeding time, and low fibrinogen levels.

■ **TREATMENT.** Identifying and treating the underlying cause usually stops DIC. In addition to treating the cause, other treatment includes heparin, an anticoagulant medication, to halt the formation of thrombi, and platelet administration to stop hemorrhage or increase clotting ability. This disorder is very difficult to manage because one administers agents both to clot and to prevent clotting at alternating intervals. The condition is usually life-threatening.

■ **PREVENTION.** A preventive measure includes getting prompt medical treatment for any condition that might bring on this disorder.

■ TRAUMA

Any traumatic injury to the bone marrow, spleen, or lymph nodes can lead to a decrease in the production of blood cells. Enlargement of the spleen or splenomegaly can lead to premature breakdown of blood cells, and chemotherapy and radiation treatments affecting bone marrow often lead to symptoms of anemia and infection related to decreased production of red cells and white cells, respectively.

■ RARE DISEASES

Thalassemia

Thalassemia is a hereditary hemolytic anemia that primarily affects people of Mediterranean descent. The RBCs are fragile and thin and form defective hemoglobin. These RBCs do not function normally and lead to symptoms of anemia. One form of thalassemia is called Cooley's anemia, or thalassemia major. This is the most severe form of the disease and presents in childhood.

Von Willebrand's Disease

Von Willebrand's disease is a hereditary, congenital bleeding disorder caused by a deficiency in clotting factor and platelet function. It is also called angiohemophilia and affects females as well as males.

Lymphosarcoma

Lymphosarcoma is a type of lymphoma also known as NHL. Symptoms are similar to those found in Hodgkin's disease and occur more frequently in males of all age groups. Prognosis is good if treatment leads to remission. Without remission, the prognosis is poor.

EFFECTS OF AGING ON THE SYSTEM

Older adults might be more prone to developing diseases of the hematologic system because of the age-related changes occurring in other systems such as the immune or digestive system, leaving them more susceptible to infections and nutritionally related blood disorders. However, total serum iron, total iron-binding capacity, and intestinal iron absorption all decrease with age. Aging does not change the number of lymphocytes, but their functioning decreases to some degree over time.

The most common disorder of the blood in the older adult is anemia. This is not usually due to a defect in the system but rather to poor nutrition (iron deficiency anemia) or inability to absorb the needed nutrients (pernicious anemia). The anemia problem often complicates other chronic diseases of the affected individual.

Some types of leukemia are more common in the older adult. Problems can arise during treatment for the condition due to decreased gastric motility and impaired circulation. These age-related changes can reduce the effectiveness of some therapies and increase the chance of experiencing side effects of the treatment.

SUMMARY

The blood and blood-forming organs (hematologic system) form the body's life fluid by transporting oxygen and nutrients to cells, removing wastes, and helping prevent infection. The main components of the system include the blood, lymph nodes, bone marrow, spleen, and liver. Common signs and symptoms of diseases of the blood and blood-forming organs are fatigue, shortness of breath, bleeding, lesions, pain, and increased susceptibility to infections. The most common disorder of the system is anemia. Although there are several types of anemia, they all have some common symptoms. WBC disorders include mononucleosis and leukemia as the most common. Disorders of platelets include the major bleeding diseases of the blood and blood-forming organs, such as hemophilia. The older adult can develop problems of the hematologic system such as anemia, but it is usually due to other problems or disorders in other systems.

REVIEW QUESTIONS

Multiple Choice

1. Which of the following are major functions of blood? (Select all that apply.)
   a. transportation of nutrients
   b. metabolism of nutrients
   c. removal of wastes
   d. protection from infection
   e. production of lymphocytes
   f. production of erythrocytes

2. Which of the following are common signs and symptoms of disorders of the blood and blood-forming organs? (Select all that apply.)
   a. inflammation
   b. fatigue
   c. shortness of breath
   d. paralysis
   e. urinary frequency
   f. bleeding

g. pain

h. lesions

3. The individual with a bleeding disorder should avoid which of the following activities?

    a. shaving with a straight razor

    b. using mouthwash

    c. eating solid foods

    d. jogging

4. The purpose of the screening test for sickle cell anemia is to determine:

    a. whether the individual is a carrier of the sickle cell trait.

    b. the presence of the sickled hemoglobin.

    c. the severity of the disease.

    d. whether the individual will eventually develop sickle cell anemia.

5. Bone marrow biopsies are performed to:

    a. determine the presence and number of platelets.

    b. diagnose cancers, anemias, and bone marrow functional disorders.

    c. diagnose vitamin B_{12} deficiency.

    d. test for antigens to prevent antigen–antibody reactions.

6. Foods recommended for the individual with a folic acid deficiency would include:

    a. milk and cheeses.

    b. beef and chicken.

    c. green and yellow vegetables.

    d. breads and grains.

7. In which of the following ways does primary polycythemia differ from secondary polycythemia (erythrocytosis)?

    a. The most common symptom of the primary type is shortness of breath, and fatigue is the most common symptom of the secondary type.

    b. The primary type responds to phlebotomy, whereas the secondary type does not.

    c. The primary form of the disease is considered to be a type of cancer, but the secondary form is not.

    d. Both red and white cell numbers are increased in the primary type, but just red cell numbers are increased in the secondary type.

8. Which of the following statements is true about hemophilia?

    a. It is most common in the older adult.

    b. It results in continuous minor bleeding internally.

    c. It is caused by a deficiency of clotting factor.

    d. It is found in male children of mothers who carry the defective gene.

9. Which of the following statements is true about leukemia?

    a. It is considered to be a group of disorders with a cancerous development occurring in the bone marrow.

    b. It is the most common cause of death in young children.

    c. Chemotherapy is ineffective against leukemia.

    d. There are several types of leukemias, but most types are diagnosed in the young or middle-aged adult.

Short Answer

10. List some of the common tests used to diagnose disorders of the blood and blood-forming organs.

11. List some diseases of the blood or blood-forming organs that are transmitted through an inherited trait.

12. Describe the common effects of a hemorrhagic disorder on an individual.

13. Why would an individual with Hodgkin's disease be instructed to avoid individuals with coughs, colds, and fever?

14. What diagnostic test would probably be used to diagnose leukemia?

15. Why are older adults with hematologic disorders more susceptible to infections?

CASE STUDIES

■ Ms. Sloan is a 27-year-old who is complaining of fatigue, shortness of breath, stomach pain, and overall weakness. She is diagnosed with iron deficiency anemia. What could you tell her about this condition? What specific nutritional needs does she have, based on her diagnosis, gender, and age?

■ Joe Butler has a friend who is having surgery and wants to donate blood for his friend in case he needs a transfusion during the surgery. Joe knows his blood type is O positive but does not know his friend's blood type. He asks you to explain to him some details about donating and receiving blood. What should you tell him? Will his blood be compatible with his friend's blood type? Which blood type is considered the universal recipient? Which blood type is considered the universal donor?

Study Tools

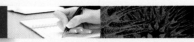

Workbook

Complete Chapter 7

Online Resources

PowerPoint® presentations

Animation

BIBLIOGRAPHY

Adams, K., & Tolich, D. (2011). Blood transfusion: The patient's experience. *American Journal of Nursing, 111*(9), 24–32.

Anionwu, E. (2011). Competence framework for treating sickle cell disease. *Nursing Standard, 25*(28), 32.

Aplastic Anemia and MDS International Foundation. (2012). *www.aamds.org/* (accessed January 2012).

Aschenbrenner, D. S. (2010). Drug watch. *American Journal of Nursing, 110*(10), 28–30.

Bilotti, E., Gleason, C. L., & McNeill, A. (2011). Routine health maintenance in patients living with multiple myeloma. *Clinical Journal of Oncology Nursing, 15*(S), 25–40.

Brown, M. (2010). Nursing care of patients undergoing allogeneic stem cell transplantation. *Nursing Standard*, *25*(11), 47–56.

Brown, S. L., & Faltus, K. J. (2011). Hematologic malignancy education for stem cell transplantation nurses. *Oncology Nursing Forum*, *38*(4), 401–402.

Centers for Disease Control and Prevention. (2012). Understanding blood disorders. *www.cdc.gov* (accessed March 2012).

Clinical digest. Patients with anemia facing blood transfusion would like more information and options. (2011). *Nursing Standard*, *26*(7), 18.

Combating infection: An inside look at infectious mononucleosis. (2010). *Nursing*, *40*(11), 66.

Faiman, B. M., Mangan, P., Spong, J., Tariman, J. D., & the International Myeloma Foundation Nurse Leadership, B. (2011). Renal complications in multiple myeloma and related disorders. *Clinical Journal of Oncology Nursing*, *15*(S), 66–76.

Foster, S. (2010). From herbs to medicines: The Madagascar periwinkle's impact on childhood leukemia: A serendipitous discovery for treatment. *Alternative & Complementary Therapies*, *16*(6), 347–350.

He, Z., Ge, W., Yue, G., Lau, C., He, M., & But, P. (2010). Anti-angiogenic effects of the fruit of *Alpinia oxyphylla*. *Journal of Ethnopharmacology*, *132*(2), 443–449.

Knight, J. (2011). The NHS saved my life. *Nursing Standard*, *25*(29), 18–19.

Koshy, M., Rich, S. E., Mahmood, U., & Kwok, Y. (2012). Declining use of radiotherapy in stage I and II Hodgkin's disease and its effect on survival and secondary malignancies. *International Journal of Radiation Oncology, Biology, Physics*, *82*(2), 619–625.

Leak, A., Mayer, D. K., & Smith, S. (2011). Quality of life domains among non-Hodgkin lymphoma survivors: An integrative literature review. *Leukemia & Lymphoma*, *52*(6), 972–985.

Lymphoma Research Foundation. (2012). *www.lymphoma.org/* (accessed February 2012).

Maloney, K., & Denno, M. (2011). Tumor lysis syndrome: Prevention and detection to enhance patient safety. *Clinical Journal of Oncology Nursing*, *15*(6), 601–603.

Milman, N. (2012). Postpartum anemia II: Prevention and treatment. *Annals of Hematology*, *91*(2), 143–154.

Peterson, C. (2011). Drug therapy of cancer. *European Journal of Clinical Pharmacology*, *67*(5), 437–447.

Smart, M. (2011). Oncology update. *Oncology Nursing Forum*, *38*(6), 739–740.

The KDH Hodgkin's Disease Foundation. *www.hodgkinsfoundation.com/* (accessed February 2012).

The Lives They Loved. (2011). *New York Times Magazine*, 50.

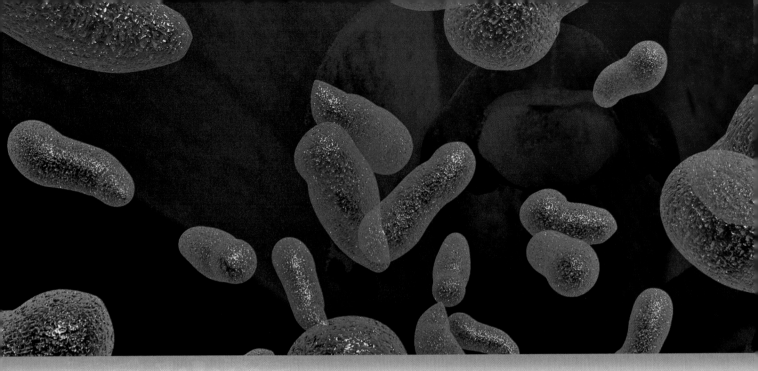

OUTLINE

- Anatomy and Physiology
- Common Signs and Symptoms
- Diagnostic Tests
- Common Diseases of the Cardiovascular System
  Diseases of the Arteries
  Diseases of the Heart
  Diseases of the Veins
- Trauma
  Hemorrhage
  Shock
- Rare Diseases
  Malignant Hypertension
  Cor Pulmonale
  Raynaud's Disease
  Buerger's Disease
  Polyarteritis Nodosa
- Effects of Aging on the System
- Summary
- Review Questions
- Case Studies
- Bibliography

KEY TERMS

Angioplasty (p. 167)
Ankle-brachial index
  (ABI) test (p. 157)
Auscultation (p. 156)
Cardiac catheterization
  (p. 156)
Cardiac palpitations (p. 154)
Cyanosis (p. 156)
Diastolic (p. 156)
Doppler (p. 156)
Electrocardiogram (p. 156)
Embolus (p. 163)
Endarterectomy (p. 165)
Exsanguination (p. 177)

Fibrillation (p. 174)
Hemothorax (p. 177)
Intermittent claudication
  (p. 165)
Ischemia (p. 154)
Lumen (p. 159)
Murmur (p. 173)
Patency (p. 156)
Perfusion (p. 177)
Plaque (p. 162)
Systolic (p. 156)
Tachycardia (p. 154)
Thrombus (p. 167)

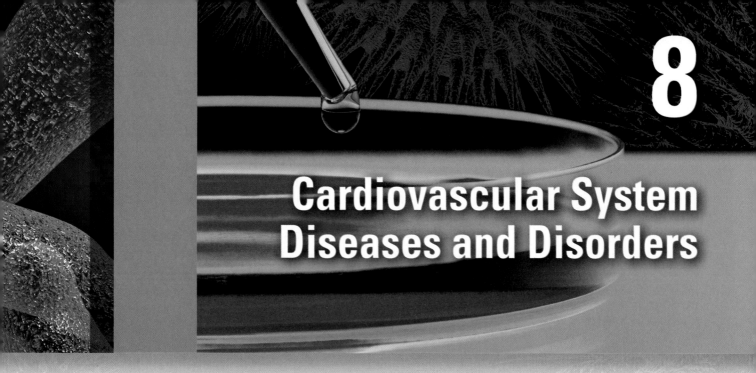

8

Cardiovascular System Diseases and Disorders

LEARNING OBJECTIVES

Upon completion of the chapter, the learner should be able to:

1. Define the terminology common to the cardiovascular system and the disorders of the system.

2. Discuss the basic anatomy and physiology of the cardiovascular system.

3. Identify the important signs and symptoms associated with common cardiovascular system disorders.

4. Describe the common diagnostics used to determine the type and cause of the cardiovascular system disorders.

5. Identify the common disorders of the cardiovascular system.

6. Describe the typical course and management of the common cardiovascular system disorders.

7. Describe the effects of aging on the cardiovascular system and the common disorders associated with aging of the system.

OVERVIEW

The cardiovascular system is often regarded as the major body system because the individual cannot live without a functioning heart and circulatory system. The heart is responsible only for pumping blood, whereas the vascular system transports the blood throughout the body. Disorders of the system often share common symptoms and problems. Other systems are affected when the cardiovascular system is malfunctioning because it is responsible for delivering necessary nutrients and oxygen to the body. Diseases of the cardiovascular system are a major cause of morbidity and mortality in all ages but especially in older adults. Heart disease is also the number one cause of death overall in women. ■

ANATOMY AND PHYSIOLOGY

The heart, arteries, and veins, along with the blood, make up the cardiovascular system. The heart is a four-chambered muscular structure. It is about the size of a man's fist and weighs about 300 grams. The heart is situated approximately in the middle of the chest, slightly to the left, behind the sternum (breastbone). The heart is composed of the cardiac muscle, the chambers, and the valves. The heart is surrounded by the pericardium, a two-layered sac with fluid between the layers. The wall of the heart is divided into three layers. The epicardium is the outermost layer, the myocardium is the middle layer, and the endocardium is the innermost layer.

The four chambers in the heart are the right atrium, right ventricle, left atrium, and left ventricle. The tricuspid valve is between the right atrium and ventricle; the mitral valve is between the left atrium and ventricle; the pulmonary valve is between the right ventricle and pulmonary artery; and the aortic valve is between the left ventricle and the aorta.

Blood enters the heart from the superior and inferior vena cava and then passes through the right atrium and the tricuspid valve into the right ventricle. It then passes through the pulmonary valve into the pulmonary artery and travels to the lungs, where carbon dioxide is exchanged for oxygen. The oxygenated blood returns to the heart through the pulmonary vein and is pumped into the left atrium through the mitral valve and into the left ventricle. It then passes through the aortic valve into the aorta and to the body (Figure 8–1). The heart itself is supplied with blood by the coronary arteries.

Cardiac muscle normally contracts continually throughout one's lifetime. Designated areas of the heart produce electrical stimulation, causing the heart muscle to contract and pump the blood to the body.

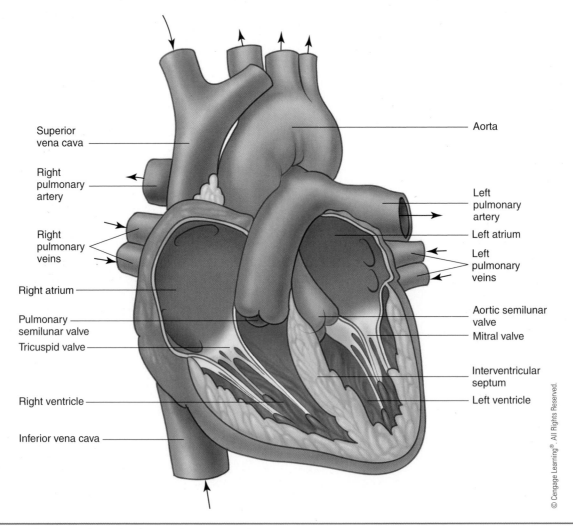

Superior vena cava

Right pulmonary artery

Right pulmonary veins

Right atrium

Pulmonary semilunar valve

Tricuspid valve

Right ventricle

Inferior vena cava

Aorta

Left pulmonary artery

Left atrium

Left pulmonary veins

Aortic semilunar valve

Mitral valve

Interventricular septum

Left ventricle

FIGURE 8–1   The heart: four chambers and great vessels.

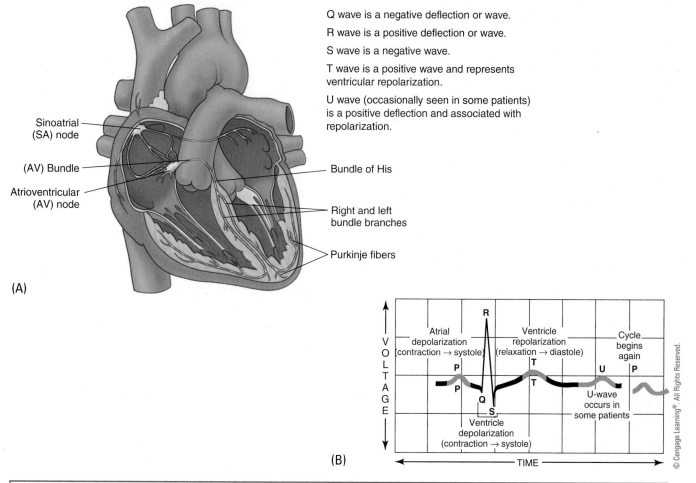

Q wave is a negative deflection or wave.

R wave is a positive deflection or wave.

S wave is a negative wave.

T wave is a positive wave and represents ventricular repolarization.

U wave (occasionally seen in some patients) is a positive deflection and associated with repolarization.

Sinoatrial (SA) node

(AV) Bundle

Atrioventricular (AV) node

Bundle of His

Right and left bundle branches

Purkinje fibers

(A)

(B)

FIGURE 8–2   (A) The conduction system. (B) ECG reading—the PQRST cycle.

This sequence of events is termed the cardiac cycle and begins in the sinoatrial (SA) node, then passes to the atrioventricular (AV) node to the bundle of HIS and the Purkinje fibers (Figure 8–2).

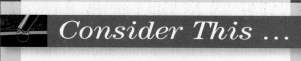

Consider This ...

The heart beats approximately 100,000 times a day, pumping 2,000 gallons of blood with enough pressure to squirt blood 30 feet into the air.

One sequence of the conduction pathway is one cardiac cycle. This is represented on the electrocardiogram as the PQRST cycle. The P wave represents the electrical stimulation beginning and passing over the atria (depolarization). The QRS wave is caused by the stimulation passing over the ventricles. The T wave represents the recovery of the ventricles (repolarization). The cardiac cycle repeats itself approximately 60–100 times per minute in the average adult. One cycle is one heartbeat. The pulsation (heartbeat) felt with the hand over the chest or the fingertips placed over an artery (such as at the wrist or neck) is called the pulse (Figure 8–3). The pulse rate is the number of pulsations felt in a minute. The closing of the heart valves produces the sounds heard when listening with a stethoscope over the heart.

Media Link

View an animation of the heart on the Online Resources.

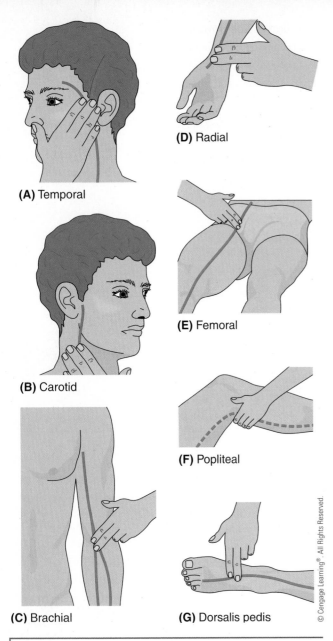

(A) Temporal

(B) Carotid

(C) Brachial

(D) Radial

(E) Femoral

(F) Popliteal

(G) Dorsalis pedis

FIGURE 8–3 Pulse points of the body.

The circulatory component of the cardiovascular system includes the arteries and veins (Figure 8–4). The three major subsystems include the portal unit, the pulmonary unit, and the systemic unit. Each of these circulatory subsystems has special functions in addition to delivering blood to the body. The portal unit, or subsystem, includes the circulation to the stomach, spleen, intestine, and pancreas. Blood from these organs goes through the liver before returning to the heart. The pulmonary subsystem includes the pulmonary artery and its divisions, leading from the heart to the lungs, the circulation through the lungs,

and the pulmonary vein leading from the lungs back to the heart. In this subsystem, nonoxygenated blood from the systemic circulation passes through the lungs, where an exchange of carbon dioxide for oxygen occurs. The oxygenated blood returns to the heart to be pumped throughout the body. The systemic subsystem includes all the arteries and veins and their capillaries not already included in the previously mentioned subsystems. This subsystem carries the oxygen and nutrients to the body cells and removes waste products.

The level of pressure of the blood pushing against the walls of the vessels as it is delivered throughout the body is referred to as blood pressure. Most individuals are familiar with the arterial blood pressure taken with a sphygmomanometer on the arm over the brachial artery. The pressure measured with this instrument is divided into two parts. The systolic pressure, caused by the contraction of the ventricles, is the first number recorded. The second number is the diastolic pressure, reflecting the relaxation of the ventricles. The average adult pressure is 120/80 mm Hg (millimeters of mercury).

COMMON SIGNS AND SYMPTOMS

Common symptoms of heart disease include chest pain, shortness of breath, fatigue, and **tachycardia** (TAK-ee-KAR-dee-ah; tachy = rapid, cardia = heart). Chest pain might be described as a severe, crushing pressure as though someone is crushing the chest, or the pain might be milder and described as a constant feeling of indigestion. Pain also can radiate down the left arm or into the jaw. Shortness of breath is also a common symptom because a lack of oxygen to the tissues stimulates the respiratory system. Individuals with heart disease often feel fatigued and experience episodes of tachycardia. Other symptoms include **cardiac palpitations** (an unusually strong, rapid, or irregular heart rate that is so abnormal that the individual "can feel" it), sweating (diaphoresis), edema in the extremities, and nausea and vomiting.

Pain, edema, and cyanosis are symptoms of diseases of the vascular system. Pain is often associated with poor blood perfusion to the tissues, leading to **ischemia** (iss-KEE-me-ah; lack of oxygen) of the organ. Edema of the extremities is commonly due to poor venous return, leading to congestion of

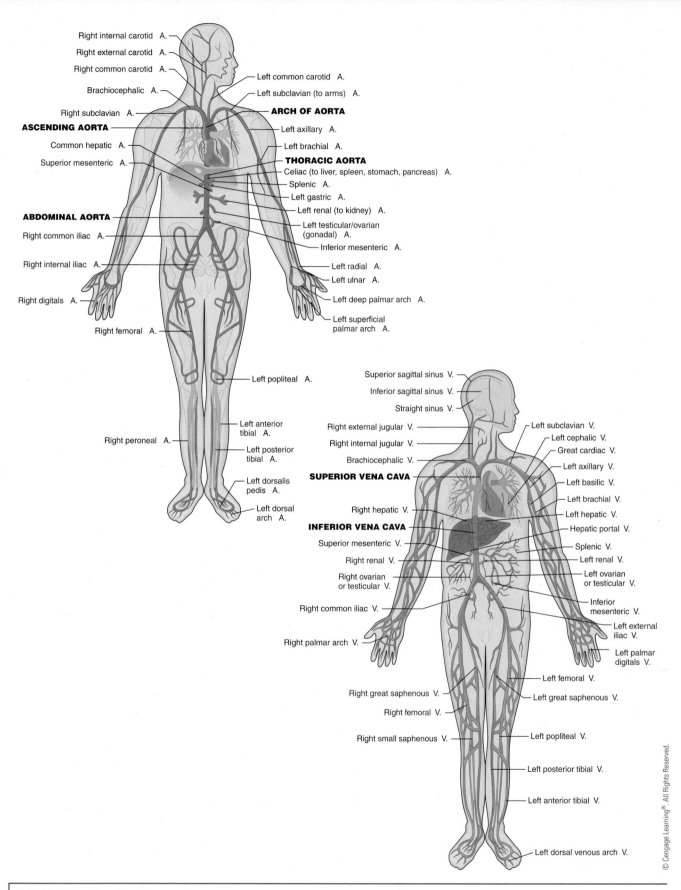

FIGURE 8–4   The circulatory system.

blood and fluids in the tissues. Tissues that lack oxygen often exhibit a characteristic blue color called **cyanosis** (SIGH-ah-NO-sis; cyano = blue, osis = condition).

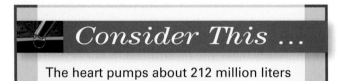

Consider This ...

The heart pumps about 212 million liters of blood in the average lifetime.

DIAGNOSTIC TESTS

Noninvasive procedures of the cardiovascular system involve listening to the heart and movement of blood in the vessels with a stethoscope in a procedure called **auscultation** (AUS-kul-TAY-shun). During auscultation, the stethoscope may be placed on the chest to listen to the heart and over various arteries to listen for blood flow. Murmurs can be auscultated in the heart area and indicate abnormal flow through the heart valves. A **Doppler** device can be placed over arteries to magnify the sound of blood flow. Decreased blood flow can be due to heart disease, vessel disease, or both.

Arterial blood pressure is simply referred to as blood pressure and is measured by a sphygmomanometer, a cuff and pressure gauge used to measure pressure when the heart beats (**systolic**; sis-TALL-ick) and when it rests (**diastolic**; dye-as-TOL-ick). Venous blood pressure is an important measure of the heart's pumping ability and can be determined by examining the individual for edema. Edema in the extremities and distention of the jugular veins in the neck are common indicators of increased venous pressure.

The action of the heart may be drawn or graphed by an electrocardiograph, a machine that receives electrical information and draws a graph of heart action. The picture produced is an **electrocardiogram** (ECG or EKG) (ee-LECK-troh-KAR-dee-oh-GRAM; electro = electrical, cardio = heart, gram = picture). The procedure involving use of a machine to make this picture is called electrocardiography. ECG or EKG is also used as an abbreviation to name the machine and the procedure. ECG is helpful in determining most cardiac diseases.

Use of ultrasound for diagnostic purposes is valuable for both heart and vessel diseases. Echocardiography (ECK-oh-KAR-dee-OG-rah-fee) and ultrasound arteriography (AR-tee-ree-OG-rah-fee) both use sound waves to produce pictures of the heart and arteries, respectively. These procedures are noninvasive.

Positron emission tomography (PET) scanning is a diagnostic test that involves imaging of radioactive positron emission. Prior to testing, a radioactive substance is administered as an intravenous injection. During imaging, different levels of tissue activity and function can be determined, and these images of the body developed by PET scanning can be used to evaluate a variety of diseases. PET scans of the heart assist in determining heart muscle function and blood flow to the heart muscle.

Cardiac catheterization (KATH-eh-ter-eye-ZAY-shun) is an invasive procedure used to sample the blood in the chambers of the heart to determine the oxygen content and blood pressure in the chambers. Cardiac output also can be checked this way. This procedure involves passing a small plastic catheter into the heart through a vein or artery. A vein is used for right-sided catheterization, and an artery is used for a left-sided approach. Vessels of the arms and legs are commonly used (Figure 8–5).

X-rays of the heart and vessels can be beneficial in determining normal structure, size, and **patency**

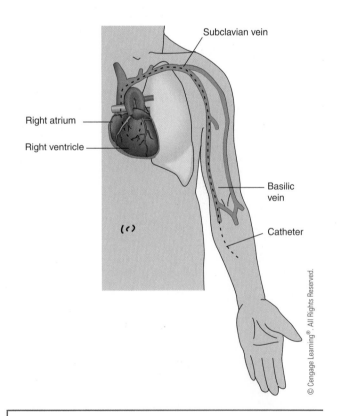

FIGURE 8–5 Cardiac catheterization.

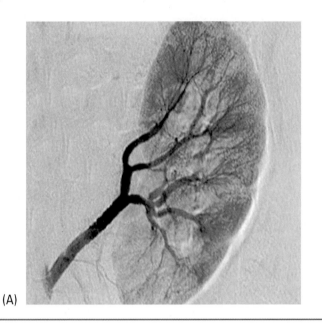
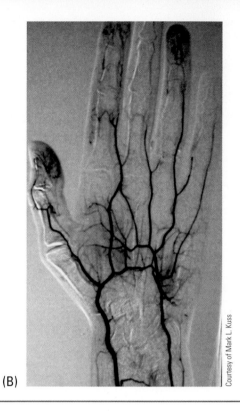

(A)　　　　　　　　　　　　　　　　(B)

Courtesy of Mark L. Kuss

FIGURE 8–6　Arteriogram. (A) Kidney (B) Hand.

(openness). These procedures involve injecting dye into the system and taking pictures of the heart and vessels. Common X-ray procedures include angiocardiography (AN-jee-oh-KAR-dee-OG-rah-fee; angio = vessel, cardio = heart, graphy = procedure), arteriography (arterio = artery, graphy = procedure),

and venography (veno = vein, graphy = procedure). The X-ray pictures produced are called angiocardiograms, arteriograms, and venograms, respectively (Figure 8–6).

The **ankle-brachial index (ABI) test** screens for peripheral arterial disease (PAD) by measuring

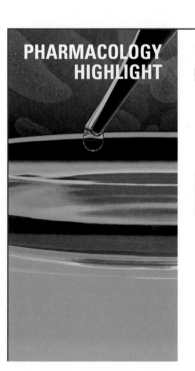

PHARMACOLOGY HIGHLIGHT

Common Drugs for Cardiovascular Disorders

CATEGORY	EXAMPLES OF MEDICATIONS
Antianginals	
Drugs used to treat angina	
Nitrates	nitroglycerin
β-Blockers	atenolol or sotalol
Calcium channel blockers	verapamil or diltiazem
Anticoagulants	
Drugs used to prevent clotting	warfarin, heparin, or dabigatran
Antihypertensives	
Drugs used to treat high blood pressure	
β-Blockers	atenolol or sotalol
Calcium channel blockers	verapamil or diltiazem
Diuretics	furosemide, hydrochlorothiazide, or spironolactone
Angiotensin-converting enzyme inhibitors	captopril or benazepril

(continued)

Common Drugs for Cardiovascular Disorders (continued)

CATEGORY	EXAMPLES OF MEDICATIONS
Angiotensin II receptor antagonists	losartan
Aldosterone antagonists	eplerenone
Vasodilators	hydralazine
α_2 Agonists	methyldopa
Antiarrhythmics Drugs used to treat abnormal heart rhythms	
	procainamide
β-Blockers	atenolol or sotalol
Calcium channel blockers	verapamil or diltiazem
Diuretics Drugs used to treat high blood pressure	furosemide, hydrochlorothiazide, or spironolactone
Vasodilators Drugs used to treat a variety of cardiovascular conditions including such disorders as high blood pressure	hydralazine or minoxidil

the blood pressure at the ankle and in the arm. The result is calculated by dividing the systolic blood pressure in the ankle by the systolic blood pressure in the arm. The normal ABI is 1.0. The blood pressure in the ankle should be the same or greater than the pressure in the arm. Less than 0.9 indicates some narrowing of the blood vessels in the legs, which can lead to PAD.

Blood tests of this system include enzyme studies that assist in determining whether the individual has had a myocardial infarction (MI) (heart attack). As the heart muscle dies, enzymes are released. The enzyme levels help determine the time and degree of the infarction. Common enzyme studies measure the levels of creatine phosphokinase (CPK) and the protein troponin (TnL) lactic dehydrogenase. In the past, lactate dehydrogenase (LDH) was usually measured, but research has shown that cardiac troponin and CPK are more specific.

COMMON DISEASES OF THE CARDIOVASCULAR SYSTEM

Cardiovascular disease (CVD) is the leading cause of death in the United States today (Figure 8–7). Approximately 800,000 people per year die with CVD at a rate of approximately 2,200 deaths per day.

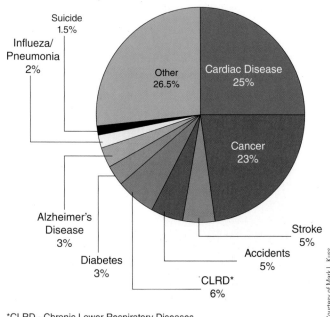

*CLRD - Chronic Lower Respiratory Diseases

Courtesy of Mark L. Kuss

FIGURE 8–7   Mortality statistics comparing cardiac disease to other diseases (Centers for Disease Control and Prevention, 2012b).

Heart disease costs approximately $444 billion a year in health care costs and lost productivity (Centers for Disease Control and Prevention, 2012b). High blood pressure accounts for most of these cases, but coronary heart disease, rheumatic heart disease, and other forms of cardiovascular disease also contribute to these staggering numbers. Education about lifestyle behavioral changes has helped decrease some individuals' risk for CVD.

Diseases of the Arteries

Arterial disorders are the most common among all the CVDs. High blood pressure (hypertension) accounts for the largest incidence of arterial disorders, but coronary artery disease (coronary heart disease) is the leading cause of death overall.

HYPERTENSION

■ **DESCRIPTION**. Most people are familiar with the basic concept that hypertension is high arterial blood pressure. Other concepts include the fact that hypertension is not only a disease process but also serves as an indicator of the development of cerebrovascular, cardiovascular, and kidney disease. Hypertension is a chronic disease affecting one in three American adults (National Heart, Lung, and Blood Institute, 2012b). It is the leading cause of stroke and heart failure. Life expectancy in all individuals, regardless of age or sex, is reduced when diastolic hypertension is greater than 90 mm Hg.

Blood pressure varies from individual to individual, but average adult blood pressure is considered to be less than 120/80 mm Hg. The top number (120) is the systolic pressure and measures the highest amount of pressure in the artery when the ventricles of the heart contract. The lower number is the diastolic pressure and measures the artery pressure when the ventricles relax. If one could view the arteries as the heart beats, one would see a wavelike pattern of blood flow related to the heart beating and resting (Figure 8–8). Medical parameters for diagnosing high blood pressure start with prehypertension at levels above 120/80. Stage I hypertension is recognized when the level reaches 140/90, and stage II begins with a blood pressure of 160/100 or greater.

In addition to heartbeat, blood vessel resistance also helps determine blood pressure. One might compare the heart and vessels to a water pump and hose: the amount of water being pumped and the width of the hose help determine the amount of water flow or water pressure. In the same way, the amount of blood the heart pumps and the resistance of the vessel, or

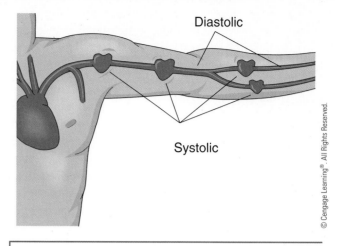

FIGURE 8–8 Systolic and diastolic blood pressure.

size of the **lumen** (LOO-men; inner open space or width), will help determine blood pressure. The larger the lumen or the more patent the vessel, the easier it is for the heart to pump blood and, generally speaking, the lower the blood pressure.

Specialized nerve receptors in the body help control pressure by bringing about vasoconstriction and vasodilation at appropriate times. For example, when an individual stands up suddenly, the blood pressure to the head drops, often causing momentary dizziness. To correct this situation, nerves react and constrict blood vessels, raising blood pressure and restoring normal pressure in the head. If blood pressure is too high, these nerve receptors dilate vessels leading to the kidneys. This increased blood flow leads to greater urine formation and output. Increased urine production decreases blood volume and thus lowers blood pressure. In this way, the kidneys play a vital role in blood pressure. If pressure is too low— as often occurs in shock—blood flow to the kidneys is diminished, urine output is minimal, blood fluid is maintained, and blood pressure is maintained or restored.

■ **ETIOLOGY**. Because blood pressure and the kidneys have such a close relationship, any disease of the kidneys can cause an alteration in blood pressure, and any change in blood pressure can have an adverse effect on the kidneys. The kidneys play a vital role in elimination of salt and water, two substances that also have a great effect on blood pressure. Retention of salt and water increases blood pressure, whereas elimination of these substances reduces blood pressure. Hypertension caused by kidney disease or some other type of disease process is called secondary

COMPLEMENTARY AND ALTERNATIVE THERAPY

Aromatherapy for Hypertension

Research studies on the use of aromatherapy for treating hypertension were reviewed for evidence of the effectiveness of this method of treatment. Some of the studies reported that aromatherapy was effective in lowering systolic and diastolic blood pressure. However, whether this therapy would work on most patients with hypertension was not determined. The summary of the systematic review of the research studies reported that there was not enough solid evidence of the positive effects of aromatherapy to support it for treatment of hypertension. It was recommended that further research on this treatment modality be conducted.

Source: Hur et al. (2012).

hypertension. Only 10% of all hypertensive cases are due to secondary problems.

Primary or essential hypertension accounts for approximately 90% of all hypertensive cases. This type of hypertension is idiopathic, or due to an unknown cause, and usually has a gradual onset over a number of years.

Some identified genetic and environmental risk factors are known to cause primary hypertension. These include:

- **Heredity** Hypertension affects black individuals twice as often as whites.

- **Diet** High salt and fat intake increases the risk of hypertension.

- **Age** Blood pressure tends to rise with age.

- **Obesity** Obesity causes an increased workload on the heart.

- **Smoking** Nicotine causes vasoconstriction.

- **Stress** Stress causes a rise in blood pressure due to vasoconstriction.

- **Type A personality traits** This type of personality tends to experience more stress.

■ **SYMPTOMS**. Symptoms usually do not occur until significant heart and vessel damage has already occurred. If left untreated, high blood pressure overworks the heart. Because the left ventricle works harder to pump blood, it is the area most often affected, leading to left ventricle hypertrophy (muscle enlargement). The vascular system, or blood supply, to the left ventricle does not increase with this enlargement of muscle, so this extra tissue does not

have adequate blood supply, often leading to bouts of angina or chest pain due to ischemia. This condition often leads to MI, or heart failure, and death.

Hypertension not only affects the heart but also adversely affects the vessels. Over a period of years, the vessels become hardened (sclerotic) and lose elasticity, a contributing factor in arteriosclerosis (arterio = artery, scler = hardened, osis = condition of). Sclerotic (hardened) vessels are also more likely to form thrombi and to rupture, which can cause damage or death to the involved organs.

■ **DIAGNOSIS**. Blood pressure screening is very important in diagnosing hypertension before the cardiovascular system is damaged. A random blood pressure of greater than 140/90 might be physiologic; thus, screening with frequent blood pressure readings under varied conditions is needed to confirm the diagnosis.

Further evaluation for hypertension consists primarily of:

1. Taking a medical and family history because hypertension tends to run in families.

2. Completing a physical examination.

3. Testing blood for:
   - Cholesterol: should be under 200
   - LDL (low-density lipoprotein—bad cholesterol): should be under 100
   - HDL (high-density lipoprotein—good cholesterol): should be over 60
   - Triglycerides (tri-GLISS-er-ides—stored energy in the cells): should be under 200

4. ECG to test the action of the heart.

Several other blood tests can be used to check kidney dysfunction, which can also cause high blood pressure.

■ *TREATMENT*. Treatment of hypertension depends on the degree of hypertension and the number of risk factors involved. If blood pressure is extremely high, antihypertensive medications might be prescribed immediately. If hypertension is discovered in a milder form, lifestyle changes or reduction of risk factors might be the initial treatment. A low-salt, low-fat diet; stress-reducing exercise; and smoking cessation might solve the problem. (See Healthy Highlight box Prevention of Hypertension and Cardiovascular Disease.)

If this treatment is ineffective or inadequate, the individual might be placed on diuretic medications. Diuretics increase urine output, thus lowering blood pressure. If further control is needed, other antihypertensive medications can be prescribed. Patient compliance with hypertension treatment is often a factor in addressing this chronic disease. Lifestyle changes and following the medication regimen for the rest of one's life are often difficult for the individual to manage.

■ *PREVENTION*. The Mayo Clinic (2012) suggests that lifestyle changes, such as those listed in the following Healthy Highlight, can aid in prevention of hypertension and cardiovascular disease.

HEALTHY HIGHLIGHT

Prevention of Hypertension and Cardiovascular Disease

To help reduce the risk of developing hypertension and CVD, practice the following lifestyle behaviors.

1. **Lose extra pounds and watch your waistline**.
   Losing just 10 pounds can help reduce blood pressure. Carrying too much weight increases the risk of high blood pressure. In general, men are at risk if their waist measurement is greater than 40 inches, and women are at risk if their waist measurement is greater than 35 inches.

2. **Exercise regularly**.
   Regular physical activity—at least 30 to 60 minutes most days of the week—can lower blood pressure by 4 to 9 mm Hg often within a few weeks. Even moderate activity for 10 minutes at a time, such as walking and light strength training, can help. Avoid being a "weekend warrior." Trying to squeeze all exercise in on the weekends to make up for weekday inactivity isn't a good strategy. Those sudden bursts of activity could actually be risky. Consult a physician before beginning any exercise program.

3. **Eat a healthy diet**.
   Eating a diet that is rich in whole grains, fruits, vegetables, and low-fat dairy products and limits saturated fat and cholesterol can lower blood pressure by up to 14 mm Hg.

4. **Reduce salt (sodium) in your diet**.
   Small reductions in dietary sodium can reduce blood pressure by 2 to 8 mm Hg. Daily intake of sodium should be 1,500 to 2,300 mg per day depending on age and health. To reach these goals one may need to:
   - **Read food labels**. If possible, choose low-sodium alternatives of the foods and beverages you normally buy.
   - **Eat fewer processed foods**. Potato chips, frozen dinners, bacon, and processed lunch meats are high in sodium.
   - **Don't add salt**. Just 1 level teaspoon of salt has 2,300 mg of sodium. Use herbs or spices, rather than salt, to add more flavor to your foods.

(continued)

5. **Limit alcohol consumption**.

   A small amount of alcohol can potentially lower blood pressure by 2 to 4 mm Hg. But that protective effect is lost if too much alcohol is consumed—generally more than one drink a day for women and men older than age 65, or more than two a day for men age 65 and younger. Drinking more than a moderate amount can raise blood pressure by several points and reduce the effectiveness of high blood pressure medications.

6. **Avoid tobacco products and secondhand smoke**.

   On top of all the other dangers of smoking, the nicotine in tobacco products can raise blood pressure by 10 mm Hg or more for up to an hour. Smoking throughout the day means blood pressure may remain constantly high. Inhaling smoke from others (secondhand smoke) increases risk of health problems, including high blood pressure and heart disease.

7. **Reduce your stress**.

   Stress or anxiety can temporarily increase blood pressure. Identify causes of stress such as work, family, finances, or illness. Once the cause is identified, consider how to eliminate or reduce stress. Stress reduction activities and support groups may also be beneficial.

8. **Monitor blood pressure at home and make regular doctor's appointments**.

   For those with high blood pressure, home monitoring is recommended. Consult a physician about home monitoring before getting started. Keep all physician follow-up appointments to assure medications and activities are effective.

9. **Get support from family and friends**.

   Supportive family and friends can help improve one's health. Encouragement and support with self-care, physician visits, and exercise programs may improve chances of success.

ARTERIOSCLEROSIS AND ATHEROSCLEROSIS

■ **DESCRIPTION**. Arteriosclerosis is a group of diseases that are characterized by a loss of elasticity and a thickening of the artery wall. Atherosclerosis is the most common form of arteriosclerosis. For this reason, these terms are often used interchangeably; *hardening of the arteries* is a lay term describing this condition. The common result of arteriosclerosis is the gradual narrowing of the vessel lumen (Figure 8–9). This narrowing leads to a slowing or complete stoppage of blood flow to the organs supplied by those vessels. Without proper blood supply, these organs become ischemic and eventually might die if blood supply is not restored.

An artery has a very smooth endothelium (inner lining), like a nonstick finish. As with nonstick cookware, food particles normally do not stick to the surface. If the endothelium is damaged, however, blood material begins sticking to the inner lining of the artery just as food particles begin sticking to scratched cookware. The artery wall surrounds this endothelium. Atherosclerosis is a condition characterized by deposits of fatty or lipid material in the wall of the artery (see Figure 8–9). These fatty, cholesterol-containing deposits, called **plaque**, damage the artery and interrupt blood flow by:

■ Pushing into the endothelium, thus damaging the inner lining. Damage to this lining allows blood material to stick to the inner lining and occlude the lumen.

■ Causing the artery wall to harden or lose elasticity. This loss of elasticity increases blood pressure and

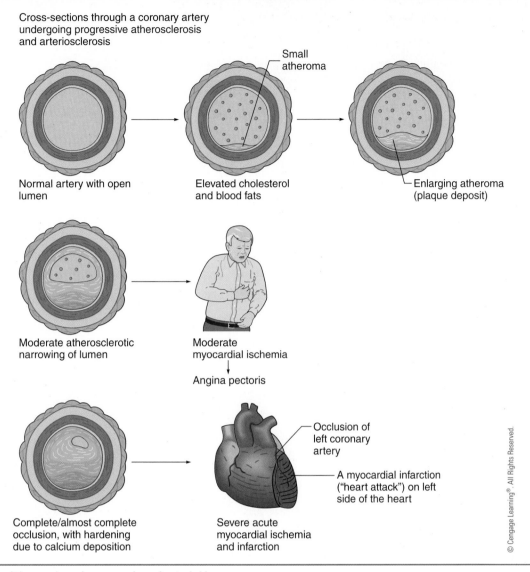

Cross-sections through a coronary artery undergoing progressive atherosclerosis and arteriosclerosis

Small atheroma

Normal artery with open lumen

Elevated cholesterol and blood fats

Enlarging atheroma (plaque deposit)

Moderate atherosclerotic narrowing of lumen

Moderate myocardial ischemia

Angina pectoris

Occlusion of left coronary artery

A myocardial infarction ("heart attack") on left side of the heart

Complete/almost complete occlusion, with hardening due to calcium deposition

Severe acute myocardial ischemia and infarction

FIGURE 8–9   Atherosclerosis: narrowing of arterial lumen.

increases workload on the heart. A hardened vessel is not able to expand and accommodate the surge of blood caused by the beat of the heart.

- Thickening the artery wall to the point that the lumen is partially or completely occluded.

- Leading to formation of plaque that often ulcerates or breaks loose, forming an **embolus** (EM-boh-lus; material floating in the blood) that can stick in a vessel and occlude or stop blood flow, leading to ischemia or death of the organs supplied by that vessel.

Narrowing of the lumen of the artery in all the aforementioned ways increases blood pressure, increases workload on the heart, and decreases blood supply to the organs. Increased blood pressure stretches the hardened arteries, causing further artery damage and further increasing workload on the heart.

Atherosclerosis can affect all arteries in the body, but four major areas are often affected by atherosclerosis, many times leading to disability or mortality (Figure 8–10).

These major areas affected are the following:

1. **Coronary arteries** These arteries feed the muscle tissue of the heart. Atherosclerosis of these arteries leads to coronary artery disease, also called coronary heart disease. Consequences of coronary artery disease can include MI (heart attack).

Affected site   **Potential complication**

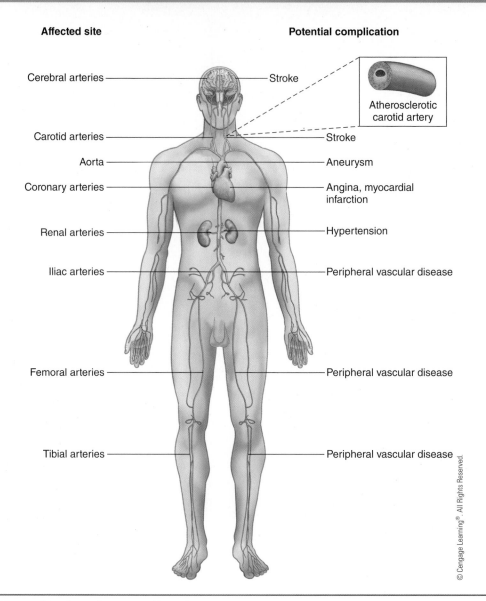

FIGURE 8–10 Atherosclerosis: major areas affected.

2. **Cerebral arteries** These arteries feed brain tissue. Atherosclerosis of these arteries can lead to a cerebrovascular accident (CVA), commonly called a stroke.

3. **Aorta** This artery is the largest artery in the body and is responsible for carrying blood to the general circulatory system. Atherosclerosis of this artery in any area can lead to aneurysms.

4. **Peripheral arteries** Peripheral arteries primarily feed the extremities (arms and legs). Atherosclerosis of these arteries can lead to peripheral vascular disease.

■ *ETIOLOGY.* The cause of atherosclerosis is unknown, but it is thought to be the result of a combination of

factors, some of which are not controllable, but many are and can be altered by a change in lifestyle. Important risk factors include the following:

NONCONTROLLABLE FACTORS

■ **Heredity** Atherosclerosis appears to run in families. This might be related to common diet or, in some instances, a clear genetic tendency to develop hypercholesterolemia (hyper = increased, cholesterol, emia = blood).

■ **Age** Atherosclerosis is considered a degenerative disease because all adults over the age of 30 have some degree of plaque formation. In general, the older the person, the more atherosclerosis is present.

- **Sex** Men have more atherosclerosis present than women until after female menopause, at which time, the incidence becomes more equal.

- **Diabetes** Individuals with diabetes have more existing atherosclerosis than those who do not have diabetes. However, if their diabetes is type 2 and related to obesity, it is considered to be a controllable factor.

CONTROLLABLE FACTORS

- **Diet** Obese individuals have more atherosclerosis present than individuals in the normal weight range. The higher the diet in carbohydrates and fats, the higher is the incidence of atherosclerosis.

- **Sedentary lifestyle** Lack of exercise increases the risk of development of atherosclerosis.

- **Cigarette smoking** This is one of the most important risk factors. Stopping smoking is 10 times more effective in reducing risk than a combination of exercise and diet control.

- **Stress** Stress increases blood pressure, but research does not support the idea that stress increases atherosclerosis.

- **Hypertension** The higher the blood pressure, the greater is the risk for development of atherosclerosis. It is difficult to determine which of these diseases occurs first. Atherosclerosis causes an increase in blood pressure, and hypertension leads to an increase in atherosclerosis. Often, hypertension and atherosclerosis occur simultaneously, each complicating the treatment of the other.

■ **SYMPTOMS**. Symptoms of atherosclerosis appear late in the disease process and vary, depending on the area affected.

■ **DIAGNOSIS**. Diagnosis of atherosclerosis is by blood pressure measurement, arteriograms, and X-ray. Doppler studies to determine blood flow also can be used.

■ **TREATMENT**. Treatment is aimed at reducing symptoms as they arise. Surgery to open the artery and remove plaque may be used. This surgical treatment is called **endarterectomy** (END-ar-ter-ECK-toh-me; endo = inside, arter = artery, ectomy = excision). If the artery is damaged, it might be bypassed with a graft.

■ **PREVENTION**. Prevention of atherosclerosis includes exercise, estrogen medication after menopause, and changing lifestyle to reduce risk factors. Detailed methods are discussed in the Healthy Highlight box Prevention of Hypertension and Cardiovascular Disease.

PERIPHERAL VASCULAR DISEASE (PVD)

■ **DESCRIPTION**. PVD refers to any disease of arteries or veins peripheral, or outside, the heart and head. By far, the most common PVD is peripheral artery (not venous) disease (PAD). Both PVD and PAD are commonly caused when vessels are partially or completely occluded or stopped up by arteriosclerotic plaque. This common connection between PVD and PAD often leads to an interchangeable use of these two terms.

PAD affects more than 8 million Americans, and it becomes more common with age, but the main risk factor is smoking (National Heart, Lung, and Blood Institute, 2012a). While PAD may affect the arteries of the arms, kidneys, and stomach, it more commonly affects the legs.

■ **ETIOLOGY**. PVD and PAD are caused by atherosclerotic plaque, primarily in the arteries supplying blood to the legs. This occlusion by plaque can be chronic or acute. Chronic occlusion is generally related to a progressive narrowing of the femoral and popliteal arteries. As these arteries become occluded, the blood supply to the leg muscles is decreased. Having PAD usually indicates the potential for arterial disease involving the coronary arteries within the brain.

■ **SYMPTOMS**. Individuals with PVD have adequate blood supply to leg muscles during minimal activity such as sitting or slow walking. If activity is increased to brisk walking or running, blood supply becomes inadequate, causing leg muscle cramps. Resting the legs will relieve the muscle cramps and allows the muscles once again to receive the needed amount of blood flow. This condition of developing muscle cramps that are relieved with rest and increase with activity is called **intermittent claudication** (KLAW-dih-KAY-shun).

■ **DIAGNOSIS**. Diagnosis is critical because people with PVD have four to five times the risk of heart attack and stroke (American Heart Association, 2011). The classic symptom of PAD is intermittent claudication. Other tests include:

- Feeling for a pulse in the foot. A Doppler flow probe can quickly pick up a pulse if one is present.

- ABI (the measurement of the blood pressure in the arm compared to the blood pressure in the leg).
- A treadmill test to attempt to induce intermittent claudication.
- Angiography and magnetic resonance imaging (MRI) to determine location and thickness of the atherosclerosis (plaque).

■ **TREATMENT.** Treatment for PAD includes management of leg pain and stopping the progression of the atherosclerosis. These goals may be accomplished with lifestyle changes. A physician-prescribed walking program may not only increase the distance walked, but also improve the body's use of oxygen. These improvements in general physical condition may decrease or eliminate the associated leg pain. People who smoke may be able to accomplish these goals by not smoking because this is the single most important lifestyle change.

If further treatment is needed, it may include medication to prevent blood clots, lower blood pressure and cholesterol, and control pain. If these treatments are ineffective, angioplasty or bypass surgery may be necessary. Chronic occlusion of the artery may be treated with a femoral popliteal bypass graft.

■ **PREVENTION.** Risk can be reduced by following the guidelines in the Healthy Highlight box Prevention of Hypertension and Cardiovascular Disease.

Acute occlusion of the peripheral arteries often involves smaller arteries supplying blood to the feet and toes. This decrease in blood supply may cause ulcers on the feet and toes, sores that do not heal, gangrene, or infections in the extremities. In some cases, amputation may be necessary.

ANEURYSM

■ **DESCRIPTION.** Aneurysm (AN-you-rizm) is a weakening in the wall of an artery that allows the vessel to bulge or rupture (Figure 8–11).

■ **ETIOLOGY.** This weakening is often due to atherosclerosis but also might be due to a congenital defect or injury.

■ **SYMPTOMS.** Aneurysms are usually asymptomatic and are often discovered accidentally during physical examinations or X-rays. The most common area affected is the abdominal aorta. Rupture of an aneurysm is a medical emergency, often causing death due to massive hemorrhage and shock.

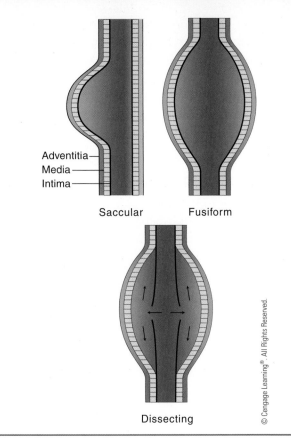

FIGURE 8–11   Three types of aneurysm.

■ **DIAGNOSIS.** A thorough physical examination can lead to the discovery of an aortic aneurysm. Placing a stethoscope on the abdomen allows a physician to hear the abnormal blood flow through the artery. Smaller aneurysms and those located in other areas are more difficult to hear and might be discovered by angiogram. Other diagnostic tests include computerized tomography (CT) and MRI scans.

■ **TREATMENT.** Treatment is aimed at repairing the aneurysm before rupture. Surgical resection and grafting are commonly performed (Figure 8–12).

■ **PREVENTION.** Preventing atherosclerosis and hypertension aids in prevention of aneurysm. Congenital aneurysms cannot be prevented.

CORONARY ARTERY DISEASE

■ **DESCRIPTION.** Coronary artery disease (CAD), often called coronary heart disease (CHD), is the narrowing of arteries that supply blood to the myocardium, the heart muscle. It is the leading cause of death in the United States today.

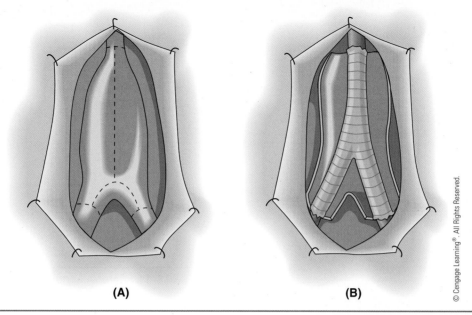

FIGURE 8–12 Abdominal aneurysm surgical resection (A) and grafting (B).

■ *ETIOLOGY*. This disease is commonly due to atherosclerosis.

■ *SYMPTOMS*. Progressive or slow narrowing of the arteries leads to ischemia of the heart muscle and symptoms of angina. Some muscle cells can actually die and be replaced with scar tissue. This scar tissue cannot function like muscle tissue, causing an increase in the workload of the remaining heart muscle. Congestive heart failure often results.

If a coronary artery becomes blocked to the point that heart muscle oxygen demands cannot be met, the heart muscle dies. Occlusion can progress slowly as plaque builds up in the vessel, or it can develop suddenly as the result of a **thrombus** (THROM-bus; a blood clot attached to a vein or artery) or embolus (traveling blood clot, free in the circulatory system, more dangerous than a thrombus). This dead muscle is called an infarct or myocardial infarct. The process of the myocardium dying is called MI.

Slow, progressive occlusion of the arteries often leads to development of collateral arteries that extend into ischemic tissue. Collateral circulation provides some protection against ischemia and infarction. For this reason, infarction caused by slow occlusion often has a better outcome than infarction caused by sudden occlusion of a vessel.

■ *DIAGNOSIS*. Diagnosis of CAD is made from a history of symptoms, ECG, and angiograms. Symptoms usually do not develop until the vessels are at least 70% occluded.

■ *TREATMENT*. Treatment of CAD is aimed at increasing blood flow or decreasing oxygen needs. Angina is often treated with rest and vasodilators. A coronary artery **angioplasty** (AN-jee-oh-PLAS-tee; angio = vessel, plasty = surgical repair) might be attempted to open the vessel by passing a catheter into the artery and inflating a balloon on the catheter to push the plaque against the vessel wall, thus widening the lumen of the vessel (Figure 8–13). Another common surgical treatment for CAD is a coronary artery bypass graft, commonly called a CABG (pronounced cabbage). This procedure bypasses the occlusion (Figure 8–14). Mammary vessels from the breast area and saphenous vessels from the legs are often used for the bypass.

■ *PREVENTION*. It is very important for individuals with CAD to reduce atherosclerotic risk factors. Diet, exercise, and a no-smoking regimen are prescribed to slow the progression of the disease.

Diseases of the Heart

Diseases of the heart are frequently due to the atherosclerotic narrowing of the coronary arteries.

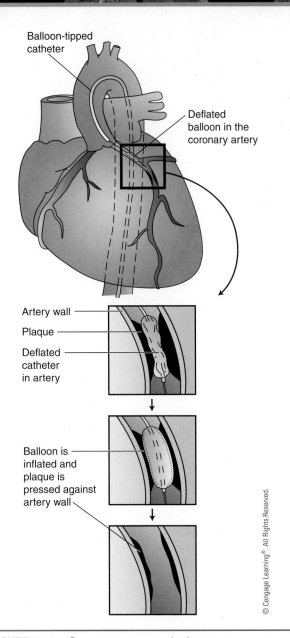

Balloon-tipped catheter

Deflated balloon in the coronary artery

Artery wall

Plaque

Deflated catheter in artery

Balloon is inflated and plaque is pressed against artery wall

© Cengage Learning®. All Rights Reserved.

FIGURE 8–13   Coronary artery angioplasty.

The result of this is usually angina, a heart attack (MI), or both. Decreasing lifestyle behaviors that contribute to the development of atherosclerosis decreases one's risk for heart disease.

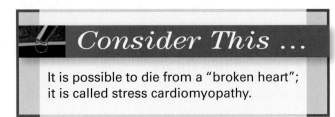

Consider This ...

It is possible to die from a "broken heart"; it is called stress cardiomyopathy.

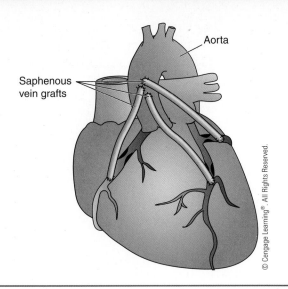

Aorta

Saphenous vein grafts

© Cengage Learning®. All Rights Reserved.

FIGURE 8–14   Coronary artery bypass graft (CABG).

CORONARY HEART DISEASE

Coronary heart disease, CAD, and arteriosclerotic heart disease are all one and the same. This disease was previously discussed as CAD. Coronary heart disease is the most common type of heart disease in the United States. The risk of this disease rises rapidly with increased age.

ANGINA PECTORIS

■ **DESCRIPTION.** Angina pectoris (an-JIGH-nah PECK-toh-riss) is commonly called chest pain.

■ **ETIOLOGY.** Angina pectoris is caused by lack of oxygen to the myocardium (heart muscle). Atherosclerosis is the leading cause of angina, although in some cases, it can be brought on by a spasm of the muscles in the arteries that restricts blood flow to the heart. Angina is commonly a symptom of impending MI.

■ **SYMPTOMS.** During an attack, the individual might complain of a suffocating tightness in the chest that radiates to the left arm, neck, and jaw (Figure 8–15). Angina usually occurs during periods of increased workload on the heart such as those experienced with physical exercise, emotional stress, or digestion of a large meal.

■ **DIAGNOSIS.** A thorough physical exam, along with blood test, electrocardiogram, and cardiac catheterization, assist in diagnosis. Blood tests include cholesterol and triglyceride blood levels. An electrocardiogram can assist in recognizing abnormal heart

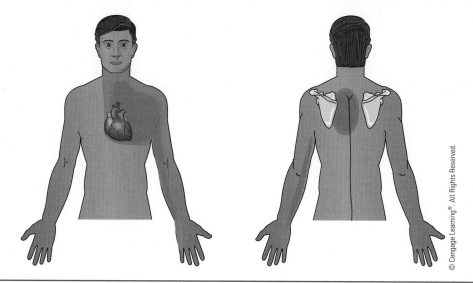

FIGURE 8–15 Patterns of angina.

function. A cardiac catheterization is the most definitive procedure to discover the cause of angina.

■ **TREATMENT.** Treatment of angina is to decrease workload on the heart by stopping the aggravating activity and increasing blood flow to the heart muscle. Vasodilatation of the coronary arteries or those that supply the heart muscle will improve blood flow and help relieve the oxygen deficit. Nitroglycerin is a vasodilator that is commonly used. It is administered sublingually (under the tongue) and usually provides immediate relief. Individuals suffering with angina need medical attention.

■ **PREVENTION.** Angina can be prevented or controlled by making healthy lifestyle choices as previously listed.

MYOCARDIAL INFARCTION

■ **DESCRIPTION.** The term *myocardial infarction* (MY-oh-KAR-dee-al in-FARK-shun) comes from the meanings of the words *myocardium* (heart muscle) and *infarction* (tissue death from lack of oxygen). It is commonly called a heart attack and often leads to cardiac arrest—stopping of the heartbeat.

■ **ETIOLOGY.** MI occurs when the heart muscle does not get adequate oxygen due to a decrease in blood supply, an increase in oxygen need, or a combination of both. The decrease in blood supply is most commonly caused by the atherosclerotic plaque of CAD. Any activity that increases the oxygen need of the heart beyond the supply level can lead to a

myocardial infarct. Such activities can include shock, hemorrhage, stress, or excessive physical exertion.

■ **SYMPTOMS.** Classic symptoms of an MI include severe chest pain with diaphoresis (sweating) and nausea. Often, the symptoms are not as obvious and can include referred pain in the left arm, neck, and jaw, along with a discomfort similar to bad or unrelieved indigestion.

According to the American Heart Association (AHA, 2012b), women often experience different symptoms than men. Women's most common heart attack symptom is also chest pain or discomfort. But often, symptoms in women may be less severe and more "flu-like" yet just as dangerous as the classic signs and may include:

■ Pain or discomfort in one or both arms, the back, or stomach

■ Shortness of breath with or without chest pain

■ Breaking out in a cold sweat, nausea, or lightheadedness

Severity of symptoms can depend on the size of the infarction. If the area is small, symptoms might be mild, and the infarction can be labeled a silent MI. If the infarcted area is large, symptoms can include cardiogenic shock and death. Mortality from MI is approximately 35%.

■ **DIAGNOSIS.** The diagnosis of MI is made by history and physical examination along with electrocardiogram and blood testing. Two specific cardiac blood tests indicative of MI are creatine phosphokinase (CPK) and troponin.

■ **TREATMENT.** Treatment of an MI involves immediate attention to prevent shock, relieve respiratory distress, and decrease workload on the heart. The individual should be assisted into a lying position. Tight or restrictive clothing should be loosened to improve respiratory function. If cardiac arrest has occurred, appropriate cardiopulmonary resuscitation (CPR) should be administered immediately, and the individual should be transported immediately to a medical facility.

Medical treatment involves the administration of oxygen and pain medication, and medication to treat arrhythmias is often needed. Intravenous thrombolytic, or clot-busting, therapy using a tissue plasminogen activator (TPA) or streptokinase might be used to open the occlusion and restore blood flow. Education following an MI is aimed at prevention by possible changes in lifestyle to reduce risk factors. Smoking cessation, dietary changes, and exercise are usually recommended.

The main site involved in an MI is the left ventricle. This is the hardest working area of the heart and has the greatest need for oxygen. Tissue changes that appear with an infarction depend on the degree or extent of oxygen deprivation suffered by the cells. Under microscopic examination, the infarcted area might take on a bull's eye appearance (Figure 8–16). The central core is made up of cells that are dead or necrotic with severely damaged cells surrounding this core. These cells might regain function within a few weeks, or they might die, thus extending the infarcted area. On the outer border of the bull's eye pattern are cells that suffered from ischemia. These cells usually live and can regain function.

Death of myocardial cells brings about a release of certain enzymes and proteins (CPK and troponin) into the general circulation. Blood tests to measure these levels assist in determining the amount of dead or necrotic tissue and the severity and time of the attack. Blood levels, along with an ECG, history, and physical examination, often confirm the diagnosis of MI.

Tissue infarction and injury naturally cause the inflammatory response. With this response comes an outpouring of polymorphonuclear cells (PMNs) and macrophages. Within the first 5 to 7 days, macrophages phagocytize the dead tissue, often leaving a thin, weak myocardial layer. Possibility of rupture and sudden death are greatest at this time. Any activity that increases the workload of the heart or increases blood pressure should be avoided. Rest is essential during this time.

Within 2 weeks, the infarcted area is healing with granulation tissue. This tissue is not made of muscle tissue; it is scar tissue. This scar will not stretch or contract like normal muscle, and it will never function as normal heart tissue. The inability of this scarred area to function increases workload on the remaining heart muscle cells for the rest of the individual's life.

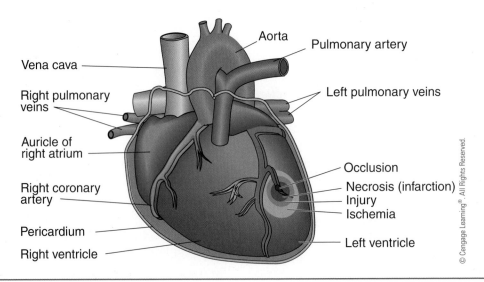

FIGURE 8–16   Myocardial infarction: areas of ischemia.

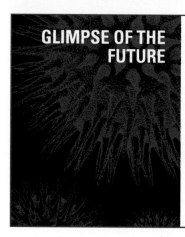

Reducing Heart Attack Risk through Weight-Loss Surgery

A recent study noted that weight-loss surgery (bariatric surgery) can reduce the patient's risk of heart attack or stroke. The subjects were those with a high body mass index (BMI) who had weight-loss surgery. The researchers followed the subjects for 14.7 years and found that the weight-loss surgery reduced the chances of dying from cardiovascular disease. However, people with abdominal obesity are more at risk for cardiovascular disease than those who have their weight in the legs and trunk of the body. In the future, people with high BMIs who are recommended for weight-loss surgery might only be those who have abdominal obesity.

Source: Roan (2012).

■ **PREVENTION.** Risk factors for MI are the same as for CAD and primarily include hypertension, cigarette smoking, a sedentary lifestyle, obesity, and a high-cholesterol diet. Controlling risk factors is the primary way to prevent MI.

HYPERTENSIVE HEART DISEASE

■ **DESCRIPTION.** Hypertensive heart disease is a group of disorders caused by hypertension. It is the number one cause of death associated with hypertension and is the result of long-term hypertension.

■ **ETIOLOGY.** Any disease or disorder that causes a chronic elevation in blood pressure can lead to hypertensive heart disease. Essential hypertension, arteriosclerosis, atherosclerosis, and kidney diseases are common causes.

■ **SYMPTOMS.** As previously discussed, chronic hypertension leads to increased workload on the heart, causing cardiac hypertrophy and, eventually, heart failure.

■ **DIAGNOSIS.** Diagnosis is made by thorough history and physical examination. X-rays revealing enlargement of the heart along with abnormal heart function as determined by an echocardiogram are indicative of this disease. Late in the course of the disease, there can be pulmonary (lung) congestion as a result of heart failure.

■ **TREATMENT.** Treatment of hypertensive heart disease is related to treating the cause of hypertension. If the hypertension cannot be cured, as with essential hypertension, then controlling blood pressure is necessary. Hypertensive heart disease, like hypertension, is not cured, only controlled.

■ **PREVENTION.** Preventing hypertensive heart disease is achieved by preventing or controlling hypertension.

RHEUMATIC HEART DISEASE

■ **DESCRIPTION.** Rheumatic heart disease refers to the cardiac symptoms related to rheumatic fever. Rheumatic fever was discussed in Chapter 5, "Immune System Diseases and Disorders," as an autoimmune disorder.

■ **ETIOLOGY.** Recall that rheumatic fever is commonly caused by a streptococcal throat infection. The immune system in a select group of individuals builds antibodies that attack the bacteria and the heart tissue. All layers of the heart might be affected, along with the valves of the heart.

■ **SYMPTOMS.** All the symptoms of rheumatic fever might be present, including joint pain and shortness of breath. Another symptom is valvular damage leading to stenosis (narrowing) of the mitral and aortic valves and then to heart murmurs.

■ **DIAGNOSIS.** A history of rheumatic fever along with a positive tropomyosin (a cardiac antibody) blood test is indicative of this disease. A chest X-ray showing an enlarged heart, lung congestion, and abnormal electrocardiogram are also positive indicators.

■ **TREATMENT.** Treatment is aimed at prevention and proper treatment of streptococcal infections. Valvular stenosis increases the workload of the heart and can cause further heart disease. During acute carditis, treatment includes bed rest, to reduce the workload on the heart, and other symptomatic treatment. Severe valve damage can lead to the need for valve surgery to correct the deformity or replace the valve.

■ **PREVENTION.** The best defense is to prevent rheumatic fever. Rapid diagnosis and proper antibiotic treatment can often prevent rheumatic fever from developing.

CONGESTIVE HEART FAILURE (CHF)

■ **DESCRIPTION.** CHF is a condition in which the heart fails to pump an adequate amount of blood to meet the body's needs. The cardiopulmonary and general vascular systems gradually become congested.

■ **ETIOLOGY.** CHF develops slowly and usually follows any type of cardiac condition that increases the workload of the heart. Such diseases include MI, hypertension, CAD, and rheumatic heart disease, to name a few.

■ **SYMPTOMS.** The individual experiences a gradual increase in shortness of breath. Tachycardia (tachy = rapid, cardia = heart) and rapid breathing occur as the body tries to compensate for decreased blood flow. As CHF progresses, fluid builds up in the vascular system, leading to neck vein distention and edema in the ankles and lower legs. Right-sided heart failure leads to congestion of the liver and spleen. Left-sided failure leads to congestion and edema of the lungs (pulmonary edema) (Figure 8–17).

■ **DIAGNOSIS.** A history and physical examination, coupled with the symptoms of shortness of breath and edema, are enough for a basic diagnosis of CHF. Further testing includes chest X-ray to show enlargement of the heart, electrocardiogram to check for irregular heart rate, and echocardiogram to view valve function.

■ **TREATMENT.** Treatment is aimed at decreasing the workload of the heart. Diuretic medications, low-salt diet, and fluid restrictions might be prescribed to increase urine output and limit fluid retention, thus reducing blood fluid volume. Cardiac medications, such as digitalis, can be prescribed to strengthen and slow the heartbeat.

■ **PREVENTION.** Adopting preventive lifestyle habits, such as smoking cessation, weight control, diet modification, and regular exercise, helps prevent this disease.

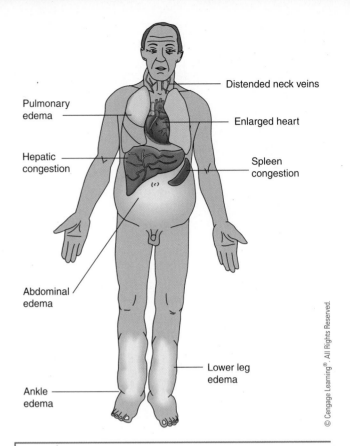

Distended neck veins
Pulmonary edema
Enlarged heart
Hepatic congestion
Spleen congestion
Abdominal edema
Lower leg edema
Ankle edema

FIGURE 8–17 Signs of congestive heart failure.

Media Link

View an animation on congestive heart failure on the Online Resources.

CARDIOMYOPATHY

■ **DESCRIPTION.** Cardiomyopathy (KAR-dee-oh-MY-OP-ah-thee; cardio = heart, myo = muscle, opathy = disease) literally is heart muscle disease. It is a deterioration of the function of the myocardium. Cardiomyopathy can be classified as primary or secondary.

■ **ETIOLOGY.** Primary cardiomyopathy is idiopathic, but a high number of cases are seen in association with alcoholism. Secondary cardiomyopathy is due to a specific cause often associated with other diseases. There are three main types of secondary cardiomyopathy: dilated, hypertrophic, and restrictive.

Dilated cardiomyopathy is the most common form. The heart is enlarged (dilated), is weak, and does not pump properly, leading to heart failure. Hypertrophic cardiomyopathy is inherited and characterized by heart muscle enlargement (hypertrophy), often causing the heart valves to leak. The least common type is restrictive cardiomyopathy, characterized by rigid muscle tissue, making it difficult for the heart to fill with blood. This type is usually seen in the elderly.

■ *SYMPTOMS.* Common symptoms for all types of cardiomyopathy include those associated with heart failure, including weakness, fatigue, shortness of breath, and swelling of the feet and legs.

■ *DIAGNOSIS.* Diagnosis of all types of cardiomyopathy is dependent on history and physical examination along with electrocardiogram and chest X-ray.

■ *TREATMENT.* Cardiomyopathies are incurable and often lead to CHF, MI, and death. Treatment is based on relieving symptoms and can include diuretic medications, heart medications, and change of lifestyle behaviors.

■ *PREVENTION.* Cardiomyopathy, in most cases, cannot be prevented. If diagnosed early, treatment can prevent worsening of the disease.

CARDITIS

■ *DESCRIPTION.* Carditis (kar-DYE-tis) is a general term describing inflammation of the heart. Forms of carditis include pericarditis, myocarditis, and endocarditis, depending on the area of the heart involved. Pericarditis affects the serous membrane on the outside of the heart as well as the pericardial sac. Myocarditis affects the heart muscle layer, and endocarditis affects the inside of the heart.

■ *ETIOLOGY.* All these inflammatory states can be due to unknown causes, bacteria, and viruses or as a result of rheumatic fever. Carditis is often secondary to a respiratory tract, urinary tract, or skin infection. It also can be related to dental infections or diseases of other systems.

■ *SYMPTOMS.* Symptoms vary, depending on the site and cause, but a common symptom includes varying degrees of chest pain.

■ *DIAGNOSIS.* Diagnosis is often difficult, but a thorough history and physical examination along with ECG, chest X-ray, and blood cultures can be helpful.

■ *TREATMENT.* Treatment of carditis generally includes bed rest to decrease the workload on the heart. Other treatments depend on the cause of the disease and can include antibiotics, analgesics, and antipyretics (anti = against, pyro = heat, or against fever).

■ *PREVENTION.* Depending on cause, many of the cases of carditis are preventable with accurate diagnosis and treatment of the cause.

VALVULAR HEART DISEASE

■ *DESCRIPTION.* Valvular heart disease is related to malfunction of the heart valves. The purpose of a valve in the heart and the vascular system is to prevent backflow of blood. Backflow causes extra workload on the heart because the heart has to re-pump the blood.

■ *ETIOLOGY.* Common causes of valvular disease can be congenital anomalies or malformations, rheumatic fever, or endocarditis. Malfunction of a valve can be due to the valvular opening being too narrow (stenotic) or being too large to close properly (valvular insufficiency). Both of these problems can affect all the heart valves and lead to heart murmurs. A heart **murmur** is an abnormal sound in the heart or vascular system. One complication of all valve defects is the vascular tendency to form clots (thrombi) on the affected areas. If the thrombus breaks loose and becomes an embolus, it might occlude arteries leading to major organs such as the lungs, brain, liver, or kidneys. Another common problem of valvular heart disease is CHF due to the increased workload on the heart.

■ *SYMPTOMS.* Symptoms include chest pain, edema (swelling) in the ankles, heart palpitations, dizziness, and weakness. The severity of the symptoms might not reflect the severity of the disease. In other words, some individuals have severe symptoms with mild disease, whereas others with severe disease might have only mild symptoms.

■ *DIAGNOSIS.* Physical examination can reveal a murmur and lung congestion. Chest X-ray showing an enlarged heart and an ECG revealing arrhythmias are indicative of this disease.

■ *TREATMENT.* Treatment depends on the cause and severity of the disease. Minor problems might not require treatment, but those with serious disease can be treated successfully with medications. Typical medication treatments include antiarrhythmics, antibiotics to prevent or treat infection, anticoagulants to prevent blood clot formation, and diuretics to assist in removal of excess fluid.

■ **PREVENTION.** Prevention is aimed at controlling heart disease by not smoking, eating a healthy diet, and daily exercise. Diseases caused by infection are prevented by quickly treating any infection. If medications are not effective, open heart surgery to repair or replace heart valves might be performed.

ARRHYTHMIAS

■ **DIAGNOSIS.** Arrhythmias (ah-RITH-me-ahs) are abnormalities in heart rhythm due to a disturbance in the conduction system of the heart.

■ **ETIOLOGY.** Often, the cause of these is unknown. Known causes include medications, ischemia of the heart muscle, and a previous MI. Auscultation and electrocardiography can diagnose arrhythmias.

■ **SYMPTOMS.** Normal heart rhythm is often called normal sinus rhythm and indicates that the rate is between 60 and 100 beats per minute, is regular, and is originating normally from the SA node. An unusually fast (up to 350 beats per minute) but regular heart rate is called flutter. If the rhythm is wild and uncoordinated, it is an arrhythmia called **fibrillation** (FIH-brih-LAY-shun). Fibrillations affect the atria or the ventricles. Atrial fibrillations are usually not serious in nature. However, ventricular fibrillations, commonly abbreviated as V fib, are serious cardiac arrhythmias that require emergency defibrillation by electrical shock.

Heart block is another group of arrhythmias caused by an interruption in the conduction system. Heart block is divided into first, second, and third degree, depending on the seriousness of the blockage. Third-degree block is treated with insertion of an artificial pacemaker.

Premature or early contractions can affect the atria or the ventricles. Premature ventricular contractions are commonly abbreviated as PVCs.

Media Link

View an animation on ventricular fibrillation on the Online Resources.

■ **DIAGNOSIS.** After physical examination, the first diagnostic test will usually be an ECG. If this shows an abnormal rhythm, the next step is often wearing a Holter monitor, a small portable ECG machine that performs a continuous monitor strip of the heart. An exercise stress test can also be useful in diagnosis.

■ **TREATMENT.** Treatment is usually unnecessary as long as the number of beats per minute is minimal and the individual is otherwise asymptomatic.

■ **PREVENTION.** Prevention is aimed at preventing heart disease in general with healthy lifestyle behaviors and at quickly treating any known heart disease.

Consider This ...

A new study shows that consumption of the chemical bisphenol A (BPA), a hormone-disrupting chemical, leads to a greater risk of developing heart disease. BPA is found in canned foods and plastic products. For this reason, it is recommended to eat less soups and canned vegetables and never reheat food in plastic containers in the microwave or eat out of plastic ware.

Diseases of the Veins

Diseases of the veins are more common in older adults. Age-related changes in the vessels and valves, along with other changes in the circulatory system, contribute to the overall general weakness of the vessels. Fluid often pools in the extremities, causing edema. Disorders of the veins are usually more serious in individuals with other chronic disorders such as diabetes mellitus.

PHLEBITIS

■ **DESCRIPTION.** Phlebitis (fleh-BYE-tis; phlebo = vein, itis = inflammation) is relatively common, especially in the veins of the arms and lower legs. Phlebitis commonly refers to inflammation of superficial (near the skin surface) veins (Figure 8–18).

■ **ETIOLOGY.** The cause of phlebitis is often unknown, but known causes can include injury, obesity, poor circulation, prolonged bed rest, and

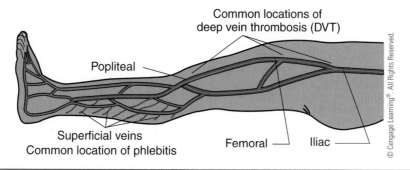

Common locations of
deep vein thrombosis (DVT)

Popliteal

Superficial veins
Common location of phlebitis

Femoral — | Iliac —

© Cengage Learning® All Rights Reserved.

FIGURE 8–18   Superficial versus deep veins in development of phlebitis and thrombosis.

infection. Injury to a vein is often a known cause of phlebitis. Intravenous medications and catheters can cause vein injury in the arms. Pooling of blood, as occurs with varicose veins or physical injury to the vessel, might lead to phlebitis in the legs.

■ **SYMPTOMS.** Symptoms of phlebitis include pain, swelling, and, often, the appearance of a red cord-like hardening that extends along the vein from the area of injury upward toward the heart. Occasionally, phlebitis in the lower leg of the mother occurs after childbirth in association with the onset of milk production. This form of phlebitis is commonly called "milk leg."

■ **DIAGNOSIS.** Phlebitis is commonly diagnosed by physical examination of veins in the legs. An ultrasound is useful to determine the extent of the disease and to look for clots and blockage of blood flow.

■ **TREATMENT.** Treatment of superficial phlebitis often includes analgesics and warm compresses to reduce pain and improve circulation. Elevation of the area above heart level will improve venous return and decrease edema. To improve venous return in the lower extremities, the use of elastic or compression stockings and exercise can be prescribed.

■ **PREVENTION.** To prevent phlebitis, participate in moderate physical exercise to maintain circulation and muscle tone and avoid smoking and sitting for long periods of time.

THROMBOPHLEBITIS

A complication of phlebitis is the development of a clot in the inflamed vessel, a condition called thrombophlebitis. Clots in superficial veins rarely embolize (break loose and travel), but clots in deep veins often do, making this condition of serious concern in a deep vein. Thrombophlebitis in the deep veins is called deep vein thrombosis.

DEEP VEIN THROMBOSIS (DVT)

■ **DESCRIPTION.** DVT primarily occurs in the lower legs, thighs, and pelvis (see Figure 8–18). Clots occurring in the femoral and pelvic veins commonly embolize.

■ **ETIOLOGY.** Risk factors for DVT include:

■ **Immobility** Early postoperative ambulation (walking) is encouraged. Prolonged bed rest greatly increases risk.

■ **Dehydration** Dehydration increases blood viscosity (thickness) and increases risk of thrombus formation.

■ **Varicose veins** Veins already weakened with disease are more likely to develop a thrombus.

■ **Leg or pelvic surgery, obesity, and pregnancy** These conditions alter venous blood flow and increase risk.

■ **SYMPTOMS.** These clots are generally asymptomatic until embolization occurs, often causing a pulmonary embolism. Pulmonary embolism is often fatal.

■ **DIAGNOSIS.** A positive Homan's test is very commonly performed as an initial indication of DVT. Homan's is performed by pulling the toes toward the knee; a positive test will cause pain in the posterior calf. If squeezing the posterior calf also elicits pain, this is indicative of DVT and is called a Pratt's sign. Ultrasonography, or ultrasound imaging of the veins, is the most widely used test to evaluate the disease.

■ **TREATMENT.** Treatment of DVT is aimed at reducing the formation of more clots and preventing embolization. Bed rest with elevation of the affected area is essential to improve blood flow. Anticoagulants are given to decrease potential thrombus formation; they will not dissolve clots, only prevent formation of new ones.

■ **PREVENTION.** Prevention is aimed at healthy lifestyle behaviors, including maintaining proper body weight, exercising, and not smoking. Wearing graduated elastic compression stockings during times of prolonged standing or sitting is also a preventive measure.

VARICOSE VEINS

■ **DESCRIPTION.** Varicose veins (VAR-ih-kohs VAYNS) are dilated, tortuous, and elongated veins commonly found in the legs. Blood in the legs must move upward against the pull of gravity. Leg muscles are primarily responsible for this movement by contracting and relaxing. This action pushes against the vessel wall and pushes blood upward. Valves are necessary to prevent backflow of blood. With varicose veins, the flow of blood is slowed, blood collects in the veins, or both, causing increased pressure on the vessel walls and the valves and eventually leading to incompetent valves (Figure 8–19). Prolonged pooling of blood in the veins stretches the vessel wall and leads to the formation of varicosities.

■ **ETIOLOGY.** Development of varicosities can be due to any activity that slows return flow and increases venous pressure. Such activities as prolonged sitting, standing, pregnancy, and obesity tend to increase the risk of developing varicose veins. Heredity also plays a part in this disorder; there appears to be an inherited vessel wall weakness.

■ **SYMPTOMS.** Varicose veins develop gradually. Initial symptoms might include leg fatigue and leg cramps, and veins often become thick, hardened, and unsightly. Poor venous blood flow causes edema and congestion of fluid in the extremities. This congestion slows arterial flow, leading to stasis dermatitis and ulceration. Stasis dermatitis is characterized by edema, dry and scaly skin, and small pinpoint hemorrhages. The skin also turns brown in color as blood pigment accumulates in the connective tissue. Stasis ulcers do not heal well and can necessitate amputation of the affected area.

■ **DIAGNOSIS.** Simply looking at the veins in the legs is often enough for a simple diagnosis. A Doppler ultrasound to evaluate blood flow can provide a more definitive diagnosis.

■ **TREATMENT.** Treatment includes improving vascular flow by elevating legs, walking, and using support or elastic hose. Surgery might be indicated to relieve discomfort and avoid recurrent thrombosis. Surgical treatment involves tying off the vessel and removing it, a procedure commonly called vein stripping. There are numerous superficial veins, so

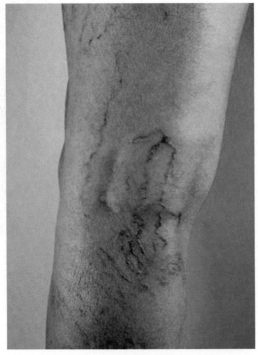
(A)

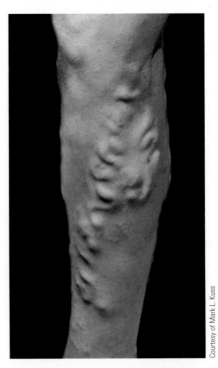
(B)

Courtesy of Mark L. Kuss

FIGURE 8–19   Varicose veins. (A) Moderate. (B) Extreme.

blood return to the heart from this area is through alternate venous routes.

■ **PREVENTION.** Wearing compression stockings, regularly elevating the legs above heart level, avoiding prolonged standing or sitting, controlling weight, and not smoking are activities that help prevent varicose veins.

■ TRAUMA

Hemorrhage

■ **DESCRIPTION.** Hemorrhage (hemo = blood, orrhage = burst forth) is an abnormal loss of blood. Hemorrhagic blood loss can be external or internal, and blood loss can be acute (sudden onset) or chronic.

■ **ETIOLOGY.** Acute blood loss is usually related to trauma, whereas chronic loss is more often related to disease processes.

External and internal blood loss, if severe enough, can lead to **exsanguination** (loss of circulating blood volume) and death. Internal blood loss can cause filling of body cavities such as **hemothorax** (hemo = blood, thorax = chest, blood in the chest cavity). Internal bleeding might not be noticeable until a large amount of blood has been lost and the individual begins to show signs and symptoms of shock.

■ **SYMPTOMS.** Hemorrhage can affect different vessels and have varying results. Hemorrhage of low-pressure vessels (the capillaries and veins) into the tissues leads to reddish to dark-purple spots on the skin and mucosa. These discolorations are called petechiae, ecchymosis, or purpura, depending on the size or cause of the discoloration. Petechiae (pee-TEE-kee-ee) are pinpoint hemorrhages. Ecchymosis (ECK-ih-MOH-sis) is a larger area of purplish color commonly called a bruise. Purpura (PUR-pew-rah) is spontaneous bleeding into the tissues related to a hemorrhagic disease that might be characterized by both petechiae and ecchymosis. Hemorrhage of the high-pressure vessels (the arteries) leads to forceful squirting of bright red (highly oxygenated) blood. The squirting of arterial blood is directly related to the beat of the heart.

Large venous and arterial hemorrhages, if not controlled, can be fatal. Blood volume varies with body size; the average adult has about 5 liters (approximately 5 quarts) of blood. Adults may lose approximately 500 ml (approximately 1 pint) of blood without any problems. This amount is equal to the amount given during a blood donation. Loss of 1 liter of blood, however, can result in hypovolemic shock. Greater losses, 1,500 ml or more, are usually lethal. Hemorrhaging in a closed cavity also can cause organ damage due to increased pressure. For example, bleeding in the head can lead to brain tissue damage or death from the resulting increase in intracranial pressure.

Chronic hemorrhages, such as those occurring in the gastrointestinal tract and female reproductive tract, commonly lead to anemia. Normal menstrual bleeding is approximately 70–80 ml. As discussed in Chapter 7, "Blood and Blood-Forming Organs Diseases and Disorders," replacement of the lost iron also can lead to iron deficiency anemia.

■ **DIAGNOSIS.** Hemorrhage is often diagnosed by a complete blood count revealing a low hemoglobin count and hematocrit. Although external hemorrhage is easy to recognize, determining the location of internal bleeding is much more difficult. Stool testing can help determine bleeding in the gastrointestinal tract. A CT scan might be needed to determine the location of internal sites.

■ **TREATMENT.** Treatment is focused on stopping the bleeding and replacing the blood volume, if needed, with blood transfusions.

■ **PREVENTION.** Although not all hemorrhages can be prevented, avoiding the causes of hemorrhage will prevent many of the occurrences.

Shock

■ **DESCRIPTION.** Shock can be defined in many ways, but basically, it is extremely low blood pressure that leads to decreased tissue **perfusion** (to pour through or supply with blood).

■ **ETIOLOGY.** This low blood pressure can be caused by one of three mechanisms:

■ Not enough blood volume

■ Inadequate pumping of blood by the heart

■ Vasodilatation that allows blood to pool in the vessels, thereby reducing circulating blood volume

Remember, the vascular system is composed of thousands of miles of vessels. If all these vessels were to open at the same time, the circulating volume of blood would be zero.

Shock can be caused by a variety of situations. Every injury brings about some degree of shock and should be treated appropriately. No matter the cause, shock leads to inadequate perfusion of tissues with blood. Inadequate perfusion can cause tissue hypoxia, anoxia, ischemia, and necrosis as discussed in Chapter 2, "Mechanisms of Disease." Types of shock include:

- **Cardiogenic shock** The leading cause of death due to shock. This type of shock results from the inability of the heart to pump blood adequately, often due to MI. Treatment can involve CPR and administration of cardiotonic and vasoconstrictor medications. (Vasoconstrictor medications cause muscle contraction of vessels, increasing blood pressure.)

- **Septic shock** The second most common cause of death due to shock. Septic shock usually results from an overwhelming septicemia (bacteria or microorganisms in the blood). Treatment can involve administration of antibiotics and vasoconstrictor medications.

- **Hypovolemic shock** Results from low fluid volume and can be due to hemorrhage (often called hemorrhagic shock), severe burns leading to loss of blood plasma, severe vomiting, and diarrhea. Treatment can involve blood transfusions and intravenous fluid volume replacement.

- **Neurogenic shock** Results from generalized vasodilatation and can be due to highly emotional situations such as fear, surprise, pain, and unpleasant sights. Medications and spinal anesthesia also can lead to neurogenic shock. Treatment can involve vasoconstrictor medications.

- **Anaphylactic shock** Results from severe allergic reactions and might be due to allergens such as contrast dyes for diagnostic tests, bee stings, medications, and blood transfusion reaction. Treatment can involve removing the allergen and administering antihistamines and bronchodilators.

■ *SYMPTOMS.* Signs and symptoms of shock vary, depending on the degree of the situation, and can include facial pallor, cool and clammy skin, cyanosis, tachycardia, tachypnea, altered mental status, syncope (fainting), unconsciousness, oliguria, and anuria.

■ *DIAGNOSIS.* Diagnosis is most often established through a thorough medical history and physical exam. Blood pressure less than 90/50 is recognized as shock.

■ *TREATMENT.* Treatment depends on the type of shock. Other treatment measures include laying the individual in a supine (on the back) position, keeping the individual warm and quiet, and elevating the feet and legs above heart level to improve vascular return.

■ *PREVENTION.* Preventing the conditions that cause shock is the best way to prevent it. Monitoring and managing these conditions can prevent progression of symptoms and thus prevent shock.

RARE DISEASES

Malignant Hypertension

Malignant hypertension is a form of essential hypertension that is considered a medical emergency. Diastolic blood pressure can reach 130–170 mm Hg. Symptoms include headache, blurred vision, and dyspnea. Without treatment, malignant hypertension is fatal.

Cor Pulmonale

Cor pulmonale is right-sided heart failure related to acute or chronic pulmonary disease. Increased pulmonary blood pressure causes hypertrophy of the right ventricle, leading to decreased pumping ability. Polycythemia develops as the body tries to compensate for hypoxemia. This increase in red blood cell number increases the viscosity of the blood, further increasing workload on the heart. Treatment involves treating the lung disease and can also include phlebotomy to decrease blood viscosity.

Raynaud's Disease

Raynaud's disease is a vasospastic disorder primarily affecting the fingers and toes. This idiopathic disease occurs most frequently in young women and is usually related to cold temperature and emotional stress. During vasospasm, the extremities can turn pale and then cyanotic before returning to normal color. As the disease progresses, small ulcers might develop on the extremities and can lead to contractures and chronic disability of the hands. Treatment is avoidance of cold and application of warmth to the extremities. Cigarette smoking is discouraged because nicotine causes further vasoconstriction.

Buerger's Disease

Buerger's disease is also known as thromboangiitis (thrombo = clot, angi = vessel, itis = inflammation) obliterans and is an inflammation of the peripheral vessels with clot formation. The affected individual often has pain in the legs and feet that is made worse with activity and improves with rest. Progression of the disease leads to muscle atrophy, ulcers, and gangrene. The primary cause of Buerger's disease is cigarette smoking. Treatment involves cessation of smoking, exercises to improve circulation, and vessel bypass surgery.

Polyarteritis Nodosa

Polyarteritis nodosa is a vasculitis that is characterized by inflammatory, necrotizing lesions in many vessels. This rare autoimmune disease is usually fatal as a result of occlusion and rupture of the involved vessels.

◼ EFFECTS OF AGING ON THE SYSTEM

Heart and blood vessel diseases are a significant cause of death and disability in the older adult. As the individual ages, the heart muscle loses some of its contractility, causing a decreased cardiac output, an increased heart rate to compensate for the changes, or both. The vessels lose elasticity and become more rigid and narrowed. The valves also lose some functioning and become thick and sclerotic. These changes add to the workload of the heart by increasing the heart rate and

the blood pressure, and the older adult can become tachycardic with minimal exercise. Although many of the changes in the system are due to the normal aging process, other changes observed in the older adult are directly due to lifestyle. Many individuals have smoked for years, been overweight, eaten a high-fat diet, endured a stressful job, and lived a fairly sedentary life. These modifiable behaviors contribute to the adverse changes in the cardiovascular system and increase the risk of chronic and acute problems in the system over time. Most older adults are at risk for hypertension, MI, angina, arrhythmias, CHF, varicosities, and other cardiovascular problems.

With age, the arteries become more rigid, causing decreased blood flow to organs and distal body tissues. The vein valves lose some of their competency, reducing good blood flow even further. Decreased peripheral circulation often results in cool or pale extremities, improper healing, and pooling of fluid (edema) in the legs and feet. Medications might not be as efficiently transmitted to the body with these changes in circulation, which can affect the therapeutic regimen for the individual.

Many older adults have postural hypotension, which can be a significant safety problem. Postural hypotension is the decrease or drop in blood pressure that occurs when the individual rises to a sitting or standing position from a reclining position. The individual usually feels very dizzy on rising and might fall. Prevention strategies should be in place to prevent injuries from postural hypotension.

SUMMARY

The cardiovascular system is responsible for pumping the blood throughout the body, delivering nutrients and oxygen to cells, and removing waste products. CVD affects millions of Americans. It is a significant cause of mortality, especially in the older adult. The risk for developing many diseases of the system can be reduced by lifestyle behavioral changes. Common symptoms of CVD include pain, fatigue, difficulty breathing, tachycardia, cyanosis, and edema. Some of the most common disorders of the system include hypertension, CAD, arteriosclerosis, and varicosities. Older adults are at greatest risk for developing heart disease, the number one cause of death in the older population.

REVIEW QUESTIONS

Multiple Choice

1. Which of the following risk factors are controllable or modifiable? (Select all that apply.)
   a. Heredity
   b. Diet

    c. Age

    d. Stress

    e. Smoking

    f. Exercise

2. Which of the following statements are correct in relation to CAD? (Select all that apply.)

    a. It is often called coronary heart disease.

    b. Slow, progressive occlusion of arteries often leads to development of collateral arteries that extend into ischemic tissue, providing some protection against infarction.

    c. It will always lead to an MI.

    d. Diagnosis of CAD is made by evaluating the history, ECG, and angiograms.

    e. CAD is not usually diagnosed in the older adult.

    f. The disease is commonly due to atherosclerosis.

Short Answer

3. Define the following terms related to hemorrhage.

    a. Petechiae

    b. Ecchymosis

    c. Purpura

4. What are the functions of the cardiovascular system?

5. Which signs and symptoms are associated with common cardiovascular system disorders?

6. Which diagnostic tests are most commonly used to determine the type, cause, or both of cardiovascular system disorders?

7. What symptoms are usually seen in CHF?

8. What is the difference between phlebitis and thrombophlebitis?

9. What are the most common signs and symptoms of shock?

10. What are some of the changes that occur in the cardiovascular system with age?

CASE STUDIES

■ Mr. Winston is a 72-year-old who has been diagnosed with CHF. He is a middle-class gentleman with a fairly broad educational background. He is a college graduate who has managed a business for 30 years. He asks you to explain his condition to him and his wife. How would you explain CHF to them? In addition, he wants to know why he is so short of breath at times, why he has edema in his ankles in the evenings, and why the physician ordered a low-sodium diet. How would you answer those questions?

■ Mrs. Marconi is a 68-year-old retired woman who volunteers 3 days per week at the hospital. A group of nursing students from the local college were holding a health fair and invited her to participate. One station was set up to check the ankle-brachial index (ABI) on the participants. Mrs. Marconi asked the students to explain what an ABI is and why she needs this test. How would you answer this question? Describe how the test is done. When should someone be referred for further testing after having the ABI checked?

Study Tools

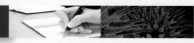

Workbook

Complete Chapter 8

Online Resources

PowerPoint® presentations

Animations

BIBLIOGRAPHY

American Heart Association (AHA). (2011). AHA statistical update: Executive summary: Heart disease and stroke statistics – 2011. *www.heart.org* (accessed August 2012).

American Heart Association (AHA). (2012a). About peripheral artery disease (PAD). *www.heart.org* (accessed August 2012).

American Heart Association (AHA). (2012b). Heart attack symptoms in women. *www.heart.org* (accessed September 2012).

Bergman, D. (2011). Preventing recurrent cerebrovascular events in patients with stroke or transient ischemic attack: The current data. *Journal of the American Academy of Nurse Practitioners 23*(12), 659–666.

Centers for Disease Control and Prevention (CDC). (2012a). Be one in a million this American Heart Month. *www.cdc.gov* (accessed May 2012).

Centers for Disease Control and Prevention (CDC). (2012b). FastStats. *www.cdc.gov* (accessed May 2012).

Drug news. (2011). *Nursing 41*(10), 24.

Gough, D. (2011). Coronary heart disease. *Practice Nurses 41*(10), 12–17.

Herning, M., Hansen, P. R., Bygbjerg, B., & Lindhardt, T. (2011). Women's experiences and behaviour at onset of symptoms of ST segment elevation acute myocardial infarction. *European Journal of Cardiovascular Nursing 10*(4), 241–247.

Hur, M., Lee, M., Kim, C., & Ernst, E. (2012). Aromatherapy for treatment of hypertension: A systematic review. *Journal of Evaluation in Clinical Practice, 18*(1) 37–41.

Jackson, M., McKenney, T., Drumm, J., Merrick, B., LeMaster, T., & VanGilder, C. (2011). Pressure ulcer prevention in high-risk postoperative cardiovascular patients. *Critical Care Nurse 31*(4), 44–53.

Kayyali, A., & Joy, S. (2011). Journal watch. *American Journal of Nursing 111*(12), 62–63.

Kuznar, W. (2011). Journal watch. High dose statins raise diabetes risk. *American Journal of Nursing 111*(11), 60.

Lawes, R. (2010). Action STAT. Acute myocardial infarction in pregnancy. *Nursing 40*(9), 72.

Marshall, K. (2011). Acute coronary syndrome: Diagnosis, risk assessment and management. *Nursing Standard 25*(23), 47–57.

Mayo Clinic. (2012). 10 ways to control high blood pressure without medication. *www.mayoclinic.com* (accessed August 2012).

National Heart, Lung, and Blood Institute (NHLBI). (2012a). About peripheral artery disease (PAD). *www.nhlbi.org* (accessed August 2012).

National Heart, Lung, and Blood Institute (NHLBI). (2012b). Risk factor spotlight: High blood pressure. *www.nhlbi.nih.gov* (accessed August 2012).

Niklasch, D. (2011). Differential diagnosis of acute heart failure: brain versus heart. *Advanced Emergency Nursing Journal 33*(4), 279–287.

Parikh, S., Shrank, W., Mogun, H., & Choudhry, N. (2010). Statin utilization in nursing home patients after cardiac hospitalization. *JGIM: Journal of General Internal Medicine 25*(12), 1293–1299.

Perez, A. (2011). Self-management of hypertension in Hispanic adults. *Clinical Nursing Research 20*(4), 347–365.

Roan, S. (2012). Weight-loss surgery reduces cardiovascular risks, study says. *Los Angeles Times* online. *www.latimes.com* (accessed January 2012).

Rosenberg, K. (2011). Heart failure process measures positively related to outpatient survival: Measures should be 'routinely incorporated into the plan of care.' *American Journal of Nursing 111*(7), 18.

Rosenberg, K. (2011). Medical management trumps stenting for intracranial arterial stenosis. *American Journal of Nursing 111*(12), 16.

Shirato, S., & Swan, B. (2010). Women and cardiovascular disease: An evidentiary review. *MEDSURG Nursing 19*(5), 282–306.

Suh, M., Chen, C., Woodbridge, J., Tu, M., Kim, J., Nahapetian, A., & Sarrafzadeh, M. (2011). A remote patient monitoring system for congestive heart failure. *Journal of Medical Systems 35*(5), 1165–1179.

Wells, M., & Kalman, M. (2011). Women & heart disease: Symptoms and treatment guidelines. *Nurse Practitioner 36*(9), 22–28.

Westerby, R. (2011). An overview of cardiovascular disease risk assessment. *Nursing Standard 26*(13), 48–55.

Wong, K. H., Li, G. Q., Li, K. M., Razmovski-Naumovski, V., & Chan, K. (2011). Kudzu root: Traditional uses and potential medicinal benefits in diabetes and cardiovascular diseases. *Journal of Ethnopharmacology 134*(3), 584–607.

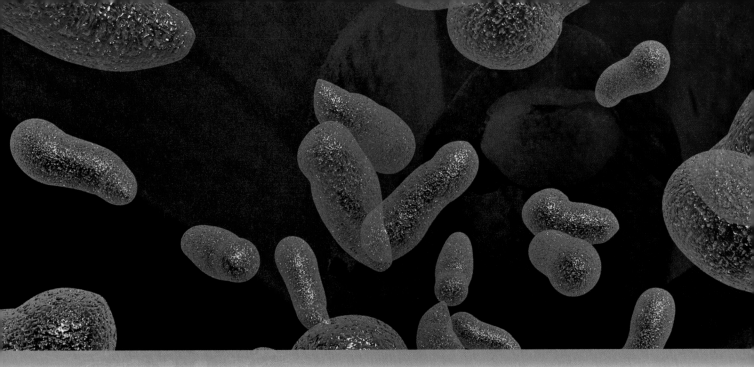

OUTLINE

KEY TERMS

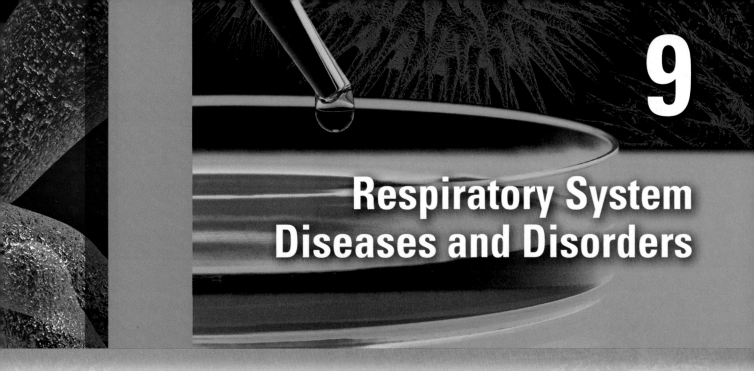

9

Respiratory System Diseases and Disorders

LEARNING OBJECTIVES

Upon completion of the chapter, the learner should be able to:

1. Define the terminology common to the respiratory system and the disorders of the system.

2. Discuss the basic anatomy and physiology of the respiratory system.

3. Identify the important signs and symptoms associated with common respiratory system disorders.

4. Describe the common diagnostics used to determine type and cause of the respiratory system disorders.

5. Identify the common disorders of the respiratory system.

6. Describe the typical course and management of the common respiratory system disorders.

7. Describe the effects of aging on the respiratory system and the common disorders associated with aging of the system.

OVERVIEW

The respiratory system includes the chest, lungs, and internal airway structures. To maintain life, the individual must breathe and have a continuous exchange of oxygen for carbon dioxide. Breathing and the exchange of gases that takes place within the system are complex processes involving the respiratory system as well as the neurologic and circulatory systems. Diseases of the respiratory system include some of the most well-known disorders such as the common cold, pneumonia, and influenza. Public health officials are worried about new strains of influenza becoming widespread. Respiratory diseases affect all ages, but older people are the most susceptible to both chronic and acute disorders of the system. ■

■ ANATOMY AND PHYSIOLOGY

The respiratory system consists of the chest (thorax), lungs, and conducting airways. The chest, or thorax, is the structure that houses the lungs and the mediastinum (heart and major vessels). The respiratory system structures in the thorax include the lungs, 12 pairs of ribs, part of the vertebral column, and the sternum. The diaphragm, a large muscle of respiration, separates the thorax from the abdomen (Figure 9–1). The lungs are two spongy organs divided into three lobes in the right lung and two lobes in the left lung. They lie in the pleural cavity, which is lined with a membrane called the pleura, in the thorax. The lungs are also covered with a second membrane or pleura. Between the two pleural membranes is a lubricating liquid that prevents friction as the process of breathing and lung expansion occurs.

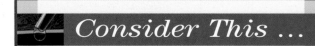

Consider This ...

If you were to roll the human lung tissue out flat, it would cover an average tennis court.

Usually, the airways of the respiratory system are divided into two parts. The upper respiratory system includes the nose (nasal cavities), mouth, sinuses, pharynx, and larynx. The lower respiratory system includes the trachea, bronchi, and bronchioles. The alveoli, grape-like clusters of air sacs that are surrounded by capillaries (Figure 9–2), are found at the distal end of the terminal bronchioles. This is where the oxygen–carbon dioxide gas exchange in the lungs occurs.

The mechanism of ventilation, the movement of air into and out of the respiratory system, and gas exchange is a complex process that requires both inhalation and exhalation to occur. Ventilation is controlled by chemosensory receptors in spinal fluid and by arterial carbon dioxide tension and oxygen deficiency in the carotid and aortic arteries. As the receptors detect increases or decreases in carbon dioxide, oxygen, or both, ventilation is increased or decreased as needed to meet body requirements. Because the respiratory control center is located in the medulla of the brain, this process can be altered by respiratory or neurologic disease.

The exchange of gases occurs both in the lungs and throughout the body at the tissue level. In the lungs, carbon dioxide is released from the capillary beds into the

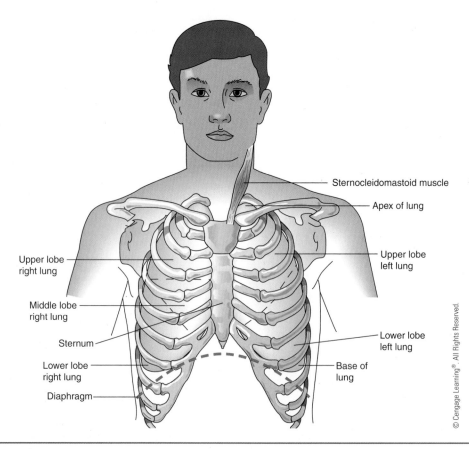

Sternocleidomastoid muscle

Apex of lung

Upper lobe right lung

Upper lobe left lung

Middle lobe right lung

Sternum

Lower lobe left lung

Lower lobe right lung

Base of lung

Diaphragm

FIGURE 9–1   The respiratory system.

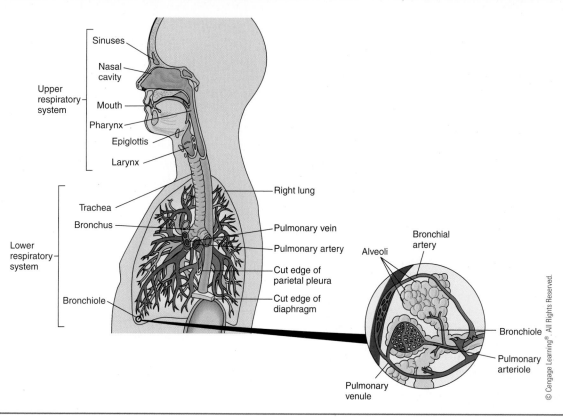

FIGURE 9–2 Airway divisions and terminal bronchiole/alveoli.

alveolar spaces by the process of diffusion. In the same way, oxygen moves from the air spaces into the capillaries for transport to the tissues. This process is reversed at the tissue level throughout the body, where oxygen moves from the bloodstream into the tissues, and carbon dioxide moves from the tissues into the blood for transport to the lungs and removal from the body (Figure 9–3).

Media Link

View an animation on respiration on the Online Resources.

COMMON SIGNS AND SYMPTOMS

There are many common signs and symptoms of respiratory disease, ranging from mild (the common cold) to severe (pneumonia). Dyspnea, orthopnea, apnea, wheezing, coughing, and nasal discharge are some of the most common symptoms.

Dyspnea (DISP-nee-ah; dys = difficulty, pnea = breathing) is a common sign of respiratory disease.

It can be in the form of **orthopnea** (or-THOP-nee-ah; ortho = straight, pnea = breathing), in which an individual has difficulty breathing in a lying position or is able to breathe with less difficulty when standing or sitting straight up. **Apnea** (ap-NEE-ah; a = without, pnea = breathing) for an extended length of time is a life-threatening emergency. Dyspnea caused by a partial obstruction of the airways will produce **wheezing**. Severe dyspnea can lead to **hypoxemia** (high-POX-SEE-me-ah; hypo = not enough, ox = oxygen, emia = blood), low blood oxygen level. A common sign of hypoxemia is **cyanosis** (SIGH-ah-NO-sis; cyano = blue, osis = condition), a blue color often observed in the nail beds and lips.

Coughing is another common symptom, caused by irritation of the airways or a buildup of fluid in the lung tissue. **Sputum** (SPYOU-tum) is fluid or secretions coughed up from the lungs, not to be confused with saliva or spit from the digestive system. A **productive cough** is one in which sputum or excessive mucus is brought up and expelled. Coughing up blood is called **hemoptysis** (he-MOP-tih-sis; hemo = blood, ptysis = saliva) and can be a sign of serious respiratory disease.

Nasal discharge is frequently present in infections, inflammation, and allergic respiratory reactions. It is the most frequent symptom of the common cold, but

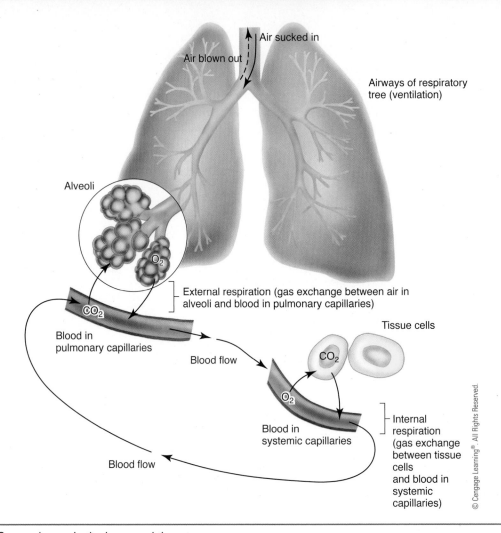

Air sucked in

Air blown out

Airways of respiratory tree (ventilation)

Alveoli

O_2

External respiration (gas exchange between air in alveoli and blood in pulmonary capillaries)

CO_2

Blood in pulmonary capillaries

Blood flow

Tissue cells

CO_2

O_2

Blood in systemic capillaries

Internal respiration (gas exchange between tissue cells and blood in systemic capillaries)

Blood flow

FIGURE 9–3   Gas exchange in the lungs and tissues.

it is also present in other respiratory disorders and can be a serious symptom of a chronic problem.

Hiccoughs, commonly called hiccups, are the result of a sudden spasm of the diaphragm. They commonly occur after eating or drinking and can be stopped by a variety of techniques, including holding the breath and drinking water through a straw. Hiccoughs might accompany disease and, in such an instance, are more difficult to eliminate.

Chronic respiratory conditions often lead to abnormal, permanent signs such as clubbing and a barrel-chested appearance. **Clubbing** is a condition of unknown pathogenesis, but it usually is related to poor distal circulation and oxygenation. It affects the distal portion of the fingers and is characterized by soft tissue enlargement and an abnormal curvature of the nail (Figure 9–4). A barrel chest appears because the individual uses accessory chest muscles over a long period of time in an effort to improve breathing.

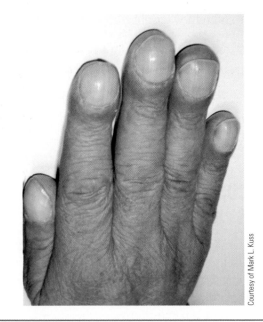

FIGURE 9–4   Clubbing.

DIAGNOSTIC TESTS

A physical examination including auscultation (listening to the chest with a stethoscope) should be completed to assess for abnormal breathing quality and rate. **Tachypnea** (TACK-ihp-NEE-ah; tachy = rapid, pnea = breathing), or rapid breathing, and abnormal breath sounds, including wheezes, rales, and rhonchi, are common with respiratory diseases. **Rales** are abnormal musical sounds heard on inspiration and are often called crackles. **Rhonchi** are dry rattling sounds in the bronchi due to obstruction of the airways.

A chest roentgenogram (X-ray) is a major diagnostic tool used to diagnose lung diseases such as tumors, tuberculosis, abscesses, and pneumonia. Sputum cultures are effective in determination of infectious disease. A tissue biopsy can be obtained as a definitive test for lung disease. Tissue biopsy is often obtained during a **bronchoscopy** (brong-KOS-koh-pee; broncho = bronchus or lung passageways, oscopy = procedure to look into the bronchus) (Figure 9–5). Lung tissue can be biopsied by using a fine-needle technique.

The best indicator of lung function is measurement of the amounts of carbon dioxide (waste) and oxygen in the blood. These measurements are done on arterial blood and are called **arterial blood gases** (ABGs). Normal arterial blood gases should be high in oxygen and low in carbon dioxide. Parameters for normal ABGs are oxygen (PaO_2) 80–100 mm Hg and carbon dioxide ($PaCO_2$) 35–45 mm Hg. The reverse of these readings is indicative of poor pulmonary function. Another important ABG is oxygen saturation (O_2Sat) with normal levels of 95–100%.

Pulmonary function tests (PFTs) are a group of tests that measure volume and flow of air by using

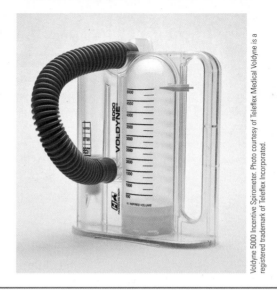

FIGURE 9–6   Spirometer: simple, for single patient use.

a spirometer. These tests are valuable in the diagnosis of a respiratory problem. PFTs can also be performed before and after bronchodilation treatment to measure treatment effectiveness. PFTs are measured against a norm for the individual's age, height, and sex. Patients are often encouraged to use a more simple model of a spirometer (Figure 9–6) to maintain and improve lung function.

COMMON DISEASES OF THE RESPIRATORY SYSTEM

Diseases of the respiratory system range from simple to very serious. The symptoms of the various disorders are often similar in the early stages, with most conditions manifesting in shortness of breath and coughing, wheezing, or both, although some disorders might not present symptoms until late in the disease development. Smoking is the number one risk behavior for developing chronic respiratory disease. Although influenza and other communicable respiratory diseases have been common for centuries, epidemics in the United States have not been as devastating as they were historically. Now public health officials are seeing new strains of respiratory viruses emerge and the threat of an epidemic is cause for concern.

Diseases of the Upper Respiratory Tract

Respiratory illnesses, which are mostly viral infections, account for approximately 50% of all acute illnesses. Respiratory infections account for approximately 55%

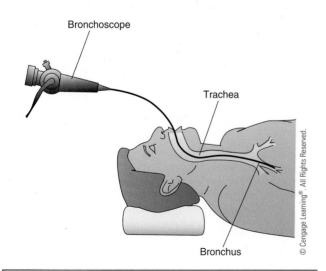

FIGURE 9–5   Bronchoscopy.

PHARMACOLOGY HIGHLIGHT

Common Drugs for Respiratory Disorders

CATEGORY	EXAMPLES OF MEDICATIONS
Antihistamines Drugs used for treatment/ prevention of allergies	carbinoxamine or levocabastine (prescription drugs), fexofenadine, cetirizine, or loratadine (over-the-counter drugs)
Antibiotics Drugs used to prevent or stop bacterial infections	ampicillin, amoxicillin, ciprofloxacin, doxycycline, erythromycin, penicillin, or tetracycline
Antivirals Drugs used to stop the action of the virus	acyclovir, imiquimod, or cidofovir
Antineoplastics Drugs used to treat cancer Alkylating agents Antimetabolites Antitumor antibiotics Hormones/antihormones Other substances	chlorambucil, cyclophosphamide, or lomustine 5-flourauracil, mercaptopurine, or methotrexate mitomycin or streptozocin estrogens, androgens, flutamide, or tamoxifen vincristine, L-asparaginase, paclitaxel, carboplatin, cisplatin, or etoposide

of all infections requiring hospitalization (Figure 9–7). Most disorders of the upper respiratory tract are not life threatening.

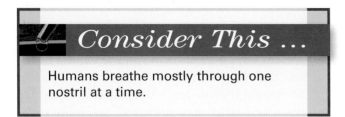

Consider This ...

Humans breathe mostly through one nostril at a time.

UPPER RESPIRATORY INFECTION (URI)

■ **DESCRIPTION.** URI is a broad term referring to several infectious diseases of the upper respiratory tract. These infections are the most common cause for lost days of work for adults.

■ **ETIOLOGY.** Most URIs (not to be confused with UTI, urinary tract infection) are caused by viruses. The most common is a group called rhinovirus.

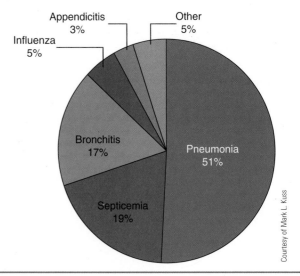

FIGURE 9–7 Frequency of infectious diseases requiring hospitalization.

Courtesy of Mark L. Kuss

■ **SYMPTOMS.** Symptoms commonly include nasal congestion, runny nose, sore throat, ear pain or fullness, sneezing, coughing, mild fever, headache, and generalized aches. Symptoms usually resolve in 7–10 days.

■ **DIAGNOSIS.** Diagnosis is usually made on the basis of a history and physical examination revealing the common signs and symptoms.

■ **TREATMENT.** General treatment for viral diseases includes rest, drinking increased amounts of fluids, and taking **antipyretics** (anti = against, pyretic = fever) and **analgesics** (an = without, algesic = pain). Antibiotics are not effective with viral infections but might be needed for secondary bacterial infection. The common cold is the most frequent URI and often leads to secondary infectious diseases.

■ **PREVENTION.** Prevention is often difficult because viruses are easily spread by droplet infection such as sneezing or coughing. These microscopic droplets are then picked up on the hands and carried to the membranes of the respiratory tract by touching or wiping the eyes and nose. The greatest preventive measure is regular hand washing. Other preventive activities include avoiding crowds, avoiding smoking, and maintaining general health.

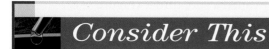

Consider This ...

It is impossible to sneeze with your eyes open due to a defensive mechanism that protects the eyes from bacteria and debris that are spread with the sneeze.

COMMON COLD (ACUTE RHINITIS)

■ **DESCRIPTION.** The common cold is an acute inflammation of the mucous membranes of the upper respiratory tract. There are several hundred virus strains that cause a cold. Developing immunity to one strain does not provide immunity to others.

■ **ETIOLOGY.** A cold is very contagious and is usually passed from one individual to another through touch and air droplets. Many individuals believe that getting chilled or wet is the cause of a cold. In actuality, these actions do not directly cause a cold; they merely lower an individual's resistance to invasion by a cold-causing virus. Children, older people, and individuals in generally poor health are at increased risk of contracting a cold.

■ **SYMPTOMS.** Most individuals are very familiar with the symptoms of runny nose, or **rhinorrhea** (rye-nor-REE-ah; rhino = nose, orrhea = run through), watery eyes, stuffy head, sore throat, sneezing, and fever.

■ **DIAGNOSIS.** Diagnosis is usually determined by physical examination and presence of signs and symptoms.

■ **TREATMENT.** Treatment involves basic comfort care, including rest, drinking increased fluids, and taking antipyretics and analgesics as prescribed.

■ **PREVENTION.** Good hand washing is the best preventive measure against a cold.

HAY FEVER (ALLERGIC RHINITIS)

Allergic rhinitis is an inflammation of the mucous membranes due to allergies. This sensitivity to an allergen

COMPLEMENTARY AND ALTERNATIVE THERAPY

Natural Immunomodulators for Upper Respiratory Infections

The use of natural immunomodulators (substances that help regulate the immune system, which helps fight infections) has become more popular with the increased acceptance of complementary or alternative therapies. The natural immunomodulators found in raw fruits and vegetables are said to enhance weak immune systems and slow down overactive immune systems. The natural immunomodulators are different from the chemical (pharmaceutical) ones such as methotrexate, which is more toxic to some patients. The natural immunomodulators do not have as many side effects as the chemical ones but more research needs to be done to understand their use in treating respiratory infections or other medical conditions.

Source: Rountree (2011).

tends to run in families. Ragweed and grasses are two common allergens. Hay fever was discussed in detail in Chapter 5, "Immune System Diseases and Disorders."

SINUSITIS

■ **DESCRIPTION.** Sinusitis is an inflammation of the mucous membrane lining the sinuses. The sinuses are air-filled cavities in the bony tissue of the head. The membranes that line the nose extend into the sinuses.

■ **ETIOLOGY.** Acute rhinitis often leads to sinusitis. It is also believed that blowing the nose too hard actually spreads infection into the sinuses. As mucous membranes become swollen, the drainage system becomes blocked. Mucus accumulates in the sinuses, causing increased pressure and often leading to sinus headaches, dizziness, and difficulty breathing. Other causes of sinusitis include tooth infections, air pollution, and nasal deformities.

■ **SYMPTOMS.** Pain in the area of the affected sinus is common. Headaches upon awakening are most common with sinus involvement. Pain in the forehead area can be related to frontal sinus inflammation. Other symptoms include tiredness, a night cough, runny nose, nasal congestion, and sore throat.

■ **DIAGNOSIS.** Diagnosis is based on clinical history, physical examination, computed tomography (CT) scan or magnetic resonance imaging (MRI), and laboratory tests to help identify the allergies.

■ **TREATMENT.** Treatment often includes antibiotics and decongestants. Because sinusitis can lead to more serious infections such as mastoiditis and encephalitis, aggressive treatment is necessary.

■ **PREVENTION.** Sinusitis in many cases cannot be prevented, although there are measures that might reduce frequency of attacks, such as use of a humidifier, avoiding cigarette smoke and other air pollutants, avoiding alcohol because it causes nasal membranes to swell, and avoiding swimming in pools due to the chlorine.

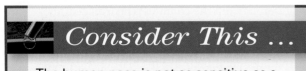

Consider This ...

The human nose is not as sensitive as a dog's nose, but it can distinguish approximately 500 different scents.

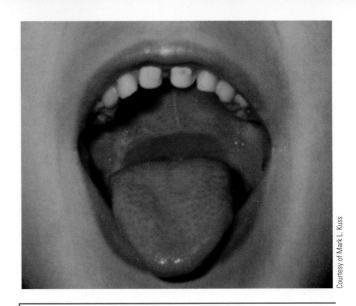

FIGURE 9–8 Pharyngitis.

PHARYNGITIS

■ **DESCRIPTION.** Pharyngitis is an inflammation of the throat (pharynx = throat, itis = inflammation) commonly called a sore throat (Figure 9–8).

■ **ETIOLOGY.** The most common cause is viral infection. Bacterial infection by *Streptococcus* can also occur and is more common in children. Irritation to the mucous membranes, such as breathing extremely hot or cold air, chemical fumes, or smoke, can also lead to pharyngitis.

■ **SYMPTOMS.** Symptoms include sore throat, fever, headache, swollen lymph glands in the neck, and pain with swallowing.

■ **DIAGNOSIS.** Physical examination, including viewing the pharynx (throat), eyes, skin, and lymph nodes is useful. A streptococcal throat swab culture might be taken to diagnosis strep infection.

■ **TREATMENT.** Treatment depends on the cause. Viral infections are treated with comfort care and throat lozenges, antiseptic or salt-water gargles, and analgesics. Bacterial infections, such as strep throat, also need antibiotic treatment. Chronic pharyngitis due to tonsillitis and adenoiditis can be treated by surgical removal of the tonsils and adenoids, called a tonsillectomy and adenoidectomy (T&A), respectively.

■ **PREVENTION.** Good hand washing, maintaining general health, and avoiding close contact with anyone who is contagious aid in prevention of pharyngitis. Using a new toothbrush after the symptoms disappear also aids in prevention.

LARYNGITIS

■ **DESCRIPTION.** Laryngitis is an inflammation of the larynx (LAR-inks) and vocal cords.

■ **ETIOLOGY.** Laryngitis can be caused by viral or bacterial infections or by breathing irritants such as extremely hot or cold air, chemical fumes, and smoke. Laryngitis frequently follows other URIs such as the common cold, pharyngitis, and sinusitis. Another cause can be overuse of the voice for an extended time.

■ **SYMPTOMS.** Most individuals are familiar with the hoarse voice quality caused by laryngitis. Other symptoms include difficulty swallowing (dysphagia), throat pain, and fever.

■ **DIAGNOSIS.** A history of a recent cold or flu followed by hoarseness is a common clue for diagnosis. A harsh wheezing sound in the throat area is usually indicative of laryngitis. A laryngoscope can be used to view the airway and vocal cords for other signs of disease.

■ **TREATMENT.** Treatment can include voice rest, increased fluid intake, analgesics, throat lozenges, and removal of causative factors.

■ **PREVENTION.** Frequent hand washing, avoiding those with infections, and avoiding breathing irritants aid in prevention.

Diseases of the Bronchi and Lungs

Diseases of the bronchi and lungs are usually more severe than diseases of the upper respiratory system. Many of these can be life threatening, such as influenza, especially in the older population.

ASTHMA

■ **DESCRIPTION.** Asthma is a hypersensitivity reaction that causes constriction of the bronchi, leading to difficulty breathing.

■ **ETIOLOGY.** Asthma, also called bronchial asthma, was discussed in detail as a hypersensitivity disorder in Chapter 5.

■ **SYMPTOMS.** Asthma is characterized by episodes of wheezing and dyspnea.

■ **DIAGNOSIS.** A diagnosis of asthma usually is based on the patient's symptoms, medical history, a physical examination, and laboratory tests that measure pulmonary (lung) function.

■ **TREATMENT.** Treatment includes avoidance of causative allergens, desensitization, education, and medications to treat symptoms.

■ **PREVENTION.** Prevention is aimed at identification and control of allergic factors and use of bronchodilators.

Media Link

View an animation on Asthma: Pathophysiology on CourseMate.

ACUTE BRONCHITIS

■ **DESCRIPTION.** Acute bronchitis is inflammation of the mucous membrane lining of the bronchus. It often involves the trachea (tracheobronchitis).

■ **ETIOLOGY.** Acute bronchitis is a short-term disorder commonly following a URI. Other causes include inhaling fumes, smoke, dust, cold air, and other irritants.

■ **SYMPTOMS.** Symptoms include fever, a tight feeling behind the sternum, and a dry cough that later progresses to a productive cough (coughing up or expectorating mucus or sputum).

■ **DIAGNOSIS.** Tests are usually unnecessary in diagnosis because this disease is easy to determine from a history and physical examination; however, an X-ray can be ordered.

■ **TREATMENT.** Treatment consists of drinking increased amounts of fluids to help liquefy secretions, rest, cough syrup, analgesics, and antipyretics. Antibiotics are helpful only if secondary bacterial infections occur. Prognosis is generally good for most individuals. Infants and small children can become seriously ill because the bronchioles are very small and can become obstructed by swollen tissue or mucus plugs. Older people and the chronically ill might have a poor prognosis because they have an increased risk for developing secondary bacterial infections such as pneumonia.

COMPLEMENTARY AND ALTERNATIVE THERAPY

Bark of Acacia Tree for Treatment of Bronchitis

The bark of the *Acacia leucophloea* has been used throughout the world for treatment of bronchitis, cough, infections, and a variety of other disorders. Research was done to justify the use of this plant for treatment of respiratory and gastrointestinal diseases and to try to find the mechanism of its action. The findings showed that the extract of the plant has some effects on spasms (relieves them) and has some bronchodilator effects. This would explain its benefit in treating bronchitis or other respiratory ailments.

Source: Imran et al. (2011).

■ **PREVENTION.** Preventive activities include:

- Washing hands frequently
- Not smoking and avoiding secondhand smoke
- Avoiding allergens such as dust and household fumes
- Not sharing eating utensils with others
- Maintaining a healthy lifestyle

INFLUENZA (FLU)

■ **DESCRIPTION.** Influenza is an acute, highly contagious respiratory infection. Influenza can be a serious disease, especially in the elderly, young children, and people with certain health conditions. Yearly flu seasons can vary from year to year in duration and in severity of illness. Flu season may be short or long, and the symptoms may range from mild to very severe. "Over a period of 30 years, between 1976 and 2006, estimates of flu-associated deaths in the United States range from a low of about 3,000 to a high of about 49,000 people" (Centers for Disease Control and Prevention, 2011b).

■ **ETIOLOGY.** Influenza is a viral infection commonly spread by coughing of respiratory secretions. There are many strains of influenza virus, the primary of which are identified as A, B, and C. Substrains, or subtypes, include H0N1, H1N1, H2N2, H3N2, and several others. Avian (bird) flu is an influenza A virus that usually does not affect humans. However, recent diagnosed cases in humans have caused concern among public health workers. Deaths have been attributed to avian influenza in children and adults. Most human infections have occurred following direct contact with infected poultry.

The flu virus has great genetic variation, and the number of strains and variations help explain how this virus causes epidemics year after year. Unfortunately, like the common cold, immunity to one viral strain does not provide immunity to another, so an individual can have the flu multiple times. Flu epidemics commonly occur in the winter and early spring.

■ **SYMPTOMS.** Influenza is characterized by sudden onset of fever, chills, headache, and back muscle pain. Other symptoms can include cough, runny nose, sore throat, sneezing, hoarseness, nausea, vomiting, and diarrhea.

■ **DIAGNOSIS.** Flu can be difficult to distinguish from many other types of common cold viruses and bacterial infections. A history and physical exam that reveals a sudden onset of symptoms can assist in diagnosis. Rapid diagnostic tests are available that can detect influenza viruses in 30 minutes.

■ **TREATMENT.** Treatment of influenza is symptomatic and can include bed rest, analgesics, and antipyretics. Oseltamivir (Tamiflu) and zanamivir (Relenza) are Food and Drug Administration (FDA)–approved antiviral medications recommended for treatment of both influenza A and B viruses. These medications must be started within 2 days of symptoms to be effective. Antibiotics are not indicated unless secondary bacterial infections occur.

■ **PREVENTION.** Vaccination is the best way to prevent influenza. Antiviral medications are also effective in prevention.

CHRONIC OBSTRUCTIVE PULMONARY DISEASE (COPD)

■ **DESCRIPTION.** COPD is the name for two distinct diseases characterized by the inability to get air into or out of the lungs. Chronic bronchitis and

HEALTHY HIGHLIGHT

Influenza Immunization (Flu Shots)

Because influenza is a viral infection, antiviral medications can be given, but there is no major treatment other than supportive treatment of symptoms in most cases. An individual is dependent on the immune system to build antibodies to kill the virus. Antibiotics can be helpful for secondary bacterial infections but do not kill the influenza virus.

The best course in dealing with flu is prevention, which includes frequent hand washing, avoiding crowds of people during flu season or when there is a local epidemic, avoiding individuals infected with influenza, and leading a healthy lifestyle to keep resistance high.

An immunization is available and is recommended for all individuals but especially for older people, those with chronic diseases, pregnant women, children, and health care workers. Reactions to the flu immunization are rare but do occur. Individuals allergic to eggs should not take the immunization because the virus is grown in eggs. Allergic hypersensitivity reactions usually occur immediately after receiving the injection, although a reaction to the antigen can occur 6 to 12 hours after the injection. Reaction symptoms mimic the flu and include fever, muscle pain, and malaise.

---

emphysema frequently coexist, hence the preference to call them, collectively, COPD. There can be pure forms of either, but usually, the individual has predominantly one or the other coexisting with the second. This term does not include other obstructive diseases such as asthma.

Both chronic bronchitis and emphysema cause excessive inflammation that leads to abnormalities in the lung that permanently obstruct airflow (thus the term *chronic obstructive*). With COPD, the loss of normal respiratory response is not unusual.

Normally, individuals are stimulated to breathe by an increase of carbon dioxide in the blood. A secondary or backup stimulus is a decrease of oxygen in the blood. Individuals with COPD commonly have high levels of carbon dioxide in the blood. Initially, the body attempts to correct this by increasing breathing in an effort to blow out excessive carbon dioxide (CO_2). When this effort fails, the respiratory system adapts to the high CO_2 levels and begins responding to the secondary stimulus of low blood oxygen levels. Giving oxygen to these individuals can be fatal because high oxygenation removes the stimulus to breathe.

Approximately 24 million people suffer from this disease, and it is the fourth most significant cause of death in United States (American Lung Association, 2012).

■ **ETIOLOGY.** Ninety percent of the time, these diseases are due to cigarette smoking. Other causes include air pollution and chronic respiratory infections. Exposure to certain industrial pollutants can also increase the risk of developing COPD.

■ **SYMPTOMS.** Symptoms of COPD occur due to lung damage. In smokers, it might take 40 to 50 years for symptoms to occur. Symptoms can occur many years after the individual actually quits smoking, quite simply because the lungs have a large amount of reserve capacity.

As we age, we normally lose lung function, but not enough to cause symptoms unless our lungs are damaged or diseased. Smokers lose function at a rate approximately five times faster than normal. Even at this rate, it commonly takes decades for a smoker to lose enough lung function to experience symptoms.

If an individual quits smoking, the loss of function slows back to approximately normal. However, if smoking has already destroyed a large portion of the lung tissue, symptoms of COPD will appear as the individual ages and continues to lose function at a normal rate. If one continues to smoke, decline continues at an accelerated rate. Quitting smoking at any time in one's life can slow loss of function and improve quality of life.

Common symptoms include the following:

- Dyspnea (difficulty breathing) is the most common symptom. Onset is usually gradual and often noticed only with exercise. As the disease progresses and the individual ages into his or her 60s and 70s, dyspnea becomes increasingly prominent as lung function declines.

- Chronic cough usually begins in the morning but slowly progresses to an all-day cough. This progression can be so slow the individual does not even recognize the fact that he or she is coughing all the time.

- Wheezing appears and is due to air passing through tight or narrow airways.

- Hemoptysis, or coughing up blood, usually occurs during acute attacks. This hemoptysis is usually blood-streaked sputum, not active bleeding. Bloody sputum in an individual with COPD also can be indicative of lung cancer.

- Cyanosis, a bluish discoloration of the skin, nail beds, and lips, is common, especially during acute attacks. Cyanosis indicates a low blood oxygen level.

- Weight loss is common because individuals with COPD work hard and burn increased calories in the activity of breathing. Shortness of breath caused by the activity of eating often interrupts meals, leading to malnutrition.

- Pursed-lip breathing is an acquired breathing pattern that forces air out of the lungs. By pursing the lips together during exhalation, the back pressure or positive pressure holds airways open to allow forced exhalation of the air through narrowed passageways. This breathing pattern is hard work, burns increased calories, and weakens the already damaged airways.

- Barrel chest describes a bulging, rounded chest that resembles the shape of a barrel. This is a symptom of late-stage COPD. The lungs are chronically overinflated with air, causing the rib cage to stay partially expanded. This change in physical structure of the chest makes breathing less efficient and leads to more shortness of breath.

■ **DIAGNOSIS.** Diagnosis of COPD is made by history and physical examination and by ruling out other pulmonary diseases. Chest X-rays, pulmonary function tests (PFTs), and ABGs help confirm the diagnosis.

■ **TREATMENT.** Symptomatic treatment includes use of bronchodilator medications, inhalers, mucolytics, and cough medications. Avoiding exposure to individuals with respiratory tract infections is important because these diseases aggravate COPD. Influenza vaccination is recommended. Cessation of smoking can slow or reverse the disease in the early stages and will ease symptoms in the later stages.

There is no cure for end-stage COPD. Individuals often become debilitated in the final stages of the disease, and prognosis is poor due to progressive deterioration of pulmonary function, often leading to respiratory failure and death.

■ **PREVENTION.** Not smoking is the best preventive action. Other preventive measures include avoiding respiratory irritants and infections and maintaining a healthy lifestyle.

CHRONIC BRONCHITIS

■ **DESCRIPTION.** Chronic bronchitis is a long-term inflammation and scarring of the lining of the bronchial tubes. It is characterized by increased mucus production with a productive cough. Chronic inflammation leads to hypertrophy of the mucus-secreting glands, thickening of the mucous membrane, and **bronchiectasis** (BRONG-kee-ECK-tah-sis), a chronic dilatation of the bronchus.

■ **SYMPTOMS.** Bronchiectasis allows mucus to pool in the bronchus, producing a foul-smelling cough. This cough is commonly called smoker's cough and occurs primarily in the morning hours. As the disease progresses, obstruction of the bronchi and bronchioles becomes more pronounced, leading to difficulty getting air into the lungs. Coughing, dyspnea, and **hypoxia** (HIGH-POCK-see-ah; hypo = low, oxia = oxygen) occur. During bouts of hypoxia, the individual often becomes cyanotic (blue condition). In the final or end stage, the symptoms are more continuous, causing lung damage, debilitation of the individual, and eventual death.

EMPHYSEMA

■ **DESCRIPTION.** Emphysema comes from the Greek word *emphysana*, meaning "to inflate." This chronic disease is characterized by an increased production of mucus, causing trapping of air in the tiny alveoli or air sacs of the lung. As air becomes trapped in the alveoli, they become overinflated, leading to destruction of the alveoli wall. Destruction of the alveoli wall allows the alveoli to fuse with other

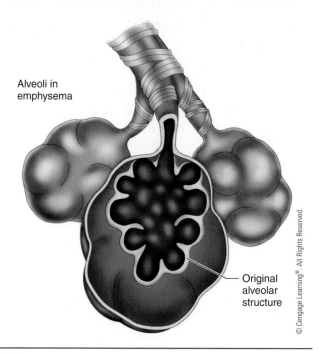

Alveoli in
emphysema

Original
alveolar
structure

© Cengage Learning®. All Rights Reserved.

FIGURE 9–9   Normal versus emphasematous alveoli.

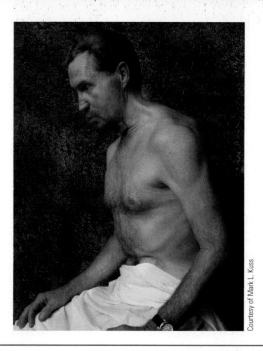

Courtesy of Mark L. Kuss

FIGURE 9–10   Pursed lips and barrel chest of emphysema.

alveoli, forming a larger air sack and trapping more air (Figure 9–9).

■ **SYMPTOMS.** The individual with emphysema is able to get air in, but the air becomes trapped and must be forced out before more air can be taken in. These enlarged alveoli have a decreased surface area, thus decreasing oxygenation of the blood. Air trapping and decreased oxygen exchange lead to dyspnea, tachypnea, wheezing, and coughing.

Individuals with emphysema often lean over a table or chair to use accessory respiratory muscles to blow out the trapped air more effectively. Pursing the lips also helps hold the alveoli open while pushing the air out (Figure 9–10). This extra pressure often causes the face and skin to become reddened. Extra pressure on the chest muscles also produces a characteristic barrel-chested appearance.

Individuals with emphysema use large amounts of energy in their respiratory efforts, so a supplemented diet is often needed. Food is eaten in small, frequent feedings to allow time for respiratory efforts. Even with a supplemented diet, these individuals are often unable to get adequate nutrition and commonly are quite thin.

ATELECTASIS

■ **DESCRIPTION.** Atelectasis (ah-tel-EK-teh-sis) is the collapse or airless state of part or all of a lung. More commonly, it affects only a small section of the lung.

■ **ETIOLOGY.** Atelectasis is often related to inadequate breathing patterns related to pain. Surgical pain and fractured ribs often cause inadequate breathing, leading to atelectasis. Blockage of the airway by a mucus plug can also cause atelectasis.

■ **SYMPTOMS.** Dyspnea, cyanosis, and anxiety are common symptoms.

■ **DIAGNOSIS.** Diagnosis is confirmed after a positive chest X-ray and physical examination.

■ **TREATMENT.** Ambulation (walking), frequent deep breathing and coughing, and analgesics for pain help open the airway, expand the alveoli, and avoid atelectasis. Prognosis is good if complications do not occur. Pneumonia is a common complication.

■ **PREVENTION.** Prevention is aimed at relieving the cause if possible.

PNEUMONIA

■ **DESCRIPTION.** Pneumonia is an inflammation of the bronchioles and alveoli due to infection by bacteria, virus, or other pathogens. Pneumonia is the term specifically related to infection. Inflammation without infection is termed *pneumonitis* and is generally caused by a hypersensitivity to dusts and chemicals.

Pneumonia can be identified in several ways. The cause might be included in the name, as in "pneumococcal," "aspiration," and "tuberculous pneumonia." The location might be identified in the name, as in "lobar," "bilateral," and "double pneumonia." Secondary pneumonia indicates a connection to another cause. Often, the location and cause can be combined to describe the pneumonia, as in "bilateral pneumococcal pneumonia."

Bacterial pneumonias tend to be the most serious, whereas viral pneumonias are the most common. People who have difficulty swallowing, as is common in those with throat surgery or stroke, are at risk for aspiration pneumonia.

Pneumonia affects millions of individuals each year and can range from mild to life threatening. It occurs more often among older people, the chronically ill, and those who are immunosuppressed and is a significant cause of death in these individuals.

■ **ETIOLOGY.** Actions that inhibit the normal protective mechanisms of the respiratory system, such as smoking, immobility, general anesthesia, and endotracheal intubation, allow the invasion of pathogens into lung tissue.

Pathogens that cause pneumonia can reach the lung tissue through the respiratory system or through the blood as a result of septicemia. Invasion of pathogens into the alveoli leads to inflammation of the alveolar tissue, causing the classic outpouring of blood fluid and white cells from the capillaries into the tissues, filling the alveolus. This causes a decrease in gas exchange, leading to hypoxia (Figure 9–11). This inflammation and infection of the lungs is pneumonia.

■ **SYMPTOMS.** Symptoms of pneumonia are related to the area involved and the amount of tissue involved. Symptoms include dyspnea, weakness, fever, chills, chest pain, and cough.

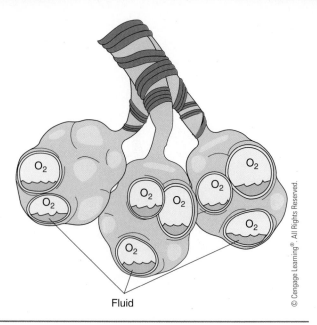

Fluid

FIGURE 9–11   Pneumonia: alveoli filling with fluid.

■ **DIAGNOSIS.** Diagnosis is made after completion of a chest X-ray, history, physical examination, and sputum culture to determine the infective pathogen.

■ **TREATMENT.** Treatment depends on cause. Bacterial infection is treated with antibiotics. Viral infection is treated symptomatically. Rest, analgesics, oxygen therapy, increased fluid intake, and high-calorie diet are common treatments for all types of pneumonia.

■ **PREVENTION.** Preventive activities include not smoking, frequent hand washing, and wearing a mask when working with fumes, dust, or mold. Vaccines can also prevent pneumonia. Pneumococcal, flu, and *Haemophilus influenzae* type B (Hib) (for children) vaccines are all effective. Taking deep breaths and use of a breathing device aid in prevention of pneumonia after surgery.

HEALTHY HIGHLIGHT

Prevent Pneumonia with Vaccines

Pneumonia can be prevented with vaccines. The Centers for Disease Control and Prevention (CDC) recommend the pneumococcal conjugate vaccine PCV13 (Prevnar 13®) for children 5 years of age or less. The CDC recommends Pneumovax® (23-valent polysaccharide vaccine [PPVSV]) for all adults over age 65, for those 2 years of age or older who are at risk because of a concurrent disease, and for adults age 19 to 64 who smoke or have been diagnosed with asthma (CDC, 2012a).

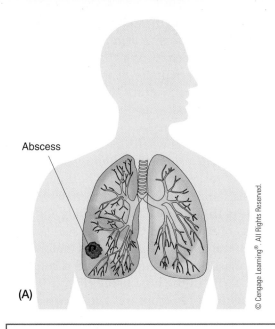 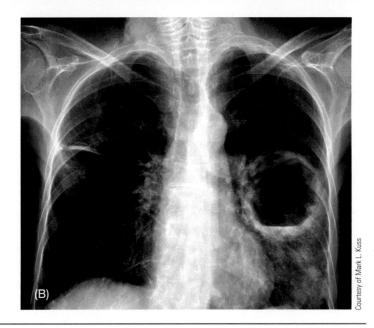

FIGURE 9–12 (A) Pulmonary abscess. (B) X-ray view of pulmonary abscess.

PULMONARY ABSCESS

■ **DESCRIPTION.** Pulmonary abscess, also called lung abscess, is a collection of infectious material contained within a capsule (Figure 9–12). Abscess formation was discussed in detail in Chapter 4, "Inflammation and Infection."

■ **ETIOLOGY.** Lung abscess is often related to a number of other diseases, including pneumonia, tuberculosis, and lung cancer. It can also be caused by aspiration of food or foreign objects.

■ **SYMPTOMS.** Symptoms include chills, fever, chest pain, and cough. Coughing of bloody or foul-smelling sputum and foul-smelling breath can also be indicative of a pulmonary abscess.

■ **DIAGNOSIS.** Diagnosis is made by completion of a history and physical examination, chest X-ray, and sputum cultures.

■ **TREATMENT.** Pulmonary abscesses are commonly treated with long-term antibiotic therapy. Surgical resection might be indicated if the abscess is quite large or if antibiotic therapy is unsuccessful.

■ **PREVENTION.** Preventing aspiration is the most important preventive measure.

PULMONARY TUBERCULOSIS

■ **DESCRIPTION.** Pulmonary tuberculosis is often called tuberculosis (TB). It is a contagious bacterial infection that mainly involves the lungs but can spread to other organs such as the kidneys, bones, and brain.

Current facts according to the World Health Organization (WHO) include the following:

■ One-third of the world's current population has been infected by TB.

■ In 2009, approximately 10 million children became orphans as a result of TB deaths among parents.

■ In 2010 alone, 8.8 million people fell ill with TB and 1.4 million died.

■ Over 95% of TB deaths occur in low- to middle-income countries.

■ TB is second only to human immunodeficiency virus (HIV)/acquired immunodeficiency syndrome (AIDS) as the greatest killer worldwide due to a single infectious agent.

In 2006, the WHO declared TB a global health emergency and developed a global plan to stop TB that aims at saving 14 million lives by the year 2015. This plan appears to be on track since the death rate has dropped 40% from 1990 to 2010 (WHO, 2012).

■ **ETIOLOGY.** TB is a bacterial infection caused by *Mycobacterium tuberculosis*. It is acquired by breathing air that is infected with the bacteria and is spread by coughing and sneezing.

Mycobacterium tuberculosis is protected in a strong coating that enables it to live outside the body for a lengthy amount of time. Infected droplets that are coughed or sneezed can dry up and remain on inanimate objects as dust but can be killed by bactericidal solutions or by direct sunlight.

TB is often prevalent in areas of overcrowding and poor sanitation. The incidence of TB was greatly reduced decades ago with the introduction of effective antibiotics. More recently, however, the number of TB cases in the United States has seriously risen due to the influx of high numbers of infected immigrants, the homeless, individuals with AIDS who have poor resistance to infection, and the development of drug-resistant bacteria.

The infection begins with a primary lesion in the lungs. *Mycobacterium tuberculosis* does not attract polymorphic nuclear cells (PMNs) and thus does not cause an acute inflammation. Lymphocytes and macrophages are attracted to these encapsulated bacteria. These immune cells begin producing antibodies and walling off the infection by forming a type of granuloma called a tubercle; hence the name, tuberculosis. The inside of the tubercle contains dead bacteria, lung tissue, and immune cells that together exhibit a cheesy appearance called caseous necrosis.

After necrosis, the tubercles change by fibrosing and calcifying. If the immune system is effective in walling off the bacteria, the disease can be arrested or rendered inactive for a long period of time (months to years). During this time, the individual is often asymptomatic and not aware that he or she has TB. If the disease is not arrested, the individual will become symptomatic with progressive primary TB. The antibodies that are produced during this time circulate in the blood for the remainder of the infected individual's life in readiness to attack future TB bacteria. These circulating antibodies are the basis for the positive reaction to a TB skin test.

Secondary TB occurs when an individual is reinfected with *Mycobacterium tuberculosis*, or the primary disease is reactivated due to a decline in the individual's resistance. Antibodies formed during the primary stage of the disease activate quickly and lead to larger areas of necrosis in the lung tissue. During secondary TB, the individual becomes symptomatic. The tubercle mass becomes liquefied and is coughed up, leaving a cavity in the lung tissue (Figure 9–13). Frequent coughing often ruptures capillaries in the lung tissue, leading to hemoptysis (coughing, spitting of blood, or both). Coughing by the infected individual fills the surrounding air with disease.

As large cavities are formed in the lung tissue, the ability of the tissue to oxygenate the blood is decreased. The individual becomes dyspneic and cachectic with a general appearance of being consumed by the disease. For this reason, historically, this disease was called consumption. During that time, individuals were placed in sanitariums to prevent the spread of TB and to provide much-needed rest. Without effective treatment, many infected individuals died from TB.

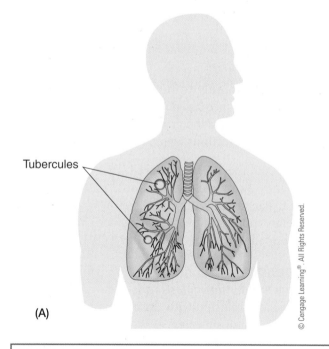

(A)

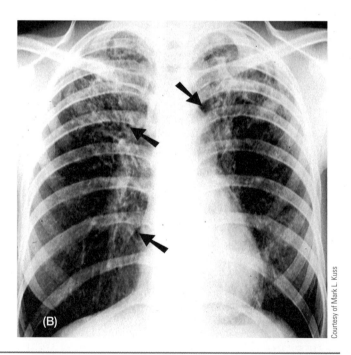

(B)

FIGURE 9–13 (A) Diagram of tuberculosis. (B) X-ray of tuberculosis cavities.

HEALTHY HIGHLIGHT

Tuberculosis Skin Test

TB skin test (TST) works on the principle that after an individual is exposed to *Mycobacterium tuberculosis*, the immune system will develop antibodies. These antibodies will be present in all cells of the body (cellular immunity) from that point on. Introduction of the bacillus or a derivative, through injection or re-exposure, will cause a cellular reaction. The Mantoux (man-TOO) test uses this principle. A small amount of purified protein derivative (PPD) is injected intradermally. PPD contains modified tuberculin bacteria that are no longer infectious. If the individual has been exposed to TB and has developed antibodies, the immune system will react. A reaction will also occur if the individual has been previously immunized with Bacillus Calmette-Guérin (BCG) tuberculin vaccine. A reaction is shown by the formation of an intradermal wheal. An 8–10 mm wheal within 48–72 hours of injection is considered a positive, now called significant, reaction. The Centers for Disease Control and Prevention (CDC) recommend using the QuantiFERON®-TB test (an interferon-gamma release assay [IGRA] test that uses whole blood) to detect TB in health care workers and suspected cases or when the patients are not compliant with returning to the clinic to get the test read. The CDC recommends using the TST for children under age 5.

After an individual has a positive skin test (significant reaction) once, that individual will always have a reaction, so a skin test is no longer beneficial in determining whether the individual has active TB. Individuals exhibiting a positive skin test need to be educated in the symptoms of TB, which include unexpected weight loss, persistent cough, night sweats, and malaise. If these symptoms occur and persist, the individual will need a chest X-ray and possible sputum culture to determine the presence of disease.

■ **SYMPTOMS.** Tuberculosis in an otherwise healthy individual is often asymptomatic, so testing is needed to determine the presence of the disease. If symptoms appear, they are often vague and include loss of weight, energy, and appetite. As the disease progresses, the individual might become symptomatic with a chronic productive cough, dyspnea, fever, and night sweats.

■ **DIAGNOSIS.** TB is diagnosed by skin testing, chest X-ray, and sputum culture.

■ **TREATMENT.** Extended antibiotic therapy is needed to rid the individual of the infection.

■ **PREVENTION.** TB is preventable with skin testing in high-risk populations or for individuals who might have been exposed, such as health care workers.

GLIMPSE OF THE FUTURE

Scientists are looking for a replacement for the TB vaccine now used throughout the world (except in the United States). The vaccine is called Bacillus Calmette-Guérin (BCG). In the past, it has been very helpful in reducing the TB rate worldwide, but now there are too many drug-resistant strains of TB. Since the WHO has set a goal to reduce the number of TB deaths, researchers are looking for a new, more effective TB vaccine.

Source: Kupferschmidt (2011).

ADULT RESPIRATORY DISTRESS SYNDROME (ARDS)

■ **DESCRIPTION.** ARDS is also called shock lung. It is a sudden, life-threatening lung failure—a syndrome, not a specific disease, that usually develops within 24 to 48 hours of a major injury or illness.

■ **ETIOLOGY.** Approximately 30% of ARDS cases are caused by sepsis, a serious infection of the blood. Other conditions that can cause the syndrome include severe chest trauma, inhalation of smoke or toxic fumes, near-drowning, fat emboli, aspiration pneumonia, major burns, massive blood transfusion, and acute pancreatitis. In most cases, these conditions do not lead to the development of ARDS. It is unclear why some people develop the syndrome but others do not.

Following the trauma, the individual might be progressing smoothly when a sudden, life-threatening attack of ARDs occurs. ARDS is characterized by fluid escaping the vascular system and filling the alveoli, leading to acute respiratory failure.

■ **SYMPTOMS.** Symptoms develop suddenly and include extreme dyspnea, severe hypoxemia, tachypnea, cyanosis, and pulmonary hypertension (high blood pressure in the pulmonary arteries).

■ **DIAGNOSIS.** History and physical examination along with a chest X-ray and ABGs aid in diagnosis.

■ **TREATMENT.** Individuals suffer extreme dyspnea and need mechanical ventilation. Even with prompt and proper treatment, ARDS has a high mortality rate. Approximately one-third of the affected individuals die within days, another third die within weeks, usually due to pneumonia and heart failure. Approximately one-third recover, but many of these individuals have permanent respiratory damage and are more prone to respiratory-related illnesses thereafter.

■ **PREVENTION.** ARDS is prevented by avoiding diseases and conditions that damage the lung, for instance, preventing aspiration, treating with as low a level of oxygen as possible, and treating infection promptly.

SUDDEN ACUTE RESPIRATORY SYNDROME (SARS)

■ **DESCRIPTION.** SARS is the first severe, easily transmissible new disease to emerge in the twenty-first century. SARS is a respiratory illness that was first reported in Asia but spread to people in Europe, South America, and North America in February 2003.

Public health officials worked quickly to halt the spread of the disease and actually contained it by July 2003. According to the WHO, 8,098 people worldwide became sick with SARS, and 774 died in the 2003 outbreak. In the United States, only eight people were infected, and all of these had traveled outside the United States to areas with SARS infection (WHO, 2008). Since 2004, there have not been any known cases of SARS reported anywhere in the world (CDC, 2012b).

■ **ETIOLOGY.** World experts have determined that SARS is caused by a previously unknown type of coronavirus, a family of viruses that usually causes only mild to moderate illness such as the common cold. This new virus has been named the SARS coronavirus.

The SARS virus appears to be spread by respiratory droplets. Persons who have close person-to-person contact with an infected individual are most at risk. Close contact is defined as having cared for or lived with someone with SARS or having direct contact with the respiratory secretions of a person with SARS. Examples of close contact include sharing drinking and eating utensils, kissing, hugging, touching, or talking to someone within 3 feet. Close contact does not include walking past an infected individual or briefly sitting across from the person in a waiting room.

The SARS virus is thought to be easily spread when an infected individual coughs or sneezes and spreads the infected respiratory droplets into the air as far as 3 feet. Infection can occur when these droplets fall on or are inhaled onto the mucous membranes of the mouth, nose, and eyes of persons nearby. The virus also can spread when a person touches an infected surface or object and then touches his or her mouth, nose, or eyes.

■ **SYMPTOMS.** SARS usually begins with a high fever. Other symptoms include malaise, chills, headache, myalgia, dizziness, rigors, cough, sore throat, and runny nose. Incubation of the SARS virus appears to be approximately 7–10 days. In many cases, patients present with headache, dizziness, and myalgia. Temperature rises and becomes excessive as the disease progresses. In more acute cases, there is rapid deterioration with low oxygen saturation and acute respiratory distress requiring ventilatory support. ARDS has been observed in a number of patients in end-stage disease.

■ **DIAGNOSIS.** Diagnosis is suspected in any person who exhibits symptoms and has a history of travel to a foreign country where SARS has been identified.

Positive chest X-rays showing small, patchy shadows that progress to generalized interstitial infiltrates are indicative of SARS. Several diagnostic test kits have been produced, but none have proved effective; thus, there is no rapid screening test for SARS.

■ *TREATMENT.* Antibiotics are ineffective against SARS because it is a viral disease. Treatment of symptoms includes antipyretic medications, oxygen administration, and ventilator support if needed. Steroids and antiviral medications have been tried but have not helped, and some research has suggested that these actually cause harm.

■ *PREVENTION.* Prevention includes avoiding contact with infected individuals and use of isolation procedures if contact is necessary. Respiratory isolation—including the use of gown, gloves, goggles, and an approved respiratory mask—are essential.

LUNG CANCER

■ *DESCRIPTION.* Lung cancer is a disease of uncontrolled cell growth in the tissues of the lung. The majority of primary lung cancers are derived from epithelial cells—cells lining the air passages. There are two types of primary tumors, called small-cell and non-small-cell.

Small-cell tumors, also called oat cell, occur less frequently (16%) but grow rapidly and are often metastatic by the time they are discovered. They usually respond better to chemotherapy and radiation but still carry a much worse prognosis than non-small-cell tumors.

Non-small-cell tumors are more frequent (80%) and are usually treated surgically. This type of lung cancer is strongly associated with smoking.

Metastatic lung cancer is common and often due to metastasis from tumors in other parts of the body. Primary lung cancers also commonly metastasize to other areas, including the brain, bone, and liver.

Lung cancer is the leading cause of cancer deaths in the United States in both men and women. Most lung cancers can be prevented because approximately 90% are due to smoking. Lung cancer claims more lives than colon, prostate, lymph, and breast cancers combined.

■ *ETIOLOGY.* Lung cancer is rare among those under 40 and, in most cases, is caused by cigarette smoking. Ninety percent of lung cancer victims are smokers. Men are affected more commonly than women, although the increase in female smokers has increased the number of female lung cancer victims.

■ *SYMPTOMS.* Lung cancer is often asymptomatic until metastasis has occurred. Often, the first symptoms are those related to other organs affected by metastasis. Discovery by metastasis makes for a very poor prognosis; approximately 10% of lung cancer victims survive 5 years. Symptoms related to the lung tumor are dyspnea, coughing, and hemoptysis.

■ *DIAGNOSIS.* Diagnosis is made by X-ray and tissue biopsy.

■ *TREATMENT.* Treatment includes chemotherapy, surgery, and radiation. If the tumor is discovered early, surgical removal might confer cure, but this is rarely the case.

■ *PREVENTION.* To never smoke or to quit smoking is the best preventive action.

Diseases of the Pleura and Chest

Diseases of the pleura and chest can be caused by infection, trauma, or other diseases. Pain and shortness of breath are the common symptoms. The severity of such disorders can range from mild to severe, depending on the cause, the individual's age, medical history, and other complicating factors.

PLEURISY (PLEURITIS)

■ *DESCRIPTION.* Pleurisy is inflammation of the membranes covering the lung (visceral pleura) and lining the chest cavity (parietal pleura).

■ *ETIOLOGY.* Pleurisy can be due to bacterial infection of the pleura. Secondary pleurisy often follows trauma, pneumonia, TB, and neoplasm.

■ *SYMPTOMS.* The main symptom of pleurisy is a sharp, chest-area pain that increases with inspiration and coughing. Pain can be so severe that it limits movement in the affected area.

■ *DIAGNOSIS.* A distinctive pain with breathing is a classic symptom of pleurisy. This symptom, combined with auscultation of a characteristic friction rub or squeaky, rubbing sound with inspiration, confirm the diagnosis. Identifying the cause of the pleurisy might be more difficult. Identification efforts can include chest X-ray, CT scan, analysis of fluid in the pleural space, and biopsy.

■ *TREATMENT.* Treatment is aimed at the cause and includes symptomatic treatment with analgesics, heat application, and taping the chest to restrict movement and, thus, decrease pain.

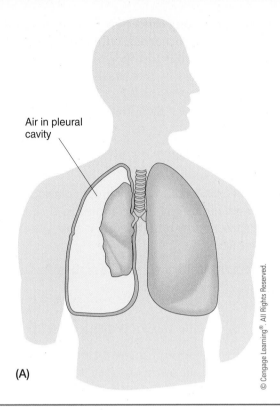

Air in pleural cavity

(A)

© Cengage Learning®. All Rights Reserved.

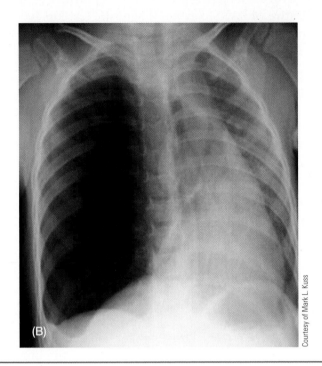

(B)

Courtesy of Mark L. Kuss

FIGURE 9–14 (A) Diagram of pneumothorax. (B) X-ray of pneumothorax.

■ **PREVENTION.** Preventing or treating the various causes, maintaining a healthy lifestyle, and avoiding respiratory allergens are helpful.

PNEUMOTHORAX

■ **DESCRIPTION.** Pneumothorax is a collection of air in the pleural cavity, often resulting in partial or complete collapse of the lung on the affected side (Figure 9–14). Spontaneous pneumothorax occurs when air is leaked into the pleural space from the inside or from the lung.

■ **ETIOLOGY.** Common causes include pulmonary disease, tumor, or pulmonary tissue tear. Traumatic pneumothorax occurs when air enters the pleural cavity from outside the chest. Causes include gunshot wound, stabbing, or crushing of the chest. A rib fracture often causes a traumatic pneumothorax.

■ **SYMPTOMS.** No matter the cause of the pneumothorax, symptoms are related to the degree of lung collapse. Complete lung collapse causes a sudden, severe chest pain, followed by severe dyspnea and symptoms of shock. Respirations are weak and shallow. Sucking breath sounds might be heard at

the site of a traumatic wound. Increased air pressure on the affected side can cause a shift of the mediastinum toward the unaffected side. The condition of mediastinal shift is a medical emergency. Emergency treatment includes placing an occlusive dressing, clean hand, or plastic material over the sucking chest wound to prevent additional air from entering the chest.

■ **DIAGNOSIS.** Auscultation of the chest reveals decreased or absent breath sounds. Diagnosis is confirmed by chest X-ray.

■ **TREATMENT.** Further treatment can include performing a **thoracentesis** (THOR-rah-sen-TEE-sis; thora = chest, centesis = puncture) to insert a chest tube to withdraw air and assist in re-expanding the lung. Oxygen therapy and analgesics might also be prescribed.

■ **PREVENTION.** Preventative measures for noninjury-related pneumothorax include not smoking and having respiratory problems treated promptly.

HEMOTHORAX

Hemothorax is the collection of blood in the chest cavity. Cause, symptoms, diagnosis, and treatments

HEALTHY HIGHLIGHT

The Harmful Effects of Smoking

The 1982 U.S. Surgeon General's Report stated that, "Cigarette smoking is the major single cause of cancer mortality in the United States." This statement is as true today as it was in 1982 (American Cancer Society, 2011).

Smoking is responsible for nearly one in five deaths in the United States. Because cigarette smoking and tobacco use are acquired behaviors—activities that people choose to do—smoking is the most preventable cause of premature death in our society.

Smoking kills more people than alcohol, AIDS, car crashes, illegal drugs, murders, and suicides combined.

The preceding facts stress how detrimental cigarette smoking is to the individual and to society. Some other harmful effects of smoking include:

- Its link to cancer, particularly cancer of the lung, larynx, esophagus, pancreas, bladder, kidney, and mouth
- Heart and cardiovascular disease, especially myocardial infarction and stroke
- Bone thinning and hip fracture
- Chronic bronchitis and emphysema
- Decreased rate of lung tissue growth
- Impaired level of lung function
- Shortness of breath, especially with exercise, and increased phlegm production
- Heartburn and peptic ulcers
- Premature birth and low birth weight if used during pregnancy
- Shortened life span with increased risk of morbidity; male smokers lose an average of 13.2 years while female smokers lose 14.5 years of life
- Addiction to nicotine

Source: American Cancer Society (2011).

---

are the same as for a pneumothorax. Blood pressure and blood loss are monitored and treated as necessary.

PLEURAL EFFUSION (HYDROTHORAX)

■ **DESCRIPTION.** Pleural effusion, or hydrothorax, is a collection of fluid in the chest cavity.

■ **ETIOLOGY.** Causes of hydrothorax can include congestive heart failure, TB, or pneumonia.

■ **SYMPTOMS.** The affected individual might be asymptomatic or can exhibit signs of dyspnea and chest or pleuritic pain.

■ **DIAGNOSIS.** Diagnosis is confirmed by X-ray.

■ **TREATMENT.** Treatment can include thoracentesis to remove the excess fluid.

■ **PREVENTION.** Correction of the condition causing hydrothorax is needed to prevent reoccurrence.

EMPYEMA

■ **DESCRIPTION.** Empyema is the collection of pus (py = pus) in the chest cavity.

■ **ETIOLOGY.** Empyema can be the result of a ruptured lung abscess or an ulcerated tumor. Empyema is not as common as it was prior to the development of antibiotics.

■ **SYMPTOMS.** Symptoms include coughing, dyspnea, and chest pain on the affected side.

■ **DIAGNOSIS.** Diagnosis is by X-ray and thoracentesis.

■ **TREATMENT.** Microbiologic cultures can be performed on the fluid to identify the infective organism. Antibiotic therapy is a common treatment for bacterial infections.

■ **PREVENTION.** Rapid and appropriate treatment of cause prevents this condition.

Diseases of the Cardiovascular and Respiratory Systems

The cardiovascular and respiratory systems are so closely related that many diseases affect both systems. The degree to which each system is affected also is often so similar that it becomes difficult to classify the disease by one system over the other. For this reason, these diseases need further consideration.

PULMONARY EMBOLISM (PE)

■ **DESCRIPTION.** PE is a sudden blockage of an artery in the pulmonary system by an embolism (Figure 9–15).

■ **ETIOLOGY.** Chapter 8, "Cardiovascular System Diseases and Disorders," discussed the pathology of an embolism. Remember that the floating material can be a blood clot, fat globule, or piece of tissue. Commonly, a blood clot or thrombus develops in the veins of the lower legs, thighs, or pelvis. This clot then breaks loose, floats in the vascular system, and sticks in a pulmonary artery, resulting in a pulmonary embolism.

■ **SYMPTOMS.** Symptoms of a PE vary greatly, depending on the size of the clot and the size of the area affected. Dyspnea, cough, chest pain, and apprehension are common symptoms. If the PE is severe, cyanosis, shock, and death can result.

Factors that contribute to the development of an embolism are immobility, dehydration, prolonged bed rest, obesity, and trauma or fractures of the legs or pelvis.

■ **DIAGNOSIS.** Diagnosis is confirmed by X-ray examination and lung scans.

■ **TREATMENT.** Treatment is aimed at maintaining cardiopulmonary function by administering oxygen and anticoagulation medications.

■ **PREVENTION.** Prevention includes ambulation, antiembolic stockings, and leg exercises to improve blood flow and prevent clotting.

PULMONARY EDEMA

■ **DESCRIPTION.** Pulmonary edema, if severe, can be a life-threatening medical emergency. It affects the tissue and air spaces of the lungs by filling them with fluid. This fluid leaks out of the vascular system due to increased vascular pressure.

■ **ETIOLOGY.** Cardiovascular disease is the common cause of pulmonary edema. It is commonly seen as a result of congestive heart failure and resulting fluid buildup, but any disease that affects blood pressure,

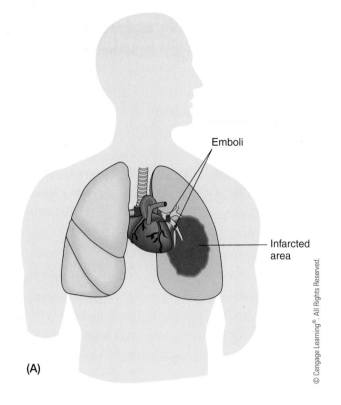

Emboli

Infarcted area

(A)

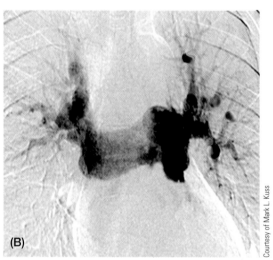

(B)

FIGURE 9–15   (A) Diagram of pulmonary emboli. (B) X-ray of pulmonary emboli.

heart function, and blood fluid levels can lead to pulmonary edema. These diseases include hypertension, pulmonary embolism, and renal failure.

■ **SYMPTOMS.** Pulmonary edema is characterized by dyspnea, orthopnea (ortho = straight, pnea = breath), or difficulty breathing when lying down, and a blood-tinged frothy sputum.

■ **DIAGNOSIS.** Diagnosis is determined by ABGs and chest X-ray. ABGs will show an increased carbon

HEALTHY HIGHLIGHT

Avoid Blood Clots while Traveling

To reduce the risk of developing blood clots:

1. **Be an active traveler**. If driving, stop every hour, walk around the car, do knee bends, or rise up and down on your toes. In a plane, try to get up and walk around the cabin every hour and perform toe rises if space permits.
2. **Avoid crossing your legs**. Crossing your legs slows blood flow.
3. **Exercise while seated**. Flex and relax different muscle groups in your legs. Rotate, flex, and extend your ankles. Ask your physician about wearing compression stockings when traveling.
4. **Drink plenty of fluids**. Immobility and dehydration can contribute to blood clot formation.

---

dioxide level, and chest X-rays will exhibit increased opacity (whiteness).

■ **TREATMENT.** Treatment is aimed at reducing pressure and blood volume. Diuretics to increase urine output, cardiogenics to increase the contraction of the heart, and morphine to bring about venous dilatation might be prescribed. Mechanical respiratory ventilation might also be needed.

■ **PREVENTION.** Pulmonary edema might not be preventable. Reducing the risk of cardiovascular disease is helpful and includes not smoking, controlling blood pressure, limiting cholesterol, limiting salt intake, exercising daily, eating a heart-healthy diet, and managing stress.

COR PULMONALE

Cor pulmonale was discussed in Chapter 8. Remember that it is a right-sided heart failure related to acute or chronic pulmonary disease. Increased pulmonary blood pressure causes enlargement of the right ventricle and decreased pumping ability. Polycythemia (poly = many, cyt = cell- red cell, emia = blood) develops as the body tries to compensate for hypoxemia (hypo = not enough, ox = oxygen, emia = blood), leading to a thickening of the blood and further increasing workload on the heart.

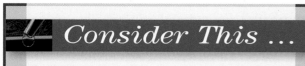

Consider This ...

Individuals inhale approximately 700,000 of their own skin flakes daily.

■ TRAUMA

Pneumothorax and Hemothorax

Pneumothorax and hemothorax often occur due to some type of trauma. Examples of trauma that often cause these conditions are fractured ribs, gunshot wounds, stabbings, and crushing chest injuries. Collapse of the lung, shock, and death are potential outcomes.

Suffocation

Suffocation is the condition of not breathing to the point of unconsciousness and, eventually, death due to the lack of oxygen and the high level of carbon dioxide in the body tissues. The brain and heart are immediately affected.

Accidental suffocation often occurs with infants and small children playing with plastic bags. Criminal suffocation of homicide victims might be a common finding in forensic pathology. Suffocation can also be caused in a variety of other ways.

■ **Aspiration** Aspiration of food that occludes or blocks the airway is common. This type of suffocation leads to the death of approximately one person a day in the United States! Treatment of food aspiration is immediate attention and can include the performance of an abdominal thrust, previously known as the Heimlich maneuver (see page 208).

■ **Strangulation** Accidental, suicidal, or criminal strangulation can occur by hanging or squeezing the neck with the hands, rope, wire, or a variety of other objects.

- **Drowning** Drowning is a common cause of accidental death, especially in children and adolescent males. Drowning may be classified as wet or dry. Wet drowning is the most common (approximately 90%) and is characterized by water entering the airways and lungs, preventing the entry of oxygen into the system. Dry drowning is less common and is characterized by a reflex laryngospasm that closes the glottis and does not allow water or air to enter. Treatment of either type of drowning is immediate resuscitation and transport to an emergency department.

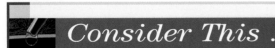

Consider This ...

If an individual is locked in a completely air-tight room, they will die of carbon dioxide poisoning before they die of oxygen deprivation.

◼ RARE DISEASES

Pneumoconioses

Pneumoconioses (new-mo-cone-ee-OH-sees) refer to a group of environmentally induced diseases that cause progressive, chronic inflammation and infection. This condition is caused by frequently inhaling the small dust particles of the offending agent for extended periods of time. Pneumoconiosis can occur within a few years, or it might take 20 or 30 years to develop. Types of pneumoconiosis, cause, and related occupations include:

- **Asbestosis**, the most frequently occurring form of the disease, related to insulating and fireproofing.
- **Anthracosis** from inhaling carbon and coal, often called coal miner's disease and black lung.
- **Silicosis** from inhaling silicone affects glass cutters, sand blasters, and stonemasons.

 HEALTHY HIGHLIGHT

Abdominal Thrust

The abdominal thrust, previously known as the Heimlich maneuver, is a technique used to remove foreign material—usually food—from the respiratory tract of a choking victim. Choking is a medical emergency. First call 911 emergency medical services and then start the procedure. If the victim is able to talk or has wheezing breath sounds, this maneuver should not be performed; the abdominal thrust is performed only on individuals who are unable to breathe. Treatment for a choking person who cannot speak, turns blue, or stops breathing is based on age. The procedure described here is for an adult. The procedure can be performed with the victim in a standing or sitting position.

To perform the abdominal thrust on a victim in a sitting or standing position, the rescuer assumes a position behind the victim. The rescuer wraps his or her arms around the victim's waist, allowing the victim's head, arms, and upper body to fall forward. The rescuer makes a fist with one hand and holds it in place with the other hand. The fist should be placed against the victim's abdomen at a point slightly above the umbilicus and below the rib cage. The maneuver calls for the rescuer to perform an upward thrust forcefully to this area. This maneuver can be repeated until the airway is cleared.

If the victim is or becomes unconscious, the rescuer should begin the steps for cardiopulmonary resuscitation (CPR).

(continued)

HEALTHY HIGHLIGHT (continued)

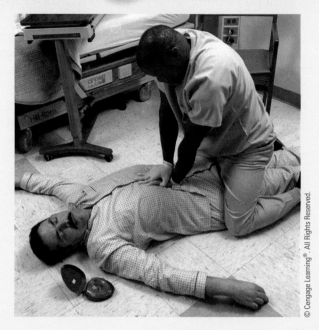

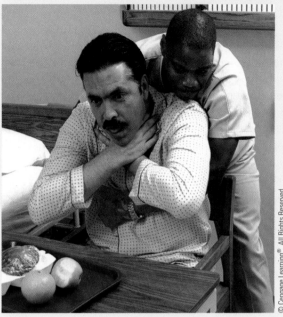

If the victim is pregnant or obese, a chest thrust can be performed. The rescuer places both hands under the victim's armpits with the thumb side of the fist on the middle of the breastbone. The fist is covered with the other hand and thrust backward until the object is coughed out. If the victim is or becomes unconscious, the rescuer should begin the steps for CPR.

Fungal Diseases

Fungal diseases affecting the lungs are caused by inhaling an airborne fungus. The lung lesions caused by fungal diseases form granulomatous inflammations like TB, but they do not cavitate (cause cavities in the lung tissue). The fungus can spread through the lung tissue and cause acute illness with symptoms of dyspnea and fever. Treatment consists of rest and antifungal medications. Two forms include:

1. Histoplasmosis, which occurs primarily in the Midwestern United States. This fungus is harbored in bird droppings such as those found in chicken houses, bat caves, and pigeon roosts.

2. Coccidioidomycosis (cox-sid-ee-OYD-o-my-co-sis), which occurs primarily in the southwestern United States. This fungus grows in hot, dry areas and produces spores that become windborne. It is also known as desert fever and valley fever.

Legionnaires' Disease

Legionnaires' disease is a bacterial pulmonary infection so named as the result of an outbreak in 1976 at a convention of the American Legion held in Philadelphia. The causative bacterium is *Legionella pneumophila*. This bacterium lives in water storage tanks and cooling systems. Legionnaires' disease can also be called Legionnaires' pneumonia because it produces typical pneumonia symptoms. It differs from other types of pneumonia in that it does not respond to the usual treatment, and it might cause permanent lung damage. Legionnaires' disease is not limited to the pulmonary system like typical pneumonia is; it can cause complications such as liver damage and renal dysfunction. Severe cases might need mechanical ventilation and can have a fatal outcome.

EFFECTS OF AGING ON THE SYSTEM

The effects of aging on the respiratory system increase the risk for the older adult to develop respiratory disease. Over time, the respiratory system loses some of its elasticity, becomes less efficient, and has less reserve. Weakened respiratory muscles contribute to the ineffectiveness of the system. It can also be adversely affected by changes in posture occurring with aging, by the long-term effects of chronic diseases such as COPD, and by the changes occurring in other systems. The older adult usually has a lower tolerance for exercise due to the increased need for oxygen during exercise and the inability of the body to meet that demand.

Changes in the immune responses that occur with aging put the older adult at increased risk for acute respiratory infections. Influenza and pneumonia are common but very serious diseases affecting older adults. Pneumonia is the leading cause of death due to infections in the older population. Another respiratory disease that older people are at increased risk of developing is TB. Their reduced immunity contributes to the high incidence of TB among older adults.

Chronic respiratory diseases are particularly difficult for older people. The nature of the disease, symptoms, effects, and treatments can all contribute to the increased respiratory dysfunction, and thus, the debilitation of the individual. Many older individuals have been heavy smokers for years. The effects of smoking might have already severely damaged respiratory function and will continue to inhibit effective breathing if the individual continues to smoke. Smoking is the major cause of the high incidence of cancer of the lung in older people.

SUMMARY

T he respiratory system is responsible for the intake of oxygen for the body and the removal of carbon dioxide. Decreased respiratory function greatly limits the ability of other systems because oxygen is necessary at the cellular level for all activities to occur. Diagnostic tests for respiratory diseases include physical examination, chest X-rays, ABGs, and PFTs. Respiratory diseases are a major cause of disability and death in the United States. Acute respiratory diseases such as the common cold, pneumonia, and influenza occur in all age groups. An increased incidence of influenza and other communicable respiratory diseases is causing concern among public health officials. Most chronic respiratory diseases are found in the older adult. Smoking is the greatest contributor to chronic respiratory disease, especially to cancer of the lung.

REVIEW QUESTIONS

Short Answer

1. What are the functions of the respiratory system?

2. Which signs and symptoms are associated with common respiratory system disorders?

3. Which diagnostic tests are most commonly used to determine the type and cause of respiratory system disorders?

4. What is the most effective preventive technique against the common cold?

5. What behavior puts an individual at highest risk for pulmonary disease?

Matching

6. Match the term on the left with the correct descriptive clause on the right.

_____	Asthma	a. Inflammation of the mucous membranes of the sinuses
_____	Pneumothorax	b. High-risk behavior for developing respiratory disease
_____	COPD	c. Best preventive behavior against respiratory infections
_____	Hemothorax	d. Hypersensitivity reaction, causing constriction of the bronchi
_____	TB	e. Bacterial infection, causing a primary lesion in the lung
_____	Sinusitis	f. Collapse of part of the lung with blood in the space
_____	Cor pulmonale	g. Group of chronic pulmonary diseases
_____	Hand washing	h. Right-sided heart failure
_____	Smoking	i. Collection of air in the pleural cavity

CASE STUDIES

■ Jake Cooper, a 37-year-old sales executive, recently returned from a business trip in Eastern Asia. He had read about avian flu while visiting clients in Hong Kong and now has some concerns for his own health. He has to return to the same area in 2 weeks and wonders whether he should cancel the trip. What can you tell him about avian (bird) flu? Might he be infected? What symptoms should he watch for? Could he infect his family or friends here? Should he see his family physician? Is there much of a threat to his health from his visit? Would you recommend that he cancel the next trip?

■ Mr. Loftin is a 78-year-old man who has been diagnosed with severe emphysema. He has been a heavy smoker since age 12 and continues to smoke. He complains about his shortness of breath, stating he cannot do much more than walk across the room without gasping for air. He has been cautioned about the effects of his continued smoking, but he responds with statements such as, "What difference does it make if I quit now? I've smoked all my life, and you can't go back and change that." How would you respond to this statement? Is it too late for him to quit and receive some benefit of that behavioral change? Is any of the damage from smoking reversible? How can you explain this to Mr. Loftin?

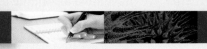

Study Tools

Workbook

Complete Chapter 9

Online Resources

PowerPoint® presentations

Animation

BIBLIOGRAPHY

Albert, J., & Chiodi, F. (2011). Towards a world free from HIV and AIDS? *Journal of Internal Medicine 270*(6), 502–508.

American Cancer Society. (2011). Learn about cancer. Cigarette smoking. *www.cancer.org* (accessed June 2012).

American Lung Association. (2012). State of the air. *http://www.stateoftheair.org* (accessed February 2012).

Aschenbrenner, D. S. (2011). Drug watch. *American Journal of Nursing 111*(3), 22–23.

Brown, J. K., Cooley, M. E., Chernecky, C., & Sarna, L. (2011). A symptom cluster and sentinel symptom experienced by women with lung cancer. *Oncology Nursing Forum 38*(6), E425–E435.

Centers for Disease Control and Prevention. (2011a). Health, United States, infectious diseases—Access and utilization of health care. *www.cdc.gov* (accessed June 2012).

Centers for Disease Control and Prevention. (2011b). Seasonal influenza (flu): Key facts about influenza (flu) and flu vaccine. *www.cdc.gov* (accessed June 2012).

Centers for Disease Control and Prevention. (2012a). Pneumonia can be prevented: Vaccines can help. *www.cdc.gov* (accessed February 2012).

Centers for Disease Control and Prevention. (2012b). Sudden acute respiratory syndrome (SARS). *www.cdc.gov* (accessed June 2012).

Clark, G. (2011). Ready to fight TB. *Nursing Standard 25*(41), 20–21.

Dobbin, K., & Howard, V. (2011). Listen closely to detect healthcare-associated pneumonia. *Nursing 41*(7), 59–62.

Edwards, M. (2011). Bronchiectasis. *Practice Nurse 41*(2), 35–38.

Glasper, A. (2011). Seasonal influenza: What every nurse needs to know. *British Journal of Nursing 20*(19), 1262–1263.

Gough, A., & Kaufman, G. (2011). Pulmonary tuberculosis: Clinical features and patient management. *Nursing Standard 25*(47), 48–56.

Greenaway, C., Sandoe, A., Vissandjee, B., Kitai, I., Gruner, D., Wobeser, W., & Schwartzman, K. (2011). Tuberculosis: Evidence review for newly arriving immigrants and refugees. *CMAJ: Canadian Medical Association Journal 183*(12), E939–E951.

Henoch, I., Lövgren, M., Wilde-Larsson, B., & Tishelman, C. (2012). Perception of quality of care: Comparison of the views of patients with lung cancer and their family members. *Journal of Clinical Nursing 21*(3/4), 585–594.

Imran, I., Hussain, L., Zia-Ul-Haq, M. M., Janbaz, K., Gilani, A. H., & De Feo, V. (2011). Gastrointestial and respiratory activities of *Acacia leucophloea*. *Journal of Ethnopharmacology 138*(3), 676–682.

Kaufman, G. (2010). Inhaled bronchodilators for chronic bronchitis and emphysema. *Nursing Standard 25*(5), 61–68.

Kelly, C. (2011). Palliative care for patients with chronic respiratory disease. *Nursing Standard 26*(5), 41–46.

Kupferschmidt, K. (2011). Taking a new shot at a TB vaccine. *Science 334*(6062), 1488–1490.

Lehto, R. H. (2011). Identifying primary concerns in patients newly diagnosed with lung cancer. *Oncology Nursing Forum 38*(4), 440–447.

Miracle, V. A. (2011). Seasonal flu. *Dimensions of Critical Care Nursing 30*(5), 302.

Morrell, N. (2010). Prone positioning in patients with acute respiratory distress syndrome. *Nursing Standard 24*(21), 42–45.

Myrianthefs, P., Ioannidis, K., Baltopoulos, G., & Tsakris, A. (2011). Treatment of hospital-acquired pneumonia. *Lancet Infectious Diseases 11*(10), 729–730.

Perry, M. (2010). Differentiating between the common cold and influenza. *Practice Nurse 40*(10), 11–15.

Pratt, R. H., Winston, C. A., Kammerer, J., & Armstrong, L. R. (2011). Tuberculosis in older adults in the United States, 1993–2008. *Journal of the American Geriatrics Society 59*(5), 851–857.

Regan, A. K., Dube, S. R., & Arrazola, R. (2012). Smokeless and flavored tobacco products in the U.S.: 2009 styles survey results. *American Journal of Preventive Medicine 42*(1), 29–36.

Rountree, R. (2011). Roundoc Rx: Immunomodulators: Fighting recurrent upper respiratory infections naturally. *Alternative & Complementary Therapies 17*(5), 255–260.

Schweon, S. J. (2011). Combating infection. Pertussis: Not just for kids anymore. *Nursing 41*(10), 61–62.

Scullion, J. E., & Holmes, S. (2011). Palliative care in patients with chronic obstructive pulmonary disease. *Nursing Older People 23*(4), 32–39.

Shapiro, A. C., & Swenson, K. K. (2011). Nutritional challenges during treatment for lung cancer. *Oncology Nursing Forum 38*(5), 515–518.

Smith, B. L., & Tasota, F. J. (2011). Smoking out the dangers of COPD. *Nursing 41*(4), 32–40.

Thornton, M. M., Parry, M. M., Gill, P. P., Mead, D. D., & Macbeth, F. F. (2011). Hard choices: A qualitative study of influences on the treatment decisions made by advanced lung cancer patients. *International Journal of Palliative Nursing 17*(2), 68–74.

World Health Organization (WHO). (2008). Sudden acute respiratory syndrome (SARS). *www.who.int* (accessed August 2012).

World Health Organization (WHO). (2012). Tuberculoses–fact sheet March 2012. *www.who.int* (accessed July 2012).

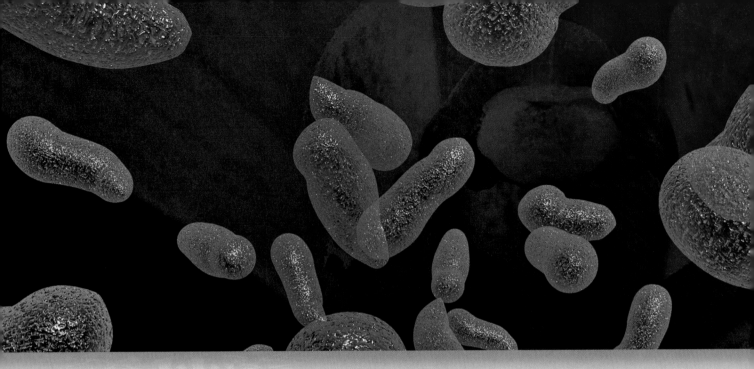

OUTLINE

- Anatomy and Physiology
- Common Signs and Symptoms
- Diagnostic Tests
- Common Diseases of the Lymphatic System
  Lymphadenitis
  Lymphangitis
  Lymphedema
  Lymphoma
  Mononucleosis
- Rare Diseases
  Kawasaki Disease
- Effects of Aging on the System
- Summary
- Review Questions
- Case Studies
- Bibliography

KEY TERMS

Lymph (p. 216)
Lymphadenopathy (p. 217)
Lymphangiography (p. 217)
Lymphangiopathy (p. 217)
Lymphocytes (p. 217)
Lymphocytopenia (p. 217)
Lymphocytosis (p. 217)

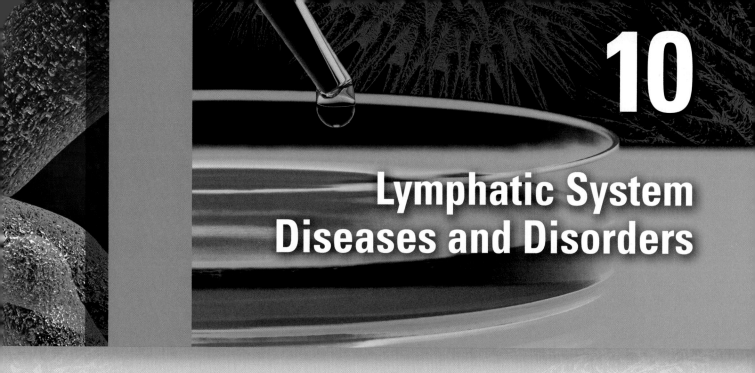

10

Lymphatic System Diseases and Disorders

LEARNING OBJECTIVES

Upon completion of the chapter, the learner should be able to:

1. Define the terminology common to the lymphatic system and the disorders of the system.

2. Discuss the basic anatomy and physiology of the lymphatic system.

3. Identify the important signs and symptoms associated with common lymphatic system disorders.

4. Describe the common diagnostics used to determine the type and cause of lymphatic system disorders.

5. Identify common disorders of the lymphatic system.

6. Describe the typical course and management of the common lymphatic system disorders.

7. Describe the effects of aging on the lymphatic system and the common disorders associated with aging of the system.

OVERVIEW

The lymphatic system is the infection-fighting system of the body. It works with the immune system to play an important role in preventing infection and maintaining one's immunity. The lymphatic system includes the lymph nodes, lymph vessels, and fluid lymph. It is a special vascular system that picks up excess tissue fluid and returns it to the blood. Disorders of the system include inflammatory conditions and neoplasms. The lymphatic system is so closely related to the immune system, the blood and blood-forming organs, and the cardiovascular system that many of the concepts and diseases of the system have already been discussed. Refer to these chapters for additional information on the lymphatic system. ■

ANATOMY AND PHYSIOLOGY

The lymphatic system includes lymph vessels, ducts, and nodes (Figure 10–1). It is important in protecting the body from infection and filters bacterial and nonbacterial products resulting from the inflammatory process. The goal of the system is to prevent these waste products from entering the general circulation, but this activity can cause some inflammation of the node filtering the waste products, causing swelling and redness of the involved node.

The lymphatic system depends, to some extent, on the vascular system because the lymphatic system returns its fluids and other materials to the vascular system. There is diffusion of fluid between the lymphatic vessels, the interstitial spaces, and the blood capillaries.

The fluid in the lymphatic system is called **lymph**, a clear liquid similar to plasma that contains many white cells. The conducting vessels of the lymphatic system include the capillaries, the smallest vessels, and the larger lymph vessels, which have valves much like the veins in the cardiovascular system. In the lymph vessels, the direction of flow is toward the thoracic cavity. The vessels meet in the right lymphatic duct or the left lymphatic duct, which drain into the venous system. The right lymphatic duct drains the lymph from the right half of the head, upper torso, and right arm. The rest of the lymph vessels in the body drain into the left lymphatic duct, also called the thoracic duct.

The lymph vessels have other functions besides the transportation of lymph. They also return important nutrients such as proteins and large particulate matter that have leaked out into the capillaries to the blood vessels (Figure 10–2). In the course of a day, approximately 3 liters of extra fluid are leaked into the tissue and not picked up by the venous system.

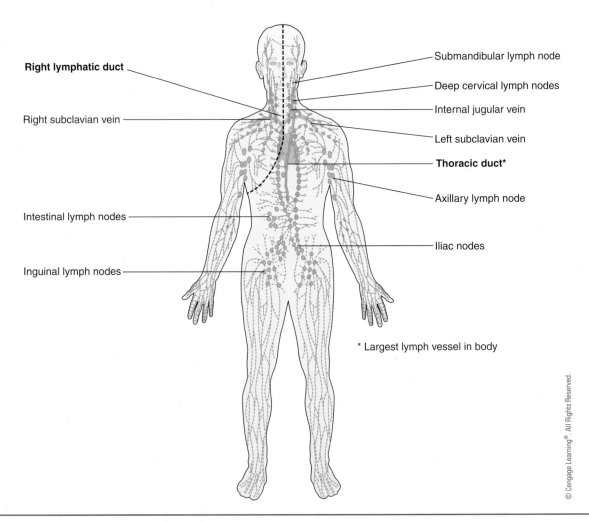

Right lymphatic duct

Right subclavian vein

Intestinal lymph nodes

Inguinal lymph nodes

Submandibular lymph node

Deep cervical lymph nodes

Internal jugular vein

Left subclavian vein

Thoracic duct*

Axillary lymph node

Iliac nodes

* Largest lymph vessel in body

FIGURE 10–1   The lymphatic system.

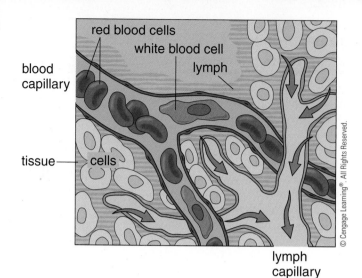

red blood cells
white blood cell
lymph
blood capillary
tissue — cells
lymph capillary

FIGURE 10–2 Exchange of fluids between the lymph and blood vessels.

The lymphatic system picks up this extra fluid and returns it to the blood. In addition, the lymph vessels transport toxic substances to the nodes for filtration. In the digestive process, the vessels are important in the absorption of fats. The nodes are important in the filtering process, but they also produce lymphocytes and protect the body by developing immunity to some diseases.

Organs related to the lymph system are the tonsils, thymus gland, and spleen. These organs also play a part in the body's immunity and protection system. See Chapter 5, "Immune System Diseases and Disorders," for a discussion on immunity.

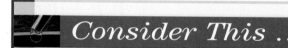

Consider This ...

In 1652, Thomas Bartholin, a Danish physician, published the first article correctly describing the lymphatic system.

Media Link

View an animation on the lymphatic system on the Online Resources.

COMMON SIGNS AND SYMPTOMS

Enlargement of the lymph glands or nodes is common and is usually due to infection somewhere in the body. Infection stimulates activity of the nodes and glands to produce more **lymphocytes** (white cells created in the lymphatic system). Fever, fatigue, and weight loss are common with lymphatic diseases.

Most disorders of the lymphatic system are related to diseases of other systems. **Lymphocytosis** (lympho = lymph, cyto = cell, osis = increase or an abnormal increase in lymphocytes) and **lymphocyto-penia** (lymphocyte = lymph cell, penia = decrease or an abnormal decrease in lymphocytes) in blood and tissue can accompany diseases of the immune system as well as of the lymphatic system.

DIAGNOSTIC TESTS

A complete blood count with white cell differential can assist in determination of inflammation or infectious diseases of the lymphatic system.

Lymphangiography (lim-FAN-jee-OG-rah-fee; lymph = lymph, angio = vessel, graphy = procedure) consists of injecting a contrast dye and taking X-rays. This procedure can be helpful in diagnosing vessel conditions. Magnetic resonance imaging (MRI) and computerized tomography (CT) can also be used.

Biopsy of lymph glands and nodes can assist in determination of lymphoma. A special connective tissue cell called a Reed–Sternberg cell confirms a diagnosis of Hodgkin's disease.

COMMON DISEASES OF THE LYMPHATIC SYSTEM

Diseases of the lymphatic system commonly include inflammatory conditions. Often, diseases of this system are the result of disease in another system. Disease of lymph glands collectively can be called **lymphade-nopathy** (lim-FAD-eh-NOP-ah-thee; lymph = lymph, adeno = gland, opathy = disease). **Lymphangiopathy** (lim-FAN-jee-OP-ah-thee; lymph = lymph, angio = vessel, opathy = disease) is a general term to describe any disease of the lymph vessels.

PHARMACOLOGY HIGHLIGHT

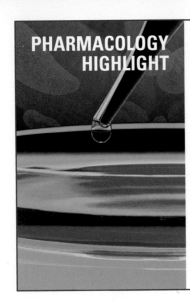

Common Drugs for Lymphatic Disorders

CATEGORY	EXAMPLES OF MEDICATIONS
Antibiotics Drugs used to prevent or stop bacterial infections	ampicillin, amoxicillin, ciprofloxacin, doxycycline, erythromycin, penicillin, or tetracycline
Antineoplastics Drugs used to treat cancer Alkylating agents Antimetabolites Antitumor antibiotics Hormones/antihormones Other substances	chlorambucil, cyclophosphamide, or lomustine 5-flourauracil, mercaptopurine, or methotrexate mitomycin or streptozocin estrogens, androgens, flutamide, or tamoxifen vincristine, L-asparaginase, paclitaxel, carboplatin, cisplatin, or etoposide

Lymphadenitis

■ **DESCRIPTION.** Lymphadenitis (lim-FAD-eh-NIGH-tis; lymph = lymph, adeno = gland, itis = inflammation) is characterized by swelling of the lymph gland, nodes, or both.

■ **ETIOLOGY.** Lymphadenitis is usually caused by infection somewhere in the body. Drainage of bacteria or toxic substances can cause the swelling. The location of the affected nodes can assist in determination of cause.

■ **SYMPTOMS.** Swelling, pain, and tenderness of the gland or node are common.

■ **DIAGNOSIS.** A physical examination revealing swollen lymph nodes is indicative of lymphadenitis. A blood culture can be performed to determine spread of infection to the bloodstream. A biopsy confirms the diagnosis.

■ **TREATMENT.** Antibiotic treatment is helpful with bacterial infections.

■ **PREVENTION.** Maintaining good general health is helpful in preventing any infection.

Lymphangitis

■ **DESCRIPTION.** Lymphangitis (lymph = lymph, angi = vessel, itis = inflammation) is a condition of swelling of the lymph vessel due to inflammation.

■ **ETIOLOGY.** This inflammation is commonly caused by infection with streptococcal bacteria following a trauma.

■ **SYMPTOMS.** Lymphangitis is often characterized by a red streak at the site of bacterial entry that extends to the area lymph nodes. Other symptoms include fever, chills, and malaise. Cellulitis (inflammation of cellular or connective tissue) and leukocytosis can also be present.

■ **DIAGNOSIS.** Diagnosis is immediate based on the high fever and the primary symptom of red streaks just below the skin surface. A blood culture can be completed to determine whether bacteria have entered the bloodstream. A biopsy can determine the type of bacteria causing the infection.

■ **TREATMENT.** Lymphangitis is commonly treated with antibiotics. Warm, moist packs and elevation of the affected area are also helpful.

■ **PREVENTION.** Good hygiene and maintaining good general health are preventive activities.

Lymphedema

■ **DESCRIPTION.** Lymphedema (lymph = lymph, edema = swelling) is an abnormal collection of lymph fluid, usually observed in the extremities (Figure 10–3).

■ **ETIOLOGY.** The most common causes are:

■ Surgery or radiation treatments for cancer, especially breast and testicular surgeries. Breast cancer surgery (mastectomy) and radiation can lead to a chronic lymphedema of the arm on the affected side. About 30% of all postmastectomy patients are affected by lymphedema.

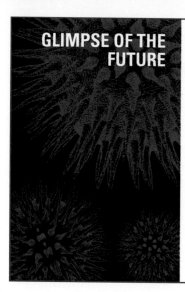
Does Obesity Increase Risk of Lymphedema after Breast Cancer Surgery?

This study looked at whether high body mass index (BMI) or obesity causes increased lymphedema in patients who had breast cancer surgery. The results showed that patients who had received treatment for breast cancer and had a high (>30) BMI at time of diagnosis and treatment did have a greater risk of developing lymphedema in 6 months or more. Those patients whose BMI increased to 30 or higher after their diagnosis and treatment did not have an increased risk of developing lymphedema. Thus, obesity prior to diagnosis and treatment for breast cancer may increase risk for developing lymphedema, but weight gain after treatment does not seem to influence the development of lymphedema. Further research needs to be done to determine how and why this occurs.

Source: Ridner et al. (2011).

- Surgery on blood vessels of the arms or legs.
- Other surgical procedures, such as liposuction.
- Other causes such as pregnancy, burns, and trauma.

■ **SYMPTOMS.** Symptoms occur in the arms and legs and include swelling and heaviness. Swelling can also extend into the fingers and toes, causing tight-fitting rings and shoes.

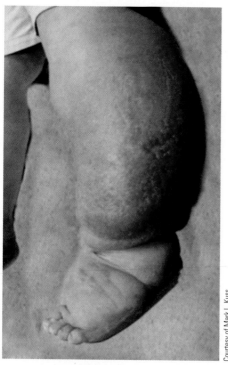

FIGURE 10–3 Lymphedema.

■ **DIAGNOSIS.** History and physical examination of the affected area along with CT and MRI scans confirm the diagnosis.

■ **TREATMENT.** Treatment is dependent on the cause. Antibiotics might be needed to treat infections that worsen with lymphedema. Placing the affected arm or leg above heart level, while resting, and exercise to increase lymph flow can decrease the edema. Procedures such as obtaining blood pressure and drawing blood samples should not be performed on the affected side because affected tissue is more prone to infection.

Pregnancy and constrictive clothing often cause an increase in venous pressure, resulting in an accumulation of fluid in the ankles and feet. Decreasing venous pressure in these cases will relieve lymphedema. To reduce venous pressure in the pregnant female, lying on the left side helps improve venous flow because the inferior vena cava is to the right of midline. Constrictive clothing should be removed or loosened when lymphedema is observed.

Compression therapy might be needed temporarily or lifelong, depending on the cause of the condition. Compression aids in pushing the excessive fluid back into the venous or lymphatic system. Compression also aids in venous return or return flow of both the lymphatic and venous system. Compression gloves, arm wraps, and leg stockings are available for this purpose.

Surgery might be needed to remove excess tissue if the affected limb becomes so large and heavy that it interferes with the ability to move and walk.

COMPLEMENTARY AND ALTERNATIVE THERAPY

Mainstream or Alternative Treatment for Lymphedema?

This study looked at the effectiveness of mainstream and alternative treatments for lymphedema after breast cancer or gynecologic cancer. Massage was the most common mainstream treatment used, followed by compression, but a variety of complementary and alternative therapy (CAT) treatments were used as well. These included the use of a Chi Machine, vitamin E supplements, yoga, and meditation. The results showed that both mainstream and CAT treatments were widely used by the participants. According to the subjects, the CAT treatments were very effective for the relief of lymphedema, as were the mainstream treatments.

Source: Finnane et al. (2011).

■ **PREVENTION.** Activities to reduce the risk of lymphedema include protecting the affected extremity (arm or leg), elevating the area while at rest, avoiding heat directly on the area, avoiding tight clothing, and keeping the extremity clean to prevent infection.

Lymphoma

Lymphoma refers to several types of neoplasms that affect lymphoid tissue (lymph nodes, tonsils, spleen, and lymph fluid). There are many types of lymphoma, but all affect normal lymphocyte production, leading to an impaired immunity. Lymphoma is the most common type of blood cancer in the United States. Lymphoma is discussed in more detail in Chapter 7, "Blood and Blood-Forming Organs Diseases and Disorders," under the heading, "Disorders of White Blood Cells."

Mononucleosis

Mononucleosis is a viral infection that affects primarily children and young adults. It is somewhat contagious and is commonly called the kissing disease. This disease is discussed in more detail in Chapter 20 under the heading "Infectious Diseases."

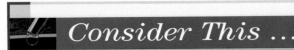

Consider This ...

Massage lowers blood pressure and assists in the movement of lymph through the lymphatic system.

■ RARE DISEASES

Kawasaki Disease

This disorder is also called mucocutaneous lymph node syndrome. It is an acute febrile disease found mostly in children and causes cervical lymphadenopathy. It resembles scarlet fever because the individual develops a rash and some edema of the hands and feet. Other symptoms include lethargy, congestion, irritability, fever, dry skin, and reddened lips, tongue, and mucous membranes. Treatment is supportive because the disease does not respond to antibiotic therapy. This disease is rarely fatal in the acute stage, but children can die quite suddenly some years later due to coronary artery disease.

■ EFFECTS OF AGING ON THE SYSTEM

As the individual ages, there is decreased ability to produce antibodies, leading to decreases in the normal immune response, which interferes with the normal ability to ward off infections. If other chronic diseases are also present, the individual can be at an even higher risk for poor healing and development of infections. In addition, as the immune response becomes less effective, the individual is more susceptible to autoimmune disorders. Many diseases of the older adult have some direct relationship to the decreased immune response. Because the lymphatic system depends, for some of its functions, on the vascular system, additional problems arise in the older person who has impaired circulation or other vascular system diseases.

SUMMARY

The lymphatic system plays an important role in the body's ability to fight infection and maintain immunity. The system is composed of lymph, lymph nodes, and vessels to transport the lymph. The lymphatic system also transports fluid that has leaked into the interstitial areas between the blood vessels.

Diseases of the system are usually caused by infections or neoplasms and can range from mild to severe. Treatment varies with the particular type of disease. Common symptoms include fever, fatigue, weight loss, and enlarged lymph nodes.

REVIEW QUESTIONS

Short Answer

1. What are the three main functions of the lymphatic system?

2. Name the four signs and symptoms associated with common lymphatic system disorders.

3. Which diagnostic tests are most commonly used to determine the type and cause of lymphatic system disorders?

True or False

4. T F   Diseases of the lymphatic system commonly include inflammatory conditions.
5. T F   Lymphangiography is a biopsy of a lymph node or several nodes.
6. T F   Lymphadenitis is characterized by a swelling of the lymph nodes.
7. T F   Lymphangitis is a condition of swelling of lymph vessels due to inflammation.
8. T F   Lymphedema is always caused by obstruction of a lymphatic vessel.
9. T F   Mononucleosis is a bacterial infection that usually affects children and young adults.
10. T F   Lymphoma affects lymphocyte production and impairs immunity.

CASE STUDIES

■ Mrs. Talik is 78 years old and has been hospitalized frequently for repeated respiratory infections. Until the past 2 years, she has been relatively healthy. She has not been diagnosed with any serious chronic diseases but does have some osteoporosis. Based on your knowledge of the aging process and lymphatic system changes, what might be contributing to the development of these repeated respiratory infections? What can she do to decrease her risk and improve her immunity to infections?

(continued)

CASE STUDIES (continued)

■ Mrs. Smithson is a 55-year-old woman who has had a mastectomy for breast cancer. She has severe lymphedema in her right arm. She had talked to her physician about treatments for this, and he recommended using compression wraps and keeping the arm elevated. Are there any other recommendations you could make to her? How would you explain the cause of her lymphedema to her? She states that she heard laser therapy would cure her condition. What should you tell her about that?

Study Tools

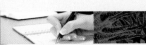

Workbook

Complete Chapter 10

Online Resources

PowerPoint® presentations

Animation

BIBLIOGRAPHY

Aschenbrenner, D. S. (2011). Drug watch. *American Journal of Nursing 111*(11), 23–24.

Biggs, T. C. (2011). Use of the absolute lymphocyte count in the diagnosis of infectious mononucleosis. *Clinical Otolaryngology 36*(5), 515–516.

Deng, J., Ridner, S. H., Dietrich, M. S., Wells, N., Wallston, K. A., Sinard, R. J., & Murphy, B. A. (2012). Prevalence of secondary lymphedema in patients with head and neck cancer. *Journal of Pain & Symptom Management 43*(2), 244–252.

Finnane, A., Liu, Y., Battistutta, D., Janda, M., & Hayes, S. C. (2011). Lymphedema after breast or gynecological cancer: Use and effectiveness of mainstream and complementary therapies. *Journal of Alternative & Complementary Medicine 17*(9), 867–869.

Leak, A., Mayer, D. K., & Smith, S. (2011). Quality of life domains among non-Hodgkin lymphoma survivors: An integrative literature review. *Leukemia & Lymphoma 52*(6), 972–985.

Lymphatic Research Foundation. (2012). *http://www.lymphaticresearch.org* (accessed February 2012).

Lymphoedema … what is it exactly? (2011). *British Journal of Community Nursing* 4–10.

Lymphoma Research Foundation. (2012). *http://www.lymphoma.org* (accessed February 2012).

Nune, S. K., Gunda, P., Majeti, B. K., Thallapally, P. K., & Forrest, M. (2011). Advances in lymphatic imaging and drug delivery. *Advanced Drug Delivery Reviews 63*(10/11), 876–885.

Ridner, S. H., Dietrich, M. S., Stewart, B. R., & Armer, J. M. (2011). Body mass index and breast cancer treatment-related lymphedema. *Supportive Care in Cancer 19*(6), 853–857.

Sylvia, M., Spera, E., Hamilton, S. M., Harrington, S., Hartford, J., & Quigley, S. (2011). Coordination of multiple services for a patient with severe lymphedema of the right lower extremity. *Critical Care Nurse 31*(4), 55–68.

Thomson, M., & Walker, J. (2011). Collaborative lymphoedema management: Developing a clinical protocol. *International Journal of Palliative Nursing 17*(5), 231–238.

Vignes, S., Porcher, R., Arrault, M., & Dupuy, A. (2011). Factors influencing breast cancer-related lymphedema volume after intensive decongestive physiotherapy. *Supportive Care in Cancer 19*(7), 935–940.

Weightlifting slashes lymphedema risk after breast cancer treatment, study suggests. (2011). *Trends in Medical Research 6*(2), 138–139.

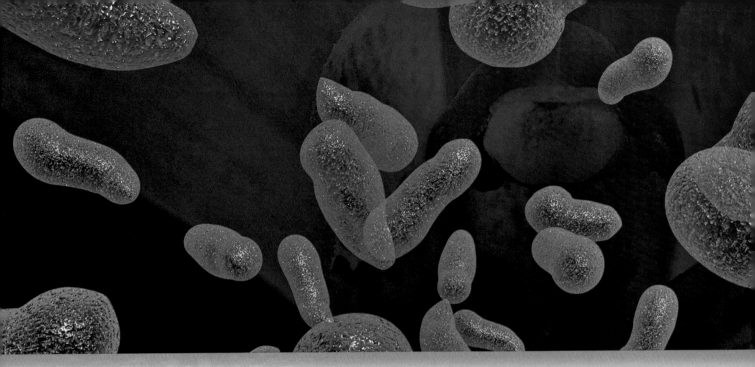

OUTLINE

- Anatomy and Physiology
- Common Signs and Symptoms
- Diagnostic Tests
- Common Diseases of the Digestive System
  Diseases of the Mouth
  Diseases of the Throat and Esophagus
  Diseases of the Stomach
  Diseases of the Small Intestine
  Diseases of the Colon
  Diseases of the Rectum
- Trauma
  Trauma to the Mouth
  Trauma to the Stomach and Intestines
- Rare Diseases
  Achalasia
  Gluten-Induced Enteropathy
  Intestinal Polyps
- Effects of Aging on the System
- Summary
- Review Questions
- Case Studies
- Bibliography

KEY TERMS

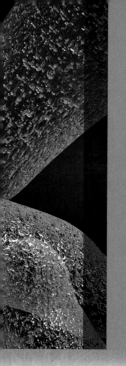

11

Digestive System Diseases and Disorders

LEARNING OBJECTIVES

Upon completion of the chapter, the learner should be able to:

1. Define the terminology common to the upper and lower digestive system and the disorders of the system.

2. Discuss the basic anatomy and physiology of the digestive system.

3. Identify the important signs and symptoms associated with common digestive system disorders.

4. Describe the common diagnostics used to determine type and cause of digestive system disorders.

5. Identify the common disorders of the digestive system.

6. Describe the typical course and management of the common digestive system disorders.

7. Describe the effects of aging on the digestive system and the common disorders associated with aging of the system.

OVERVIEW

The digestive system provides nutrients for the body through the processes of ingestion, digestion, and absorption and eliminates waste products from the system. Diseases or disorders of the digestive system are some of the most common medical problems. Because there are many differences in eating patterns, lifestyle behaviors, and inherited traits, digestive system problems vary considerably among individuals. Some digestive system problems are caused by poor nutritional habits, whereas others might be due to structural problems or a particular disease process. ■

ANATOMY AND PHYSIOLOGY

The digestive system has been described as a long tube running through the body. It has two main purposes: (1) to change the food we eat into simpler substances so they can be absorbed into the blood and carried to all cells of the body and (2) to eliminate waste products from the body. The two major parts of the digestive system are the alimentary canal and the accessory organs, including the tongue, teeth, salivary glands, gallbladder, pancreas, and liver.

The alimentary canal (Figure 11–1) is a continuous tube running from the mouth to the anus. The term *gastrointestinal (GI) tract* technically refers only to the stomach and intestines but is often used as a synonym for the alimentary canal. The alimentary canal is approximately 30 feet, or 9 meters, in length, but most of it is coiled up in the abdomen and surrounded by the peritoneum. The peritoneum is a large, serous membrane covering the organs in the abdomen and lining the walls of the abdominal cavity. It secretes fluid to prevent friction between organs in the abdomen as they move during the process of digestion. The alimentary canal starts at the mouth, where ingested food begins to be broken down to supply the body with needed nourishment. The teeth begin the process by breaking the food into smaller parts. The tongue, the organ of taste, assists the process by helping move the food in the mouth. The salivary glands, located outside the mouth with ducts leading from the glands to the mouth, secrete about 1,500 milliliters of saliva per day. The saliva continues the process of breaking down food and moistening it to make it easier to swallow. At the back of the mouth lies the pharynx, the channel for food to pass from the mouth to the esophagus.

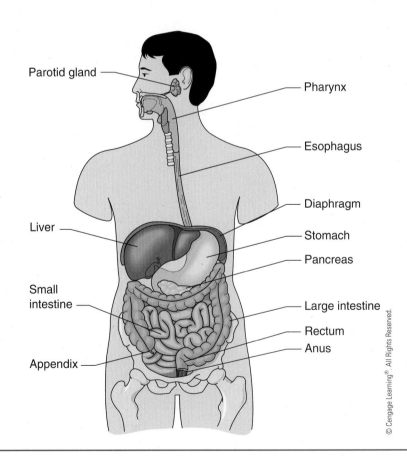

Parotid gland

Pharynx

Esophagus

Liver

Diaphragm

Stomach

Pancreas

Small intestine

Large intestine

Rectum

Anus

Appendix

FIGURE 11–1   The digestive system.

Consider This ...

If saliva can't dissolve the food, it can't be tasted. In order for the taste buds to taste something, it must be dissolved by saliva.

The esophagus is a tube (about 9 inches in length) that extends from the pharynx to the stomach. The walls of the esophagus are very muscular. Movement of these muscles is called peristaltic contraction. These contractions, the process called **peristalsis**, move the food from the pharynx to the stomach.

The stomach is a sac-type receptacle that lies just under the diaphragm in the upper abdomen. The esophagus connects to the stomach at the cardiac orifice (opening). A thick ring of smooth muscle called the cardiac, or gastroesophageal, sphincter surrounds this opening. The upper portion of the stomach, at the cardiac orifice end, is called the fundus, and the middle portion of the stomach is called the body. Food is broken down in the stomach by a process of chemical changes from the action of pepsin—an enzyme—and hydrochloric acid secreted by cells in the stomach. Food is mixed with these chemicals by the contractions of the stomach. The lining of the stomach also secretes a substance called the **intrinsic factor**, which is necessary for the absorption of vitamin B_{12}. At the lower portion of the stomach, called the pyloric region, the stomach is connected to the first part of the small intestine, called the duodenum. The opening at this end of the stomach is the pyloric orifice, which is surrounded by the pyloric sphincter. Sphincter muscles control the cardiac and pyloric openings.

Consider This ...

The stomach of the average-sized adult will produce approximately 2 liters of hydrochloric acid per day.

The small intestine extends from the pyloric orifice to the ileocecal valve at the beginning of the large intestine. It is divided into three sections. The first section, the duodenum, is about 10 inches, or 25 centimeters, in length, the shortest of the three sections. The duodenum receives bile from the liver and pancreatic juices from the pancreas, which aid in the digestive process. The duodenum connects the stomach to the jejunum (jay-JUNE-um), the second section of the small intestine, on the left side of the upper abdomen. The jejunum extends from the duodenum to the ileum. It is about 7.5 feet, or 2 meters, in length and is coiled throughout the abdomen. The ileum is the third section of the small intestine, attaching to the jejunum at its beginning and ending at the ileocecal (il-ee-oh-SEE-cal) valve, the beginning of the large intestine.

The major function of the small intestine is digestion and absorption of food and fluids. Material is moved through the small intestine by muscular action (peristalsis). Most of digestion takes place in the small intestine. Finger-like projections called villi, containing lymph vessels and blood capillaries, are located on the inside surface of the intestine. Additional extensions called microvilli cover the villi, forming a velvety surface that greatly increases the surface area of the small intestine. As a result of this increased surface area, nutrient absorption is greatly increased. Nutrients pass into the vascular capillaries for delivery to the body cells.

The large intestine connects to the small intestine at the ileocecal valve in the lower-right portion of the abdomen. The first section of the colon is called the cecum. The appendix is attached to the cecum near the ileocecal valve. The large intestine, also called the colon, is about 5 feet, or 1.5 meters, long. Each section of the colon is named according to its anatomical position. The colon begins in the lower-right quadrant of the abdomen (cecum), rises to the mid-level (ascending colon), crosses the abdomen at the umbilicus level (transverse colon), and descends on the left side (descending colon) into the pelvic cavity, where it is called the sigmoid colon. The sigmoid colon forms an S-shaped tube that extends into the lower pelvic region, ending at the rectum and anus. The process of digestion and absorption continues in the large intestine, but the most important function of the large intestine is the absorption of water and electrolytes and the elimination of **feces**, the material not absorbed by the intestines.

Media Link

View an animation on digestion on the Online Resources.

COMMON SIGNS AND SYMPTOMS

Diseases of this system usually result in signs and symptoms related to hemorrhage, **perforation**, and altered **motility** (movement) in the system. Hemorrhage can be mild or severe and can originate at any site along the system. Terms identifying bleeding are **hematemesis** (HEM-ah-TEM-eh-sis; hemat = blood, emesis = vomiting), **hematochezia** (HEM-at-toe-KEE-zee-ah, bright red blood in the feces), and **melena** (meh-LEE-nah, dark, tarry **stool**) due to the presence of blood.

Perforation in any area of the tract can be life-threatening due to the contaminating contents of the tract and the ease of spread in the abdominal cavity. Perforation in the stomach or intestines allows spillage of contents into the abdominal cavity, causing **peritonitis** (PER-ih-toe-NIGH-tis; an inflammation of the peritoneum), of which pain is a common symptom. Spilled gastric contents are high in gastric acid and are corrosive to abdominal organs, and intestinal contents have a normally high bacterial count. Spilling intestinal contents into the abdominal cavity causes infection, which can lead to **septicemia** (SEP-tih-SEE-me-ah; septic = dirty, emia = blood or bacteria in the bloodstream). Causes of perforation can include peptic ulcer, injury from gunshot or stab wounds, and untreated appendicitis.

Alteration in motility, or movement of food along the tract, commonly leads to a variety of signs and symptoms, including nausea, vomiting, diarrhea, or constipation. Diarrhea is a disorder characterized by frequent, watery stools. Irritability of the intestinal lining causes hyperactivity of muscle contractions (peristalsis), causing a rushing of the watery contents in the small intestine through the large intestine. This rushing denies the large intestine the time needed to reabsorb the water. The primary concern with diarrhea, especially in young children and older people, is loss of fluids, leading to dehydration. Causes of diarrhea include a sudden increase in stress or nervous condition, bacterial or viral infection, or food poisoning.

Constipation is the opposite of diarrhea. The stool in the colon remains for an extended period of time, too much water is reabsorbed, and the stool becomes hard, dry, and difficult to pass. Constipation is commonly caused by poor dietary and elimination habits. Avoiding the urge to **defecate** (have a bowel movement) increases the amount of time the stool remains in the colon and, thus, increases constipation.

DIAGNOSTIC TESTS

Diagnostic tests for the digestive system commonly include radiologic (X-ray) examinations and endoscopic (looking into the cavity with a lighted scope) examinations. An upper GI series, also called a barium swallow, allows visualization of the esophagus, stomach, and upper portion of the small intestine. In preparation for such an examination, the individual must be N.P.O. (*non per os*—nothing by mouth) for a minimum of 8 hours. Prior to the examination, the individual drinks a barium solution, which coats the inside of the upper tract, allowing visualization by X-ray. The physician can view a series, or several X-rays, to detect problems of the upper tract (Figure 11–2).

HEALTHY HIGHLIGHT

Good Elimination Habits

To avoid constipation, defecation should be allowed to occur when reflexes are the strongest, usually early in the morning following breakfast, although elimination habits differ from individual to individual. Some people might have bowel movements after every meal; others will have a bowel movement daily or every 2 or 3 days. Other good elimination habits include a diet high in fiber (fruits, vegetables, grains, and cereals), daily exercise, and adequate intake of fluids. Laxatives and enemas should be avoided because these artificially stimulate the bowel and can alter its normal elimination pattern. Regular use of laxatives produces dependence on them for bowel elimination.

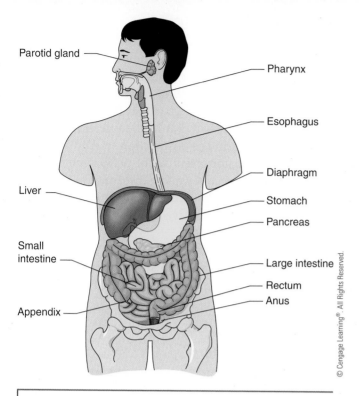

Parotid gland

Pharynx

Esophagus

Diaphragm

Liver

Stomach

Pancreas

Small
intestine

Large intestine

Rectum

Anus

Appendix

FIGURE 11–2   Upper GI; yellow area is visualized.

A lower GI series, also called a barium enema, provides visualization of the large intestine. In preparation for this radiologic examination, the individual is given an enema or laxatives the day before the examination to rid the colon of fecal material, and the diet is restricted to clear liquids. The day of the examination, an enema of barium solution is administered to coat the lower tract and allow X-ray visualization of the large intestine (Figure 11–3).

Endoscopic examination allows the physician to look directly into the digestive organs through a lighted scope (Figure 11–4). The name of each procedure is identified by naming the organ being scoped: stomach (gastroscopy), colon (colonoscopy), sigmoid colon (sigmoidoscopy), and entire upper GI area (esophagogastroduodenoscopy, EGD). During an endoscopic examination, a physician might obtain a biopsy (small piece of tissue for examination) to determine the presence of a neoplasm or other disease processes.

Video capsule endoscopy has recently been added as a diagnostic test. In this test, a capsule containing a miniature video camera is swallowed and travels

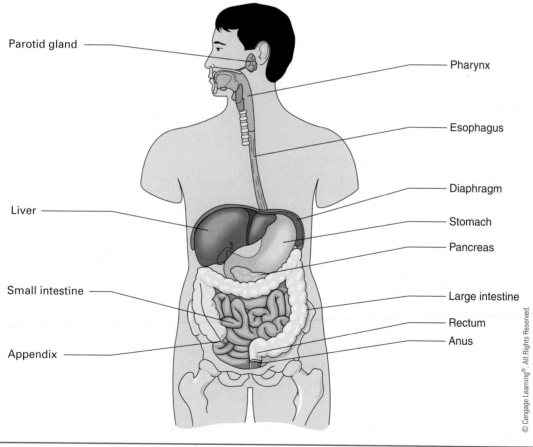

Parotid gland

Pharynx

Esophagus

Diaphragm

Liver

Stomach

Pancreas

Small intestine

Large intestine

Rectum

Anus

Appendix

FIGURE 11–3   Lower GI; yellow area is visualized.

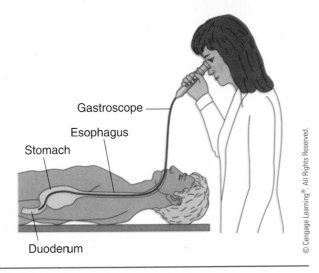

Gastroscope

Esophagus

Stomach

Duodenum

© Cengage Learning®. All Rights Reserved.

FIGURE 11–4 Esophagogastroduodenoscopy.

through the small intestine. As it travels along, it sends video images of the lining to a receiver worn on a belt at the waist. The images can then be downloaded and viewed on computer. The value of this test is the ease of viewing even very small or mild abnormalities. A disadvantage of this camera is that it cannot be used in patients with obstruction in the intestine because it might get stuck in the obstruction.

Several laboratory tests can be performed to assist in diagnosis of digestive system diseases. One of these is the occult stool test, which tests stool for **occult (hidden) blood**. A positive occult stool test can be indicative of colon cancer.

Another laboratory test is an **ova and parasite (O&P)**, an examination of a stool specimen for the presence of adult parasites or their eggs (ova). Parasites

PHARMACOLOGY HIGHLIGHT

Common Drugs for Gastrointestinal Disorders

CATEGORY	EXAMPLES OF MEDICATIONS
Antacids Drugs used to reduce stomach acidity	
Phosphate binders	sodium bicarbonate, calcium carbonate, magnesium carbonate, magnesium hydroxide, or aluminum hydroxide
H₂ receptor antagonists	cimetidine, ranitidine, famotidine, or nizatidine
Proton pump inhibitors	omeprazole, lansoprazole, or esomeprazole
Antibiotics Drugs used to prevent or stop bacterial infections	ampicillin, amoxicillin, ciprofloxacin, doxycycline, erythromycin, penicillin, or tetracycline
Anti-inflammatories Drugs used to reduce inflammation	
Steroids	hydrocortisone, beclomethasone, or amcinonide
Nonsteroidal	acetaminophen, aspirin, or ibuprofen
Antidiarrheals Drugs used to treat diarrhea	bismuth subsalicylate, loperamide, or octreotide
Antineoplastics Drugs used to treat cancer	
Alkylating agents	chlorambucil, cyclophosphamide, or lomustine
Antimetabolites	5-flourauracil, mercaptopurine, or methotrexate
Antitumor antibiotics	mitomycin or streptozocin
Hormones/antihormones	estrogens, androgens, flutamide, or tamoxifen
Other substances	vincristine, L-asparaginase, paclitaxel, carboplatin, cisplatin, or etoposide
Laxatives Drugs used to treat constipation	docusate, bisacodyl, senna, or methylcellulose

identified by an O&P might include roundworms, tapeworms, pinworms, or hookworms and protozoa such as *Giardia lamblia*. Stool or fecal cultures can be used to determine bacterial infections in the colon.

■ COMMON DISEASES OF THE DIGESTIVE SYSTEM

Diseases of the Mouth

The primary function of the mouth is to begin the breakdown of food into smaller particles. Diseases of the mouth include those related to inflammation and tumors.

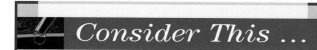

Consider This ...

The lifespan of a taste bud is about 10 days, and before it dies, it is replaced with a new taste bud.

DENTAL CARIES

■ **DESCRIPTION.** Dental caries is an infectious disease that damages the teeth; it primarily affects children and young adults.

■ **ETIOLOGY.** Microorganisms in the mouth attack the teeth, producing dental cavities. The cause of caries is twofold, requiring bacteria along with a diet high in carbohydrates (sugars). Left untreated, the disease can lead to infection, pain, and tooth loss.

■ **SYMPTOMS.** The bacteria stick to the tooth surface in a tough, sticky material called **dental plaque**. Acids produced by the bacteria erode the tooth surface.

■ **DIAGNOSIS.** Diagnosis involves inspecting the teeth for plaque, followed by X-rays revealing cavities.

■ **TREATMENT.** Treatment can range from simple dental fillings to oral surgery, depending on the extent of the caries.

■ **PREVENTION.** Prevention is based on frequently removing dental plaque by brushing and flossing

HEALTHY HIGHLIGHT

The Tongue Tells All

The tongue can tell a great deal about the health of a person. The tongue helps in chewing and swallowing. About 15% of the population has some disorder in which the tongue is directly involved. It is important for individuals to be aware of the tongue and any changes that might be observed.

Growths and ulcerations such as cold sores, ulcers (canker sores), benign lesions, or oral cancer are common. The tongue can also be enlarged in some case of hypothyroidism or in allergic reactions. In fact, a thick or enlarged tongue might be one of the first signs of an anaphylactic reaction, which is a medical emergency.

Color changes such as white patches may indicate an infection, a suppressed immune system, or a precancerous condition. A "hairy tongue" (black tongue) is common to persons who drink large amounts of coffee or tea or use tobacco. A pale tongue may indicate anemia, but a reddened tongue may indicate inflammation or infection or other dietary insufficiencies.

Pain in the tongue usually indicates sores or ulcers that need to be reviewed for the underlying cause. Pain may also occur in women during menopause and can be treated with some lozenge medications.

Some problems of the tongue will disappear without treatment, but others need medical intervention. The tongue can tell the physician some important factors about the patient's health. Individuals should report any abnormalities to their health care provider.

Source: eDocAmerica (2010).

the teeth. A decrease in carbohydrate (sugar) intake is also helpful. The use of fluoride in drinking water and toothpaste also reduces the incidence of caries.

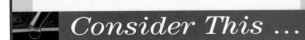

Consider This ...

Enamel is the hardest substance in the human body.

PERIODONTAL DISEASE

■ **DESCRIPTION.** Periodontal disease affects the supporting structures of the teeth such as the gums. It is a disease that affects adults and incidence increases with aging. Most adults have some degree of periodontal disease, the main reason for tooth loss in an adult.

■ **ETIOLOGY.** Dental plaque, poor oral hygiene, and inadequate diet are common factors leading to this disease.

■ **SYMPTOMS.** Dental plaque sticks on the tooth at the gum line, often leading to **gingivitis** (inflammation of the gums with painful bleeding) (Figure 11–5).

■ **DIAGNOSIS.** A dentist can make a diagnosis by inspecting the gums and measuring the pocket depth of the teeth. Redness, puffiness, and bleeding along with a pocket depth of 3 millimeters indicate disease.

■ **TREATMENT.** Treatment involves removing the plaque and treating the inflammation.

■ **PREVENTION.** Prevention is based on frequent brushing and flossing of the teeth with special attention given to the gum line, regular dental care to remove plaque, and an adequate diet.

Consider This ...

Individuals with gum disease are twice as likely to have a stroke or heart attack as those without gum disease.

CANCER OF THE MOUTH

■ **DESCRIPTION.** Tumors of the mouth can occur on the lip, cheek, gum, palate, or tongue. A common oral cancer is squamous cell carcinoma of the lip.

■ **ETIOLOGY.** This tumor usually occurs on the lower lip of men and is related to exposure to sunlight, chewing tobacco, and smoking pipes or cigars (Figure 11–6).

■ **SYMPTOMS.** The common symptom is a small, pale-colored, painless lump on the tongue, lip, or other mouth area.

■ **DIAGNOSIS.** A tissue biopsy of the lump is the most definitive diagnostic test.

■ **TREATMENT.** Radiation therapy and surgical excision are usually quite effective in treating this cancer.

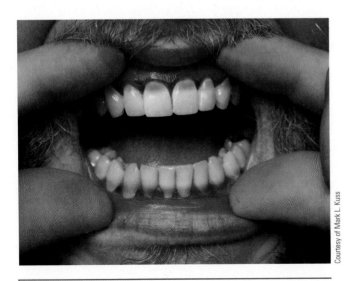

Courtesy of Mark L. Kuss

FIGURE 11–5   Gingivitis (inflamed gingiva).

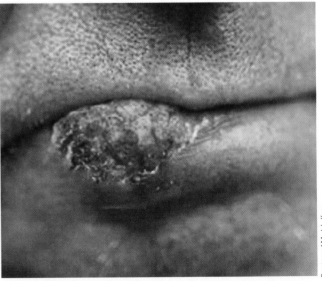

Courtesy of Mark L. Kuss

FIGURE 11–6   Cancer of the lip.

■ **PREVENTION.** Decreasing exposure to sunlight by using SPF sunscreen, wearing hats to shade the face, and eliminating the use of tobacco products aid in prevention.

Diseases of the Throat and Esophagus

There are many diseases of the throat and esophagus, ranging from mild to severe and acute to chronic. Infections and inflammatory conditions are some of the most common. Pharyngitis is often categorized as a respiratory problem because the pharynx can be considered part of the respiratory system as well as part of the digestive system.

Consider This ...

Another word for the esophagus is "gullet" from the Latin word *gula* meaning throat.

PHARYNGITIS

■ **DESCRIPTION.** Pharyngitis is commonly called a sore throat.

■ **ETIOLOGY.** Viral or bacterial microorganisms are common causes of pharyngitis.

■ **SYMPTOMS.** The most frequent and earliest symptom of pharyngitis is a sore throat. Visual examination reveals redness in the area. A common type of pharyngitis is an inflammation of the tonsils called tonsillitis, in which the tonsils form crypts of pus, which give the tonsils a whitish appearance. (See Chapter 9, Figure 9–8, for a picture of pharyngitis.)

An acute type of pharyngitis is called **strep throat**, caused by **virulent** (VIR-u-lent; infectious, difficult to kill) bacteria, *Streptococci*. These bacteria can spread into the bloodstream and produce other diseases such as scarlet fever, rheumatic fever, glomerulonephritis, and endocarditis.

■ **DIAGNOSIS.** Diagnosis is made by examination and throat culture.

HEALTHY HIGHLIGHT

Get Rid of Halitosis

Halitosis (bad breath) is often caused by food particles in the mouth or from a health problem.

To prevent or reduce bad breath:

1. **Clean your teeth after you eat.** Brushing is best, but if this is not an option, then swishing mouth wash or even water alone helps rid the mouth of food particles.
2. **Floss your teeth at least once a day.** Flossing removes decaying food from between your teeth.
3. **Clean the back of your tongue. Either brush your tongue or scrape it with a tongue scraper.**
4. **Drink water or chew gum.** Water and saliva help wash away dead cells and food particles.
5. **If you wear dentures, clean them daily.** Dentures can also harbor decaying food particles.
6. **Limit foods and beverages that may cause bad breath.** This includes garlic, onion, coffee, and alcohol. These are easily absorbed through the lungs and then exhaled.
7. **See your doctor or dentist.** If these simple measures do not help, then the halitosis may be related to a health problem such as a sinus infection or abscessed tooth.

TREATMENT. Treatment of strep throat includes identification of the organism through laboratory cultures, followed by antibiotic treatment and follow-up culture to check effectiveness of antibiotic treatment. Antibiotic treatment is quite effective if taken as prescribed.

PREVENTION. Frequent and thorough hand washing is one of the best preventive methods, along with avoiding contact with people who are sick. Using a new toothbrush after an infection prevents reinfection.

REFLUX ESOPHAGITIS

DESCRIPTION. Reflux esophagitis, more recently called gastroesophageal reflux disease (GERD), is an inflammation of tissue at the lower end of the esophagus.

ETIOLOGY. GERD is caused by a reflux (backflow) of stomach acids through the cardiac sphincter upward into the esophagus.

SYMPTOMS. The most common symptom of reflux esophagitis is heartburn, a burning sensation in the mid-chest or epigastric (epi = above, gastric = stomach) area. Long-term reflux can lead to bleeding, ulceration, and scarring of the esophagus, which can cause stricture and difficulty swallowing.

DIAGNOSIS. Diagnosis is usually made by barium swallow X-ray (upper GI). If further diagnostic testing is needed, an EGD with biopsy can be performed.

TREATMENT. Treatment is directed at reducing reflux and can include recommendations to avoid large meals, spicy foods, caffeine, and tight clothing. Medications such as stool softeners, laxatives, and antacids might be helpful. Several drugs specifically

HEALTHY HIGHLIGHT

Tips about Strep Throat

Sore throats need to be tested routinely to diagnose the *Streptococcus* infection commonly called strep throat. Practitioners cannot determine this condition by simply viewing the throat. The most accurate diagnostic test is a throat culture. Some practitioners use a rapid strep test (RST) that produces results within 15 minutes, while a routine culture takes 2 days. The main disadvantage of an RST is that it may give a false negative. Symptomatic patients with negative tests are often then cultured and thus are charged for two tests. Although an RST allows an antibiotic to be started faster, thus decreasing the contagious state and allowing return to work or school earlier, it is felt there is some advantage to waiting 48 hours to start an antibiotic to allow the body to build up some of its own disease-fighting immunity (Pickering, 2009).

It is recommended that antibiotics be started within 9 days of the appearance of symptoms in order to prevent rheumatic fever and other streptococcal-related diseases. Parents of children who have recurrent attacks of strep throat should also have throat cultures because they might be carriers of the strep infection. Strep throat is usually treated effectively with antibiotics.

Antibiotics should be taken as prescribed. They should always be taken until all tablets or capsules are gone. Even if the affected individual begins to feel better, the medication should be continued until completed because discontinuing the antibiotic or saving some medicine for later can lead to bacterial resistance. If an individual does not take the prescribed number of tablets, it is possible for many bacteria to survive the short dosage time and actually build up a resistance to that antibiotic. These bacteria can then cause another attack of strep throat that cannot be treated or cured with the previously prescribed antibiotic. Taking all antibiotics as prescribed should destroy all the bacteria and eliminate the risk of bacterial resistance.

for reflux problems are also available, some over the counter and others requiring a prescription. Activities that increase abdominal pressure might be restricted. Sleeping with the head of the bed elevated is often helpful. Surgery on the incompetent sphincter is usually not recommended and considered only in extreme cases.

■ **PREVENTION.** Preventive measures include controlling weight and avoiding smoking, caffeine, carbonated beverages, chocolate, and high-fat foods as well as late-night meals.

HIATAL HERNIA

■ **DESCRIPTION.** Hiatal hernia is a sliding of part of the stomach into the chest cavity.

■ **ETIOLOGY.** The stomach slides upward through the natural hole in the diaphragm where the esophagus passes through to the stomach (Figure 11–7). This herniation can increase in frequency with age and weakening of the cardiac sphincter.

■ **SYMPTOMS.** Many hiatal hernias are **asymptomatic** (a = without, symptomatic = symptoms), but those that do cause discomfort are usually related to esophageal reflux.

■ **DIAGNOSIS.** Hiatal hernias are diagnosed by an upper GI X-ray.

■ **TREATMENT.** Treatment is often the same as for reflux esophagitis.

■ **PREVENTION.** Although it is difficult to prevent hiatal hernias totally, risk can be reduced by maintaining a healthy weight, avoiding heavy lifting, and not smoking.

ESOPHAGEAL VARICES

■ **DESCRIPTION.** Esophageal varices are extremely dilated varicose veins located in the esophagus (Figure 11–8).

■ **ETIOLOGY.** Unusually high pressure in the veins of the esophagus causes them to enlarge and become tortuous, resulting in esophageal varices. This increased venous pressure is due to blockage or reduced flow of blood into the liver, causing poor venous return from the esophagus. (For more information on liver disease, see Chapter 12, "Liver, Gallbladder, and Pancreatic Diseases and Disorders.") Any condition that leads to venous congestion in the liver can lead to esophageal varices, but they are most commonly related to cirrhosis of the liver. The most common cause of cirrhosis is excessive alcohol consumption. Hemorrhage of the varices can be a life-threatening condition.

■ **SYMPTOMS.** Symptoms include vomiting blood, black stools, and, on endoscopic examination, dilated esophageal blood vessels.

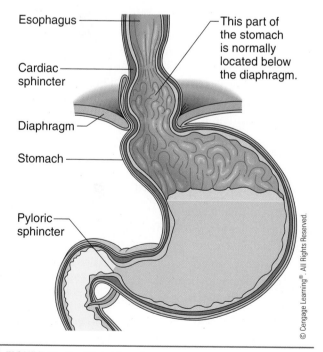

FIGURE 11–7 Hiatal hernia.

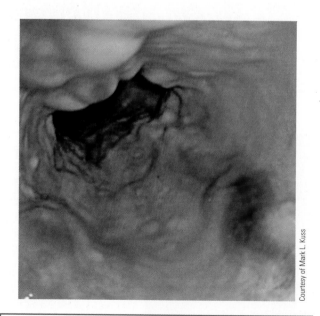

FIGURE 11–8 Esophageal varices.

■ **DIAGNOSIS.** Physical examination can reveal low blood pressure, bloody stools, and signs of chronic liver disease. Diagnosis is confirmed with an EGD.

■ **TREATMENT.** The goal of treatment is to decrease venous pressure by methods such as portal vein bypass surgery and medication to lower blood pressure. Other treatments include limiting the diet to soft, nonirritating foods and the use of stool softeners to prevent straining, which increases esophageal venous pressure. Chronic bleeding of the vessels can be treated with a sclerosing agent that hardens or destroys the vessel. Treatment for acute bleeding includes instillation of cold saline washings, the application of pressure to the site through a nasogastric tube, or both.

■ **PREVENTION.** Treating or preventing liver disease can prevent this disease.

Diseases of the Stomach

Diseases of the stomach are common problems in the digestive system. Complaints of stomach pain, especially after eating, are frequently voiced to the physician. This problem increases with age due to age-related changes in the system and is also complicated by other chronic diseases. Disorders of the stomach range from mild acute gastritis to more serious diseases such as cancer of the stomach.

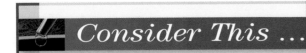

Consider This ...

When an individual's face blushes, the color of their stomach tissue turns red, too.

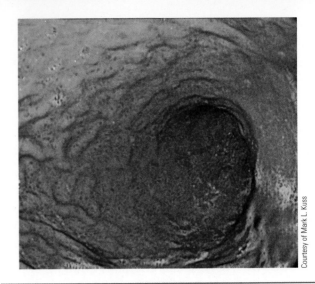

FIGURE 11–9 Gastritis.

Courtesy of Mark L. Kuss

GASTRITIS

■ **DESCRIPTION.** Gastritis is not a specific disease but a condition that results from several problems that all cause inflammation of the stomach (Figure 11–9).

■ **ETIOLOGY.** Common causes are use of anti-inflammatory medications or nonsteroidal anti-inflammatory drugs (NSAIDS), such as aspirin or ibuprofen, smoking, alcohol consumption, and infection with bacteria such as *Helicobacter pylori* (*H. pylori*).

H. pylori are corkscrew-shaped bacteria that commonly live and multiply within the mucous layer that lines the stomach and small intestine (Figure 11–10). About half of the world's population is infected with *H. pylori* (Mayo Clinic, 2011). These bacteria are usually picked up during childhood and do not cause symptoms in the majority of people. Those persons

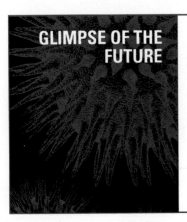

GLIMPSE OF THE FUTURE

Kudzu Root for Diarrhea and Other GI Disorders

Kudzu root is the dried part of a perennial vine found in Southeast Asia. It has been used in Chinese herbal medicine for the treatment of dysentery, diarrhea, and other GI disorders, as well as diabetes and cardiovascular diseases. The root contains many phytochemicals that have an effect on these diseases. Further study needs to be done to determine which phytochemicals and how much should be used to treat each disorder. In the future, kudzu root might be found to be an effective treatment for a variety of GI illnesses.

Source: Wong et al. (2011).

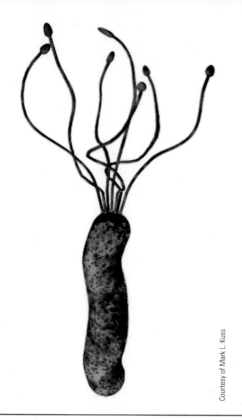

FIGURE 11–10 Helicobacter pylori.

kill off ingested bacteria. Achlorhydria also leads to loss of intrinsic factor (a protein produced by the gastric mucosa), leading to pernicious anemia. (See Chapter 7, "Blood and Blood-Forming Organs Diseases and Disorders," for more information on anemia.)

■ *SYMPTOMS.* The most common symptom is abdominal pain. Other symptoms include nausea, belching, and vomiting.

■ *DIAGNOSIS.* Diagnosis is made using several tests. Urea breath tests determine presence of the bacteria in the stomach. A stool antigen test determines whether there is antigen present that triggers the immune system. An upper GI endoscopy or EGD may be used for visual confirmation or to obtain a stomach biopsy.

■ *TREATMENT.* Medications to reduce stomach acid help relieve symptoms and promote healing. Treatment for *H. pylori* involves treatment with antibiotics. Avoiding irritating foods, medications, smoking, and alcohol is also helpful. Treating and resolving the underlying cause usually leads to resolution of gastritis.

■ *PREVENTION.* Avoiding irritating factors and promptly treating those who are symptomatic with *H. pylori* aid in prevention of gastritis.

PEPTIC ULCER

■ *DESCRIPTION.* An ulcer is an area of tissue that has eroded, leaving a crater-like appearance (Figure 11–11). Peptic ulcers are those ulcers found in the stomach and duodenum that are caused, in part, by the action of pepsin. Peptic ulcers found in the

affected often have pain and gastric ulceration as the *H. pylori* weakens the protective mucous lining of the stomach, allowing acid to contact the sensitive tissues underneath. Why the bacteria cause ulcers in some people and not in others is not known.

Gastritis also increases with age. As people age, the number of acid-producing cells decreases, thus leading to atrophic gastritis, or **achlorhydria** (AH-klor-HIGH-dree-ah; no hydrochloric acid), because there is not enough hydrochloric acid to

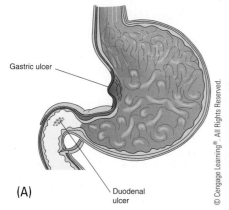

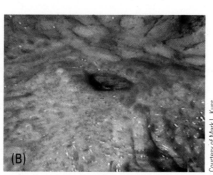

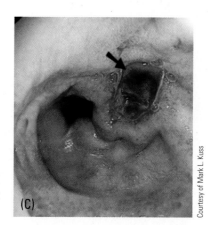

FIGURE 11–11 Peptic ulcers. (A) Location. (B) Gastric ulcer. (C) Duodenal ulcer.

COMPLEMENTARY AND ALTERNATIVE THERAPY

Reducing the Bloated Feeling

There are a variety of ways to reduce bloating after eating using complementary or alternative treatments as opposed to using medications. One article suggested trying relaxation strategies or exercise to relieve stress that might interrupt proper digestion. Also recommended was the use of acupuncture treatments. Several herbal supplements are available over the counter that relieve digestion and bloating. Another suggestion was preventative in nature—chew food 20 times per bite before swallowing.

Source: Acosta et al. (2011).

---

stomach are called gastric ulcers, and those located in the duodenum are called duodenal ulcers.

■ *ETIOLOGY.* As many as 50% of these ulcers are associated with *Helicobacter pylori* (National Digestive Diseases Information Clearinghouse, 2012). Other contributing factors include severe stress, heavy intake of drugs (such as aspirin, steroids, and alcohol), and smoking.

The stomach lining is normally protected by a thick mucous membrane lining. Pepsin is an enzyme secreted in the stomach that breaks down protein, but this same enzyme, to some degree, breaks down the stomach's lining, causing ulcers.

■ *SYMPTOMS.* Ulcer pain is caused by the hydrochloric acid in the stomach irritating the raw ulcerated area. Complications of peptic ulcers are massive bleeding, perforation, and obstruction.

■ *DIAGNOSIS.* Diagnosis is based on symptoms and the results of a gastroscopy or visual examination of the inside of the stomach

■ *TREATMENT.* Treatment is aimed at reducing the gastric acidity and healing the stomach lining. Antibiotics are also used to treat ulcers caused by *Helicobacter* bacteria. Other treatments include reduction or elimination of contributory factors. Antacids to neutralize gastric acids and other gastric medications might be helpful. Surgery is warranted in severe cases that might lead to hemorrhage, perforation, obstruction, or extreme pain.

■ *PREVENTION.* Infection with *H. pylori* is thought to occur during childhood through water, food, or kissing someone who has the bacteria. At this time, routes of infection are unproven, and the fact that

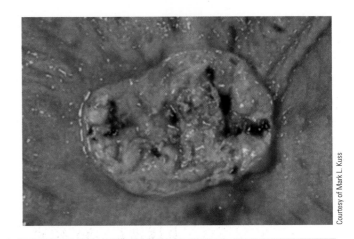

Courtesy of Mark L. Kuss

FIGURE 11–12   Stomach cancer.

many people with *H. pylori* do not develop peptic ulcers makes this cause unpreventable. Quick treatment of *H. pylori*, when discovered as an irritant, along with avoiding other irritants, is beneficial.

CANCER OF THE STOMACH

■ *DESCRIPTION.* Cancer of the stomach often spreads through the stomach tissue to nearby organs such as the pancreas, intestine, and esophagus (Figure 11–12). These cancer cells can also spread through the blood and lymphatic system to the liver, lungs, and lymph nodes all over the body. Often, this cancer goes undiagnosed until after it spreads outside the stomach and into other organs.

■ *ETIOLOGY.* The cause of stomach cancer is unknown, although research has proven certain causative factors. These include some correlation to food additives and foods that are smoked, salted, and pickled. Cigarette smoking is another risk factor along with gender, in that men are more affected than women.

■ *SYMPTOMS.* Symptoms are often vague and include loss of appetite, general stomach distress, and heartburn. Prognosis is good if the cancer is discovered early.

■ *DIAGNOSIS.* Diagnostic testing includes upper GI studies, endoscopy, and biopsy. Biopsy is the most definitive diagnostic test.

■ *TREATMENT.* Treatment can include surgical resection, chemotherapy, and radiation.

■ *PREVENTION.* Preventing causative factors might help in prevention.

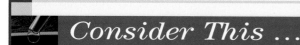

Consider This ...

The stomach produces a new layer of mucus every 2 weeks in order to prevent it from digesting itself.

Diseases of the Small Intestine

The small intestine, consisting of the duodenum, jejunum, and ileum, secretes enzymes and absorbs nutrients for cellular functions. Disorders of the small intestine frequently manifest themselves by pain that radiates across the abdomen, although this symptom alone is not enough to diagnose the specific disease process. Additional evaluation is needed, such as X-ray or computerized tomography (CT) scan. The disorders of the small intestine can range from mild intestinal upset to more severe chronic problems such as ulcers or regional enteritis.

DUODENAL ULCER

A duodenal ulcer, also called a peptic ulcer of the duodenum, was discussed previously under "Peptic Ulcer."

MALABSORPTION SYNDROME

■ *DESCRIPTION.* The primary purpose of the small intestine is to absorb nutrients. Malabsorption syndrome occurs when this process is altered and nutrients are not adequately absorbed into the blood.

■ *ETIOLOGY.* Persons with malabsorption syndrome can be unable to absorb nutrients (especially fat) and minerals. Other diseases such as diabetes mellitus, cystic fibrosis, pancreatic deficiencies, lactose intolerance, and gluten enteropathy can also lead to malabsorption syndrome. Malabsorption syndrome can range from mild intestinal upset to more severe chronic problems such as ulcers or regional enteritis.

■ *SYMPTOMS.* Symptoms include anemia, diarrhea, edema, muscle cramping, and weight loss. Heart arrhythmias can result from potassium deficiency, and blood clotting disorders can also occur. Children who are affected might exhibit signs of failure to grow.

■ *DIAGNOSIS.* Diagnosis is often very difficult and requires extensive testing. Basic testing will include a thorough medical and physical examination followed by a variety of blood tests, X-rays, stool samples, endoscopies, ultrasound, and CT and magnetic resonance imaging (MRI) scanning. All these tests aid in measuring abnormalities of the GI tract.

■ *TREATMENT.* Most treatments include diet therapy for control. One of the complications of the disorder is a bleeding tendency due to the lack of vitamin K absorption.

■ *PREVENTION.* Many of the malabsorption syndromes are hereditary, so there are no preventive solutions. Genetic screening followed by early detection through routine physical exams and testing is of benefit. Prevention, in some cases, is as easy as avoiding the foods or substances that cause problems.

REGIONAL ENTERITIS (CROHN'S DISEASE)

■ *DESCRIPTION.* Regional enteritis is a chronic inflammatory disease most commonly affecting the small intestine, but it can also affect the large intestine. It is characterized by bouts of **remission** (slowing or stopping of symptoms) and **exacerbation** (x-AS-er-BAY-shun; flaring up of symptoms) (Figure 11–13) and is commonly classified as inflammatory bowel disease (IBD) until complete diagnosis is made. As regional enteritis progresses, the intestinal wall thickens, resulting in a narrowing of the lumen.

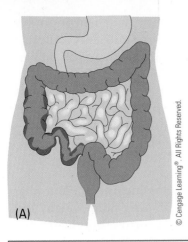
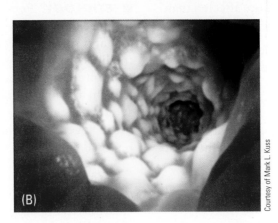
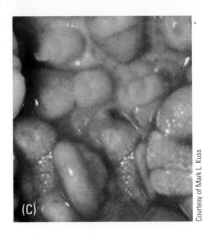

(A)

© Cengage Learning®. All Rights Reserved.

(B)

Courtesy of Mark L. Kuss

(C)

Courtesy of Mark L. Kuss

FIGURE 11–13   (A) Regional enteritis. (B) Regional enteritis: view through endoscope. (C) Regional enteritis.

■ **ETIOLOGY.** The cause of the disease has not yet been determined, although genetic, immunologic, infectious, and psychological factors have been considered.

■ **SYMPTOMS.** Symptoms include anorexia, flatulence, abdominal pain, diarrhea, and constipation. Individuals with regional enteritis tend to experience relapse or exacerbations of the condition during periods of stress or emotional upset, factors that support the psychogenic theory. Young females are most often affected by regional enteritis.

■ **DIAGNOSIS.** Symptoms, along with blood tests, upper GI series, CT scanning, and colonoscopy, help determine the diagnosis. Recently, video capsule endoscopy has been added to diagnostic testing.

■ **TREATMENT.** Treatment is supportive but not likely to be curative. Approaches can involve a low-residue diet and medications to control diarrhea, inflammation, infection, and depression. Surgical resection is not curative and is performed to treat complications such as perforation and obstruction.

■ **PREVENTION.** Because Crohn's is thought to have some inherited tendency, there are no known preventive measures. To prevent flare-ups, maintaining a healthy diet and reducing stress are helpful.

GASTROENTERITIS

■ **DESCRIPTION.** Gastroenteritis (gastro = stomach, entero = intestines, itis = inflammation), as its name suggests, is inflammation of both the stomach and intestines (Figure 11–14).

■ **ETIOLOGY.** Causes can include bacterial, viral, or parasitic invasion; ingestion of tainted food; lactose intolerance; allergic reaction to food or drugs; and stress.

■ **SYMPTOMS.** Gastroenteritis can have an acute and violent onset with nausea, vomiting, abdominal cramping, and diarrhea, leading to rapid fluid and electrolyte loss. Or symptoms may be less violent, with stomach rumbling, **malaise** (ma-LAZ; general ill feeling), nausea, and mild diarrhea.

■ **DIAGNOSIS.** The symptoms usually help identify this illness. Identifying the cause might require stool samples to examine for viruses, bacteria, and parasites.

■ **TREATMENT.** Treatment focuses on symptoms and can include antinausea medication, antidiarrhea medication, antibiotics, fluids, and nutritional support and stress management. Prognosis is generally good.

■ **PREVENTION.** If the gastroenteritis is caused by a virus, it probably cannot be prevented. With bacterial gastroenteritis, the best preventive measures include hand washing and properly preparing and storing food because bacteria easily grow and multiply in poultry, egg, and cream products. Keeping foods such as potato and chicken salad refrigerated, especially during warm weather, is helpful. Avoiding contaminated food and water, especially in underdeveloped countries, also prevents gastroenteritis.

If stress is the cause of the upset, then controlling this with stress reduction, healthy diet, and regular exercise will help with prevention.

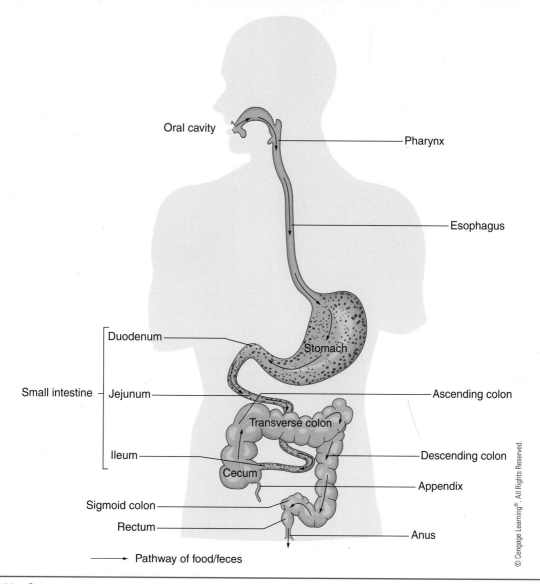

Oral cavity

Pharynx

Esophagus

Duodenum

Stomach

Small intestine — Jejunum

Ascending colon

Transverse colon

Ileum

Descending colon

Cecum

Appendix

Sigmoid colon

Rectum

Anus

→ Pathway of food/feces

FIGURE 11–14   Gastroenteritis.

INGUINAL HERNIA

■ **DESCRIPTION.** An inguinal hernia is a common problem that affects the digestive system.

■ **ETIOLOGY.** A pouching of the small intestine and the peritoneum (abdominal cavity lining) into the groin area (Figure 11–15) causes this condition. Inguinal hernias are more common in males, perhaps due to a congenital defect that developed as the testes descended from the abdomen into the scrotum, thus pulling part of the peritoneum into the inguinal area. Inguinal hernias also develop in both sexes due to a weakness in the abdominal wall.

The portion of the intestine that herniates can become caught and twisted, thus cutting off blood supply to the organ. If this occurs, it is called a strangulated hernia, which can be life-threatening and needs immediate surgical intervention.

■ **SYMPTOMS.** Symptoms include a bulge in the groin or scrotum and groin pain that increases with bending or lifting and is relieved by lying down. If there is sudden pain, nausea, and vomiting, chances are the hernia has become strangulated.

■ **DIAGNOSIS.** Diagnosis depends on a thorough history and physical exam of the groin area. Ultrasound and CT scans can be used to finalize the diagnosis.

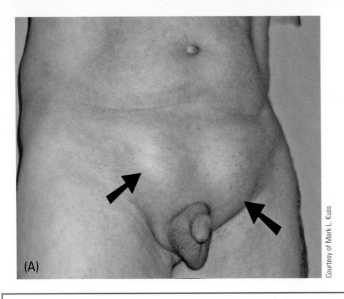
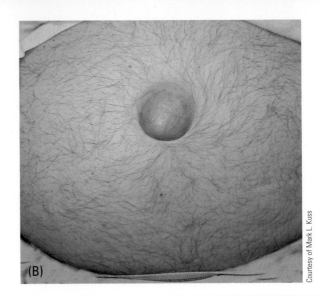

FIGURE 11–15   Hernias. (A) Inguinal–bilateral. (B) Umbilical hernia.

■ *TREATMENT.* Fortunately, inguinal hernias can be repaired surgically to prevent this potentially life-threatening situation.

Portions of the small intestine can also herniate through other openings in the body such as the femoral canal or the umbilicus. The femoral hernia, like the inguinal hernia, is more common in males. The umbilical hernia is most common in infants. Like the inguinal hernia, both are corrected surgically to prevent complications.

■ *PREVENTION.* Preventive measures include maintaining proper body weight, stopping smoking, using proper body mechanics during lifting, and avoiding constipation because straining to have a bowel movement increases abdominal pressure and can lead to a hernia.

Diseases of the Colon

Diseases of the colon or large intestine are common to all ages but are found most frequently in the middle-aged and older adult with the exception of appendicitis. Some colon diseases may require surgical removal of part or all of the colon, called colon resection.

Resection is a major surgery and involves removing part of the colon (partial or hemicolectomy) or the entire colon (colectomy). If only part of the colon is removed, reconnecting the two healthy bowel ends together is possible and is called an anastomosis; however, if a large amount of the colon is removed, an anastomosis might not be possible. In this case, a permanent or temporary opening called a colostomy might be required.

COMPLEMENTARY AND ALTERNATIVE THERAPY

Turmeric for Colon Cancer

The Chinese herbal medicine turmeric (*Curcuma longa L.*) has been used for centuries for colon, pancreatic, and endocrine disorders. It has antioxidant, anti-inflammatory, and other pharmacologic properties. Curcumin, one of turmeric's properties, has been found to be effective in cancer treatment in recent studies. It may have great potential for diseases like colon cancer. The safety and use of the herbal product are still being tested in clinical trials.

Source: Rui et al. (2010).

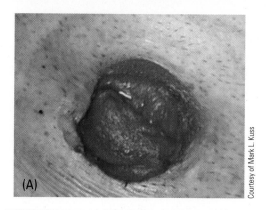

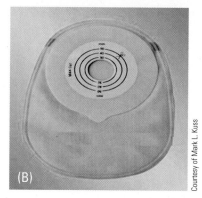

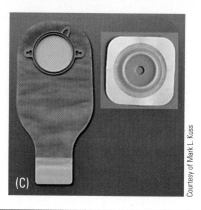

Courtesy of Mark L. Kuss

Courtesy of Mark L. Kuss

Courtesy of Mark L. Kuss

FIGURE 11–16   (A) Ostomy stoma. (B) Ostomy: one-piece appliance. (C) Ostomy: two-piece appliance.

A colostomy is developed by bringing the end of the colon through an opening in the abdominal wall. The new opening is called a stoma (Greek word for mouth), so named because it is pink in color like the inside of the mouth (Figure 11–16). This stoma will excrete feces. Management of a stoma requires education and special supplies. The basic supplies are a face plate that sticks to the skin and a collection bag for the feces. These supplies come in one- and two-piece systems. The system used depends on the thickness of the stool excreted and patient preference.

APPENDICITIS

■ **DESCRIPTION.** The appendix is located near the junction of the small and large intestines, and although it is primarily composed of lymphoid tissues, the exact function is yet unknown.

■ **ETIOLOGY.** Appendicitis is the inflammation of the **vermiform** (VER-my-form; worm-like) appendix. Infection or obstruction usually causes appendicitis. The position of the appendix near the colon allows bacteria-laden fecal contents to drop into the appendix, causing obstruction and infection. The inflamed appendix swells (Figure 11–17), decreasing circulation and potentially leading to gangrene.

■ **SYMPTOMS.** The pain of appendicitis usually begins with generalized abdominal pain that shifts to the lower right quadrant. Other signs and symptoms include nausea, vomiting, fever, and leukocytosis. This combination of signs and symptoms also mimics other abdominal diseases such as kidney stones, pelvic inflammatory disease, and pancreatitis, which can lead to an incorrect diagnosis.

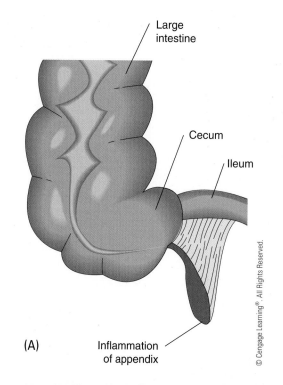

Large intestine

Cecum

Ileum

(A)

Inflammation of appendix

© Cengage Learning®. All Rights Reserved.

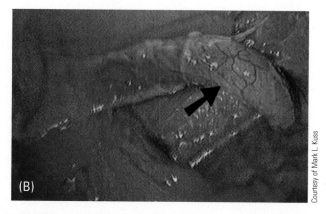

(B)

Courtesy of Mark L. Kuss

FIGURE 11–17   Appendicitis. (A) Location. (B) Inflammation of appendix.

As appendicitis progresses, the wall of the appendix thins and can rupture. Rupture of the appendix usually relieves the pain for a short time but leads to the more severe complication of peritonitis. Before the development of antibiotics, peritonitis was usually fatal.

■ **DIAGNOSIS.** A physical examination revealing increased pain when gentle pressure is applied in the area of the appendix and then released, called rebound tenderness, is helpful in diagnosis. Blood tests revealing an elevated white blood cell count, along with a urinalysis to rule out bladder infection, are helpful. Ultrasound and CT are used to confirm the diagnosis.

■ **TREATMENT.** Surgical removal of the appendix, preferably before rupture occurs, is the common treatment.

■ **PREVENTION.** There is no proven way to prevent appendicitis, but eating a healthy diet, including fruits and vegetables, might aid in prevention.

INTESTINAL OBSTRUCTION

■ **DESCRIPTION.** Intestinal obstruction may be classified as a symptom of a disease process or as a disease itself.

■ **ETIOLOGY.** Regardless of the classification, it is identified as an inability to move intestinal contents through the bowel. An obstruction can be due to a blockage of the intestine or to a disease or **ileus** (ILL-ee-us; absence of peristalsis).

Blockage can occur due to tumors, hernias, or **adhesions** (ad-HE-zhuns) (Figure 11–18). Adhesions are areas within the colon that abnormally link together, resulting from a previous abdominal surgery or from inflammation. Blockage also can occur if the colon becomes twisted (**volvulus**; VOL-view-lus) (Figure 11–19). If the colon telescopes on itself, the condition can lead to a blockage called **intussusception** (IN-tus-sus-SEP-shun).

A decrease or absence of peristalsis that causes intestinal obstruction is classified as a **paralytic obstruction**—colon action is paralyzed (unable to move). This type of obstruction can be a postoperative complication or a result of peritonitis.

■ **SYMPTOMS.** Symptoms depend on the type and severity of the obstruction. The individual might experience mild to severe abdominal pain and distention, nausea, and vomiting.

■ **DIAGNOSIS.** Barium enema, abdominal CT scan, upper GI, and abdominal films all aid in the diagnosis.

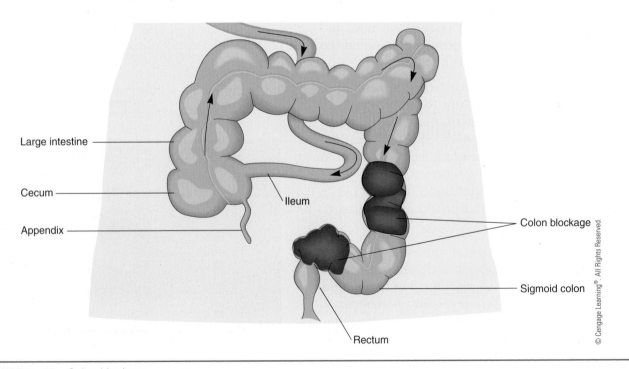

FIGURE 11–18 Colon blockage.

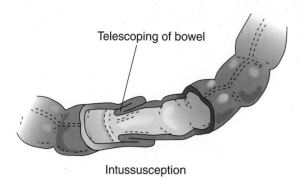

Telescoping of bowel

Intussusception

180-degree twisting of bowel

Volvulus

© Cengage Learning®. All Rights Reserved.

FIGURE 11–19   Volvulus and intussusception.

■ **TREATMENT.** Intestinal obstruction can be relieved by nasogastric suctioning, but more commonly, surgery is required.

■ **PREVENTION.** Prevention depends on the cause. If the condition is related to adhesions, intussusception, or volvulus, intestinal obstruction might not be preventable. Treatment of other causes, such as tumors and hernias, is helpful in prevention of intestinal obstruction.

ULCERATIVE COLITIS

■ **DESCRIPTION.** Ulcerative colitis is a chronic inflammation of the colon (Figure 11–20) that causes inflammation and ulcers in the lining of the rectum and colon. Like regional enteritis, it is commonly called inflammatory bowel disease until diagnosis is confirmed.

■ **ETIOLOGY.** The cause of ulcerative colitis is unknown. Exacerbations of the disease often occur during stressful times, leading to the belief that a psychogenic factor is involved. Other causative theories include hereditary, autoimmune, and dietary factors. Patients with ulcerative colitis are at high risk for developing colon cancer.

■ **SYMPTOMS.** The colon and rectum have multiple ulcerations that lead to lower abdominal pain, blood in the stools, anemia, and diarrhea.

■ **DIAGNOSIS.** Diagnostic tests include blood tests to check for anemia, stool sample, CT scan, and colonoscopy. A colonoscopy is the best test to confirm the diagnosis.

■ **TREATMENT.** Treatment can include dietary limitations, stress reduction, mild sedatives, and anti-inflammatory medications. Surgery is usually considered only if conservative treatment fails.

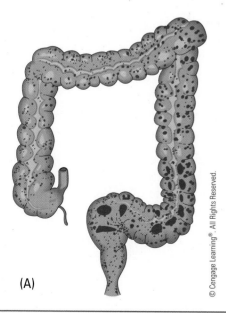

(A)

© Cengage Learning®. All Rights Reserved.

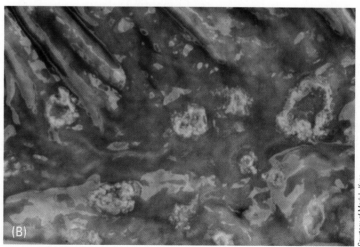

(B)

Courtesy of Mark L. Kuss

FIGURE 11–20   Ulcerative colitis. (A) Location. (B) Internal view.

HEALTHY HIGHLIGHT

Food Poisoning

Microorganisms that we ingest (eat) can cause GI upset in a variety of ways. Most microorganisms that we ingest are easily incapacitated and destroyed by the acid in the stomach. Some microorganisms will cause illness only if we ingest great numbers of them at a time. Ingestion of these great numbers allows a large number of microorganisms to escape the acid environment, invade the small intestine, and cause illness. An example of this type of microorganism is *Salmonella* (SAL-moh-NEL-ah). For *Salmonella* to make us ill, we must eat food that has been tainted with it. The bacteria reproduce in the food product before we eat it, thus providing the circumstances for ingestion of a large number of bacteria at one time. *Salmonella* bacteria invade the lining of the small intestine and bring about symptoms, usually 24 to 48 hours after ingestion of the food. *Salmonella* food poisoning can be prevented by refrigerating foods and by cooking foods thoroughly. *Salmonella* food poisoning is determined by a stool culture.

Other types of microorganisms also are very virulent and are thus able to withstand the stomach's acid environment. Ingestion of even small numbers of these will allow passage into the small intestine and cause illness. These organisms include viruses, amoebae, and *Shigella*, which are frequently spread by a fecal–oral route.

Another way that microorganisms make us ill is by producing a toxin (poisoning). The bacteria themselves do not cause the harm, but the **enterotoxin** (intestine poison) they produce does the damage. Staphylococcal food poisoning is of this type. Staphylococcal organisms contaminate nonrefrigerated food and release enterotoxins. When these enterotoxins are ingested, they quickly invade the lining of the stomach and small intestine, leading to symptoms within 1 to 4 hours. Staphylococcal food poisoning can be prevented by proper refrigeration of food products. This type of food poisoning is determined by a food culture. Prognosis is good, and symptoms usually resolve within 24 hours.

Observing the following measures can prevent most GI upset caused by contaminated food:

- Always wash your hands before and after preparing food.
- Wash your hands before and after a meal.
- Keep eating utensils and plates clean and stored until ready for use.
- Cover and refrigerate food properly.
- Cook foods thoroughly, especially meats and seafood.

Surgical intervention often results in a colostomy (opening in the colon), either temporary or permanent (Figure 11–16). If the colostomy is permanent, a portion of the colon might be removed.

■ **PREVENTION.** Since the cause is unknown, prevention is not possible. Taking steps to reduce stress is helpful in reducing the severity of the symptoms.

INFLAMMATORY BOWEL DISEASE (IBD)

IBD refers to both regional enteritis (Crohn's disease) and ulcerative colitis. Both diseases (as previously discussed) are chronic in nature with undetermined etiology. However, a general diagnosis of IBD can be used until a definite diagnosis of another bowel disorder is made.

IRRITABLE BOWEL SYNDROME (SPASTIC COLON)

■ **DESCRIPTION.** Irritable bowel syndrome (IBS) is the most common intestinal disorder and commonly can be confused with IBD, but they are not the same. IBS is an inflammation of the bowel with chronic lesions. Inflammation and lesions do not occur in IBS.

■ **ETIOLOGY.** The cause of IBS is unknown, but a strong psychogenic factor has been considered. IBS is chronic, and onset usually occurs in the young adult. Frequent recurrence over the years is very frustrating to the affected individual and the physician.

■ **SYMPTOMS.** IBS is a functional disorder of motility and can cause a group of symptoms, including abdominal pain and altered motility. Typically, an individual suffering from IBS has bouts of diarrhea, constipation, or both.

Spicy foods, caffeine, alcohol, and seasonings can irritate the colon and bring about symptoms of IBS. Stress also has an adverse effect and often causes alterations in intestinal motility.

■ **DIAGNOSIS.** Tests to assist in diagnosis include stool sampling, blood test, X-rays, and endoscopy. Colonoscopy is the most helpful in confirming the diagnosis.

■ **TREATMENT.** Avoidance of causative factors and stress reduction techniques often allow the colon to return to its normal functional state.

■ **PREVENTION.** IBS cannot be prevented, but symptoms can be reduced. Avoiding causative agents along with stress reduction techniques will help prevent symptoms. Stress reduction techniques include counseling, biofeedback, regular exercise, yoga, meditation, deep breathing, and hypnosis.

DYSENTERY

■ **DESCRIPTION.** Dysentery is a general term for a group of GI disorders characterized by acute inflammation. Dysentery commonly affects those in underdeveloped countries and those who travel to these countries. According to the Centers for Disease

Control and Prevention (CDC), most cases in the United States occur in immigrants, in those who live in inner-city housing, in frequent travelers, in children in day care, and in people in nursing homes.

■ **ETIOLOGY.** Invasion of microorganisms into the lining of the colon causes dysentery, usually as a result of ingestion of contaminated food, water, or both due to poor sanitary conditions.

■ **SYMPTOMS.** The main symptom is massive bloody or watery diarrhea along with severe abdominal pain and cramping. Dysentery is the disease and should not be confused with diarrhea, the symptom.

■ **DIAGNOSIS.** Diagnosis is based on stool samples showing the presence of causative microorganisms.

■ **TREATMENT.** Treatment depends on the cause of the disease. Antibiotics are usually effective for dysentery caused by a bacterial infection.

■ **PREVENTION.** Dysentery is spread by poor hygiene. Preventive steps include hand washing and not sharing eating utensils and straws. If traveling to an underdeveloped country, do not drink the water, use ice cubes, or eat salad or any fresh fruit or vegetables.

DIVERTICULOSIS/DIVERTICULITIS

■ **DESCRIPTION.** Diverticulosis is a condition of having diverticula, or little pouches, in the colon (Figure 11–21), especially in the sigmoid colon. It can be asymptomatic (without symptoms) until the pouches become packed with fecal material and become irritated and inflamed. Once inflamed, the condition is called diverticulitis.

■ **ETIOLOGY.** Diverticulitis increases in incidence with age and has been associated with poor dietary habits, lack of physical activity, and poor bowel habits.

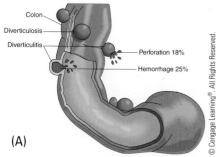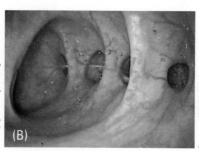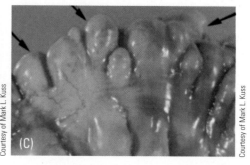

FIGURE 11–21   (A) Diverticulosis. (B) Colon diverticulosis: internal view of pockets. (C) Colon diverticulosis: external view.

■ **SYMPTOMS.** Low abdominal pain and cramping are indicative of diverticulitis. Because this inflammatory disease progresses, it can lead to hemorrhage, perforation, or narrowing of the lumen of the colon and, thus, obstruction.

■ **DIAGNOSIS.** Diagnosis is easily made by performing a colonoscopy and visualizing the pouches.

■ **TREATMENT.** Increasing the amount of fiber in the diet is usually effective in relieving symptoms and preventing complications. Foods high in fiber include fruits, vegetables, beans, potatoes, rice, and cereals. Fiber keeps the stool soft, allowing it to move more easily through the colon. Antibiotics might be needed if acute diverticulitis develops.

■ **PREVENTION.** A high-fiber diet can aid in prevention of diverticulosis. Some believe that avoiding any foods with seeds and nuts is helpful, although this concept has not been proven.

COLON POLYPS

■ **DESCRIPTION.** A **polyp** (PAH-lip) is an inward projection of the mucosal lining of the colon (Figure 11–22).

■ **ETIOLOGY.** Polyps can be due to an inflammatory reaction or caused by a benign or malignant neoplasm.

■ **SYMPTOMS.** Colon polyps can cause rectal bleeding, but most commonly, they are asymptomatic.

■ **DIAGNOSIS.** These growths are often diagnosed during a routine colonoscopy (colon = colon, oscopy = procedure to look into) or sigmoidoscopy (sigmoid = sigmoid portion of the colon).

■ **TREATMENT.** Suspicious polyps can be excisionally biopsied during these procedures. Cancerous polyps are removed by excisional biopsy or surgical resection, depending on the number and type of polyps present.

■ **PREVENTION.** Colon polyps might not be preventable, but making healthy lifestyle changes and lowering certain risk factors is helpful. Preventive activities include the following: eat healthy, limit fat intake, limit alcohol consumption, stop smoking, maintain a healthy body weight, and exercise.

CARCINOMA OF THE COLON AND RECTUM

■ **DESCRIPTION.** Commonly called **colorectal** cancer, this classification covers a variety of carcinomas that arise in the colon and rectum. These tumors are usually adenocarcinomas that arise from the mucosal lining. Colorectal cancer commonly affects both sexes (Figure 11–23).

■ **ETIOLOGY.** The cause of colorectal cancer is unknown. Some identified predisposing factors include ulcerative colitis, familial polyposis (many colon polyps), and a diet high in red meat and low in fiber.

■ **SYMPTOMS.** Signs and symptoms of colorectal cancer depend on the site of the malignancy. Common symptoms can include a change in bowel habits (diarrhea or constipation), pencil-sized stools, blood in the stools, anemia (due to tumor bleeding), abdominal discomfort, and obstruction.

Adenocarcinomas (the most common type found in colorectal cancer) tend to grow slowly.

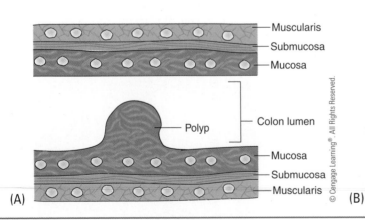

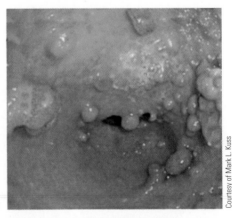

FIGURE 11–22   (A) Colon polyps. (B) Colon polyps: internal view.

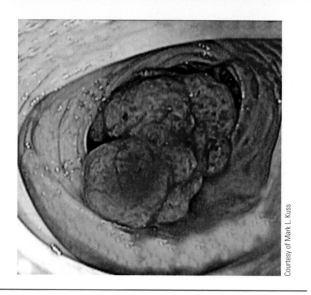

FIGURE 11–23   Colon cancer.

Eventually, the tumor can grow large enough to obstruct the lumen and spread through the colon wall. After it has spread through the colon wall, it can gain access to the lymphatic and vascular systems and spread throughout the body. The most common site of metastasis is the liver. Prognosis is good if the carcinoma is detected before metastasis; after metastasis, prognosis is poor.

■ **DIAGNOSIS.** Diagnosis of colorectal cancer can be made by stool examinations for occult blood, colonoscopy, and barium enema. Some rectal tumors also can be palpated by digital examination.

■ **TREATMENT.** Colorectal carcinoma is one of the leading causes of death from cancer in the United States. If detected early, it is potentially curable by surgical resection (Figure 11–24).

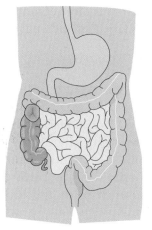

Ascending colostomy

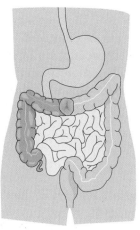

Transverse colostomy

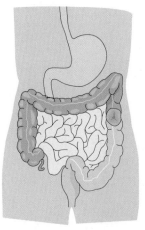

Descending colostomy

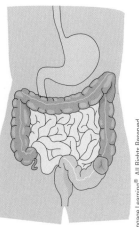

Sigmoid colostomy

FIGURE 11–24   Colostomy locations (blue section may be surgically removed if colostomy is permanent).

Does Marriage Affect Cancer Survival by Gender and Stage?

Whether you are married or not may affect your risk for cancer according to the literature. Most of the studies have looked at breast cancer, but recent research reviewed the association of colon cancer with marital status. The results showed that married persons tended to be diagnosed earlier than nonmarried persons or those who were separated or divorced. The 5-year survival rate was also lower for the single person who was diagnosed with colon cancer than the married person. Thus, it seems that persons who are married and diagnosed with colon cancer do much better overall through the treatment and recovery, and thus have a longer life expectancy. Further research needs to be done in this area to determine all the factors that support better outcomes for married persons.

Source: Wang et al. (2011).

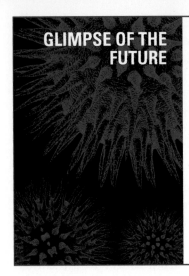

Other treatments for colon cancer include chemotherapy and radiation. These can be used in conjunction with surgery or used separately, depending on the treatment plan and prognosis.

■ **PREVENTION.** Prevention of colorectal cancer focuses on dietary changes. These include a decrease in red meat consumption and an increase in the consumption of fiber. It is also recommended that stool examination be performed on individuals annually, beginning at age 50.

Diseases of the Rectum

The rectum is the terminal or end part of the digestive system. The most common rectal problem is hemorrhoids. Rectal fissures and other minor problems can also occur, but cancer of the rectum is one of the most serious diseases of the rectum. Cancer of the rectum is more commonly diagnosed in the older adult than at any other age.

HEMORRHOIDS

■ **DESCRIPTION.** Hemorrhoids are varicose veins, either internal or external, in the rectum (Figure 11–25). Internal hemorrhoids can be examined by a physician using a proctoscope (procto = rectum, scope = instrument used to view). Internal hemorrhoids are located on the rectal wall; external hemorrhoids are located externally around the anus.

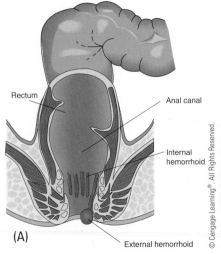

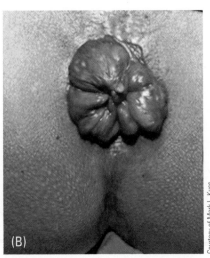

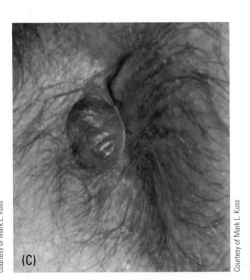

FIGURE 11–25   Hemorrhoids. (A) Location. (B) Hemorrhoids: internal protruding to outside. (C) Hemorrhoid: external.

Colon Cancer Prevention

Colon cancer commonly occurs after age 50. It is, therefore, recommended that everyone age 50 and older should have an annual clinical exam, including a stool examination for occult blood. This relatively easy examination can assist with early detection of colon cancer. If the individual is at risk, if something is found at the clinical exam, or if the occult blood test is positive, a colonoscopy is recommended. If nothing is found during the colonoscopy, another one is not necessary for 10 years if the yearly exam and occult blood test continue to be negative. If any abnormality is found during the colonoscopy, another one should be done in 3 years. Prognosis for colon cancer is good if it is discovered in its early stages.

Internal hemorrhoids cannot be seen unless they prolapse or get pushed through the anal opening. External hemorrhoids are the ones commonly known as hemorrhoids and can be viewed around the anal opening. External hemorrhoids are bluish in color and might bleed with straining during bowel movements.

■ *ETIOLOGY.* Factors that increase the risk of developing hemorrhoids include any activity that increases pressure in the anal area such as straining to have a bowel movement, frequent bouts of constipation, prolonged standing, prolonged sitting, pregnancy, and childbirth. Other causes can be related to heredity and loss of muscle tone.

■ *SYMPTOMS.* The most common symptoms are itching, bleeding with bowel movements, and rectal pain.

■ *DIAGNOSIS.* External hemorrhoids are easily diagnosed by physical examination including a digital rectal exam. During this exam, the physician uses a gloved, lubricated finger to feel for abnormalities. Internal hemorrhoids might need visual inspection with an anoscope (lighted tube to examine the anus) or proctoscope (lighted tube to examine the rectum).

■ *TREATMENT.* Treatment of hemorrhoids can include medications and warm sitz baths to ease the pain. Manual reduction, cryosurgery, and hemorrhoidectomy can be optional treatments, depending on the severity of the disease.

■ *PREVENTION.* Preventive measures are focused on softening the stool (which decreases constipation and straining with bowel movements). These measures include good bowel habits (defecating when reflexes are strong), adequate fluid intake, increased fiber intake, exercise, and avoiding laxative use.

CARCINOMA OF THE RECTUM

See "Carcinoma of the Colon and Rectum."

■ TRAUMA

Trauma to the Mouth

Trauma to the mouth can be due to motor vehicle accidents, falls, abuse, burns, or any other blunt or perforating injury. The result can be broken teeth or jawbones or lesions and lacerations. Depending on the severity of the injury and the treatment needed, the individual might have difficulty eating. If the jaw is broken, the individual might need to have the jaw wired closed for a period of time, requiring a special liquid nutrition program to maintain adequate intake of fluids, vitamins, and minerals. Burns and lacerations also interfere with the normal oral intake of fluid and food. The individual might need alternate feeding methods such as parenteral (intravenous) or enteral (tube feeding) nutrition.

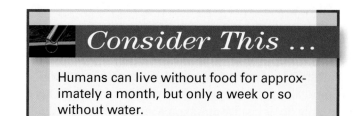

Consider This ...

Humans can live without food for approximately a month, but only a week or so without water.

Trauma to the Stomach and Intestines

Trauma to the digestive system other than to the mouth is usually due to perforation (a hole through the organ), which can be the result of a stabbing, gunshot wound, or piercing by some other kind of object. This is a medical emergency because the contents of the stomach or intestines can spill out into the abdominal cavity, causing peritonitis. Commonly, the wound is surgically repaired and the individual is given antibiotics for the infection.

■■ RARE DISEASES

Achalasia

Achalasia (eh-cha-LAY-see-ah) is a disorder of the esophagus that causes pain with swallowing. The peristaltic movement of the lower portion of the esophagus does not function properly. The cause of the disorder is unknown. Treatment might involve surgery, drug therapy, or both.

Gluten-Induced Enteropathy

This disease is also called celiac disease and is an immune problem that sensitizes the individual to gluten proteins. These proteins are found mainly in wheat and rye products but also in oat and barley foods. Individuals with gluten-induced enteropathy have impaired absorption of some vitamins and proteins, fats, and carbohydrates. Gluten-induced enteropathy is treated by a dietary measure, restricting all gluten-containing foods.

There has been a fourfold increase in celiac disease in the last 50 years. This rapid increase is being questioned by many researchers. Many feel there is a true increase in celiac disease due to the growing amount of processed gluten products in the American diet. Others feel there is a false increase in the condition related to marketing of the benefits of gluten-free diets coupled with self-diagnosis. People who suffer the side effects of abdominal bloating, tiredness, and irregular bowel movements often find relief with gluten-free diets and thus self-diagnose as having celiac disease.

Intestinal Polyps

Intestinal polyps are benign (noncancerous) tumors found along the lining of the intestine. Although they usually do not cause any symptoms for the individual, they are often surgically removed as a preventive treatment because polyps can increase the risk of cancer.

■■ EFFECTS OF AGING ON THE SYSTEM

Disorders of the digestive system are common in the aging population, so the incidence of problems increases with age. Some of the problems occurring with age in the system are caused by changes in the cardiovascular or neurologic system, which causes disruptions in the functioning of the digestive system. In the upper digestive system, the most common problem with aging is related to loss of teeth. Preventive dentistry has lessened teeth and gum problems in recent years, but it is still a significant factor in the older adult. Further, the sense of taste becomes less sensitive, and the motility in the esophagus decreases and can cause some distress, but it is generally asymptomatic.

Changes in the lining of the stomach and decreased secretion of hydrochloric acid increase the likelihood of digestive disorders in the older adult. Decreased circulation to the stomach increases the incidence of ulcer disease.

Consider This ...

By age 70, most individuals produce only 15% of the hydrochloric acid and only 50% of the digestive enzymes that they did at age 20.

Lower digestive disorders are common in the older adult. The lower intestinal lining is affected much like the stomach lining. Absorption of some nutrients such as vitamin B_{12} and fats can decrease. Decreased circulation to the intestines can cause ischemia and pain in the abdomen, and decreased motility can contribute to constipation problems. The development of inflammatory disease and hemorrhoids is common to the aging process but also can be caused by earlier problems or other predisposing factors.

Consider This ...

By age 60, most people have lost approximately half of their taste buds.

SUMMARY

The digestive system is a long, hollow tube that extends from the mouth to the anus. Its purpose is the ingestion, digestion, and absorption of fluids and nutrients and elimination of wastes. Accessory organs of the digestive system include the liver, pancreas, and gallbladder. The most common diseases of the system are infections, ulcers, and cancer. Physiologic and lifestyle changes in older adults put them at higher risk for diseases of the digestive system.

REVIEW QUESTIONS

Short Answer

1. What are the functions of the digestive system?

2. Which signs and symptoms are associated with common digestive system disorders?

3. Which diagnostic tests are most commonly used to determine type and cause of the digestive system disorders?

Matching

4. Match the disorders listed in the left column with the correct region of the digestive system in the right column:

_____	Pharyngitis	a. Small intestine
_____	Gastritis	b. Mouth
_____	Hemorrhoids	c. Colon
_____	Periodontal disease	d. Throat or esophagus
_____	Regional enteritis	e. Rectum
_____	IBS	f. Stomach

Multiple Choice

5. Which of the following behaviors might contribute to digestive system problems? (Select all that apply.)
   a. Eating four to six small meals per day
   b. Improperly cooking food
   c. Failure to wash hands after toileting
   d. Poor dietary habits
   e. Straining with bowel movements
   f. Drinking plenty of fluids daily
   g. Frequent use of laxatives and enemas

True or False

6. T F   The alimentary canal is a continuous tube from the mouth to the anus.

7. T F   Strep throat should always be treated because it can lead to rheumatic heart disease.

8. T F   The main function of the large intestine (colon) is the digestion of food.

9. T F   The *Helicobacter* bacteria are contributing factors in the development of peptic ulcers.

10. T F   The effects of aging put the older adult at an increased risk for digestive system problems.

CASE STUDIES

■ Stacey Erin is a 32-year-old accountant who has just been diagnosed with peptic ulcer disease. She would like some information about her disorder and to find out what to expect in the future and how to cope with it. What would you tell her about peptic ulcer disease? How can she prevent continued problems with her ulcer?

■ Mr. Montgomery was recently diagnosed with colon cancer. He is 67 years old and was recently widowed. He has no family members nearby to assist him during the ordeal of coping with the diagnosis, surgical treatment, and postoperative care. He asks you to explain the treatment and the care that he will need after surgery. He was told that his cancer has not metastasized, so the surgeon will just do a resection of the colon. What would you tell him? How can you help Mr. Montgomery with his questions and fear for his future? What resources can you give him for more information and support?

Study Tools

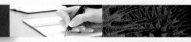

Workbook

Complete Chapter 11

Online Resources

PowerPoint® presentations

Animation

BIBLIOGRAPHY

Acosta, K., Lee, R., Perry, A., & Raden, K. (2011). How can I feel less bloated? *Natural Health 41*(3), 28.

Ardilio, S. (2011). Calculating nutrition needs for a patient with head and neck cancer. *Clinical Journal of Oncology Nursing 15*(5), 457–459.

Chiocca, E. M. (2011). Action STAT epiglottitis. *Nursing 41*(3), 72.

Chung-Yuan, H., Delclos, G. L., Wenyaw, C., & Xianglin L. D. (2011). Post-treatment surveillance in a large cohort of patients with colon cancer. *American Journal of Managed Care 17*(5), 329–336.

Eccles, D. M. (2011). Development of genetic testing for breast, ovarian and colorectal cancer predisposition: A step closer to targeted cancer prevention. *Current Drug Targets 12*(13), 1974–1982.

eDocAmerica. (2010). What the tongue says about health. *www.edocamerica.com* (accessed February 2012).

Fasano, A. (2011). Should we screen for coeliac disease? *BMJ: British Medical Journal 1339*(27), 998–999.

Ford, O. (2011). Cook receives FDA approval for evolution GI stent. *Medical Device Daily 15*(195), 1–5.

Hassan, I., & Advani, V. (2010). Single incision laparoscopic colon surgery. Is the ride worth the curve? *Colorectal Disease 12*(9), 847–848.

Hawley, P., Barwich, D., & Kirk, L. (2011). Implementation of the Victoria Bowel Performance Scale. *Journal of Pain & Symptom Management 42*(6), 946–953.

Holdstock, R. (2011). What you need to know about bowel cancer. *Practice Nurse 41*(18), 13–18.

Imran, I., Hussain, L., Zia-Ul-Haq, M. M., Janbaz, K., Gilani, A. H., & De Feo, V. (2011). Gastrointestinal and respiratory activities of *Acacia leucophloea*. *Journal of Ethnopharmacology 138*(3), 676–682.

Jonker, D. J., Spithoff, K. K., & Maroun, J. J. (2011). Adjuvant systemic chemotherapy for stage II and III colon cancer after complete resection: An updated practice guideline. *Clinical Oncology 23*(5), 314–322.

Jullumstrø, E. E., Wibe, A. A., Lydersen, S. S., & Edna, T. H. (2011). Colon cancer incidence, presentation, treatment and outcomes over 25 years. *Colorectal Disease 13*(5), 512–518.

Kelly, P. P. (2011). Colorectal cancer family history assessment. *Clinical Journal of Oncology Nursing 15*(5), E75–E82.

Kindt, S. S., Imschoot, J. J., & Tack, J. J. (2011). Prevalence of and impact of pantoprazole on nocturnal heartburn and associated sleep complaints in patients with erosive esophagitis. *Diseases of the Esophagus 24*(8), 531–537.

MacKenzie, M. M., Spithoff, K. K., & Jonker, D. D. (2011). Systemic therapy for advanced gastric cancer: A clinical practice guideline. *Current Oncology 18*(4), 202–209.

Masoomi, H., Buchberg, B., Dang, P., Carmichael, J., Mills, S., & Stamos, M. (2011). Outcomes of right vs. left colectomy for colon cancer. *Journal of Gastrointestinal Surgery 15*(11), 2023–2028.

Mayo Clinic. (2011). *H. pylori* infection. *www.mayoclinic.com* (accessed May 2012).

McCaughan, E., Parahoo, K., & Prue, G. (2011). Comparing cancer experiences among people with colorectal cancer: A qualitative study. *Journal of Advanced Nursing 67*(12), 2686–2695.

Mroczkowski, P. P., Kube, R. R., Schmidt, U. U., Gastinger, I. I., & Lippert, H. H. (2011). Quality assessment of colorectal cancer care: An international online model. *Colorectal Disease 13*(8), 890–895.

National Digestive Diseases Information Clearinghouse (NDDIC). (2012). *H. pylori* and peptic ulcers. *www.digestive.niddk.nih.gov* (accessed May 2012).

Ohlsson-Nevo, E., Andershed, B., Nilsson, U., & Anderzén-Carlsson, A. (2012). Life is back to normal and yet not: Partners' and patients' experiences of life of the first year after colorectal cancer surgery. *Journal of Clinical Nursing 21*(3–4), 555–563.

O'Shea, L. (2010). Diagnosing indigestion. *Practice Nurse 40*(10), 17–25.

Pavlidis, T. E., Pavlidis, E. T., & Sakantamis, A. K. (2010). Current management of diverticular disease of the colon. *Techniques in Coloproctology 14*(Suppl), 79–81.

Pickering, L. P. (2009). Group a streptococcal infections. *Red Book: 2009 Report of the Committee on Infectious Diseases*. 28th ed. Grove Village, IL: American Academy of Pediatrics, 616–628.

Rhoads, K. F., Cullen, J., Ngo, J. V., & Wren, S. M. (2012). Racial and ethnic differences in lymph node examination after colon cancer resection do not completely explain disparities in mortality. *Cancer 118*(2), 469–477.

Rui, L., Cheng, X., Xing, Z., De-An, G., & Min, Y. (2010). Chemical analysis of the Chinese herbal medicine turmeric (*Curcuma longa* L.). *Current Pharmaceutical Analysis 6*(4), 256–268.

Saleeby, Y. M. (2011). Colon cancer screening. *American Fitness 29*(6), 53–54.

Shaw, S. Y., Blanchard, J. F., & Bernstein, C. N. (2011). Association between the use of antibiotics and new diagnoses of Crohn's disease and ulcerative colitis. *American Journal of Gastroenterology 106*(12), 2133–2142.

Shehzad, A., Ha, T., Subhan, F., & Lee, Y. (2011). New mechanisms and the anti-inflammatory role of curcumin in obesity and obesity-related metabolic diseases. *European Journal of Nutrition 50*(3), 151–161.

Stephen-Haynes, J. (2010). Dressing choice: A practical guide to clinical outcomes. *Practice Nurse 40*(8), 27–31.

Vestergaard, P. (2011). Occurrence of gastrointestinal cancer in users of bisphosphonates and other antiresorptive drugs against osteoporosis. *Calcified Tissue International 89*(6), 434–441.

Vítor, J. B., & Vale, F. F. (2011). Alternative therapies for *Helicobacter pylori*: Probiotics and phytomedicine. *FEMS Immunology & Medical Microbiology 63*(2), 153–164.

Wang, L., Wilson, S. E., Stewart, D. B., & Hollenbeak, C. S. (2011). Marital status and colon cancer outcomes in US Surveillance, Epidemiology and End Results registries: Does marriage affect cancer survival by gender and stage? *Cancer Epidemiology 35*(5), 417–422.

Wasnik, S., & Parmar, P. (2011). The design of colon-specific drug delivery system and different approaches to treat colon disease. *International Journal of Pharmaceutical Sciences Review & Research 6*(2), 167–177.

Wong, K. H., Li, G. Q., Li, K. M., Razmovski-Naumovski, V., & Chan, K. (2011). Kudzu root: Traditional uses and potential medicinal benefits in diabetes and cardiovascular diseases. *Journal of Ethnopharmacology 134*(3), 584–607.

Zielinski, M., Merchea, A., Heller, S., & You, Y. Y. (2011). Emergency management of perforated colon cancers: How aggressive should we be? *Journal of Gastrointestinal Surgery 15*(12), 2232–2238.

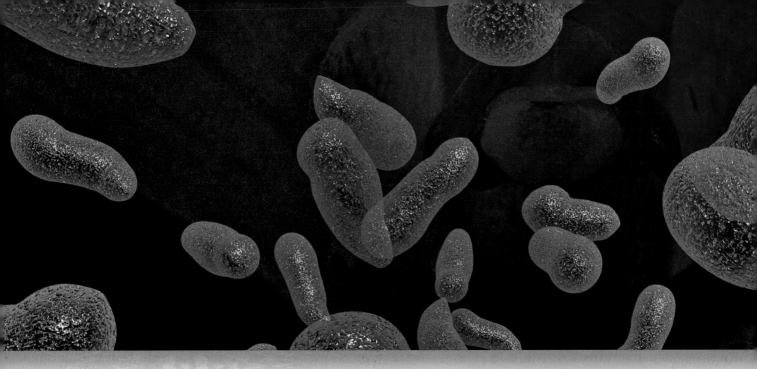

OUTLINE

KEY TERMS

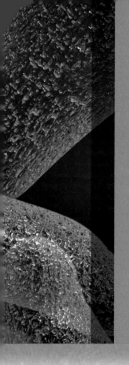

12

Liver, Gallbladder, and Pancreatic Diseases and Disorders

LEARNING OBJECTIVES

Upon completion of the chapter, the learner should be able to:

1. Define the terminology common to the liver, gallbladder, and pancreas and the disorders of the organs.

2. Discuss the basic anatomy and physiology of the liver, gallbladder, and pancreas.

3. Identify the important signs and symptoms associated with common liver, gallbladder, and pancreas disorders.

4. Describe the common diagnostics used to determine the type and cause of liver, gallbladder, or pancreas disorders.

5. Identify common disorders of the liver, gallbladder, and pancreas.

6. Describe the typical course and management of the common liver, gallbladder, and pancreas disorders.

7. Describe the effects of aging on the liver, gallbladder, and pancreas and the common disorders associated with aging of the organs.

OVERVIEW

The liver, gallbladder, and pancreas are the accessory organs of digestion. Although these organs are not considered part of the digestive system, they have important roles in the digestive process as well as in many other functions in the body. Disorders of the liver, gallbladder, or pancreas can cause serious digestive problems and many other systemic disorders. ■

ANATOMY AND PHYSIOLOGY

The liver is the largest solid organ of the body, taking second place only to the skin as the largest organ overall (Figure 12–1). The liver has many functions, most of which are related to its chemical actions. It plays a role in digestion, absorption, metabolism, blood clotting, the manufacture of important chemicals, and storage of nutrients. The liver is composed of two lobes, weighs about 3.5 pounds, and lies in the right upper quadrant of the abdomen. Some of the most important functions of the liver include:

- Production and secretion of bile used for fat digestion.
- Production of cholesterol.
- Oxidation of fatty acids and glycerol used for body energy.
- Metabolism of carbohydrates, fats, and protein.
- Conversion of glucose to glycogen for storage and the reverse process for energy.
- Synthesis of amino acids.
- Detoxification of many drugs and other toxins.

- Storage of vitamins and other minerals.
- Production of fibrinogen and prothrombin for blood clotting.

The liver receives blood from the portal system through the portal vein and the hepatic artery. About 1,450 ml of blood flows through the liver every minute. The blood returns to the circulatory system through the hepatic vein to the inferior vena cava.

Bile to emulsify, or break down, lipids in the intestine is continually produced in the liver and conducted through the hepatic duct to the duodenum. When bile is not needed in the digestive process, excess bile is stored in the gallbladder until needed by the intestine in the digestive process.

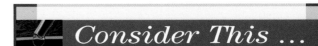

Consider This ...

If the liver were to totally stop working, without medical intervention, the individual would die within 24 hours.

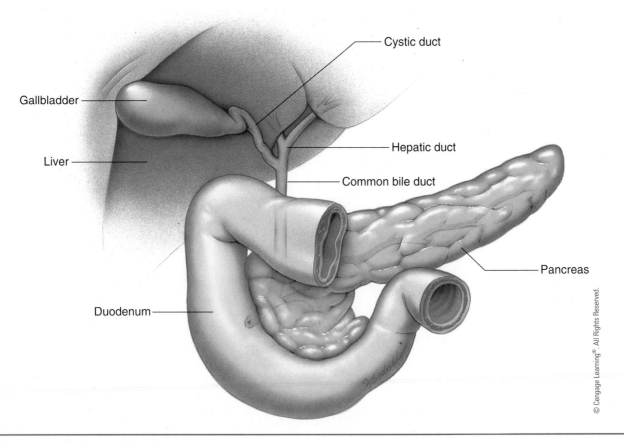

FIGURE 12–1 The liver, gallbladder, and pancreas.

The gallbladder is a small, pear-shaped organ lying just under the liver (see Figure 12–1). Bile travels from the gallbladder to the duodenum via the cystic duct and the common bile duct.

The pancreas lies in the abdomen behind the stomach between the duodenum and the spleen (see Figure 12–1); it is both an endocrine gland (the islet cells secrete hormones) and an exocrine gland, producing and secreting most of the digestive enzymes. The pancreas secretes intestinal juices consisting of chymotrypsin and trypsin, which break down proteins; amylase, which breaks down starch; and lipase, which breaks down fats. The pancreatic juices exit the gland by way of the pancreatic duct to the duodenum.

Media Link

View an animation on the pancreas on the Online Resources.

COMMON SIGNS AND SYMPTOMS

Jaundice (JAWN-dis, a yellowish discoloration of the skin) is an obvious symptom of liver disease and can be secondary to gallbladder disease as well. If a bile duct is blocked, for instance, the bile backs up into the liver and leads to jaundice.

Jaundice is caused by high levels of bilirubin in the blood. Bilirubin is a by-product of the breakdown of heme, the main component of hemoglobin in red blood cells. The liver filters bilirubin out of the blood and excretes it in bile. If the liver is unable to filter bilirubin and excrete it, hyperbilirubinemia (hyper = too much, bilirubin, emia = blood), or excessive bilirubin in the blood, occurs. This excess leaks into the tissues, and the individual's skin, mucosa, and sclera (white part of the eye) become yellowish in color.

Bilirubin can be broken down in the skin by exposure to sunlight or direct lighting, which explains the use of bili lights to clear bilirubin in a jaundiced newborn infant. Excessive bilirubin is also filtered out of the blood by the kidneys, causing dark brown urine.

Pain is a common symptom of gallbladder disease, pancreatitis, and end-stage pancreatic cancer. With gallbladder disease, right-sided abdominal pain commonly occurs following a meal containing fat. Acute abdominal pain occurs with pancreatitis and pancreatic cancer.

DIAGNOSTIC TESTS

Liver function tests are blood tests to measure levels of bilirubin, albumin (blood protein), and alkaline phosphatase (enzyme). Impaired liver function will lead to elevated bilirubin and alkaline phosphatase levels and low albumin levels.

Ultrasound is used to evaluate the liver, gallbladder, and pancreas for size, shape, and position. X-ray examinations of the gallbladder and the vessels of the gallbladder (cholecystogram and cholangiogram, respectively) use radiopaque dye to show the presence of gallstones, tumors, and function of the gallbladder. Ultrasonography is used more often than the previously mentioned radiologic examinations.

Computer axial tomography (CAT or CT) scans can be performed to visualize the liver, gallbladder, and pancreas. Visualization of these organs aids in diagnosis of hepatic and pancreatic cancer. A liver biopsy can be performed by needle biopsy or during laparoscopic surgery. Biopsy is the most reliable test for determination of chronic hepatitis, cirrhosis, and cancer.

Blood tests to measure pancreatic function commonly include serum amylase and lipase. Amylase and lipase are digestive enzymes produced by the pancreas that break down carbohydrates and fats, respectively.

COMMON DISEASES OF THE ACCESSORY ORGANS OF DIGESTION

Diseases of the accessory organs of digestion can seriously affect the digestion and metabolism of nutrients. Symptoms of these disorders reflect an interference with the particular organ's function. Over 30 million individuals—1 in 10—in the United States have been diagnosed with liver disease (American Liver Foundation, 2012).

Liver Diseases

Liver diseases can range from mild inflammation to those that destroy the liver and result in liver failure. Any disease of the liver can have serious consequences by interfering with the many functions of the liver.

HEPATITIS

■ **DESCRIPTION.** Hepatitis is inflammation of the liver that can lead to abnormal function and other diseases or conditions.

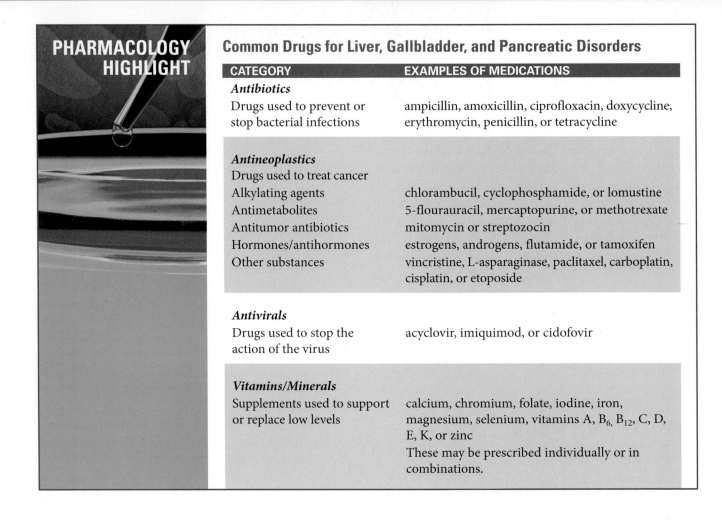

PHARMACOLOGY HIGHLIGHT

Common Drugs for Liver, Gallbladder, and Pancreatic Disorders

CATEGORY	EXAMPLES OF MEDICATIONS
Antibiotics Drugs used to prevent or stop bacterial infections	ampicillin, amoxicillin, ciprofloxacin, doxycycline, erythromycin, penicillin, or tetracycline
Antineoplastics Drugs used to treat cancer Alkylating agents Antimetabolites Antitumor antibiotics Hormones/antihormones Other substances	 chlorambucil, cyclophosphamide, or lomustine 5-flourauracil, mercaptopurine, or methotrexate mitomycin or streptozocin estrogens, androgens, flutamide, or tamoxifen vincristine, L-asparaginase, paclitaxel, carboplatin, cisplatin, or etoposide
Antivirals Drugs used to stop the action of the virus	acyclovir, imiquimod, or cidofovir
Vitamins/Minerals Supplements used to support or replace low levels	calcium, chromium, folate, iodine, iron, magnesium, selenium, vitamins A, B_6, B_{12}, C, D, E, K, or zinc These may be prescribed individually or in combinations.

■ *ETIOLOGY.* Hepatitis might be caused by the chemical action of drugs or toxic substances. Chronic alcoholism often leads to hepatitis prior to the functional changes seen with cirrhosis, but the most common cause of hepatitis is a group of viruses. This form of hepatitis is often called viral hepatitis and is the form most commonly thought of when one considers hepatitis.

Viral hepatitis is the most prevalent liver disease in the world and is often asymptomatic. When symptoms do occur, they can be so vague that the disease is misdiagnosed, which explains why approximately 40% of Americans have antibodies to hepatitis A and 10% have antibodies to hepatitis B, yet these individuals do not recall ever having hepatitis.

Viral hepatitis occurs in five basic types. A different virus causes each type. The types of hepatitis are A, B, C, D, and E.

Hepatitis A (HAV)

The most benign or harmless form of hepatitis. Total recovery occurs 98% of the time. This virus is spread by fecal–oral route and commonly affects children and young adults, especially in areas where there is poor sanitation and overcrowding. Symptoms are usually very vague and similar to flu, often leading to misdiagnosis. The virus is shed in the feces, and the affected individual does not become a carrier of the disease. HAV never leads to chronic hepatitis or cirrhosis. A vaccine is available and is recommended for those traveling or living in a high-risk area.

Hepatitis B (HBV)

A serious form of hepatitis formerly called serum hepatitis. It was once thought that HBV was spread only by contact with blood, as occurs with blood transfusions and contaminated needles. However, it is now known that saliva, urine, feces, and semen can spread the virus, which also qualifies it as a sexually transmitted disease. HBV is 100 times more infectious than human immunodeficiency virus (HIV), the virus that causes acquired immunodeficiency syndrome (AIDS) (Hepatitis Foundation International, 2012).

HBV also can be spread transplacentally (across the placenta from mother to unborn infant). This virus is a major health problem, with over 350 million individuals infected worldwide. Another major concern is the fact that individuals can unknowingly become carriers of the virus and carry it for years or even a lifetime. Carriers are not only a threat to others, but also are at high risk for developing chronic hepatitis and cirrhosis. About 1 out of every 250 persons is a carrier of HBV. Approximately 40,000 new infections occur every year in the United States (Centers for Disease Control and Prevention [CDC], 2012). It is estimated that 1 in every 20 people in the United States will become infected with HBV at some time during their life. The good news is that the number of new cases of HBV has decreased 80% over the past 20 years primarily due to childhood vaccinations. Those at high risk for HBV are drug addicts, homosexuals, blood recipients, and health care workers. The best prevention is to get vaccinated. The HBV vaccine is 95% effective in prevention of the disease.

Hepatitis C (HCV)

Similar to HBV because it also is spread by blood or sexual contact but differs from HBV in that it attacks the RNA of a cell, whereas HBV attacks the DNA. After HCV was distinguished from HBV, it was found to be the cause of most cases of hepatitis following blood transfusion (posttransfusion hepatitis). HCV is more likely to become chronic hepatitis than HBV, with approximately 50% of those affected with HCV developing chronic hepatitis and cirrhosis. HCV progresses very slowly and may take 10 to 40 years before serious liver damage is discovered. Approximately 3% of the world's population, or some 170 million individuals, are infected with HCV (Hepatitis Foundation International, 2012).

Hepatitis D (HDV)

Also called the delta virus. It requires the presence of HBV to replicate. Infection with both HBV and HDV can cause more prominent symptoms and a greater risk of developing chronic and **fulminant** (FULL-ma-nant; to occur suddenly and with great intensity) hepatitis.

Hepatitis E (HEV)

Similar to HAV in that it is spread through the fecal–oral route. It is commonly due to water contamination. Chronic hepatitis does not develop with HEV, but this virus can be fatal in pregnant women.

■ *SYMPTOMS.* Jaundice is often the first symptom that signals a liver problem, although not all individuals become yellow. Interestingly, those who become more jaundiced are more likely to have a good recovery than those who are less jaundiced. Individuals with mild jaundice are more likely to develop chronic hepatitis. Other symptoms include malaise, anorexia, myalgia (myo = muscle, algia = pain), fever, and abdominal pain. Physical examination might reveal **hepatomegaly** (HEP-ah-toh-MEG-ah-lee; hepato = liver, megaly = enlargement). Dark-colored urine and clay- or light-colored stools are related to the inability of the liver to form normal bile.

■ *DIAGNOSIS.* A blood test showing hepatitis virus antibodies is adequate for diagnosis.

■ *TREATMENT.* Treatment for HAV in most cases is symptomatic. Antivirals are also used, especially for HBV and HCV. General treatment includes adequate rest and good nutrition, which are essential for all types. Approximately 85% of affected individuals with HAV recover in 6 weeks. The most serious complications with hepatitis are development of chronic hepatitis and fulminant hepatitis. Chronic hepatitis develops

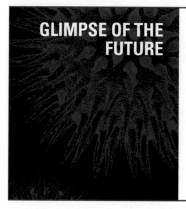

GLIMPSE OF THE FUTURE

Using Antiviral Medications for Hepatitis C

Chronic hepatitis C is a major global liver disease affecting millions of people. The present treatment includes the use of antiviral medications in various combinations. More research needs to be done to find adequate treatments for patients who have co-infections with HIV or other diseases and for transplant patients. In the future, if researchers can find the right combination of antiviral medications to treat HCV, it might be the first chronic viral infection that is eliminated throughout the world.

Source: Asselah & Marcellin (2012).

in one out of four cases and often leads to cirrhosis of the liver. Fulminant hepatitis is an acute hepatitis that causes extensive necrosis of liver tissue. Symptoms include a high fever, hemorrhages from the skin and mucous membranes, confusion, and stupor. Coma often develops and leads to death. Even with prompt and supportive care, fulminant hepatitis is 90% fatal.

■ **PREVENTION.** Prevention of hepatitis involves good hygiene and special care when handling needles and body secretions.

Other activities that aid in prevention include:

- Avoiding excessive alcohol consumption.
- Avoiding use of illegal drugs or snorting cocaine.
- Avoiding unprotected sex, especially with multiple partners.
- Receiving the hepatitis vaccines, especially for those in a high-risk group.

OTHER DISEASES OF THE LIVER

CIRRHOSIS

■ **DESCRIPTION.** Cirrhosis (sir-ROH-sis) of the liver is a chronic, irreversible, degenerative disease also known as end-stage liver disease. It is characterized by the replacement of normal liver cells with nonfunctioning, fibrous scar tissue, giving the surface of the liver a nodular appearance known as hobnail liver (Figure 12–2). This change in structure and function of the liver cells leads to impaired blood flow and altered function of the liver.

■ **ETIOLOGY.** The most common cause of cirrhosis is chronic alcoholism. Cirrhosis is more common in

males than females. It also can be idiopathic or the end result of other diseases such as chronic hepatitis and congestive heart failure. The development of the disease often takes years. Symptoms usually do not appear until serious structural and functional changes in the liver tissue have occurred. If symptoms occur, they are usually mild and nonspecific and might include loss of appetite, nausea, indigestion, weakness, and weight loss.

As the disease progresses, the abnormal scar tissue alters blood flow through the liver and leads to a variety of complications such as blood backing up in the hepatic portal vein. The relationship of the liver, the hepatic portal system, and the digestive system is as follows:

- The purpose of the hepatic portal system is to carry venous blood from the spleen and digestive organs (esophagus, stomach, and intestines) to the

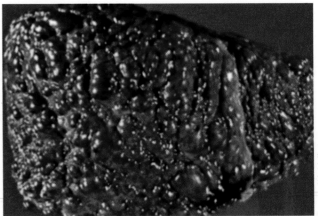

FIGURE 12–2 Hobnail liver.

Courtesy of Mark L. Kuss

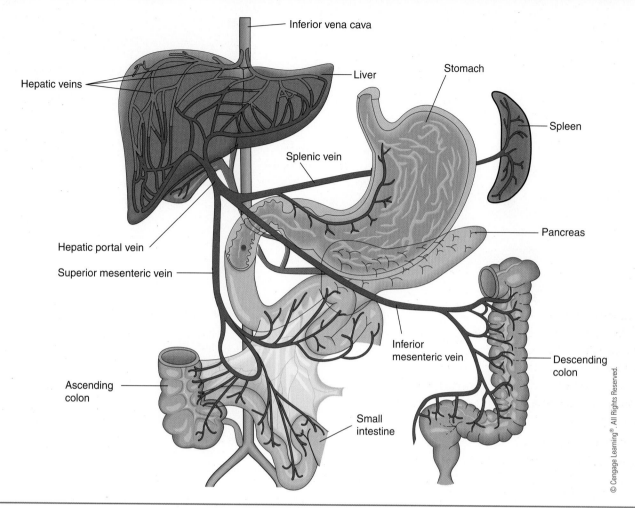

Inferior vena cava

Liver

Stomach

Spleen

Hepatic veins

Splenic vein

Pancreas

Hepatic portal vein

Superior mesenteric vein

Inferior mesenteric vein

Descending colon

Ascending colon

Small intestine

© Cengage Learning® . All Rights Reserved.

FIGURE 12–3   Hepatic portal system.

liver (Figure 12–3). The liver plays a major role in the digestive system by detoxifying and metabolizing nutrients before releasing them into the systemic blood in the inferior vena cava. For example, if an individual consumes a meal with an alcoholic beverage, these nutrients are absorbed into venous blood in the small intestine and transported to the liver to be filtered, detoxified, and stored. The liver's responsibility, in part, is to keep blood glucose levels from soaring when an individual eats a high-carbohydrate meal. Nutrients are filtered, metabolized, stored, and released as needed into the systemic circulation by the liver. Toxins such as alcohol are detoxified. If alcohol consumption is too great or outpaces the liver's ability to detoxify the blood, the blood alcohol level will rise.

■ If the liver is obstructed for any reason, blood will back up in this portal system. As blood backs up, pressure increases in the portal vein and is called **portal hypertension**.

■ **SYMPTOMS.** Complications of severe cirrhosis can include:

1. **Varicosities** Portal hypertension causes varicosities (varicose veins) of the veins of the digestive system organs. Varicosities are commonly located in the esophagus (**esophageal varices**) (Figure 12–4). Esophageal varices (VAIR-ah-SEEZ) are prone to rupture, leading to massive hemorrhage, shock, and death. Other sites of varicosities include the rectum (hemorrhoids) and anterior abdominal wall. Varicosities across the front of the abdomen are often quite tortuous and unsightly, a condition called **caput medusae** (Medusa's head) because the physician who named the condition was reminded of Medusa's head when observing the varicosities (Figure 12–5). Medusa, in Greek mythology, was a woman who had snakes on her head in place of hair.

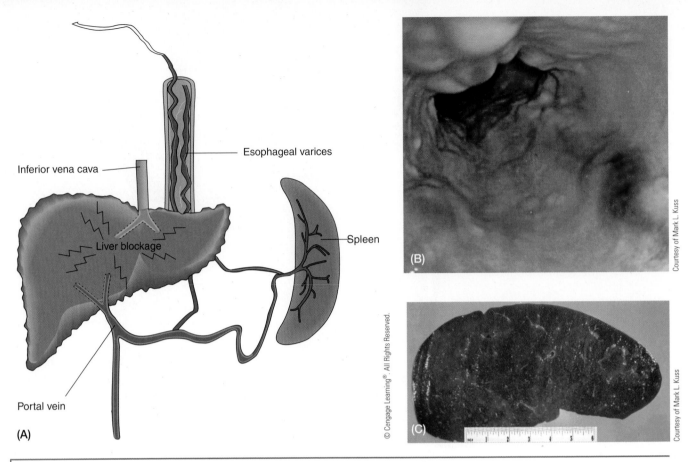

FIGURE 12–4   (A) Esophageal varices and splenomegaly. (B) Esophageal varices—internal view. (C) Splenomegaly.

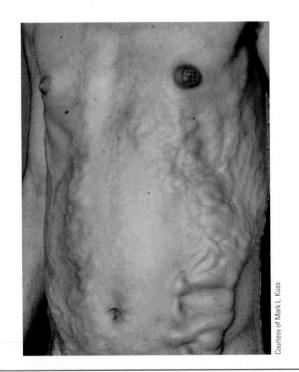

FIGURE 12–5   Caput medusae.

2. **Splenomegaly** Portal hypertension also causes increased pressure on the organs that are connected to or drained by the portal system. Often, this passive congestion in the spleen leads to **splenomegaly** (SPLEE-no-MEG-ah-lee; spleno = spleen, megaly = enlarged). The normal spleen weighs approximately 150 g (1/3 pound) and is 11 cm (4 inches) long. With this condition, the spleen may increase in size and length by four times its original size (see Figure 12–4). Splenomegaly often causes increased blood cell destruction, leading to anemia, leukopenia, and thrombocytopenia. Thrombocytopenia (thrombo = clot, cyto = cell, penia = decrease) increases the risk of bleeding.

3. **Gastrointestinal hemorrhage** This condition occurs due to thrombocytopenia and inability of the liver to secrete blood proteins essential for clotting. **Hematemesis** (HEM-ah-TEM-eh-sis; hema = blood, emesis = vomiting) is often the first symptom of severe cirrhosis.

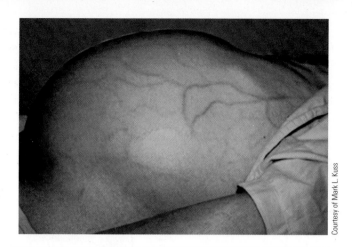

FIGURE 12–6 Ascites.

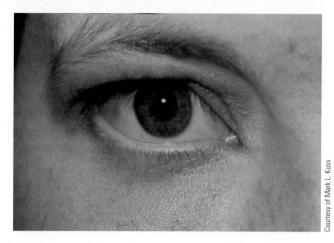

FIGURE 12–7 Jaundice.

4. **Ascites** (ah-SIGH-teez) This is an accumulation of fluid in the abdominal cavity that develops as a result of liver failure and portal hypertension. The increased pressure on the veins of the portal system causes leaking of serum into the abdomen. Often, this fluid enlarges the abdomen to the point of causing difficult breathing (Figure 12–6). Excessive abdominal fluid can be drained by piercing the abdominal wall with a large-bore needle, a procedure called **abdominocentesis** (ab-DOM-ih-no-sen-TEE-sis; abdomino = abdomen, centesis = puncture). The malnutrition of cirrhosis leads to spindly arms and legs despite the bloated abdomen.

5. **Edema** This often develops in the ankles and feet as a result of liver failure. The normal liver produces a blood protein called **albumin** (AL-byou-men), which is responsible for the osmotic pressure of blood, the movement of fluid from the blood through the capillaries to the tissues and back into the blood. Without osmotic pressure, blood fluid tends to leak into the tissues and remain there. A decrease in albumin allows this to occur, leading to edema in the feet and ankles.

6. **Jaundice** This usually results from the obstruction of the bile ducts as normal tissue is replaced by fibrous scar tissue, a characteristic of cirrhosis (Figure 12–7).

7. **Altered sex hormone metabolism** The normal liver inactivates small amounts of estrogen secreted by the adrenal glands in both the male and female. The cirrhotic liver is not capable of inactivating estrogen; thus, the male develops characteristics related to excessive estrogen. Such characteristics include:

- **Gynecomastia** (GUY-neh-koh-MAS-tee-ah) An enlargement of the breasts (Figure 12–8)

- **Palmar erythema** Palms of the hands become reddened in color (Figure 12–9)

- **Spider angiomas** Small dilated blood vessels on the face and chest (Figure 12–10)

- **Female hair distribution** Absent or reduced chest and pubic hair (see Figure 12–5)

- **Testicular atrophy** Decrease in testicle size

8. **Hepatic encephalopathy** The liver is often unable to detoxify the blood of nitrogenous waste products such as ammonia. This waste product can circulate in the blood and can affect the brain, causing mental confusion, stupor, and a

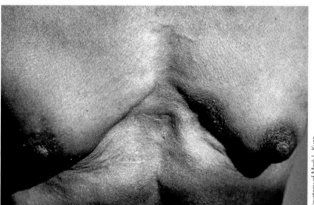

FIGURE 12–8 Gynecomastia.

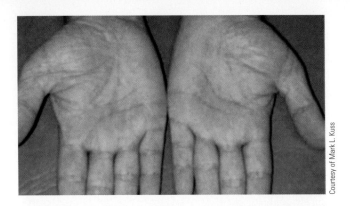

FIGURE 12–9   Palmar erythema.

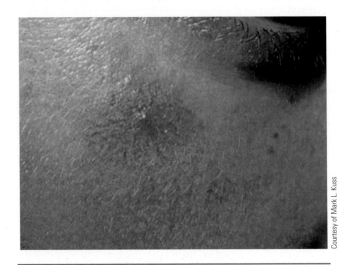

FIGURE 12–10   Spider angiomas: facial.

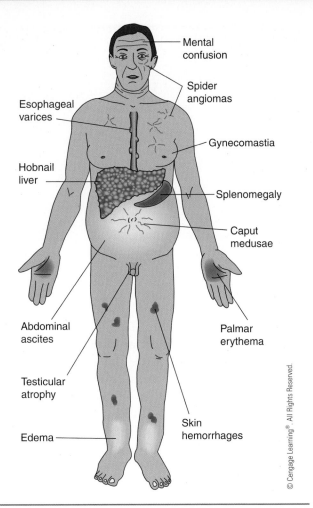

Mental confusion

Spider angiomas

Esophageal varices

Gynecomastia

Hobnail liver

Splenomegaly

Caput medusae

Abdominal ascites

Palmar erythema

Testicular atrophy

Skin hemorrhages

Edema

FIGURE 12–11   Clinical features of cirrhosis of the liver in the male.

characteristic shaking or tremor. This shaking, combined with hallucinations, is called **delirium tremens** (dee-LIR-ee-um TREE-mens) or DTs. Further depression of the nervous system can lead to hepatic coma and, ultimately, death. The clinical features of cirrhosis of the liver in the male are shown in Figure 12–11.

■ **DIAGNOSIS.** An examination revealing the physical characteristics described in Figure 12–11, along with blood testing, including elevated liver enzymes, elevated bilirubin, low serum albumin, and enlarged liver seen on abdominal X-ray, are all indicative of liver cirrhosis. A liver biopsy will confirm the diagnosis.

■ **TREATMENT.** Treatment of cirrhosis is directed at the cause in an attempt to prevent further liver damage. Alcohol is strictly prohibited regardless of the cause of the cirrhosis. Adequate nutrition and rest are necessary. Vitamins, minerals, and diet supplements might be needed to prevent malnutrition. Diuretics might be necessary to reduce edema and ascites.

Cirrhosis has an unfavorable prognosis, with most individuals surviving only 10 to 15 years after diagnosis. The appearance of ascites is a prognostic indicator because a majority of individuals with cirrhosis die within 5 years after the onset of ascites. Individuals usually die of massive bleeding from esophageal varices, hepatic encephalopathy, and other metabolic disorders.

■ **PREVENTION.** Although not all cases of cirrhosis are preventable, preventive measures include avoiding alcohol and exposure to all types of hepatitis and obtaining vaccinations for hepatitis A and B.

LIVER CANCER

■ **DESCRIPTION.** Primary and benign tumors (or those arising directly from liver tissue) are rare. When primary tumors do develop, they are more likely to

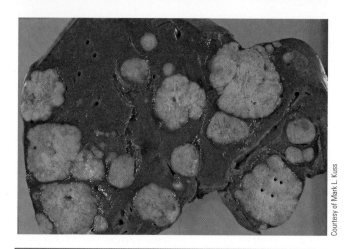

FIGURE 12–12   Liver cancer.

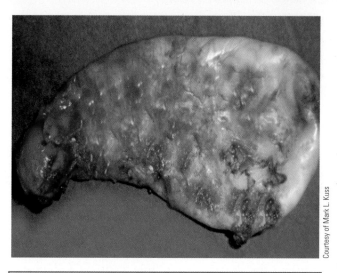

FIGURE 12–13   Cholecystitis.

occur in individuals with cirrhosis (Figure 12–12). Men are five times more likely to develop liver cancer than women. Secondary liver tumors (those that metastasize from other organs) are the most common and usually are the result of cancers in the breast, digestive system, and lungs.

■ **ETIOLOGY.** The cause of liver cancer, like most cancers, is not fully understood.

■ **SYMPTOMS.** Liver cancer is usually discovered late or at end stage because symptoms of anorexia, weight loss, and abdominal discomfort are so nonspecific.

■ **DIAGNOSIS.** Diagnosis is confirmed by biopsy.

■ **TREATMENT.** Treatment of liver cancer can involve surgery, chemotherapy, and radiation. Even with aggressive treatment, prognosis is very poor, with only 10% of affected individuals living 5 years after diagnosis.

■ **PREVENTION.** In many cases, avoiding the spread of cancer from other organs is not possible. The best prevention is to avoid hepatitis, cirrhosis, and other liver diseases by reducing risks for these diseases.

Gallbladder Diseases

Gallbladder disorders usually cause symptoms related to indigestion when eating fatty foods. Nausea, pain, and excessive gas are the most common symptoms. Nutritional changes and a variety of surgical procedures can be used to treat the disease.

CHOLECYSTITIS

■ **DESCRIPTION.** Cholecystitis (KOH-lee-sis-TYE-tis; chole = bile or gall, cyst = bladder, itis = inflammation) is inflammation of the gallbladder (Figure 12–13).

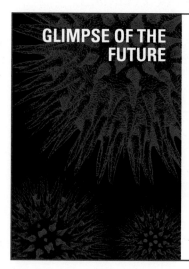

GLIMPSE OF THE FUTURE

Individuals with Diabetes: Increased Risk of Liver Cancer with Cirrhosis or Hepatitis

Patients with cirrhosis and hepatitis are at increased risk of developing liver cancer if they also have diabetes. In recent research, results have shown that patients with diabetes should be monitored for signs or symptoms of liver cancer, especially if they have hepatitis C. Their risk of developing liver cancer was twice that of patients who did not have diabetes. Researchers are looking at medications used to treat diabetes to see if they have an effect on this problem. In the future, studies need to be done to determine ways to better monitor these patients, to discover earlier diagnostic tests for liver cancer, and to determine if diabetes medications are causing the development of liver cancer.

Source: Douglas (2011).

■ *ETIOLOGY.* Cholecystitis is usually caused by obstruction of bile flow due to a gallstone. When bile flow is obstructed, bile in the gallbladder becomes overly concentrated and irritates the lining of the gallbladder, leading to inflammation. When a fatty meal is eaten, fat in the duodenum stimulates the gallbladder to contract and release bile.

■ *SYMPTOMS.* This contraction of the inflamed gallbladder causes mild to severe pain in the upper right quadrant of the abdomen. This pain, combined with a history of nausea and vomiting after meals, is indicative of cholecystitis.

■ *DIAGNOSIS.* Ultrasound and cholecystogram confirm the diagnosis of cholecystitis. Cholecystogram involves swallowing a dye that is absorbed by the liver and excreted into the bile. Radiographic pictures can confirm the presence of stones.

Complications of cholecystitis include rupture of the gallbladder, leading to peritonitis. Chronic cholecystitis can cause bile to back up into the liver, leading to liver damage and cirrhosis.

■ *TREATMENT.* Treatment for cholecystitis is aimed at the cause. Gallstones often obstruct the gallbladder or one of its ducts. Treatment of choice for cholecystitis caused by stones is surgical removal by a procedure called **cholecystectomy** (KOH-lee-sis-TECK-toh-me; chole = bile or gall, cyst = bladder, ectomy = removal).

Cholecystectomy can be performed using an abdominal incision or by using a laparoscope (laparo = abdomen, scope = scope). Removal of the gallbladder using a laparoscope is called laparoscopic cholecystectomy (LAP-ah-row-SKOP-ic KOH-leh-sis-TECK-toh-me). Laparoscopic cholecystectomy is performed by passing a small, thin tubular scope through a small cut made just below the umbilicus (navel), allowing the surgeon to view the gallbladder during surgery. Three other small incisions are made in the abdomen to insert surgical tools. The gallbladder is also removed through one of these incisions. This type of procedure drastically reduces pain, hospital stay, length of recovery, and missed workdays compared to surgery with a larger abdominal incision.

After a cholecystectomy, the bile continues to be excreted by the liver into the common bile duct and simply drips into the duodenum as it is produced. As long as the individual does not take in an excessive amount of fatty foods, the amount of bile will be sufficient to break down the consumed fat, and normal digestion will occur.

■ *PREVENTION.* Preventive measures include maintaining a healthy body weight and eating a diet high in fiber, including vegetables and fruit.

CHOLELITHIASIS

■ *DESCRIPTION.* Cholelithiasis (KOH-lee-lih-THIGH-ah-sis; chole = bile or gall, lith = stone, iasis = condition) is the presence of gallstones in the gallbladder or bile ducts (Figure 12–14). Gallstones affect 1 in 5 women and 1 in 10 men—approximately 25 million people. In the United States, there are approximately one million new cases per year, with 500,000 undergoing surgery for removal of the stones (HealthGuidance, 2012).

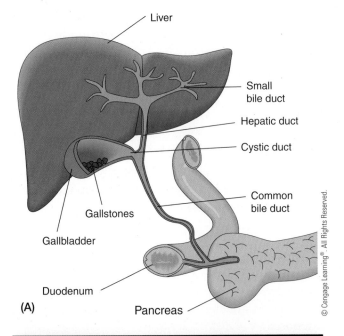

Liver

Small bile duct

Hepatic duct

Cystic duct

Common bile duct

Gallstones

Gallbladder

Duodenum

(A)

Pancreas

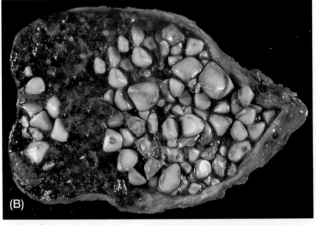

(B)

FIGURE 12–14 (A) Location of gallbladder. (B) Cholelithiasis.

■ **ETIOLOGY.** Gallstones form from bile salts and cholesterol and can vary in size, shape, number, color, and composition. Cholesterol stones are by far the most common and are formed when a change in the composition of bile occurs. When bile becomes highly saturated with cholesterol, it crystallizes and forms a stone.

The three most important risk factors for developing gallstones include excessive body weight, increasing age, and being female. In general, individuals developing cholelithiasis have several factors in common, called the five Fs of cholelithiasis: (1) Female, (2) Fair complexion, (3) Fat or obese, (4) Fertile or has had children, and (5) Forty years of age or older.

■ **SYMPTOMS.** Gallstones are often asymptomatic. If symptoms do occur, they are usually related to blocking the outflow of the gallbladder or of its ducts. Symptoms can include nausea, vomiting, and upper-right quadrant pain following meals containing fat. Complications of cholelithiasis include cholecystitis and jaundice.

■ **DIAGNOSIS.** A cholecystogram and ultrasound, along with a positive history, will confirm the diagnosis.

■ **TREATMENT.** Extracorporeal shockwave lithotripsy (litho = stone, tripsy = destruction) (ESWL) can be performed to break up the stones so they can be passed. If this procedure is not effective or is not recommended, cholecystectomy is performed.

■ **PREVENTION.** Decreasing fat intake in the diet will not aid in dissolving stones, but may be helpful in prevention.

Pancreatic Diseases

Diseases of the pancreas are often quite advanced by the time symptoms appear. Some pancreatic disorders are associated with alcoholism. Replacement or supplements of pancreatic enzymes and insulin might be necessary when the pancreas is not functioning properly or is surgically removed.

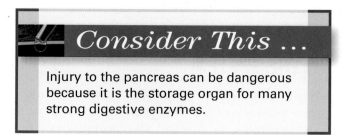

Consider This ...

Injury to the pancreas can be dangerous because it is the storage organ for many strong digestive enzymes.

PANCREATITIS

■ **DESCRIPTION.** Pancreatitis is an inflammation of the pancreas that can range from mild to fatal. With pancreatitis, the pancreas becomes inflamed, edematous, hemorrhagic, and necrotic.

Pancreatitis differs from inflammation of other organs because of the powerful digestive enzymes the pancreas produces. As this organ becomes diseased, these enzymes often escape the pancreatic cells and ducts, causing digestion of the pancreas (**autodigestion**) and the surrounding tissues. If this destruction extends into blood vessels, hemorrhage occurs, leading to severe pain and shock. Acute hemorrhagic pancreatitis usually follows an alcohol-drinking spree and is often fatal despite emergency medical attention.

■ **ETIOLOGY.** This disease is similar to cirrhosis of the liver in that most cases of severe pancreatitis are due to alcoholism.

Pancreatitis can also be caused by blockage of pancreatic ducts by gallstones. Many cases of pancreatitis are idiopathic (of unknown cause).

■ **SYMPTOMS.** An acute attack of pancreatitis causes sudden, severe abdominal pain that often radiates to the back. The individual may find some relief by drawing the knees up toward the abdomen. Other symptoms exhibited during an acute attack are nausea, vomiting, diaphoresis (sweating), and tachycardia.

Individuals with chronic pancreatitis might complain of constant back pain and frequent bouts of mild symptoms similar to those of an acute attack. As the disease progresses, the pancreatic tissues are replaced with fibrous tissues, and function is lost. As endocrine function is lost, the individual exhibits symptoms of diabetes mellitus. Digestive disorders, including malabsorption, occur when exocrine function is impaired.

■ **DIAGNOSIS.** Diagnosis of pancreatitis is often made based on the individual's history and is confirmed by blood testing. A high blood **amylase** (pancreatic enzyme) is indicative of pancreatitis.

■ **TREATMENT.** Treatment and prognosis of pancreatitis depend on the cause. If it is caused by gallstones, it is treated successfully by removing the gallbladder and the involved stones. Treatment for idiopathic and alcohol-related pancreatitis is palliative because there is no cure. Individuals must stop drinking alcohol and are treated with analgesics and nutritional support. Prognosis for these types of pancreatitis is poor.

■ **PREVENTION.** In some cases, pancreatitis might not be preventable. Actions that reduce risk include the following:

- Limit alcohol intake. If any symptoms of pancreatitis develop, alcohol should be avoided completely.

- Stop smoking. Tobacco use increases the risk of pancreatitis.

- Eat a healthy, low-fat diet. Increased consumption of fat increases the risk of gallstones and, thus, increases the risk of pancreatitis.

PANCREATIC CANCER

■ **DESCRIPTION.** Pancreatic cancer is usually an adenocarcinoma that occurs in the head of the pancreas. This cancer spreads very rapidly, and its poor prognosis makes it a leading cause of cancer death (Figure 12–15).

■ **ETIOLOGY.** The cause of this tumor is unknown, but known carcinogens include cigarette smoking, high coffee consumption, chemical exposure, and consumption of a high-fat diet.

■ **SYMPTOMS.** Symptoms usually do not occur until late in the disease process, after metastasis has already occurred. As pancreatic tissue is destroyed, the individual can experience abdominal pain, back pain, nausea, vomiting, loss of appetite, weakness, jaundice, and fatigue.

■ **DIAGNOSIS.** Ultrasound, CT, and magnetic resonance imaging (MRI) can be helpful in making a diagnosis. A biopsy is the definitive test.

■ **TREATMENT.** Treatment can include surgical resection, chemotherapy, and radiation. This tumor usually responds poorly to all therapies, and prognosis is very poor. Supportive care can be provided, including pain management and nutritional support.

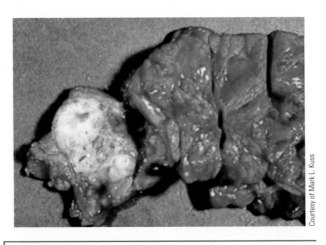

Courtesy of Mark L. Kuss

FIGURE 12–15 Pancreatic cancer.

■ **PREVENTION.** There is no proven prevention. Activities to reduce risk include not smoking, maintaining a healthy weight, eating a healthy diet, and exercising regularly.

■ RARE DISEASES

Primary Biliary Cirrhosis

Primary biliary cirrhosis is a chronic liver disease that gradually destroys the bile ducts in the liver. The cause is unknown, but it might be related to immune system dysfunction. Destruction of bile ducts decreases bile excretion from the liver and causes a chronic inflammation, resulting in cirrhosis. The disease is much more common in middle-aged females than in males. Signs and symptoms of the disease include jaundice, edema, itching, and abnormal liver function studies. Treatment is directed at relieving the symptoms. A liver transplant might be necessary.

Gilbert's Syndrome

Gilbert's syndrome is a congenital liver disorder that usually has its onset in the teenage or young adult years and is more common in males. Symptoms include increased serum bilirubin and jaundice, but it is usually left untreated because it does not seem to affect liver function adversely.

Hemochromatosis

Hemochromatosis is a disorder in which the body absorbs and stores excessive amounts of iron. It is the most common inherited disease, affecting approximately one million people in the United States (CDC, 2011). Eventually, damage to the liver can occur. It is diagnosed by blood tests for iron levels, and treatment requires blood (about 1 to 2 units) to be removed weekly until iron levels return to normal. This regimen must be continued every 4 months for life to keep the iron levels within normal limits.

■ EFFECTS OF AGING ON THE SYSTEM

The older adult who develops hepatitis usually undergoes a more severe infection than a younger person does with the same disease. The mortality rate for hepatitis increases with age. Older people can be at an increased risk for developing hepatitis if any of the following factors are present:

- A depressed immune system
- Increased contact with a variety of caregivers
- Poor nutrition
- Increased intake of medications
- Poor hygiene
- Multiple blood transfusions

Cirrhosis in an older person can be of unknown etiology or due to chronic alcohol intake. It is usually progressive and severe, and the prognosis is poor. Bile stones are also seen more frequently in the older adult. Surgery is usually the treatment of choice but might not be an option due to the age of the individual and other complicating disorders. Pancreatic disease is also common in the older adult population, so replacement of pancreatic enzymes might be needed if the pancreas is not producing adequate amounts.

SUMMARY

Diseases of the liver, gallbladder, and pancreas have serious effects on digestion and metabolism. The liver has many functions in the body, so when it is diseased, a variety of other disorders can result. If the liver fails completely, a transplant is necessary. Hepatitis is the most common liver disorder and is usually viral in nature. Cirrhosis of the liver is a chronic, progressive disease most commonly related to alcohol ingestion.

Gallbladder disease, most commonly caused by gallstones, affects thousands of individuals annually. Pancreatic disorders are often not diagnosed until late in the disease process because early symptoms are often not apparent. If the pancreas is not functioning properly, pancreatic enzymes and hormones might need to be supplemented. The older adult is at increased risk for developing disorders of the liver, gallbladder, and pancreas.

REVIEW QUESTIONS

Short Answer

1. What are the functions of the liver, gallbladder, and pancreas?

2. Which signs and symptoms are associated with common liver, gallbladder, and pancreatic disorders?

3. Which diagnostic tests are most commonly used to determine the type and cause of liver, gallbladder, or pancreatic disorders?

Multiple Choice

4. Which of the following is the cause of jaundice?
   a. Increased levels of amylase in the blood
   b. Decreased levels of pancreatase in the blood
   c. Increased levels of bilirubin in the blood
   d. Decreased levels of lipase in the blood

5. Impaired liver function reveals an elevation in which of the following tests?

   a. Bilirubin and alkaline phosphatase

   b. Albumin and bilirubin

   c. Alkaline phosphatase and amylase

   d. Amylase and albumin

6. Diseases of the liver, gallbladder, or pancreas generally have an adverse effect on which of the following?

   a. The immune system

   b. Digestion and metabolism

   c. The inflammatory process

   d. The endocrine system

7. Which of the following types of hepatitis is the most common?

   a. Hepatitis A

   b. Hepatitis B

   c. Hepatitis C

   d. Hepatitis D

8. Individuals at high risk for developing HBV include which of the following?

   a. Drug addicts

   b. Blood recipients

   c. Health care workers

   d. All of the above

9. Which of the following is the best definition of cirrhosis?

   a. A chronic, degenerative disease of the pancreas

   b. An acute irreversible disease of the liver

   c. An abnormality of the liver caused by alcoholism

   d. A chronic, degenerative, irreversible disease of the liver

10. Ascites is an accumulation of fluid in the abdominal cavity, usually due to which of the following conditions?

    a. Pancreatic cancer

    b. Liver failure and portal hypertension

    c. Cholelithiasis

    d. Cirrhosis

True or False

11. T F   Gallbladder disorders usually cause symptoms related to indigestion when eating high-fat foods.

12. T F   A cholecystogram is a radiographic exam used to diagnose cholecystitis.

13. T F   Gallstones are most commonly found in obese, middle-aged men.

14. T F   A high serum amylase is usually diagnostic for pancreatitis.

15. T F   The older adult who develops hepatitis usually experiences a much milder episode of the disease than does a young person.

CASE STUDIES

■ Ms. Fisher is a 68-year-old woman with the classic symptoms of gallbladder disease. She is diagnosed with gallstones and is scheduled for surgery in 2 weeks. She asks you about the cause of gallstones and why she would develop them. How would you respond to her? What typical factors put an individual at risk for developing gallstones?

■ Mr. Swicky came to the clinic with complaints of abdominal pain, sweating, fever, and anorexia. His physician sent him to the hospital for an in-depth evaluation. He was diagnosed with viral hepatitis A. Mr. Swicky's wife is very concerned about his condition. What can you tell her about type A hepatitis? Should she be vaccinated for hepatitis A now? Are there other treatments? What precautions should the family practice to prevent transmitting hepatitis? Where can she find more information about hepatitis?

Study Tools

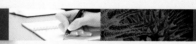

Workbook

Complete Chapter 12

Online Resources

PowerPoint® presentations

Animation

BIBLIOGRAPHY

American Liver Foundation. (2012). *www.liverfoundation.org* (accessed February 2012).

Asselah, T., & Marcellin, P. (2012). Direct acting antivirals for the treatment of chronic hepatitis C: One pill a day for tomorrow. *Liver International Supplement*, 88–102.

Blacklaws, H., Gardner, A., & Usher, K. (2011). Irritability: An underappreciated side effect of interferon treatment for chronic hepatitis C? *Journal of Clinical Nursing* 20(9/10), 1215–1224.

Brenner, Z. R., & Krenzer, M. E. (2010). Understanding acute pancreatitis. *Nursing* 40(1), 32–37.

Britt, R. C., Bouchard, C., Weireter, L. J., & Britt, L. D. (2010). Impact of acute care surgery on biliary disease. *Journal of the American College of Surgeons* 210(5), 595–599.

Carr, R., & Traufler, R. (2011). Immune reconstitution inflammatory syndrome in HIV-infected patients. *Dimensions of Critical Care Nursing* 30(3), 139–143.

Centers for Disease Control and Prevention. (2011). Iron overload and hemochromatosis. *www.cdc.gov* (accessed August 2012).

Centers for Disease Control and Prevention. (2012). Hepatitis B. *www.cdc.gov* (accessed August 2012).

Craig, M., & Infante, S. (2011). Abdominal mysteries: Pain, peritonitis, pancreatitis, pseudocyst. *Nephrology Nursing Journal* 38(2), 173–186.

Douglas, D. (2011). Cirrhosis tied to increased risk of liver cancer in diabetics. Reuters Health Information. *www.reutershealth.com* (accessed January 2012).

Drug news. (2011). *Nursing* 41(10), 24.

Forbes, S. J., & Newsome, P. N. (2012). New horizons for stem cell therapy in liver disease. *Journal of Hepatology* 56(12), 496–499.

Ghosh, N., Ghosh, R., Mandal, V., & Mandal, S. C. (2011). Recent advances in herbal medicine for treatment of liver diseases. *Pharmaceutical Biology* 49(9), 970–988.

Graziadei, I. W. (2011). The clinical challenges of acute chronic liver failure. *Liver International 31*(8), 24–26.

Habib, H. A., & Saunders, M. (2011). The yellow bird of jaundice: Recognizing biliary obstruction. *Nursing 41*(10), 28–36.

HealthGuidance (2012). Digestive diseases: The facts. *www.healthguidance.org* (accessed August 2012).

Hepatitis Foundation International. (2012). *www.hepfi.org* (accessed February 2012).

Hepatitis Foundation International. (2012). The ABCs of hepatitis. *www.hepfi.org* (accessed August 2012).

Hull, D., & Armstrong, C. (2010). Managing patients receiving sorafenib for advanced hepatocellular carcinoma: A case study. *International Journal of Palliative Nursing 16*(5), 249–254.

Hytiroglou, P., Snover, D. C., Alves, V., Balabaud, C., Bhathal, P. S., Bioulac-Sage, P., & van Leeuwen, D. J. (2012). Beyond "cirrhosis." *American Journal of Clinical Pathology 137*(1), 5–9.

Lee, J., Kim, J., & Shin, H. (2011). Therapeutic effects of the oriental herbal medicine Sho-saiko-to on liver cirrhosis and carcinoma. *Hepatology Research 41*(9), 825–837.

MacIntyre, J. (2011). Metastatic pancreatic cancer: What can nurses do? *Clinical Journal of Oncology Nursing 15*(4), 424–428.

Marchiondo, K. (2010). Acute pancreatitis. *MEDSURG Nursing 19*(1), 54–55.

Mason, M. (2011). Positives of testing. *Nursing Standard 25*(50), 23.

National Liver Foundation. (2012). *www.nlfindia.com* (accessed February 2012).

Storer, A. (2011). A 54-year-old woman with a rare case of drug-induced pancreatitis. *Advanced Emergency Nursing Journal 33*(1), 23–28.

Tingting, Z., Yuan, L., Qingqing, X., Yaping, H., & Jun, L. (2011). Care strategies for patients with severe drug-induced hepatitis. *Health (1949–1998) 3*(4), 228–232.

Wong, F. (2012). Management of ascites in cirrhosis. *Journal of Gastroenterology & Hepatology 27*(1), 11–20.

Yarnell, E., & Abascal, K. (2010). Herbal medicine for viral hepatitis. *Alternative & Complementary Therapies 16*(3), 151–157.

Zucker, D. M., Choi, J., & Gallagher, E. R. (2012). Mobile outreach strategies for screening hepatitis and HIV in high-risk populations. *Public Health Nursing 29*(1), 27–35.

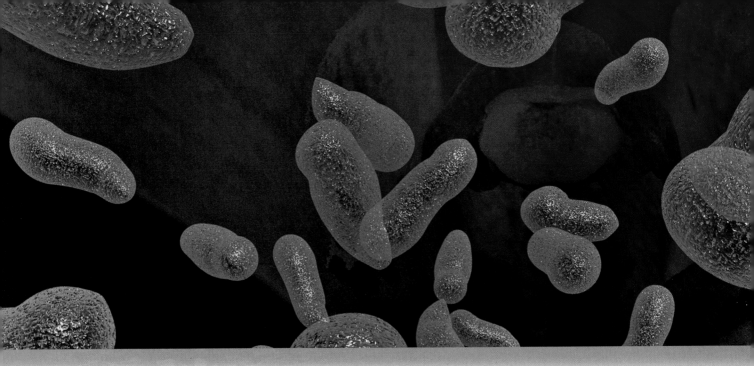

OUTLINE

KEY TERMS

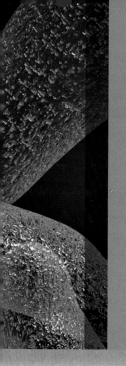

13

Urinary System Diseases and Disorders

LEARNING OBJECTIVES

Upon completion of the chapter, the learner should be able to:

1. Define the terminology common to the urinary system and the disorders of the system.

2. Discuss the basic anatomy and physiology of the urinary system.

3. Identify the important signs and symptoms associated with common urinary system disorders.

4. Describe the common diagnostics used to determine the type and cause of urinary system disorders.

5. Identify common disorders of the urinary system.

6. Describe the typical course and management of the common urinary system disorders.

7. Describe the effects of aging on the urinary system and the common disorders associated with aging of the system.

OVERVIEW

The urinary system maintains homeostasis in the body by excreting and reabsorbing important electrolytes, compounds, and water. It also excretes wastes from the body in the form of urine. Disturbances in other systems such as the circulatory or nervous systems can adversely affect the functioning of the urinary system. Urinary disorders range from mild infections to very serious diseases such as cancer of the bladder or kidneys. ■

ANATOMY AND PHYSIOLOGY

The urinary system includes the kidneys, ureters, bladder, and urethra (Figure 13–1). The kidneys are located behind the intestines at the mid-back level; each is about the size of a man's fist and weighs about 150 grams. The kidneys are responsible for removing waste products from the bloodstream. Every minute, about one-fourth of the blood circulating in the body passes through the kidneys, where toxic wastes and unused nutrients are filtered and pass out of the body as urine. The kidneys also regulate fluid, electrolyte, and acid–base balances, assist in the metabolism of calcium, and help regulate blood pressure. The kidneys are composed of nephrons that act as filters, selectively filtering, excreting, or reabsorbing what is needed by the body to maintain homeostasis. They monitor the amount of salts and other chemicals needed for proper body functioning. The kidneys also produce an active form of vitamin D necessary for strong bones.

The ureters are tubules that run from the kidney to the bladder (see Figure 13–1) and transport the urine from the renal pelvis to the bladder, where it is stored until emptied, usually voluntarily by the individual. The bladder, the muscular organ that holds urine, can usually store about 350–500 ml. This amount varies from individual to individual and is affected by many other factors, especially bladder tone, neurologic disease, and urologic disorders. Micturition is the process of voiding, or emptying, the bladder. This usually occurs in response to stimuli to the pelvic nerves.

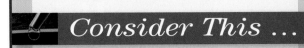

Consider This ...

A full human adult bladder is about the size of a softball.

The urethra is a hollow tube, significantly longer in males than in females, running from the bladder to the external opening (the meatus) for excretion (see Figure 13–1). The urethra serves as the passageway for urine in the female and for both urine and semen ejaculation in the male.

Urine is normally clear, slightly yellow to gold in color, and free of sediments. Some drugs can change the color of urine. Urine has its own distinct odor but is not foul-smelling unless disease is present. Some foods, however, will change the odor of urine as their by-products are excreted, such as asparagus. Urine has a normal specific gravity of 1.005–1.030 and a pH of about 6. Changes in these values can indicate disease.

Media Link

View an animation on urine formation on the Online Resources.

COMMON SIGNS AND SYMPTOMS

Common signs and symptoms of urinary tract diseases include any abnormality in urine or in the ability to urinate. Some of these include:

- **Hematuria** (hem-ah-TOO-ree-ah; hema = blood, uria = urine), blood in the urine.

- **Pyuria** (pye-YOU-ree-ah; py = pus, uria = urine), pus in the urine.

- **Proteinuria**, protein in the urine. A specific protein, albumin, can be identified, revealing **albuminuria**.

Inferior vena cava

Hilum

Inferior vena cava

Urinary bladder

Meatus

Descending aorta

Left kidney

Left renal artery

Left renal vein

Aorta

Left ureter

Left common iliac artery

Urethra (lined with sphincter muscle)

FIGURE 13–1   The urinary system.

- **Dysuria** (dis-YOU-ree-ah; dys = difficult or painful, uria = urine), difficulty or pain with urination.

- **Nocturia** (nock-TOO-ree-ah; noc = night, uria = urine), increased voiding at night.

- **Oliguria** (OL-ih-GOO-ree-ah; olig = scanty or few, uria = urine), a decrease in urine output.

- **Anuria** (ah-NEW-ree-ah; an = without, uria = urine), no urine output.

- **Frequency**, urinating frequently.

- **Urgency**, the need to urinate immediately.

Varying degrees of pain in the low back or flank area also can indicate urinary disease; other symptoms include nausea, vomiting, malaise, and fatigue. Urinary system diseases also can affect the cardiovascular and respiratory systems, leading to hypertension, edema, and shortness of breath.

▣ DIAGNOSTIC TESTS

A **urinalysis** (YOU-rih-NAL-ih-sis; urine analysis) is the most common test performed to diagnose urinary system diseases. This test is important because the results can confirm the presence of various urinary tract disorders. It consists of physical, chemical, and microscopic examinations. It tests a urine sample for pH; specific gravity; and presence of protein, glucose, and blood cells. A urine test may also check

for other urine contents such as bilirubin or urobilinogen. Some of these tests require a urine sample collected over period of time, such as a 2-hour or 24-hour urine sample. The urine test also includes a microscopic examination to determine the presence of bacteria, crystals, and casts (tube-shaped particles made up of red cells, white cells, and kidney cells). The specific test, normal findings, abnormal findings, and pathologies are summarized in Table 13–1.

A **urine culture and sensitivity (C&S)** test can be performed in the laboratory if the urinalysis shows an abnormal number of white cells or bacteria in the urine. If the pure culture bacteria count is greater than 100,000 bacteria per ml or cc of urine, a diagnosis of urinary tract infection is confirmed. A smaller number can indicate a contaminated specimen or the presence of a mild infection. A culture helps determine the type of bacteria present, and a sensitivity test will help determine the most effective antibiotic to prescribe for treatment.

A urine specimen collected for a culture can be obtained by the **clean catch** method or by sterile technique. The clean catch method involves cleaning the urethral meatus, voiding a moderate amount of urine to flush out the urethra, and then catching a urine specimen in a sterile container. Catching the specimen after urinating as described above is considered a mid-stream catch and is part of the proper technique of obtaining a clean catch specimen. A sterile technique involves placing a sterile urinary catheter into the bladder to obtain a sterile urine specimen.

TABLE 13–1 Urinalysis Values

Urinalysis	Normal Values	Abnormal Results
Color	Clear amber	Very light or very dark; cloudy
Odor	Pleasantly aromatic	Offensive, unpleasant
Albumin (protein)	Negative	Albuminuria
Acetone	Negative	Ketonuria
Red blood cells	2–3/HPF	Hematuria
White blood cells	4–5/HPF	White, cloudy urine
Bilirubin	Negative	Bilirubinuria
Urobilinogen	0–8 mg/dl	Higher than normal
Glucose	Negative	Glycosuria
Specific gravity	1.005–1.030	Higher or lower than normal
Bacteria	Negative	Present
Casts	Rare	Present, several to many
pH	4.6–8.0	Higher or lower than normal

HPF, high-power field.

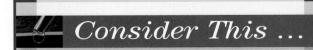

Consider This ...

Lab tests can detect traces of alcohol in urine 6–12 hours after a person has stopped drinking.

Blood tests can be performed to determine whether waste products are being filtered out adequately by the glomerulus, thus checking kidney function. The two most common nitrogenous waste products normally filtered from the blood are **urea** and **creatinine**. A **blood urea nitrogen (BUN)** test will determine the levels of urea nitrogen or waste product in the blood. A **creatinine clearance test** is a blood test to determine the ability of the renal glomeruli to filter creatinine out of the blood after creatinine is ingested by the subject. The condition of high levels of waste products in the blood is called **uremia** (you-REE-me-ah; ur = urine, emia = blood), a toxic condition of the blood.

Radiologic examinations of the urinary system include **kidneys-ureter-bladder (KUB)**, **intravenous pyelogram (IVP)**, and **cystogram**. A KUB is a common X-ray of the structures of the urinary tract to determine abnormalities. An IVP is an X-ray taken after injecting dye into the individual's bloodstream. The dye accumulates in the urinary tract, improving the ability to visualize and identify obstructions, tumors, and deformities. A cystogram (cysto = bladder, gram = picture) is an X-ray taken of the bladder after a radiopaque dye is instilled into the bladder by using a urinary catheter; the procedure is called a cystography (cysto = bladder, ography = procedure to graph or take a picture). A cystogram helps determine shape and function of the bladder.

Cystoscopy (sis-TOS-koh-pee; cysto = bladder, scopy = procedure to look) is an invasive procedure to look into the urethra and bladder by using a lighted scope (Figure 13–2). Stones, tumors, and areas of infection and inflammation can be viewed with a cystoscope. Additional instruments might be used to allow the physician to obtain a tissue biopsy or to crush bladder stones.

Biopsies of the kidney and bladder are often performed to determine the presence of disease. Bladder biopsies are often obtained by using a cystoscope as previously mentioned; renal biopsies are often obtained by using X-ray technique to guide a fine needle through the flank area to remove a core of renal tissue.

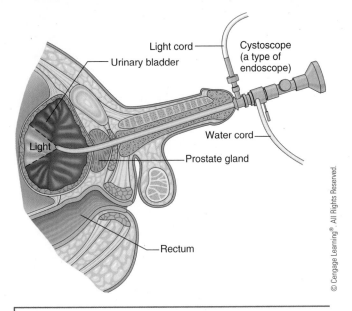

FIGURE 13–2   Cystoscopy.

Catheterization of the urinary bladder is a sterile procedure. Sterile technique must be maintained to prevent urinary tract infections. A soft catheter is passed through the urethra and into the bladder to instill fluids or medication into the bladder or to remove urine. Urinary catheterization to remove urine can be performed to relieve urinary retention, to empty the bladder prior to a procedure, to obtain a sterile urine specimen for testing, or as a treatment for incontinence.

If the catheter is removed as soon as the urine is drained, the catheterization is temporary and is called an **in and out catheterization**. If the catheter is placed for a longer period of time, as commonly occurs for urinary incontinence, a balloon on the end of the catheter is inflated after placement to hold the catheter in the bladder, and the catheterization is called an **indwelling catheter**. If the catheter is inserted surgically through the pelvic wall, as is often done after urinary tract surgeries, it is called a **suprapubic catheter** (Figure 13–3).

COMMON DISEASES OF THE URINARY SYSTEM

Diseases of the urinary system can affect either gender at any age. Urinary tract infections are the most common disorders of the system. Many of the diseases of the urinary system, such as dysuria, oliguria, and frequency of urination, have similar symptoms in their early stages of development.

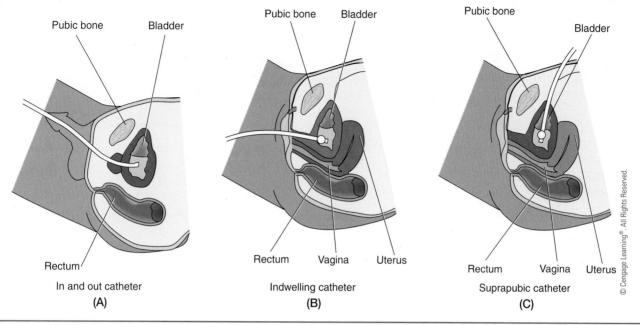

Pubic bone   Bladder

Rectum

In and out catheter
(A)

Pubic bone   Bladder

Rectum   Vagina   Uterus

Indwelling catheter
(B)

Pubic bone   Bladder

Rectum   Vagina   Uterus

Suprapubic catheter
(C)

FIGURE 13–3   Types of urinary catheters.

PHARMACOLOGY HIGHLIGHT

Common Drugs for Urinary Disorders

CATEGORY	EXAMPLES OF MEDICATIONS
Antibiotics	
Drugs used to prevent or stop bacterial infections	ampicillin, amoxicillin, ciprofloxacin, doxycycline, erythromycin, penicillin, or tetracycline
Antihypertensives	
Drugs used to treat high blood pressure	
β-Blockers	atenolol or sotalol
Calcium channel blockers	verapamil or diltiazem
Diuretics	furosemide, hydrochlorothiazide, or spironolactone
Angiotensin-converting enzyme inhibitors	captopril or benazepril
Angiotensin II receptor antagonists	losartan
Aldosterone antagonists	eplerenone
Vasodilators	hydralazine
α₂ Agonists	methyldopa
Antineoplastics	
Drugs used to treat cancer	
Alkylating agents	chlorambucil, cyclophosphamide, or lomustine
Antimetabolites	5-flourauracil, mercaptopurine, or methotrexate
Antitumor antibiotics	mitomycin or streptozocin
Hormones/antihormones	estrogens, androgens, flutamide, or tamoxifen
Other substances	vincristine, L-asparaginase, paclitaxel, carboplatin, cisplatin, or etoposide

(continued)

Common Drugs for Urinary Disorders (continued)

CATEGORY	EXAMPLES OF MEDICATIONS
Diuretics Drugs used to treat high blood pressure	furosemide, hydrochlorothiazide, or spironolactone
Vitamins/Minerals Supplements used to support or replace low levels	calcium, chromium, folate, iodine, iron, magnesium, selenium, vitamins A, B_6, B_{12}, C, D, E, K, or zinc; these may be prescribed individually or in combinations.

Urinary Tract Infection (UTI)

■ *DESCRIPTION.* UTI is a broad diagnosis covering any infection of the urinary tract, including the urethra, bladder, and kidneys (Figure 13–4A).

■ *ETIOLOGY.* UTIs can be caused by a virus or fungus, but by far, the most common infection is due to bacteria.

Bacteria can reach the urinary tract through the blood (hematogenous infection) or by entering the tract through the urethra (ascending infection). Hematogenous infection is less common and is usually the result of septicemia. In this case, the urinary tract is a site of secondary infection. Primary infection might begin in the respiratory or

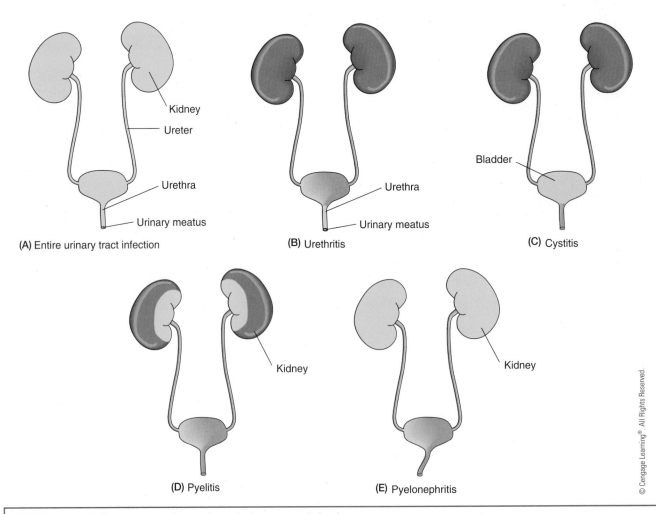

(A) Entire urinary tract infection — Kidney, Ureter, Urethra, Urinary meatus

(B) Urethritis — Urethra, Urinary meatus

(C) Cystitis — Bladder

(D) Pyelitis — Kidney

(E) Pyelonephritis — Kidney

FIGURE 13–4   Yellow areas indicate sites of urinary tract infections.

gastrointestinal tract and be carried to the urinary tract through the blood.

The most common route for infection of the urinary tract is the ascending route by which bacteria enter the urethra and climb, or ascend, upward toward the kidneys, infecting the various organs as they progress.

Approximately 80% of the time, the bacteria causing ascending infection are *Escherichia coli* (*E. coli*). This bacterium is a normal flora of the intestine and is commonly found in large numbers around the anal and perineal area. Sexual intercourse, bladder catheterization, and surgical procedures increase the risk of ascending infection.

UTIs in males are quite rare and are usually related to obstruction of the tract by an enlarged prostate or a sexually transmitted disease. Ascending UTIs are far more common in females than in males for the following reasons:

- Anatomically, the female urethra is shorter than the male urethra, allowing bacteria to ascend more easily.

- Anatomically, the female urethral opening is closer to the rectal area than that of the male, allowing migration of bacteria from the rectal area to the urethra.

- Improper female toileting habits or wiping improperly from the back (rectal area) toward the front (vulva area) pulls rectal bacteria toward and into the urethral opening.

- Vaginal secretions can harbor bacteria and contaminate the urethral area.

- Sexual intercourse can cause trauma to the urethra and bladder, leading to inflammation and potential infection.

- Pregnant females are more susceptible to infection due to the pressure of the heavy uterus on the urinary tract and because pregnancy hormones tend to relax the organs of the urinary tract, allowing easier entry by bacteria.

- Male prostatic secretions have an antibacterial effect, reducing the risk of UTI.

SYMPTOMS. Signs and symptoms of UTI can include dysuria, flank pain, urinary frequency and urgency, hematuria, and low back pain.

DIAGNOSIS. UTIs are commonly diagnosed by urinalysis and culture of a urine specimen. Bacterial counts of 100,000 bacteria or greater per milliliter of urine confirms UTI.

TREATMENT. Antibiotic treatment is usually effective. A bacterial sensitivity test helps in the selection of the most effective antibiotic for treatment.

PREVENTION. There are several natural preventive measures against UTIs. The act of urination actually washes most bacteria out of the urethra. A low pH (acidity) and the presence of urea in the bladder have

HEALTHY HIGHLIGHT

Preventing Urinary Tract Infections

Females who suffer frequent UTIs might find the following measures helpful to prevent them.

- Drink six to eight glasses of water a day.
- Drink cranberry juice to lower the pH or acidify the urine.
- Follow correct female toileting habits—wiping front to back.
- Avoid tight-fitting jeans and body suits.
- Wear underwear and pantyhose with absorbent cotton perineal panels.
- Avoid perfumed soaps, bubble baths, douches, and feminine deodorants.
- Cleanse the genital area before and after sexual intercourse.
- Urinate before and after sexual intercourse.
- Use a water-soluble lubricant if needed during sexual intercourse.
- Remove a contraceptive diaphragm or sponge as soon as possible.

As previously discussed, UTI includes infection of any of the organs of the urinary tract. Types of urinary tract infection include urethritis, cystitis, pyelitis, and pyelonephritis. A brief discussion of each follows.

a bactericidal effect. Also, the ureters close off during urination to prevent urine from refluxing up the ureter to the kidney. Other preventive measures are discussed in the preceding Healthy Highlight.

URETHRITIS

Urethritis (YOU-reh-THRIGH-tis; urethri = urethra, itis = inflammation) is more common in males than in females as a symptom of gonorrhea (Figure 13–4B). In females, urethritis can also be the result of irritation from tight clothing, application of soaps or powders to the genital area, or sexual intercourse. Urethritis commonly occurs in conjunction with cystitis. In males and females, it can be a symptom of herpes genitalis or chlamydia. Symptoms of urethritis can include swelling of the urethra, dysuria, and a urethral discharge.

CYSTITIS

Cystitis (sis-TYE-tis; cyst = bladder, itis = inflammation) is commonly called a bladder infection (Figures 13–4C and 13–5). Cystitis, occurring in females as they become sexually active, is called honeymoon cystitis. Antibiotic treatment is usually effective. Antispasmodic medications might be prescribed in addition to antibiotics to decrease the discomfort of bladder spasms. Pyridium (phenazopyridine) is often prescribed to relieve the pain, burning, and increased urge to urinate. Individuals taking Pyridium should be warned that this medication normally stains the urine a reddish orange, which will permanently stain clothing. After treatment is completed, a follow-up urinalysis and culture are important to ensure complete elimination of all bacteria because recurrent infections are common.

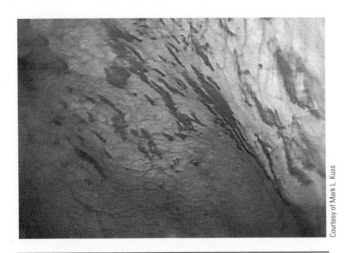

Courtesy of Mark L. Kuss

FIGURE 13–5   Cystitis: view through cystoscope.

PYELITIS

Pyelitis (PYE-eh-LYE-tis; pyelo = pelvis of kidney, itis = inflammation) is a fairly common disease among young female children (Figure 13–4D). It is usually the result of an ascending infection from the bladder (cystitis) but also can be spread by blood (hematogenous infection). Rapid diagnosis and treatment must be initiated to prevent the spread of infection to adjacent tissue, which can cause pyelonephritis.

PYELONEPHRITIS

Pyelonephritis (PYE-eh-loh-neh-FRY-tis; pyelo = pelvis of kidney, nephr = kidney, itis = inflammation) can be due to an ascending or a hematogenous infection and can affect one or both kidneys (Figure 13–4E). Obstruction or urine flow blockage in the urinary tract caused by pregnancy, prostate enlargement, stones, or tumors increases the risk of pyelonephritis. Commonly, abscesses form in the kidney and rupture, filling the kidney pelvis with pus and leading to pyuria (pyo = pus, uria = urine). Other symptoms include a sudden onset of fever and chills with flank pain and hematuria. Pyelonephritis is usually treated effectively with antibiotics, but repeated bouts of acute pyelonephritis or chronic pyelonephritis lead to scarring of the kidney. Chronic pyelonephritis can eventually lead to uremia and kidney failure.

Diseases of the Kidney

Diseases of the kidney affect the filtering system of the body. This, in turn, affects the homeostatic balance of fluids and electrolytes, and if left untreated, kidney diseases can affect all other body systems and interrupt their functioning. Therefore, symptoms of kidney disease can first appear in an affected system rather than in the urinary system. An example of this is an elevated blood pressure caused by inappropriate reabsorption of sodium and water.

GLOMERULONEPHRITIS (ACUTE)

■ **DESCRIPTION.** Acute glomerulonephritis is an inflammation of the glomerulus, or filtering unit, of the kidney. It is the most common disease of the kidney.

■ **ETIOLOGY.** This disease usually affects children and young adults within 1 to 4 weeks following a strep throat infection. Other *Streptococcus* infections such as scarlet fever and rheumatic fever also can cause this problem. Glomerulonephritis with this etiology also may be called acute poststreptococcal glomerulonephritis. In addition to *Streptococcus* bacterial infections, viruses, other bacteria, and parasites can lead to this disease.

Glomerulonephritis is nonsuppurative, or in other words, it is not associated with bacterial infection and pus formation. Inflammation in this case is the result of tissue destruction caused by the individual's immune system. Glomerulonephritis is a type of allergic or immune disease caused by an antigen–antibody reaction. The causative agent (bacteria, virus, or parasites) produces antigen that stimulates the individual's immune system to produce antibodies. These antibodies stick to the antigen, thus producing large antigen–antibody complexes that circulate in the bloodstream until they become trapped in the tiny capillaries of the glomerulus, thus blocking the glomerulus. This leads to increased pressure, irritation, and the inflammatory response.

The outpouring of neutrophils and serum as part of the inflammatory response increases pressure and decreases blood flow to the glomerulus. Ultimately, the glomerulus weakens and becomes permeable, allowing red blood cells and blood plasma proteins to leak into Bowman's capsule and appear in the urine.

■ **SYMPTOMS.** Signs and symptoms of glomerulonephritis are flank pain, fever, loss of appetite, and malaise (general ill feeling). The eyes and ankles might appear edematous (swollen). Oliguria and hematuria are frequent signs of glomerulonephritis. A urinalysis can show albuminuria (albumin = a blood protein, uria = urine) and casts (proteins that mold to the shape of the kidney tubules).

■ **DIAGNOSIS.** A routine urinalysis can show red blood cells, indicating possible damage to the glomeruli; white blood cells, indicative of infection; and increased protein, which might indicate nephron damage. Blood tests revealing increased levels of creatinine or urea are also positive indicators of the condition. An X-ray, ultrasound, and computerized tomography (CT) of the kidney can also be completed. A biopsy confirms the diagnosis.

■ **TREATMENT.** Treatment is usually supportive. Antipyretic (anti = against, pyretic = fever) and diuretic (to increase urine output) medications can be prescribed. Dietary management might include restrictions of salt, protein foods, and fluids. If a secondary bacterial infection occurs, antibiotics can be prescribed.

■ **PREVENTION.** Prevention is aimed at proper antibiotic treatment for streptococcal infections. Proper treatment of strep throat in children and young adults decreases the number of antigen–antibody complexes, thus reducing the risk of developing glomerulonephritis.

Prognosis for glomerulonephritis is generally good. Children usually recover at a slightly better rate than adults. Those who do not recover may progress into chronic glomerulonephritis.

GLOMERULONEPHRITIS (CHRONIC)

■ **DESCRIPTION.** Chronic glomerulonephritis occurs when there is a slow, progressive destruction of the kidney's glomeruli. This chronic condition is among the leading causes of chronic kidney failure and end-stage kidney disease and often leads to chronic hypertension.

■ **ETIOLOGY.** Repeated bouts of acute glomerulonephritis can lead to a chronic condition that might extend over several years with periods of remission and exacerbation. During this time, a number of the glomeruli are destroyed, leading to an inability of the kidney to produce urine. This decrease in urine output leads to edema, an increase in fluid volume in the blood, retention of salt, and, ultimately, hypertension.

Approximately 25% of people with this condition have no prior history of kidney disease. In most of these cases, the cause of the condition is unknown, but it is thought to be related to an unidentified abnormality of the immune system.

■ **SYMPTOMS.** Symptoms of chronic glomerulonephritis include those mentioned in the acute disease plus hypertension. Uremia (you-REE-me-ah; ur = urine, emia = blood or urine waste in the blood) and kidney failure can occur during late stages of the disease.

■ **DIAGNOSIS.** Diagnosis is based on testing and symptoms. An abnormal urinalysis, complete blood count (CBC), BUN, and creatinine, along with symptoms of anemia and uremia, may be indicative of the disease. A CT scan and kidney ultrasound might also be completed; biopsy confirms the diagnosis.

■ **TREATMENT.** The primary treatment goal is control of symptoms. High blood pressure can be difficult to control and is often the most important aspect of treatment. Various medications can be tried to control high blood pressure. Dietary restrictions of salt, protein, and fluids might be recommended to help control hypertension and prevent kidney failure. Steroids and immunosuppressive medications can treat some forms of glomerulonephritis. End-stage disease might require hemodialysis or kidney transplant to control symptoms and sustain life.

■ **PREVENTION.** There is no specific prevention for most cases of chronic glomerulonephritis, but prompt treatment of the acute form might be beneficial.

HYDRONEPHROSIS

■ **DESCRIPTION.** Hydronephrosis (HIGH-droh-neh-FROH-sis; hydro = water, nephro = kidney, osis = condition of) is a collection of urine in the renal pelvis, due to some type of obstruction. This accumulation of urine leads to dilation and distention of the kidney pelvis.

■ **ETIOLOGY.** Causes of obstruction include congenital defects in urinary tract structure, kidney stones, tumors, enlarged prostate, and urinary tract infections. If the obstruction is unrelieved, permanent damage can occur, and the kidney pelvis will become nonfunctioning.

■ **SYMPTOMS.** Symptoms of hydronephrosis depend on whether the obstruction is acute or chronic. One or both kidneys can be affected, depending on the position of the obstruction (Figure 13–6).

If one kidney is affected, the disease can go undetected because the other kidney continues to function adequately. A symptom that occurs regardless of where the obstruction lies is loin or flank pain. An enlarged kidney might be palpable on physical examination. If both kidneys are involved, anuria and uremia can develop.

■ **DIAGNOSIS.** Blood tests can show elevated creatinine and electrolyte imbalance. Diagnosis is confirmed by pyelogram.

■ **TREATMENT.** Treatment involves immediate draining of the kidney pelvis by surgical intervention and immediate relief of the obstruction.

■ **PREVENTION.** The causes of hydronephrosis usually cannot be prevented. Prompt treatment of conditions that may lead to hydronephrosis, such as kidney failure, reduces the risk of complications.

RENAL CALCULI

■ **DESCRIPTION.** Renal calculi are commonly called kidney stones. These stones are often composed of calcium salts and other substances. Size, location, and number of stones can vary (Figure 13–7). Urinary stones are more common in males than in females and commonly occur between ages 30 and 50.

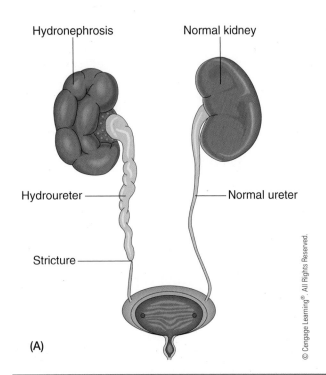

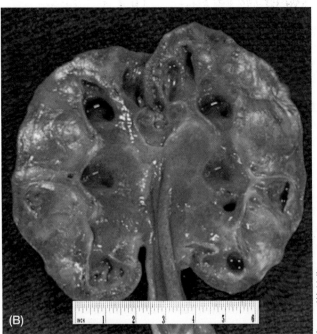

FIGURE 13–6 (A) Hydronephrosis. (B) Hydronephrosis—internal view.

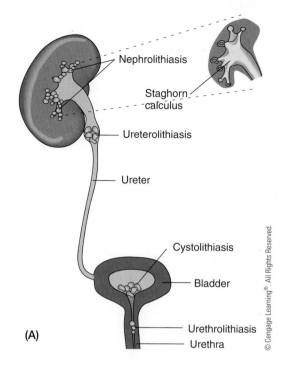

(A)

© Cengage Learning®. All Rights Reserved.

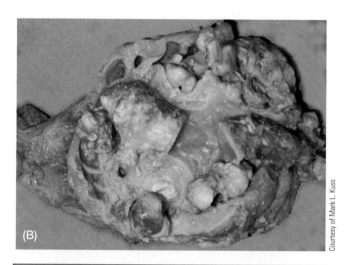

(B)

Courtesy of Mark L. Kuss

FIGURE 13–7   (A) Types and location of renal calculi. (B) Renal calculi—internal view.

■ *ETIOLOGY.* Cause of stone formation is unknown in most cases, but some precipitating factors include dehydration, chronic urinary tract infection, and immobility or prolonged bed rest, leading to release of calcium from the bones. Less commonly, stones are the result of metabolic disorders such as hyperparathyroidism, severe bone disease, and gout.

Staghorn calculi are one of the more common types of stones. These form in the pelvis of the kidney and can become so large that they fill the entire kidney pelvis. Calculi commonly form in the kidney,

but they also can form in the urinary bladder. Bladder stones cause difficulty with emptying the bladder, often leading to frequent or chronic bladder infections. Individuals can frequently form small kidney stones that easily pass through the urinary tract unnoticed, and stones can be present in the kidney yet cause no problems. It is only when stones become caught in the ureters or obstruct the urinary tract that problems and symptoms arise.

■ *SYMPTOMS.* Typical symptoms of kidney stones are hematuria and renal or urinary colic. Urinary colic is an extreme, spasmodic flank pain caused by the contraction of an obstructed ureter. This pain is often described as "the worst pain I've had in my entire life."

■ *DIAGNOSIS.* Diagnosis is commonly confirmed by using an IVP. A KUB and renal ultrasound also can be beneficial for diagnosis.

■ *TREATMENT.* Treatment during an acute attack of kidney stones includes administering pain medication and increasing fluid intake with the hope the stone will pass in the urine. Urine is often strained through a filtering device in an effort to catch the stone for identification. Even though stones feel like they should be quite large to the individual passing them, the ones that are voided and filtered are usually quite small, ranging in size from a grain of salt to a small piece of rice.

If the urinary tract is totally obstructed, emergency surgery must be performed to prevent hydronephrosis and kidney damage. Surgery called a stone basket procedure can be performed in which a retrieval instrument is passed through the urethra, bladder, and ureter to remove the stone. Another method is to break the stones into pieces for retrieval or in hopes that the pieces can be passed. This breaking of the stone is called **lithotripsy** (litho = stone, tripsy = breaking). During lithotripsy, the affected individual is placed in a tub of water and external shock waves are emitted into the water, shattering the hard stones (Figure 13–8).

■ *PREVENTION.* Prevention of further stone development can include medications, correcting any causative metabolic conditions, and increasing water intake.

POLYCYSTIC DISEASE

■ *DESCRIPTION.* Polycystic kidney disease (PKD) causes massive enlargement of both kidneys

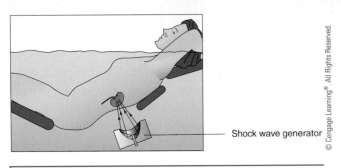

Shock wave generator

FIGURE 13–8 Lithotripsy.

due to development of multiple grape-like cysts (Figure 13–9). These cysts can cause the kidneys to increase to a weight of 20 or 30 pounds. Polycystic disease is a slow, progressive disease that affects teenagers and young adults, usually leading to renal failure by age 30 or 40. There is no cure for the disease.

■ *ETIOLOGY.* PKD is an inherited disorder. Most commonly, it is autosomal dominant, meaning if one parent has the disease, there is a 50% chance that the disease gene will pass to a child.

■ *SYMPTOMS.* As the disease progresses, kidney tissue is destroyed and function becomes increasingly impaired. Hypertension generally develops as the kidneys fail. Symptoms include lumbar pain, hematuria, and recurrent UTIs.

■ *DIAGNOSIS.* Diagnosis includes a family and clinical history. CT scan, especially when combined with dye infusion, is one of the most sensitive tests available and confirms the diagnosis.

■ *TREATMENT.* Treatment involves management of hypertension and UTIs. Dialysis and kidney transplant are often needed for end-stage treatment.

■ *PREVENTION.* PKD is an inherited disease and is not preventable.

RENAL FAILURE

■ *DESCRIPTION.* Renal failure is the failure of the kidneys to cleanse the blood of waste products. The primary method of cleansing the body of waste involves the formation of urea in the liver, which the kidneys filter out of the blood and excrete in urine. When the kidneys fail, the urea remains in the blood. A high urea level in the blood is called uremia, meaning, literally, urine in the blood. Urea is eventually converted to ammonia, leading to

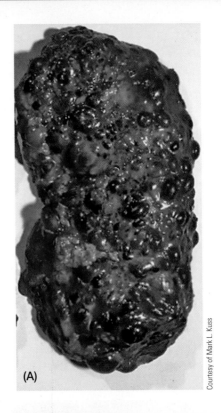

(A)

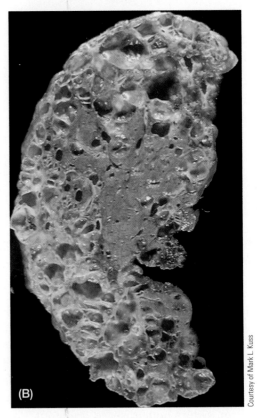

(B)

FIGURE 13–9 Polycystic kidney. (A) Exterior view of kidney. (B) Internal view of kidney.

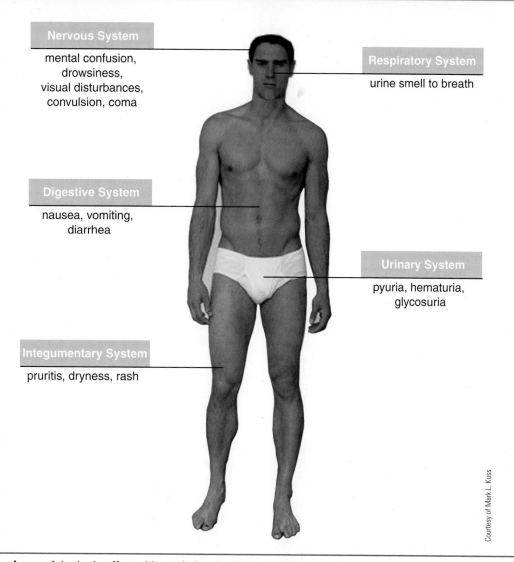

Nervous System
mental confusion, drowsiness, visual disturbances, convulsion, coma

Respiratory System
urine smell to breath

Digestive System
nausea, vomiting, diarrhea

Urinary System
pyuria, hematuria, glycosuria

Integumentary System
pruritis, dryness, rash

Courtesy of Mark L. Kuss

FIGURE 13–10   Areas of the body affected by toxic levels of circulating ammonia.

toxicity and related symptoms in all systems of the body (Figure 13–10).

■ *ETIOLOGY.* Acute renal failure is usually related to decreased blood flow to the kidneys due to conditions such as hemorrhagic or surgical shock, embolism, congestive heart failure, and dehydration. Blockage of urine flow, caused by tumors, stones, or enlarged prostate, also can lead to acute failure. Reversal of acute renal failure, which involves treating the cause of the failure, is usually quite successful. Dialysis might be needed temporarily to remove toxic wastes from the individual's blood until kidney function is restored. Individuals in acute renal failure are placed on a limited diet to allow the kidneys to rest and regenerate function.

Chronic renal failure occurs slowly and is usually the result of chronic kidney disease such as glomerulonephritis, pyelonephritis, renal hypertension, and PKD. Long-term substance abuse, alcoholism, and diabetes also can cause chronic renal failure.

■ *SYMPTOMS.* Symptoms of renal failure are not significant until approximately 75% of kidney function has been destroyed. Symptoms can include those of acute failure and problems of infertility; impotence; and bone weakness, leading to pain and fractures.

■ *DIAGNOSIS.* History and physical exam along with blood testing assist in diagnosis. Elevated blood creatinine levels along with an elevated BUN are indicative of kidney failure.

■ *TREATMENT.* Treatment includes management of the related cause of the failure, limiting protein and sodium in the diet, and monitoring fluid intake and urine output. Medications can include antihypertensives, diuretics, and antibiotics as needed. Dialysis and kidney transplantation might be options for long-term treatment.

Dialysis is a procedure that cleanses the blood of waste products when the kidneys have failed or are failing to perform this function. There are two types of dialysis; both require the same components: the patient's blood, a semipermeable membrane, and a washing or dialyzing solution. In both types of dialysis, the waste products in the individual's blood pass through the semipermeable membrane by diffusion to enter the dialyzing solution, thus cleansing the blood.

The most common type of dialysis is hemodialysis (Figure 13–11). During hemodialysis, the individual's blood is routed out of an artery (usually the brachial or radial artery) and through an artificial kidney machine, or hemodialyzer, which mechanically cleans the blood. This machine is filled with semipermeable, cellophane-like material and dialyzing solution. As blood passes through the machine, the waste products diffuse through the membrane into the dialyzing

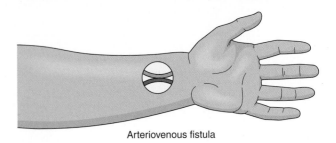

Arteriovenous fistula

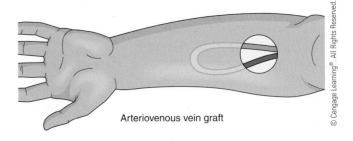

Arteriovenous vein graft

FIGURE 13–12   Hemodialysis sites: AV shunts.

solution to cleanse the blood. The clean blood reenters the patient through a venous access.

One common problem with hemodialysis is maintaining vascular access. Usually, an arteriovenous (AV) shunt is created by placing catheters in the needed artery and vein (Figure 13–12), which are then connected (shunted) with silicone rubber tubing. Complications of AV shunts include infection and clotting.

The other type of dialysis is peritoneal dialysis. This procedure involves performing a paracentesis to instill dialyzing solution into the peritoneal cavity. This type of dialysis uses the membrane that lines the peritoneal cavity to act as the semipermeable membrane. The dialyzing solution is allowed to stay in the abdomen for varying amounts of time (dwell time), during which waste products diffuse out of the peritoneal capillaries and into the dialyzing solution. Solution is then drained and disposed of. Peritoneal dialysis can be performed by several methods such as the following:

- **Continuous ambulatory peritoneal dialysis (CAPD)** is a self-dialysis that does not use a machine. Solution drains by gravity into and out of the peritoneal cavity by way of a permanently connected catheter into a bag worn around the individual's waist. CAPD is performed several times a day and usually once at night (Figure 13–13).

- **Continuous cycling peritoneal dialysis (CCPD)** uses a cycling machine and proceeds while the individual sleeps.

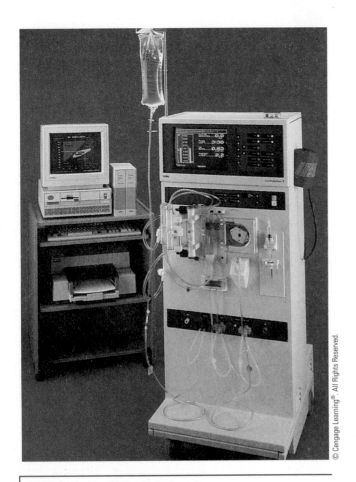

FIGURE 13–11   Hemodialysis unit.

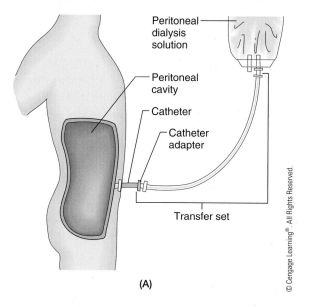

(A)

© Cengage Learning®. All Rights Reserved.

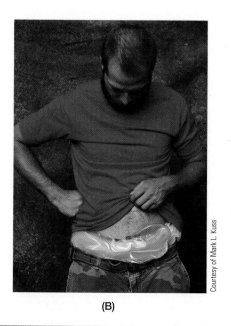

Courtesy of Mark L. Kuss

(B)

FIGURE 13–13 Continuous ambulatory peritoneal dialysis. (A) Infusion of solution. (B) Empty solution container is rolled up and hidden under clothing.

■ **Intermittent peritoneal dialysis (IPD)** is performed several times a week, usually in a medical clinic.

Hemodialysis is a much faster and more efficient process than peritoneal dialysis, but it is also much more expensive and more time-consuming. Also, access to an artificial kidney machine might be limited to large metropolitan areas.

Renal transplantation is a procedure to transplant a kidney of a donor into a recipient. This is a relatively simple surgical procedure performed on individuals with chronic renal failure commonly due to diabetes, hypertension, and glomerulonephritis.

Best results from kidney transplants are obtained when the donor and recipient are close human leukocyte antigen (HLA) matches or are histocompatible. An identical twin provides the greatest probability of match, with a fraternal twin, sibling, parent, and biological child the next best matches, in that descending order. The greatest problems with renal transplant are obtaining a kidney that is histocompatible with the recipient and dealing with postoperative organ rejection and complications with lifelong administration of immunosuppressant medications.

■ **PREVENTION.** Some causes of kidney failure might not be preventable. Controlling risk factors and conditions that cause kidney failure is the best preventive method. Because kidney disease is often caused by hypertension and diabetes, keeping these under control is important. Other preventive activities include not smoking, maintaining a healthy weight, eating healthy, and exercising regularly.

ADENOCARCINOMA OF THE KIDNEY

■ **DESCRIPTION.** Cancer of the kidney is relatively uncommon. When it does occur, the most common type is renal cell carcinoma or renal cell adenocarcinoma (Figure 13–14). These tumors are more common in men than in women and usually affect men 55 years of age or older.

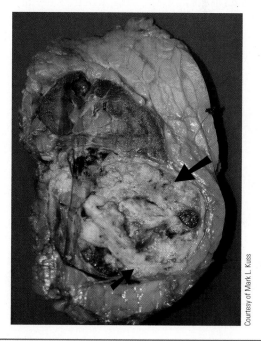

Courtesy of Mark L. Kuss

FIGURE 13–14 Adenocarcinoma of the kidney.

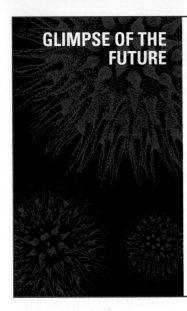

A Relationship between Red Meat and Kidney Cancer?

Eating large amounts of red meat may increase one's risk of developing kidney cancer according to recent research. The study discovered that persons who ate large amounts of red meat were 19% more likely to develop kidney cancer than those who ate very little red meat. Previous studies have not found strong evidence of the same link between red meat and kidney cancer, but they have found a link between barbecued/grilled meat and kidney cancer (because of the chemicals in the meat). Even if eating red meat does not lead to kidney cancer, it may lead to other health issues such as increased plaque in arteries. The federal guidelines suggest individuals should eat more lean meat, poultry, and seafood. More research on the effect of red meat needs to be done in the future to determine specifically who this might affect and how much red meat ingestion is necessary to increase the risk of developing kidney cancer.

Source: Pittman (2011).

■ **ETIOLOGY.** The cause of this tumor is unknown, although cigarette smoking is considered to be a risk factor. Adenocarcinoma of the kidney frequently metastasizes to the liver, brain, and bone before symptoms appear.

■ **SYMPTOMS.** The most common initial symptom is painless hematuria. Later, as the tumor increases in size, the individual experiences flank pain and fever.

■ **DIAGNOSIS.** A KUB, IVP, CT scan, and biopsy of the kidney can confirm the diagnosis.

■ **TREATMENT.** Treatment, whether metastasis has occurred or not, is **nephrectomy** (neh-FRECK-toh-me; nephr = kidney, ectomy = excision or removal). If metastasis has occurred, chemotherapy and radiation also might be employed, but prognosis varies with the extent of spread. Cure might be possible if no metastasis has occurred, but with metastasis, prognosis is poor.

■ **PREVENTION.** Kidney cancer might not be preventable, but controlling risk factors by living a healthy lifestyle, including not smoking, eating more fruits and vegetables, staying active, maintaining normal body weight, and controlling blood pressure, might be helpful in prevention.

Diseases of the Bladder

With the exception of incontinence, diseases of the bladder are relatively uncommon compared to the many other disorders of the urinary system. However,

COMPLEMENTARY AND ALTERNATIVE THERAPY

An Herbal Medicine for Kidney Disease

Palicourea coriacea (Cham.) K. Schum is the name of a species in the genus *Palicourea* (family Rubiaceae) that has been used for centuries in South America as a traditional medicine treatment for kidney diseases. Locally, the plant is known as "douradinha do campo" or "congonha do campo." Research was recently completed on the effects of the medicine and its properties. The study tried to determine the effectiveness of the plant as a diuretic, which is what it has been most frequently used for, as well as a few other ailments. The research found that *Palicourea* did act as a diuretic agent, so it might be helpful for some disorders, but further research needs to be completed to determine the amount needed and the potential side effects.

Source: Freitas et al. (2011).

incontinence is very common, especially in the older adult. It can cause many physical and psychological problems for an individual.

URINARY INCONTINENCE

■ **DESCRIPTION.** Urinary incontinence is the loss of control of urine flow. It is estimated that more than 15 million people have this disorder, and 85% of them are female. Forty percent of females age 60 and older suffer from urinary incontinence.

■ **ETIOLOGY.** Pregnancy, childbirth, hysterectomy, and menopause can all affect female continence. Males are also affected by incontinence but not nearly as often as females. As males age, the prostate is often enlarged, leading to urinary dribbling, the inability to control flow. Prostate surgery also can affect continence.

■ **SYMPTOMS.** Incontinence affects all areas of an individual's life by disrupting sleep, physical activity, travel plans, and sexual activity. Often, the fear of urinary accidents drives affected individuals away from social activity and into a life of seclusion.

There are several types of incontinence. Stress incontinence is the inability to hold urine when the bladder is stressed by coughing, sneezing, or laughing. Urge incontinence occurs with a sudden uncontrollable urge to empty the bladder. Overflow incontinence is caused by the bladder not properly emptying and leaking when overfilled.

■ **DIAGNOSIS.** A complete medical history and physical exam, including a voiding diary, are helpful in diagnosis. Diagnostic testing can include urinalysis and CBC to determine any underlying infections. Specialized urodynamic testing uses cystometry to measure anatomic and functional status of the bladder and urethra. Postvoid residual volumes of the bladder use a urinary catheter placed into the bladder to measure any urine remaining in the bladder after voiding. Cystoscopy might help identify the presence of bladder tumors, cysts, or foreign bodies.

■ **TREATMENT.** Incontinence can be managed by wearing sanitary napkins, incontinence pads, adult diapers, or waterproof briefs. Males also might use external appliances to catch the urine.

Stress incontinence can be improved by different treatments, depending on the cause of the incontinence. A common noninvasive treatment employs frequently emptying the bladder and exercising the

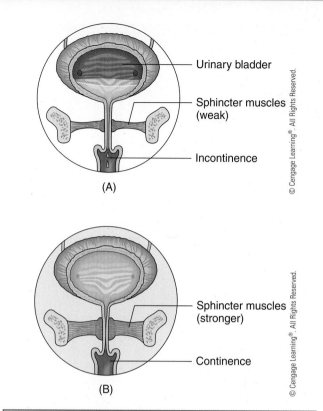

FIGURE 13–15   Kegel exercises: (A) Before exercises, pelvic muscles are thin, the sphincter is weak, and the urethra cannot close. (B) After exercises (3 months), the muscles are thicker and stronger, closing the sphincter.

pelvic muscles and external sphincter to strengthen these structures. Exercises of these muscles are called Kegel exercises. These exercises are performed by tightening or contracting the pelvic muscles as one would do to hold or stop urine flow. Performing repetitions of 20 to 40 Kegel exercises several times a day can be quite effective in controlling some types of stress incontinence (Figure 13–15).

Another treatment for stress incontinence involves collagen injections near the external sphincter to narrow the urethra (Figure 13–16). Laparoscopic bladder suspension also might be a treatment of choice. Another surgical procedure performed to suspend the bladder neck and urethra to correct urinary incontinence is called Marshall-Marchetti-Krantz (MMK). Female stress incontinence can be improved with estrogen therapy because low estrogen levels weaken the urethral sphincter.

Overflow incontinence can be controlled with medications, self-catheterization, or both. If the bladder has herniated through the pelvic floor or if there is vaginal prolapse, surgery might be necessary.

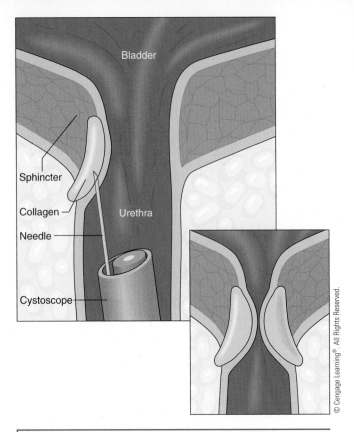

FIGURE 13–16   Collagen injection for incontinence.

Urge incontinence can be improved by bladder training. Bladder training consists of emptying the bladder every hour for 7 to 10 days and then gradually increasing the length of time until one is toileting every 3 hours. Kegel exercises also might help. Surgery is usually a last alternative because it is quite expensive.

In males, urinary incontinence is common following prostate surgery. To control this incontinence, exercise is necessary. If exercise does not control the incontinence, collagen injections might be needed. Another treatment option is surgical insertion of an artificial sphincter. This artificial device has a valve that an individual can activate to control urine flow.

Urinary incontinence in both sexes can be related to other diseases such as stroke and UTI. Sleeping pills, antihistamines, muscle relaxants, and medications to control hypertension also might cause urinary incontinence.

■ **PREVENTION.** Incontinence is not always preventable. Decreasing risk involves maintaining a healthy weight, not smoking, performing Kegel exercises, avoiding bladder irritants such as coffee, eating more fiber, and remaining physically active.

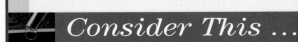

Consider This …

The average adult goes to the restroom to urinate about six times a day.

TRANSITIONAL CELL CARCINOMA OF THE BLADDER

■ **DESCRIPTION.** Bladder cancer is the most common neoplasm of the urinary tract. It usually occurs in males after age 60 and is three times more common in males than in females. Transitional cell carcinoma arises from the lining of the bladder. Bladder cancer commonly metastasizes before symptoms appear, making it highly malignant (Figure 13–17).

■ **ETIOLOGY.** The cause of these tumors is unknown. The most important risk factor is cigarette smoking, which increases the chance of cancer proportionate to the number of cigarettes smoked during the life of the affected individual. Other predisposing factors include exposure to industrial chemicals and chronic cystitis.

■ **SYMPTOMS.** Symptoms include hematuria, dysuria, and nocturia, but these symptoms do not usually appear until late in the course of the disease.

■ **DIAGNOSIS.** Diagnosis can be confirmed by cystoscopy and biopsy.

■ **TREATMENT.** Treatment depends on the stage of the tumor. **Transurethral resection (TUR)** (trans =

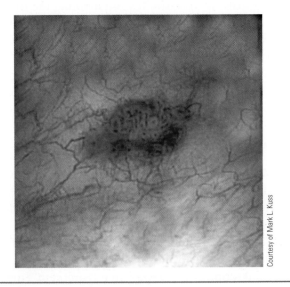

Courtesy of Mark L. Kuss

FIGURE 13–17   Bladder cancer.

through, urethral = urethra; resection = partial excision) can be performed to remove the tumor, or, more frequently, a **radical** (radical = a treatment that seeks to cure; aggressive, not palliative or conservative) **cystectomy** (sis-TECT-toh-me; cyst = bladder, ectomy = excision or removal) is performed. If metastasis has occurred, radiation and chemotherapy also might be used. Prognosis depends on the stage of the tumor when discovered. Usually, discovery is late in the course of the disease, and prognosis is poor.

■ **PREVENTION.** Prevention consists of not smoking, avoiding exposure to industrial chemicals, and promptly treating cystitis.

■ TRAUMA

Straddle Injuries

Straddle injuries commonly cause injury to the urethra. This type of injury occurs when an individual accidentally falls in a straddling position. These injuries are more common in males. Instances when straddle injuries can occur include walking a fence or roof beam or, in some cases, riding a horse or motorcycle. Treatment varies, depending on the severity of the injury.

Neurogenic Bladder

■ **DESCRIPTION.** Neurogenic bladder is dysfunction of the bladder due to some type of injury to the nervous system supplying the urinary tract or bladder.

■ **ETIOLOGY.** A common trauma that causes neurogenic bladder is a spinal cord injury such as those sustained in motor vehicle accidents or diving accidents. Other traumatic causes include cerebrovascular accidents, strokes, tumors, and herniated lumbar disks. Diabetes, dementia, and Parkinson's disease are metabolic disorders that often lead to neurogenic bladder.

■ **SYMPTOMS.** Symptoms of neurogenic bladder vary, depending on the nerves involved. Individuals might have no feeling of the need to void, or they might feel like they need to void all the time. Other symptoms are mild to severe urinary incontinence, difficulty or inability to empty the bladder, and bladder spasms.

■ **DIAGNOSIS.** Neurogenic bladder is difficult to diagnose. A detailed history, physical and neurologic examinations, and a series of urologic studies might be needed to confirm a diagnosis.

■ **TREATMENT.** Treatment goals are aimed at prevention of UTIs and controlling incontinence. Indwelling urinary catheters can control incontinence. Intermittent self-catheterization can be taught to individuals unable to empty the bladder to prevent hydronephrosis and possible renal failure.

The prognosis of neurogenic bladder depends on the possibility of reversing the nerve damage. Herniated lumbar disks that cause neurogenic bladder are commonly repaired and rapidly restore bladder function. If nerve damage is permanent, neurogenic bladder will also be permanent.

■ **PREVENTION.** Neurogenic bladder, in many cases, is not preventable. In other cases, prevention is aimed at rapid diagnosis and treatment of the cause.

■ RARE DISEASES

Goodpasture Syndrome

Goodpasture syndrome is an autoimmune disorder characterized by glomerulonephritis and pulmonary hemorrhage. For some unknown reason, the body's own antibodies attack the membranes of the kidneys and lungs, leading to symptoms of hemoptysis (he-MOP-tih-sis; hemo = blood, ptysis = saliva), or coughing or spitting up blood; dyspnea (dys = difficulty, pnea = breathing); chest pain; and anemia. Goodpasture syndrome usually results in renal failure and, ultimately, death.

Interstitial Cystitis

Interstitial cystitis is a chronic nonbacterial cystitis due to inflammation of the inner lining of the bladder. Typically, this disease affects young women and is thought to be autoimmune in nature.

The inflammation and swelling of the inner lining of the bladder decrease the capacity of the bladder, leading to the need to urinate frequently. Often, the lining is ulcerated, leading to hematuria. Other symptoms include pain above the pubic area and lower abdomen, bladder fullness, and urgency.

Treatment includes instillation of liquid medications into the bladder to distend the bladder and treat the disorder. Treatment can be needed for up to 12 weeks, but response to treatment is generally good.

EFFECTS OF AGING ON THE SYSTEM

The most common problem of the urinary system in the older adult is urinary incontinence. It is frequently due to changes in other body systems in the aging process rather than to the urinary system. Because the urinary elimination process is primarily controlled by the nervous system, changes with aging or diseases of this system can affect the individual's ability to control urine flow. Individuals with Alzheimer's disease, brain tumor, or other disorders of the nervous system might not be aware of the urge to urinate or be able to communicate the need to urinate.

In older males, benign prostatic hypertrophy is a common disorder that often causes urinary frequency, dribbling, pain or burning with urination, and difficulty starting the urine flow. In older females, the changes in estrogen levels can cause a decrease in vaginal muscle tone and, along with the changes in structure, cause increased frequency and some urine incontinence. Changes in lower abdomen muscle tone, usually the result of multiple pregnancies or obesity, also contribute to some urinary incontinence in the older adult female. (See Chapter 17, "Reproductive System Diseases and Disorders," for more information on changes in the female and male reproductive systems.)

Older individuals with other common system disorders such as stroke or severe circulatory impairment might not feel the urge to urinate and, thus, have urinary incontinence. Chronic UTIs also can affect bladder function so that the result over time is urinary incontinence.

Urinary problems in the older adult might not be due to the aging process at all, however, but to many other events occurring in the individual's life. For instance, fecal impactions that are common in the institutionalized older individual also can cause urinary incontinence.

Some medications can cause changes in the ability of the bladder to empty thoroughly, causing overflow incontinence. Many older adults take medications such as antidepressants, narcotic pain relievers, or cardiac drugs that can cause some urinary retention, eventually resulting in incontinence.

Older adults who have mobility problems frequently have urinary incontinence. Individuals who have some difficulty rising from a chair or bed, or who walk slowly, often have periods of incontinence simply because they cannot get to the restroom in time. Lack of mobility causes the individual to be dependent on others for toileting, and this frequently leads to urinary incontinence problems. This is a common problem for the institutionalized older adult.

SUMMARY

The urinary system includes the kidneys, ureters, bladder, and urethra. This system maintains homeostasis in the body by excreting and reabsorbing important electrolytes, compounds, and water. Urinary disorders range from mild infections to very serious diseases such as cancer. The most common signs and symptoms of urinary dysfunction include an abnormality in the urine or in the individual's ability to urinate. The most common disorders of the urinary system include infections and incontinence.

Some diseases are diagnosed by urinalysis or urine culture and sensitivity, but radiologic examinations are also used. A cystoscopy can be performed for diagnostic or treatment purposes. In the older adult, urinary incontinence is the most frequent problem of the system. Urinary disorders can be the result of urinary system pathology or of disease or malfunction of other body systems.

REVIEW QUESTIONS

Short Answer

1. What are the functions of the urinary system?

2. Which signs and symptoms are associated with common urinary system disorders?

3. Which diagnostic tests are most commonly used to determine the type and cause of urinary system disorders?

4. What is the most common urinary problem in the older adult population?

Matching

5. Match the disorders listed in the left column with the correct definition in the right column:

_____ Urethritis	a. Most commonly used diagnostic test for urinary system disorders
_____ Pyuria	b. Pus in the urine
_____ Oliguria	c. An inflammation of the filtering components of the kidney
_____ Anuria	d. Difficulty urinating
_____ Nocturia	e. Excision of the kidney
_____ Cystectomy	f. Inflammation of the urethra
_____ Dysuria	g. Frequent urination at night
_____ Nephrectomy	h. Surgical removal of the bladder
_____ Urinalysis	i. Scanty urine output
_____ Pyelonephritis	j. Absence of urine output
_____ Glomerulonephritis	k. Inflammation of the kidney pelvis

CASE STUDIES

■ Ms. Hayden, age 55, has been noticing a small amount of urine leakage at intervals when she participates in her low-impact aerobics class. She has noticed this problem for about a year now, but thinks it is nothing to worry about. She tells you that this occurs every time she does aerobics and asks what you think the cause might be. She is also embarrassed to ask her physician about it. How would you respond to Ms. Hayden? Do you think this is a problem for concern? Should she seek medical advice?

■ Jeremy is a 30-year-old truck driver who has had several episodes of kidney stones. Although he states the episodes are extremely painful, he has been able to pass the stones each time he has been afflicted and has not had to have surgery or lithotripsy treatment. He asks you how he might be able to prevent kidney stones from developing in the future. Are there some lifestyle interventions he can institute to prevent the recurrence of kidney stones? What would you tell him? Where could he find additional information about this?

Study Tools
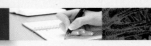

Workbook

Complete Chapter 13

Online Resources

PowerPoint® presentations

Animation

BIBLIOGRAPHY

Baldwin, S. (2011). Helping patients manage hypertension. *Nursing 41*(8), 60–63.

Borch, M., Baron, B., Davey, A., Hattala, P., Kiernan, M., Rust, K., & Yovanovich, J. (2011). Management of patients with interstitial cystitis: A case study. *Urologic Nursing 31*(3), 183–189.

Busuttil-Leaver, R. (2011). Chronic diseases and incontinence. *Practice Nurse 41*(14), 32–36.

Castner, D. (2011). Management of patients on hemodialysis before, during, and after hospitalization: Challenges and suggestions for improvements. *Nephrology Nursing Journal 38*(4), 319–330.

Cutrell, J., & Reilly, R. (2011). Miscellaneous stone types. *Clinical Reviews in Bone & Mineral Metabolism 9*(3/4), 229–240.

Donovan, K. A., Boyington, A. R., Ismail-Khan, R., & Wyman, J. F. (2012). Urinary symptoms in breast cancer. *Cancer 118*(3), 582–593.

Drug news. (2011). *Nursing 41*(8), 16.

Fassett, R., Robertson, I., Mace, R., Youl, L., Challenor, S., & Bull, R. (2011). Palliative care in end-stage kidney disease. *Nephrology 16*(1), 4–12.

Freitas, P. M., Pucci, L. L., Vieira, M. S., Lino, R. S., Oliveira, C. A., Cunha, L. C., & Valadares, M. C. (2011). Diuretic activity and acute oral toxicity of *Palicourea coriacea* (Cham.) K Schum. *Journal of Ethnopharmacology 134*(2), 501–503.

Geraghty, J. (2011). Introducing a new skin-care regimen for the incontinent patient. *British Journal of Nursing 20*(7), 409–415.

Hobson, K., Gomm, S., Murtagh, F., & Caress, A. (2011). National survey of the current provision of specialist palliative care services for patients with end-stage renal disease. *Nephrology Dialysis Transplantation 26*(4), 1275–1281.

Hooton, T. M., Bradley, S. F., Cardenas, D. D., Colgan, R., Geerlings, S. E., Rice, J. C., & Nicolle, L. E. (2010). Diagnosis, prevention, and treatment of catheter-associated urinary tract infection in adults: 2009 international

clinical practice guidelines from the Infectious Diseases Society of America. *Clinical Infectious Diseases 50*(5), 625–663.

Kell, S. (2011). Renal cell carcinoma: Treatment options. *British Journal of Nursing 20*(9), 536–539.

Leaver, R. (2011). Essential guide to urinary incontinence. *Practice Nurse 41*(8), 33–36.

National Kidney Foundation. (2012). *www.kidney.org* (accessed February 2012).

Newman, D. K., & Willson, M. M. (2011). Review of intermittent catheterization and current best practices. *Urologic Nursing 31*(1), 12–48.

Noble, H. (2011). An aging renal population: Is dialysis always the answer? *British Journal of Nursing 20*(9), 545–547.

Paramanandam, G., Prommer, E., & Schwenke, D. C. (2011). Adverse effects in hospice patients with chronic kidney disease receiving hydromorphone. *Journal of Palliative Medicine 14*(9), 1029–1033.

Pittman, G. (2011). Red meat lovers have more kidney cancer. Reuters News. *www.reuters.com* (accessed December 2011).

Steiber, A. L. (2010). Renal nutrition update. *Renal & Urology News 9*(11), 21.

Team care in preparing patients with stage 4 chronic kidney disease for renal replacement therapy. (2011). *Nephrology Nursing Journal 38*(2), 193.

Thompson, J. A. (2009). Metastatic renal cell carcinoma. *Clinical Journal of Oncology Nursing 13*(Suppl), 8–12.

Tuckett, A., Hodgkinson, B., Hegney, D., Paterson, J., & Kralik, D. (2011). Effectiveness of educational interventions to raise men's awareness of bladder and bowel health. *International Journal of Evidence-Based Healthcare 9*(2), 81–96.

Ward-Smith, P. (2011). Quality versus quantity of life: What is the appropriate treatment outcome? *Urologic Nursing 31*(6), 375–381.

Yaklin, K. M. (2011). Acute kidney injury: An overview of pathophysiology and treatments. *Nephrology Nursing Journal 38*(1), 13–19.

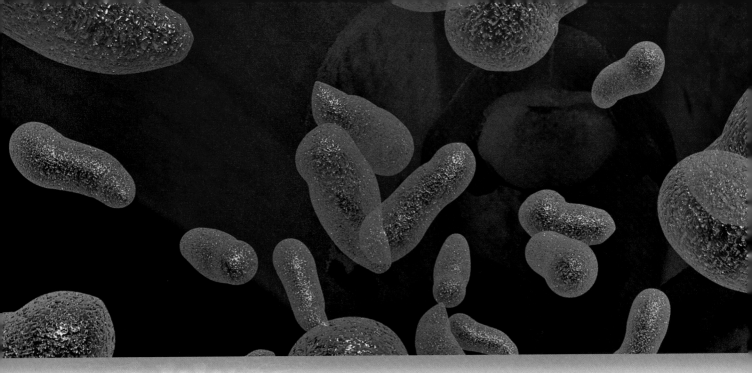

OUTLINE

KEY TERMS

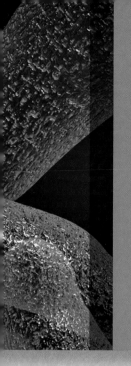

14

Endocrine System Diseases and Disorders

LEARNING OBJECTIVES

Upon completion of the chapter, the learner should be able to:

1. Define the terminology common to the endocrine system and the disorders of the system.

2. Discuss the basic anatomy and physiology of the endocrine system.

3. Identify the important signs and symptoms associated with common endocrine system disorders.

4. Describe the common diagnostics used to determine the type and cause of endocrine system disorders.

5. Identify common disorders of the endocrine system.

6. Describe the typical course and management of the common endocrine system disorders.

7. Describe the effects of aging on the endocrine system and the common disorders associated with aging of the system.

OVERVIEW

*T*he endocrine system is a highly complex system of glands that secrete important hormones for a variety of body functions. The glands of the system work in harmony, discharging the hormones into the bloodstream as needed. The disorders of the system can be caused by problems in the primary gland or in another gland whose secretions control the primary gland. Disorders of the endocrine system can be related to oversecretion or undersecretion of the gland's hormones. ■

ANATOMY AND PHYSIOLOGY

The endocrine system consists of many glands located throughout the body (Figure 14–1). It includes the following glands:

1. Hypothalamus—located beneath the thalamus in the area of the third ventricle of the brain

2. Pituitary or hypophysis—located at the base of the brain

3. Pineal—located behind the midbrain

4. Thymus—located in the mediastinal cavity under the sternum, near the heart

5. Thyroid—located in the neck on each side of the trachea

6. Parathyroids—usually four glands, embedded in the posterior part of the thyroid

7. Adrenals—two glands, one on top of each kidney

8. Pancreatic islets—embedded in the pancreas

9. Ovaries (female) and testes (male)—one ovary on each side of the uterus and one testis in each side of the scrotal sac

Each of these glands has a unique function and delivers its secretion as needed into the bloodstream. Table 14–1 lists the glands, their hormones, and the functions of each hormone. The mechanism known as negative feedback controls the amount of hormones secreted into the bloodstream. Although the hypothalamus monitors the hormone secretions, negative feedback regulates the amount secreted. In the negative feedback system, levels of the particular hormone in the bloodstream trigger the release of the hormone as needed. If the concentration of the hormone in the blood is low, the sequence of events stimulates the

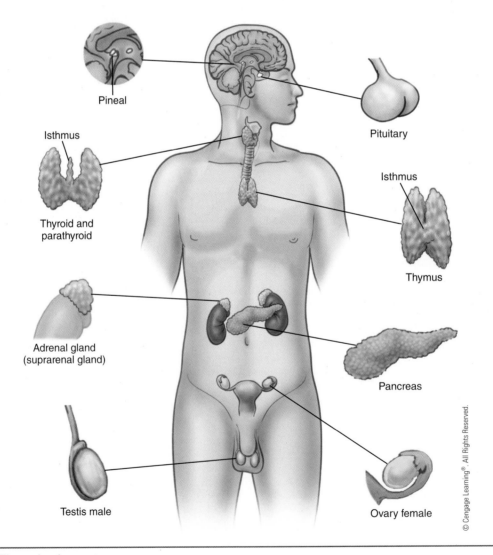

Pineal

Isthmus

Thyroid and parathyroid

Adrenal gland (suprarenal gland)

Testis male

Pituitary

Isthmus

Thymus

Pancreas

Ovary female

FIGURE 14–1   The endocrine system.

TABLE 14–1 The Endocrine Glands: Their Hormones and Hormone Functions

Endocrine Gland	Hormone	Hormone Function
Hypothalamus	Inhibiting hormones and releasing hormones	Inhibits or releases hormones from the anterior pituitary
Hypophysis (Pituitary)		
Adenohypophysis (Anterior Pituitary)	Thyrotropin hormone (TSH)	Stimulates release of thyroid gland hormones
	Adrenocorticotropin hormone (ACTH)	Stimulates release of adrenal cortex hormones
	Somatotropin hormone (STH)	Stimulates growth
	Melanocyte-stimulating hormone (MSH)	Stimulates melanin production
	Lactogenic hormone (prolactin)	Stimulates mammary glands and lactation
	Follicle-stimulating hormone (FSH)	Induces ovulation in females and testosterone secretion in males
	Luteinizing hormone (LH; also called interstitial cell–stimulating hormone, ICSH)	Stimulates estrogen production in females and testosterone production in males
Neurohypophysis	Antidiuretic hormone (ADH)	Increases reabsorption of water in the distal tubules of the kidneys
(Posterior Pituitary)	Oxytocin	Stimulates uterine contraction and the initiation of breast milk flow in females and increases the ejection of sperm into the seminal fluid in males
Pineal	Melatonin	Affects circadian rhythms
Thymus	Thymopoietin	Causes immune response development in the newborn and maintains it in the adult
Thyroid	Triiodothyronine (T_3)	Stimulates growth and development
	Thyroxine (T_4)	Regulates metabolism
	Calcitonin	Increases calcium deposits into the bones
Parathyroid	Parathormone (PTH)	Regulates calcium and phosphate levels and increases reabsorption of calcium from the bones
Adrenals		
Adrenal Cortex	Glucocorticoids	Affect stress reactions; promote protein and fat use to raise blood sugar; affect sodium and water reabsorption
	Mineralocorticoids	Promote sodium and water reabsorption
	Sex hormones	Develop secondary sex characteristics
Adrenal Medulla	Epinephrine	Fight or flight response
		Increases blood pressure and metabolism
	Norepinephrine	Causes vasoconstriction and increases blood pressure
Pancreas Islets		
Alpha Cells	Glucagon	Increases blood glucose levels and is counter-regulatory to insulin
Beta Cells	Insulin	Regulates protein, carbohydrate, and fat metabolism
Delta Cells	Somatostatin	Counterregulatory to insulin, glucagon, and somatotropin (STH)
Ovaries	Estrogen	Regulate development, maturation, secondary sex characteristics, and the reproductive cycle in females
	Progesterone	
Testes	Testosterone	Regulates growth and development, maturation, secondary sex characteristics, and the reproductive system in males

gland to secrete more hormones. In like manner, if the concentration of the hormone in the blood is higher than normal, the feedback mechanism triggers the gland to suppress the release of more hormones.

The hypothalamus, located in the third ventricle area of the brain, contains neurosecretory cells that secrete hypothalamic hormones. These hormones regulate the function of the anterior pituitary gland. The hypothalamus also produces the two hormones stored in the neurohypophysis or posterior pituitary gland.

The pituitary gland, also known as the hypophysis gland, is divided into two distinct parts. The adenohypophysis, or anterior part of the gland, produces several hormones that affect other endocrine glands. These include adrenocorticotropin hormone (ACTH), thyrotropin hormone (TSH), somatotropin hormone (STH), melanocyte-stimulating hormone (MSH), lactogenic hormone (prolactin), follicle-stimulating hormone (FSH), and luteinizing hormone (LH; also called interstitial cell–stimulating hormone, ICSH).

The posterior pituitary, also called the neurohypophysis, stores two hormones that are secreted by the hypothalamus. Oxytocin (Pitocin) helps the progress of labor in the pregnant female and causes uterine contractions after childbirth. It also affects the cells in the breasts, causing a release of milk during lactation. Antidiuretic hormone (ADH), also known as **vasopressin**, is also released from the neurohypophysis. It affects the reabsorption of water from the renal tubules.

The pineal gland, located behind the midbrain, secretes melatonin. It might also secrete other hormones that interact with the hypothalamus and the pituitary gland to cause the secretion of hormones from other glands.

The thymus gland, located just below the clavicle behind the sternum, secretes thymopoietin, a hormone that stimulates the development of lymphocytes. Lymphocytes are important for immunity development and prevention of infections.

The thyroid gland, located in the neck on either side of the trachea, secretes thyroxine (T_4), triiodothyronine (T_3), and calcitonin. These hormones are released as needed in response to the thyroid-stimulating hormone secreted by the pituitary gland. T_4 and T_3 increase metabolic activity. Calcitonin affects the regulation of calcium and works in opposition to the hormone secreted by the parathyroid gland.

Embedded in the posterior part of the thyroid gland are the parathyroid glands. There are usually four of these, but there can be more. The parathyroid glands secrete parathormone, important in the regulation of calcium and phosphorus in the body.

The adrenal glands, located on top of each kidney, have two distinct parts. The cortex, the outer part, secretes **mineralocorticoids**, **glucocorticoids**, and **androgens**. The mineralocorticoids promote sodium retention. The glucocorticoids affect the metabolism of protein, glucose, and fats. **Cortisol** is the main glucocorticoid and is important for metabolism of carbohydrates. The androgens enhance masculinization. The most common androgen hormone is testosterone. The adrenal medulla or middle section secretes epinephrine and norepinephrine.

The beta cells located in the pancreas secrete **insulin**, another important hormone. Insulin is most important in the metabolism of glucose, but it also promotes fatty acid synthesis and amino acid entry into cells. Insulin secretion is regulated by the feedback mechanism and by counterregulatory hormones such as **glucagon**, cortisol, epinephrine, and the growth hormone.

The ovaries and testes secrete the sex hormones, as they are commonly known. The ovaries secrete **estrogen** and **progesterone**, important for development and maturation and maintaining the functions of the reproductive system. The testes secrete testosterone, important for growth and development, secondary sex characteristics, and maintaining the reproductive system functions. See Chapter 17, "Reproductive System Diseases and Disorders," for more information about the reproductive system.

Consider This ...

There are about 30 hormones in our body being produced by the various glands of the endocrine system.

Media Link

View an animation on the endocrine system on the Online Resources.

COMMON SIGNS AND SYMPTOMS

Most endocrine disorders are due to hypo- or hypersecretion by a gland; diagnosis depends on matching the signs and symptoms with the hormone dysfunction. The difficulty in diagnosing endocrine disorders is related to tracking the problem to the correct source. For instance, a pituitary dysfunction can easily lead to signs and symptoms of multiple gland disorders; a decreased secretion of thyroid-stimulating hormone from the pituitary might initially lead one to believe that the thyroid gland itself is dysfunctional. Some common signs and symptoms of endocrine system disorders include mental abnormalities, lethargy or fatigue, and tissue atrophy.

DIAGNOSTIC TESTS

The only endocrine glands that can be physically examined are the thyroid glands and testes; enlargement or atrophy of these glands can be felt, and severe enlargement can be seen. Assessment of proper function of the endocrine organs can be accomplished with blood or urine testing for the hormones they produce. Blood glucose and hemoglobin A1C (HbA1C) are used to diagnose diabetes mellitus and to monitor the progression of the disease. Computerized tomography (CT) and magnetic resonance imaging (MRI) can be used to check for presence of tumors or alteration in organ size.

COMMON DISEASES OF THE ENDOCRINE SYSTEM

Endocrine diseases are the result of abnormally high or low hormone secretion by endocrine glands. Abnormal secretion might be due to the size of the gland: abnormally large or hypertrophied glands tend to produce abnormally high hormone levels, whereas abnormally small or atrophied glands tend to produce abnormally low levels. Abnormal gland size can be the result of injury to the gland by surgery, trauma, infection, or radiation. Abnormal function of endocrine glands leads to many physical and mental abnormalities. Abnormalities vary with the amount of hormone secreted (hypersecretion or hyposecretion) and the age of the individual involved.

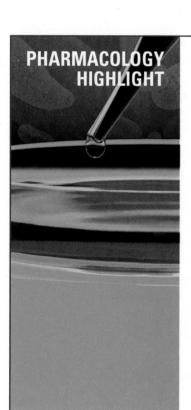

PHARMACOLOGY HIGHLIGHT

Common Drugs for Endocrine Disorders

CATEGORY	EXAMPLES OF MEDICATIONS
Antidiabetics (also known as hypoglycemic or antihyperglycemic agents) Drugs used to treat diabetes	
Hormones	Insulin (many types; rapid acting, intermediate acting, and long acting)
Peptide analogs	exenatide, liraglutide, or alogliptin
Biguanides	metformin
Thiazolidinediones	pioglitazone
Sulfonylureas	tolazamide or glimepiride
Dipeptidyl peptidase-4 inhibitors	sitagliptin
Meglitinides	repaglinide
Hormones Drugs used to treat low hormone levels or other types of endocrine disorders	hydrocortisone, fludrocortisone, prednisone, prednisolone, triamcinolone, methimazole, levothyroxine, oxytocin, pramlintide, Premarin, progesterone, testosterone, desmopressin, or vasopressin

Consider This ...

The physician specialist of the endocrine system is called an endocrinologist.

Pituitary Gland Diseases

The anterior pituitary gland produces tropic (going toward or changing) hormones. These hormones stimulate target organs to grow or produce specific hormones. Growth hormone (GH or somatotropin) promotes growth and development of all body tissues. Other target organs are the thyroid, adrenal gland, testes, and ovaries.

The posterior pituitary gland produces ADH and oxytocin. Diseases of the posterior gland are rare. One worth mentioning is syndrome of inappropriate antidiuretic hormone secretion (SIADH). It is usually related to head trauma, brain tumors, or stroke and is characterized by excessive release of ADH, resulting in water retention and elevated sodium levels.

HYPERPITUITARISM

■ **DESCRIPTION.** Hyperpituitarism is an abnormal increase in the activity of the pituitary gland. This oversecretion especially affects GH production, leading to excessive growth of bones and tissues.

■ **ETIOLOGY.** The most common cause is benign pituitary tumors, which lead to excessive secretion of the adenohypophyseal trophic hormones. Carcinoid tumors can also cause hyperpituitarism. This condition often affects other areas controlled by the pituitary such as thyroid and prolactin hormones.

■ **SYMPTOMS.** If hyperpituitarism occurs before puberty, **giantism** occurs (Figure 14–2). Children affected with hyperpituitarism can grow as much as 6 inches in a year. Sexual development is usually slowed; mental development might be normal or slowed.

If hyperpituitarism occurs in an adult, **acromegaly** (ACK-roh-MEG-ah-lee; acro = extremity, megaly = enlargement) occurs: the long bones are unable to grow in length, but the small bones of the hands, feet, and face enlarge. Common symptoms include large, doughy hands and large feet. Abnormal facial features

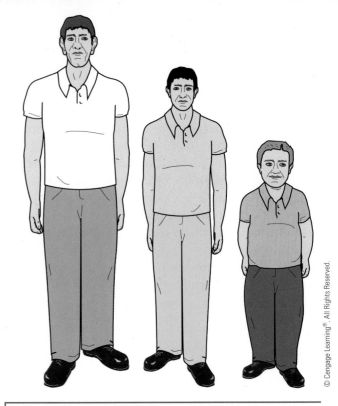

FIGURE 14–2   Giantism and dwarfism. (Right) A dwarf. (Left) A giant. A normal sized individual is in the center.

include enlarged jaw with widely spaced teeth, tongue enlargement leading to slurred speech, large forehead, and oily, tough skin with skin pigmentation changes—darker or lighter. Females can also have excessive hair growth.

Acromegaly is a chronic, disfiguring disease that usually shortens life expectancy and often leads to congestive heart failure and respiratory and cerebrovascular diseases.

■ **DIAGNOSIS.** Diagnosis is made through examination of physical characteristics of abnormal or excessive growth in children and acromegaly in adults. Blood testing reveals high levels of GH, thyroid, and prolactin. MRI often reveals a pituitary tumor.

■ **TREATMENT.** In children, microsurgical removal, radiation, and drug therapy can decrease the secretion of GH and slow the growing process. Prognosis for giantism is usually good. In adults, surgical removal of pituitary tumors often leads to hypopituitarism, and these tumors tend to recur.

■ **PREVENTION.** There is no known prevention for hyperpituitarism except to prevent injury or trauma to the gland.

HYPOPITUITARISM

■ **DESCRIPTION.** Hypopituitarism is an abnormal decrease in the activity of the pituitary gland, leading to a deficiency or absence of any or all of the tropic hormones.

■ **ETIOLOGY.** A common cause is a tumor on the pituitary gland. As the tumor increases in size, damage to the gland interferes with hormone production. Other diseases and traumas can also damage the pituitary, including radiation treatments, head injuries, stroke, brain surgery, brain tumors, and infection.

■ **SYMPTOMS.** Because the pituitary gland is the master gland, hypopituitarism can lead to a variety of problems involving the function of all target organs (Figure 14–3). GH and gonadotropin are the most common deficiencies in hypopituitarism. The degree of hypopituitarism can range from mild to severe.

A decrease in growth hormone leads to impaired growth of all body tissues with the most severe decreases causing **dwarfism** (see Figure 14–2). Children affected with dwarfism are proportionately small and underdeveloped sexually and might or might not suffer from mental challenges. Gonadotropin deficiency can lead to abnormal development or absence of secondary sexual characteristics.

In adult women, this deficiency can cause amenorrhea and infertility. Adult men might have a lowered testosterone level, decreased libido (la-BE-doe; sex drive), and abnormal loss of facial and body hair. A decrease in ACTH and TSH can lead to metabolic disorders.

If the pituitary gland is destroyed or nonfunctional, a condition called **panhypopituitarism** (pan = all, hypo = decreased) exists and can lead to all the preceding disorders and result in fatal complications.

■ **DIAGNOSIS.** Diagnosis and area of dysfunction can be confirmed by clinical history and blood testing. The dysfunction could involve the pituitary, the individual target organ, or both. Specific blood hormone tests to determine pituitary function can include each tropic hormone (GH, TSH, FSH, LH, and ACTH). Target organ function can be assessed by testing blood levels of each individual organ hormone (T_3, T_4, estrogen, progesterone, testosterone, and cortisol).

■ **TREATMENT.** Treatment of hypopituitarism involves hormone replacement of needed hormones. Constant monitoring and adjusting of hormone levels is needed for optimum results.

■ **PREVENTION.** There is no known prevention for hyperpituitarism except to prevent injury or trauma to the gland.

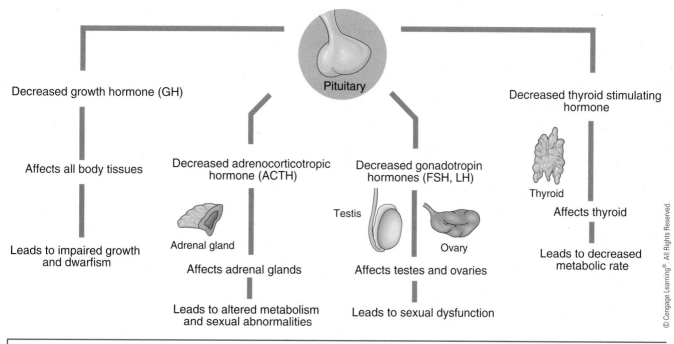

FIGURE 14–3 Effects of hypopituitarism.

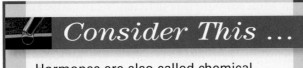

Consider This ...

Hormones are also called chemical messengers.

DIABETES INSIPIDUS (DI)

■ **DESCRIPTION.** *Diabetes* is a general term meaning "passing through," and describes a variety of disorders characterized by **polyuria** (POL-ee-YOU-ree-ah; poly = many, uria = urine), excessive urination. There are several types of diabetes, but diabetes mellitus, a disorder of the pancreas, is the disease most often thought of as diabetes. Diabetes mellitus and gestational diabetes will be discussed later in the chapter.

DI is a disorder characterized by severe thirst and polyuria. There are two types of insipidus, depending on the cause, central DI (pituitary related) and nephrogenic DI (kidney related).

■ **ETIOLOGY.** Central DI is caused by a decrease in the release of vasopressin, or ADH, by the posterior portion of the pituitary gland. The cause is damage to the pituitary gland by tumor, surgery, traumatic head injury, or infection.

Nephrogenic DI occurs when there is a defect in the kidney tubules leading to inability of the kidney to respond to ADH. The defect can be an inherited (genetic) disorder or related to chronic kidney disease or kidney damage caused by certain medications. In many cases, the cause is unknown.

■ **SYMPTOMS.** Without antidiuretic (anti = against, di = run through, uri = urine) hormone, the individual has excessive polyuria and might urinate between 2 and 15 gallons of urine in 24 hours. The urine quality is colorless and dilute. The individual experiences excessive **polydipsia** (POL-ee-DIP-see-ah; poly = many, dipsia = thirst or drinking) in an effort to overcome dehydration. Other symptoms include hypotension, dizziness, and constipation.

■ **DIAGNOSIS.** Testing for DI includes a urinalysis and a water restriction test. The urinalysis of an affected individual will show colorless urine with a very low specific gravity. The water restriction test includes limiting the suspected individual's water intake for several hours while measuring the urine output, blood pressure, and urine concentration. After several hours, the individual is given vasopressin

medication. If the medication decreases urine output and increases urine concentration, the diagnosis of DI is confirmed. MRI of the kidney and pituitary gland assists in locating the cause.

■ **TREATMENT.** Central DI can be controlled with vasopressin administered as either a nasal spray or as tablets. Nephrogenic DI is treated with fluid intake to match urine output and drugs that lower urine output. Prognosis is generally good.

■ **PREVENTION.** Many cases might not be preventable. Prompt treatment of infections, injuries, and tumors can reduce risk, however.

Thyroid Gland Diseases

The activity of the thyroid gland affects the entire body. The hormone released by the thyroid gland (T_4) regulates metabolism, the rate at which calories are used. In this way, T_4 also regulates body heat, ensuring that the body is kept warm even in a cold environment. T_4 also stimulates the gastrointestinal system by increasing gastric secretions and peristalsis. To make T_4, the thyroid gland requires iodine. Diseases of the thyroid gland are primarily those of hypersecretion and hyposecretion.

HYPERTHYROIDISM

■ **DESCRIPTION.** Hyperthyroidism occurs when the thyroid gland secretes excessive T_3 and T_4. This condition is also known as overactive thyroid and is a type of thyrotoxicosis.

■ **ETIOLOGY.** The cause of hyperthyroidism can be idiopathic (unknown), but there are several known causes of hyperthyroidism, including tumors or **adenoma** (AD-eh-NO-ma; adeno = gland, oma = tumor), heredity, excessive dietary intake of iodine (found in seaweed and liver), and taking too much thyroid hormone medication.

The most common cause is an autoimmune condition called Graves' disease. In this condition, antibodies stimulate the thyroid, leading to glandular hypertrophy. Graves' disease commonly affects young women.

■ **SYMPTOMS.** No matter the cause, the thyroid gland becomes enlarged and produces a characteristic **goiter** (GOI-ter), a noticeable protrusion of the thyroid gland (Figure 14–4). Overproduction of T_4 increases metabolism, leading to symptoms of

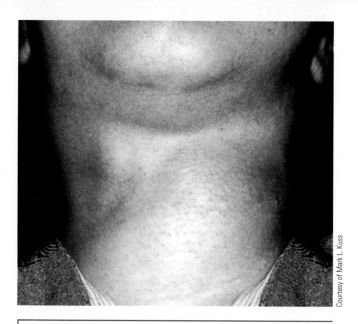

Courtesy of Mark L. Kuss

FIGURE 14–4 Goiter.

tachycardia, nervousness, hyperactivity, weakness, and excessive excitability. The individual has a tremendous appetite but loses weight to the point of extreme thinness. Diarrhea is common because T_4 speeds up peristalsis of the gastrointestinal tract. High metabolic rate causes high heat production, leading to excessive sweating and an intolerance to heat. The skin can be moist, and the individual might have extreme thirst due to this water loss.

One very distinguishing characteristic of hyperthyroidism is a stare in the eyes due to **exophthalmos** (ECK-sof-THAL-mos; abnormal protrusion of the eyeballs) (Figure 14–5) from edema in the tissues

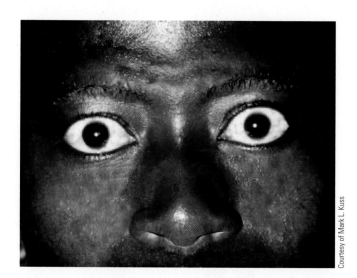

Courtesy of Mark L. Kuss

FIGURE 14–5 Exophthalmos in Graves' disease.

behind the eyes. It can be so severe that the eyelids will not close. Unfortunately, this condition might not totally resolve when the hyperthyroidism is corrected.

■ **DIAGNOSIS.** A diagnosis is made based on history and physical examination and is confirmed with blood tests. An elevated thyroid-stimulating hormone is usually all that is needed to confirm the diagnosis.

■ **TREATMENT.** Hyperthyroidism can be treated with medication, radiation of the thyroid, or surgical removal of all or part of the gland. If the entire gland receives eradication radiation or is surgically removed, hormone replacement medication will be needed for the life of the individual.

A sudden, life-threatening exacerbation of all symptoms of hyperthyroidism is called thyroid storm. This condition can occur in an individual with severe hyperthyroidism or during the immediate postoperative period following a thyroidectomy (ectomy = excision or removal of). Symptoms of **thyroid storm** include severe tachycardia with heart rates reaching 200 beats per minute, tachypnea, and loss of temperature regulation characterized by a rapid and steady increase in body temperature. Emergency medical intervention must be initiated to save the individual's life.

■ **PREVENTION.** There are no general preventive measures for hyperthyroidism, but people who smoke are more likely to develop Graves' disease and ophthalmopathy than people who do not smoke.

SIMPLE GOITER

■ **DESCRIPTION.** Simple goiter is an enlargement of the thyroid gland. It occurs as the thyroid attempts to produce adequate amounts of T_4.

■ **ETIOLOGY.** Causes of goiter include:

- A family history of goiter incidence.

- Eating large amounts of **goitrogenic** (goiter-producing) foods that inhibit production of thyroid hormone. These include soy, peanuts, peaches, spinach, turnips, cabbage, Brussels sprouts, seaweed, and millet.

- Regular use of medications that affect thyroid production, including lithium and propylthiouracil.

- Iodine deficiency is rare in the United States due to the use of iodized table salt, but some people in other parts of the world have iodine deficiency.

■ **SYMPTOMS.** This condition usually affects females and can be asymptomatic until the thyroid gland enlarges to the point of forming a noticeable mass at the front of the neck. If the gland is extremely enlarged, it can cause pressure on the trachea and esophagus and cause dyspnea and dysphagia (dys = difficulty, phagia = swallowing). The main symptom is a swollen thyroid gland. The size can range from a single small nodule to a large neck lump.

■ **DIAGNOSIS.** A physical examination including palpation (feeling the enlarged thyroid gland) and blood tests, ultrasound, and fine-needle biopsy help confirm the diagnosis.

■ **TREATMENT.** Treatment includes administration of potassium iodide initially, followed by increasing iodine in the diet with iodized salt. If the cause is related to goitrogenic foods or drugs, avoidance of these often leads to cure. If the goiter is unresponsive to treatment, surgery might be needed to reduce the size of the gland. Treatment is aimed at stopping the enlargement of the gland, but it will not reduce the current size of the gland. Surgery also might be needed to improve physical appearance and decrease difficulty with breathing and swallowing.

■ **PREVENTION.** Monitoring dietary intake of goitrogenic foods and medications, along with ensuring adequate intake of iodine, helps prevent some types of goiter.

HYPOTHYROIDISM

■ **DESCRIPTION.** Hypothyroidism is the decrease in normal T_4 production.

Advanced hypothyroidism in an adult is called **myxedema** (MICK-seh-DEE-mah). Myxedema commonly occurs in middle-aged women.

Hypothyroidism in infants is rare in the United States. It is caused when any part of the fetus's thyroid fails to develop properly. Congenital hypothyroidism is called **cretinism**. It can be quite devastating, leading to mental and physical growth challenges in the infant and young child.

■ **ETIOLOGY.** There are two fairly common causes of hypothyroidism. The first and most common natural cause is an autoimmune disorder called Hashimoto's disease. This condition occurs most frequently in women. It is believed that lymphocytes react with thyroid tissue, leading to destruction of the thyroid gland tissue. This loss of tissue leaves the thyroid unable to produce adequate amounts of thyroid hormone.

The second cause is the result of medical treatments. Often, treatments to cure hyperthyroidism lead to destruction of part or all of the thyroid gland, leading to hypothyroidism.

In underdeveloped countries, congenital hypothyroidism is more common and is due to an iodine deficiency during the mother's pregnancy.

The symptoms, diagnosis, and treatment plan for hypothyroidism are quite similar regardless of the cause.

■ **SYMPTOMS.** Symptoms of hypothyroidism are the opposite of those for hyperthyroidism. The affected individual is fatigued, drowsy, and sensitive to cold temperature; has thin nails and brittle hair; and gains excessive weight. The individual becomes sluggish, mentally and physically.

An individual with myxedema can exhibit all these symptoms as well as a characteristic swelling or bloating of the facial tissue, thickened tongue, and puffy eyelids.

Children with hypothyroidism, cretins, are dwarfed with a short, stocky body build and a protruding tongue and abdomen. The face is abnormal, with a broad nose, puffy eyelids, and small eyes. Sexual organs fail to develop (Figure 14–6). Muscle growth is slowed to the point that the child is unable to stand or walk. The earlier this condition is discovered,

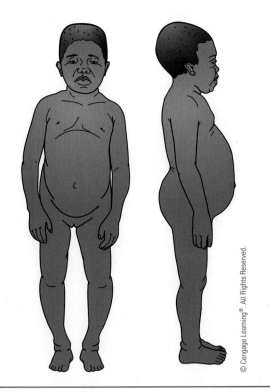

FIGURE 14–6   Cretinism.

the better the prognosis. For this reason, many states mandate a thyroid blood test on newborns.

■ **DIAGNOSIS.** Diagnosis is confirmed by review of symptoms along with thyroid hormone blood test, including T_4, T_3, and free T_4 index (FTI).

■ **TREATMENT.** This condition responds well to treatment with thyroxine hormone replacement. Symptoms usually disappear after a few months of treatment.

■ **PREVENTION.** Most cases of hypothyroidism in the United States are caused by Hashimoto's thyroiditis and cannot be prevented.

Parathyroid Gland Diseases

Parathyroid glands regulate blood calcium levels. Most of the body's calcium (approximately 99%) is stored in the bones, but the remaining 1% circulates in the blood. Blood calcium plays a vital role in blood clotting and muscle contraction, thus affecting heart function. If blood calcium levels drop, parathyroid hormone (parathormone, PTH) increases the level by increasing calcium absorption in the digestive tract, releasing calcium from bone stores, and saving calcium excretion in urine. When blood calcium levels are restored to normal, parathormone is no longer released. Like other endocrine glands, most endocrine diseases of the parathyroid are related to hypersecretion or hyposecretion.

HYPERPARATHYROIDISM

■ **DESCRIPTION.** Hyperparathyroidism is a condition of overproduction of parathormone by one or more of the four parathyroid glands.

■ **ETIOLOGY.** Oversecretion is usually due to a glandular tumor or idiopathic hyperplasia of the gland. Excessive parathormone production causes excessive blood calcium levels called hypercalcemia (hyper = excessive, calc = calcium, emia = blood).

■ **SYMPTOMS.** As previously discussed, this calcium is pulled from the bones, leading to bone weakness and spontaneous fractures. Hypercalcemia also leads to kidney stones because the urinary system—under the influence of parathormone—retains calcium, further increasing blood calcium levels. The digestive system increases absorption of calcium, leading to abdominal pain, vomiting, and constipation. Hypercalcemia also leads to hyperactivity of cardiac muscle, thus causing arrhythmias.

■ **DIAGNOSIS.** Blood tests for parathormone levels assist with diagnosis.

■ **TREATMENT.** Treatment of hyperparathyroidism is directed at the cause. Removal of a tumor or removal of the parathyroid glands might be necessary. Only half of one parathyroid gland is necessary to maintain normal parathormone levels. Other treatments include diuretics to increase urine output, thus forcing excretion of calcium, and limiting dietary intake of calcium. Prognosis is generally good with adequate treatment, although cardiac arrest can occur with severe hyperparathyroidism.

■ **PREVENTION.** There is no known way to prevent primary hyperparathyroidism.

HYPOPARATHYROIDISM

■ **DESCRIPTION.** Hypoparathyroidism is a decrease in the normal amount of parathormone secreted, which leads to abnormally low blood calcium levels.

■ **ETIOLOGY.** This condition is usually the result of surgical removal of all parathyroid glands in an effort to treat hyperparathyroidism or following a thyroidectomy.

■ **SYMPTOMS.** Low blood calcium levels (hypocalcemia) cause irritability to muscles, called **tetany**. Tetany should not be confused with the infectious disease tetanus (lockjaw). The tetany associated with hypoparathyroidism affects the face and hands primarily, causing uncontrolled contraction of these muscles.

■ **DIAGNOSIS.** Physical examination reviewing for symptoms, along with blood tests revealing low blood calcium level and low parathyroid hormone level, aid in diagnosis. Testing for hypocalcemia and hypoparathyroidism may also include checking for Chvostek's (VOHS-tecks) and Trousseau's (true-SOHs) signs (Figure 14–7).

■ **TREATMENT.** Treatment with calcium and vitamin D, which controls absorption of calcium from the gastrointestinal tract, will cure the problem.

■ **PREVENTION.** There are no preventive measures for hypoparathyroidism.

Adrenal Gland Diseases

The adrenal glands, also called the suprarenals because they sit atop the kidneys, have two distinct parts that function quite differently. The inner part,

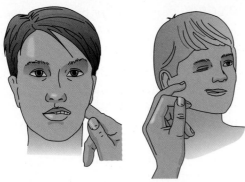

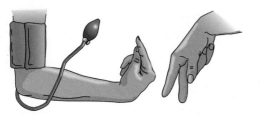

(A) Positive Chvostek's sign. Tapping over facial nerve causes facial muscle spasm.

(B) Positive Trousseau's sign. Pressure to nerves and vessels of upper arm causes muscle spasm.

FIGURE 14–7   Tetany of the hand and face: (A) Chvostek's sign. (B) Trousseau's sign.

called the medulla, releases two hormones, epinephrine (adrenaline) and norepinephrine, when stimulated by the nervous system. These hormones have a direct effect on the vascular system and are known as fight-or-flight hormones. The cortex, or outer part of the adrenal gland, is controlled by the pituitary gland's release of ACTH. The adrenal cortex secretes several hormones.

- **Mineralocorticoids** The primary hormone is **aldosterone**, which regulates salt balance.
- **Glucocorticoids** The primary hormone is cortisol (**cortisone**), or **hydrocortisone**, which regulates carbohydrate metabolism.
- **Sex hormones** The primary ones are androgens and estrogens, which provide male and female characteristics, respectively. Males and females have both of these androgenic sex hormones.

Cortisone is a hormone frequently used to treat inflammatory diseases such as arthritis because it acts as an anti-inflammatory agent. Cortisone does not cure the inflammatory condition; it only relieves the inflammation and the associated pain. Prolonged use of cortisone is avoided whenever possible because it has some detrimental side effects including

hypertension, ulcers, puffy face called moon face, and drowsiness. The anti-inflammatory properties of cortisone reduce the body's inflammatory response. This alteration in the immune system can mask the symptoms of an infection, allowing it to go unnoticed until it is in advanced stages. This side effect of prolonged cortisone use can be potentially life-threatening.

HYPERADRENALISM

Hyperadrenalism is the oversecretion of hormones by the adrenal cortex. The specific forms of hyperadrenalism depend on which hormones are secreted in excess. Three syndromes identified with hyperadrenalism are Conn's, Cushing's, and androgenital syndromes.

CONN'S SYNDROME

■ **DESCRIPTION.** Conn's syndrome, also called hyperaldosteronism, is due to an overproduction of aldosterone, a mineralocorticoid that plays an important role in maintaining blood volume pressure and electrolyte balance. It affects people between ages 30 and 50 and is more common in women than in men.

■ **ETIOLOGY.** This form of hyperadrenalism is most often due to an adrenal cortex tumor.

■ **SYMPTOMS.** Symptoms include hypokalemia (low potassium levels), alkalosis (increased blood pH), and hypertension.

■ **DIAGNOSIS.** Conn's should be suspected in those with hypertension that is resistant to standard treatment. Diagnosing Conn's is important because it represents a cause of hypertension that might be curable. Blood testing for the two hormones that play a role in stimulating aldosterone is helpful and includes aldosterone and rennin testing. Positive testing reveals high aldosterone and low rennin levels.

■ **TREATMENT.** Removal of the tumor usually leads to a good prognosis.

■ **PREVENTION.** There is no known prevention for most causes of hyperaldosteronism.

CUSHING'S SYNDROME

■ **DESCRIPTION.** Cushing's syndrome is due to an overproduction of the cortisol glucocorticoid.

■ **ETIOLOGY.** Cushing's might be caused by a tumor on the pituitary gland or on the adrenal cortex. Prolonged administration of large doses of glucocorticoid steroids (cortisone) will also cause this syndrome.

■ **SYMPTOMS.** Classic symptoms include a round, moon-shaped face and a buffalo hump on the upper back. Other symptoms include fatigue, weakness, poor wound healing, a rotund abdomen with pencil-thin arms and legs, hypertension, and **striae** (stretch marks) on the skin (Figure 14–8).

■ **DIAGNOSIS.** Blood test to measure cortisol levels and MRI to view tumors aid in diagnosis.

■ **TREATMENT.** Surgical removal of the tumor or the adrenal cortex may correct the condition. Lifetime hormone therapy to replace this hormone is then needed. Cushing's syndrome may develop in individuals receiving long-term glucocorticoid steroids. These individuals need to be carefully monitored for symptoms of Cushing's syndrome.

■ **PREVENTABLE.** Cushing's syndrome may be prevented by early detection and treatment of the associated symptoms.

ANDROGENITAL SYNDROME

■ **DESCRIPTION.** Androgenital syndrome is due to an overproduction of sex hormones by the adrenal cortex. It is also known as adrenal **virilism** (masculinization or feminization), depending on the excessive hormone.

■ **ETIOLOGY.** Androgenital syndrome is hereditary. Most of these conditions involve excessive, or hypersecretion of, androgen.

■ **SYMPTOMS.** Increased androgen leads to premature sexual development in male children, also called **precocious** (early development) puberty. In female children, overproduction of androgen leads to excessive hair growth on the legs, chest, and abdomen; an enlarged clitoris; a deepened voice; and **amenorrhea** (ah-MEN-oh-REE-ah; a = without, menorrhea = menses).

If adrenal feminization occurs due to excessive estrogen production, female children experience premature sexual development (precocious puberty). Male children with an overproduction of estrogen experience **gynecomastia** (GUY-neh-koh-MAS-tee-ah; excessive breast development), testicular atrophy, and decreased libido.

Virilism in the adult female leads to symptoms of **hirsutism** (HER-soot-izm), or abnormal hair on the face and body; decreased breast size; and amenorrhea.

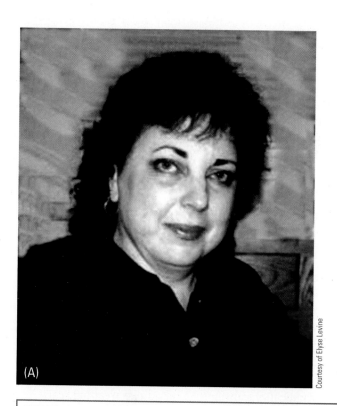 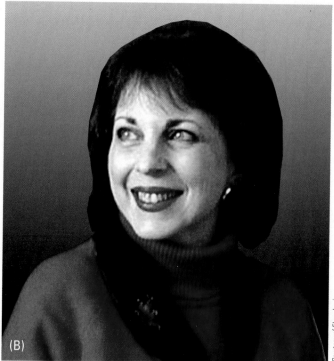

FIGURE 14–8 Cushing's syndrome. (A) Individual affected with Cushing's. (B) Same individual after treatment.

■ **DIAGNOSIS.** Physical exam of symptoms and blood testing for elevated ACTH aid in diagnosis.

■ **TREATMENT.** Treatment of adrenal cortex tumors usually involves surgical removal of the tumor.

■ **PREVENTION.** Because this is a hereditary disease, it is not preventable.

OTHER DISEASE OF THE ADRENAL GLANDS

HYPOADRENALISM

■ **DESCRIPTION.** Hypoadrenalism, Addison's disease, is an uncommon undersecretion of hormones by the adrenal cortex.

■ **ETIOLOGY.** Causes of Addison's disease include an autoimmune disorder, tumor of the pituitary gland, tuberculosis, and prolonged steroid hormone therapy. As much as 90% of the adrenal cortex can be destroyed before hyposecretion occurs.

■ **SYMPTOMS.** Symptoms of Addison's disease can be mild to life-threatening. Lack of mineralocorticoids allows depletion of sodium, leading to diarrhea and dehydration. Deficiency in glucocorticoids affects blood sugar levels, leading to **hypoglycemia** (HIGH-poh-gly-SEE-me-ah; hypo = decreased, glyc = glucose, emia = blood). Increased ACTH levels by the pituitary lead to a hyperpigmentation, or increased skin coloring, ranging from yellow to dark brown. This increased skin color affects the palms, elbows, scars, and skin folds and the areola of the nipples.

■ **DIAGNOSIS.** Diagnosis is based on medical history, symptoms, physical examination, and blood tests, including cortisol and ACTH.

■ **TREATMENT.** Treatment includes a combination of glucocorticoids and mineralocorticoids to replace the adrenal insufficiency.

■ **PREVENTION.** There are no guidelines for preventing Addison's disease.

Pancreatic Islets of Langerhans Diseases

The pancreas is both an exocrine and endocrine gland. As an exocrine gland, it secretes digestive juices through ducts into the digestive system. As an endocrine gland, it secretes two hormones—insulin and glucagon—directly into the blood. Both of these hormones are secreted by specialized tissue called

HEALTHY HIGHLIGHT

Using Steroids Therapeutically

■ Anabolic steroids are synthetic derivatives of testosterone that have anabolic (tissue-building) effects. These drugs were initially used by athletes to increase strength and endurance, but because of their potential for abuse, steroids have been placed in the Controlled Substance Act in category C-III. General uses include treatment for chronic infections, some types of anemia, extensive burns, and severe trauma.

■ Use of steroids to enhance athletic performance is not recommended and has been banned in professional athletics. Serious irreversible side effects occur with long-term use of steroids and include kidney damage, increased risk of liver tumors, and increased risk of heart disease. Long-term steroid users exhibit increased irritability and aggressive behavior. In women, masculinization occurs as evidenced by hirsutism, menstrual difficulties, male patterned baldness, and a deepening of the voice. Males experience a decrease in testosterone production, leading to testicular atrophy, decrease in sperm production, and impotence. Individuals taking steroids need to follow the following recommended guidelines:
  ■ A well-balanced diet, including adequate proteins and carbohydrates, should be followed during steroid therapy.
  ■ Never share steroid medications with others.
  ■ Do not stop taking these medications abruptly. A scheduled weaning regimen should be determined and monitored by a qualified physician.

islets of Langerhans that are scattered throughout the pancreas; however, insulin and glucagon have an antagonistic relationship. Insulin lowers blood sugar, whereas glucagon raises it. The overall effect of these hormones maintains a normal blood sugar level (80–120 mg/dl).

When blood sugar levels rise, for instance after a meal, insulin is secreted. Insulin assists in moving sugar out of the blood and into the tissues, thus decreasing the blood sugar level (Figure 14–9). Without adequate insulin, the blood sugar level rises, and the tissues are depleted of sugar.

Sugar, or glucose, is the primary source of energy for all tissue cells. Without glucose, cells must burn fats and proteins for energy. When tissue cells burn fat and protein, they produce a waste product called **ketones**. Ketones are picked up by the blood to be filtered and excreted by the kidneys. Acetone, a part of this ketone waste, is excreted by the respiratory system, giving the affected individual a fruity- or sweet-smelling breath. This condition of having ketones in the blood, breath, and urine is called ketosis. Chemically, a large part of ketones is acidic in nature, which leads to metabolic acidosis, or a low pH, in the body tissues. For this reason, ketosis is often called **ketoacidosis**.

When carbohydrates or sugars are eaten, the extra sugar, the amount not needed for immediate energy, is stored, primarily, in the liver as **glycogen**. If blood sugar levels drop, for instance during exercise, the pancreas secretes glucagon. Glucagon circulates in the blood and stimulates the liver to release glycogen in the form of glucose, thus raising the blood sugar to normal.

DIABETES MELLITUS (DM)

■ **DESCRIPTION.** DM, commonly known simply as diabetes, is the most common major disease of the endocrine pancreas.

■ **ETIOLOGY.** DM is a chronic disease affecting carbohydrate, or sugar, metabolism due to inadequate production of insulin by the pancreatic islets of Langerhans.

■ **SYMPTOMS.** Diabetes is characterized by symptoms of polyuria (excessive urination), polydipsia (excessive thirst), and polyphagia (excessive eating). **Glycosuria** (GLYE-koh-SOO-ree-ah; glyco = glycogen or sugar, uria = urine), or the spilling of sugar in the urine, is also a common symptom. The excessive sugar in the blood, known as **hyperglycemia** (hyper = excessive, glyc = glycogen or glucose, emia = blood), causes the kidney to filter out part of the excess, resulting in glycosuria. Hyperglycemia indicates that sugar is not being pulled into the tissues, and cells are using fat for energy, resulting in the formation of ketones (the waste product of fat metabolism). Ketones can be found in the blood and urine and smelled on the breath.

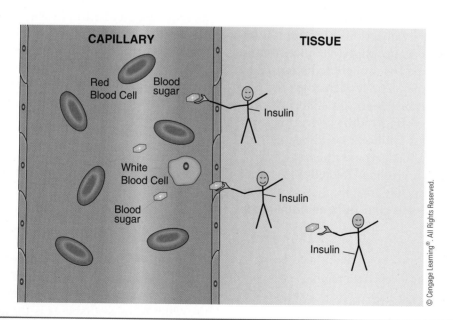

FIGURE 14–9   Effect of insulin on blood sugar. Insulin assists in moving sugar out of the blood and into the tissues, thus decreasing blood sugar levels. Think of insulin as "offering a hand" in pulling blood sugar levels down.

HEALTHY HIGHLIGHT

Assessing Risk for Diabetes

The American Diabetes Association (ADA) recommends that individuals be checked for diabetes every 3 years after age 45. Individuals who might be at higher risk for diabetes (overweight, family history, etc.) should be checked earlier than age 45 and more frequently. In assessing for risk, the individual should:

- Assess overall health status:
  - Review current health status with a health care provider.
  - Check body mass index (BMI).
- Assess environment:
  - Review how the home environment might affect the individual's health status and eating habits.
  - Review food shopping habits.
  - Look at work environment and how it supports or discourages healthy living and eating patterns.

A "Changing Health Habits Assessment" can be found on the ADA Web site. It also contains helpful information for making a plan to reduce one's risk for developing diabetes.

Source: Modified from the American Diabetes Association (2012).

There are two types of DM:

Type 1

Formerly known as insulin-dependent diabetes mellitus (IDDM) or juvenile-onset diabetes. This form of diabetes is the most serious and usually occurs quite suddenly. It affects children and young adults before age 25 and requires daily injections of insulin. Insulin must be injected because digestive juices would destroy oral forms. Type 1 is thought to be caused by an autoimmune disorder. The tendency for the disease also is thought to be genetically inherited. The immune system, when triggered by a virus or some other stressor, develops antibodies and begins warring against the islets of Langerhans, thereby destroying the insulin-secreting cells. Affected individuals generally do not secrete any insulin, making regulation of blood glucose levels quite difficult. Individuals with type 1 must:

- Follow a strict diet
- Monitor blood sugar levels on a regular basis
- Administer the needed amounts of insulin

Exercise and stress can alter insulin needs and must be considered as part of the treatment plan.

Type 2

Formerly known as noninsulin-dependent diabetes mellitus (NIDDM) or adult onset-diabetes. This is the more common form of DM. Until recently, this type of diabetes was seen primarily in obese females over age 40, but due to the dramatic increase in childhood and adolescent obesity, the trend is changing. Obesity has led to a dramatic increase in the incidence of type 2 diabetes among children and adolescents over the past two decades. The Centers for Disease Control and Prevention (2012) reports that:

- Childhood obesity has more than tripled in the past 30 years!
- Children age 6 to 11 years in the United States who are obese increased from 7% in 1980 to nearly 20% in 2008.
- Adolescents age 12 to 19 years who are obese increased from 5% to 18% over the same period.

These drastic increases raise concern about the future of Americans' health. It is well known that obesity increases the risk of many diseases, including type 2 diabetes.

This form of diabetes is thought to be due to a wearing out of the pancreatic islets of Langerhans. It is believed that excessive carbohydrate consumption over the life of the individual places such a heavy demand on the pancreas to produce the needed insulin. This increased demand literally wears out the pancreatic cells, leading to type 2 diabetes. Type 2 is usually controlled with diet, exercise, and oral and/or injectable medications that stimulate insulin secretion.

Complications of DM may be classified as immediate or long term. Immediate and life-threatening complications of type 1 diabetes include diabetic coma and insulin shock. Both of these complications occur as a result of improper insulin administration, either too much or not enough insulin. Diabetic coma can occur as a result of not administering enough insulin or taking in too many carbohydrates in the diet. Symptoms of diabetic coma are those related to *hyperglycemia* and include:

- Polyuria
- Polydipsia
- Dehydration
- Ketoacidosis

Diabetic coma usually progresses rather slowly. The affected individual becomes lethargic and, if untreated, slips into a coma. The individual in a coma will have a slow deep-breathing pattern and fruity- or sweet-smelling breath. The individual requires emergency medical treatment with insulin and intravenous fluids.

Insulin shock occurs quite rapidly and is the result of taking too much insulin, not eating enough food, or participating in excessive exercise. The affected individual becomes *hypoglycemic* with symptoms of:

- Diaphoresis (sweating)
- Light-headedness
- Trembling

Without treatment, the affected individual progresses quite rapidly into a state of confusion followed by coma. Individuals in insulin shock need immediate emergency medical treatment with intravenous glucose to raise blood sugar levels (Table 14–2).

Long-term complications of diabetes usually appear gradually after many years. With improper carbohydrate metabolism, **lipids** or fats are pulled into the bloodstream for cellular energy. This increase in lipids in the vascular system leads to atherosclerosis.

TABLE 14–2 Emergency Treatment of Diabetic Coma or Insulin Shock

Step 1: Determine a Need for Intervention

Unfortunately, it is usually difficult to determine whether an affected individual is suffering from diabetic coma or insulin shock, especially if found in a comatose state. The best rule to follow in this case is, "when in doubt—sugar." Raising an already elevated glucose level is not as life-threatening as allowing the blood sugar level to remain low or to drop even further.

Step 2: Administer Glucose

If the individual is still alert, drinking fruit juice with sugar added can be effective in raising blood sugar level. If juice is not available, candy of any type will help. If the individual is unconscious and emergency medical assistance is not available, turn the individual on his or her side and place table sugar or hard candy in the lower cheek of the mouth to help raise blood sugar. Emergency medical assistance should be sought immediately.

Additional Important Information

Individuals with diabetes should wear a diabetic alert tag and should carry some type of carbohydrate treat with them at all times for use during a hypoglycemic reaction. If an incident occurs, the tag alerts the medical responder or other individuals aiding the person that he or she is diabetic and, thus, could be having a hypoglycemic or hyperglycemic reaction. This saves time between assessing the victim for probable cause of the problem and treating the person. The diabetic alert tag also helps those who are assisting the individual to recognize the fruity breath of a hyperglycemic diabetic as ketone breath rather than mistaking it as alcohol breath. Allowing a hyperglycemic individual to sleep it off can be a fatal mistake.

Atherosclerosis leads to a variety of complications, including myocardial infarction, cerebrovascular accidents or strokes, and peripheral vascular disease. The poor circulation caused by peripheral vascular disease is the cause of diabetic gangrene in the feet and legs, which can lead to amputation, and poor wound healing.

Atherosclerosis also affects the vessels of the eyes and kidneys. The retinas of the eyes become damaged, causing **diabetic retinopathy** (retino = retina, opathy = disease) and leading to blindness. Damage to the kidney leads to kidney failure, a frequent cause of death in individuals affected with diabetes.

■ *DIAGNOSIS.* Diagnosis is confirmed by a positive history of symptoms along with blood glucose testing including a 3-hour glucose tolerance test. This test starts with a baseline blood glucose test. Next the fasting individual drinks a glucose-concentrated drink. Blood testing is completed every hour after the drink is consumed to determine how quickly it is cleared from the blood.

■ *TREATMENT.* Diabetes cannot be cured. Management of the disease is dependent on education and a lifetime commitment to following the treatment regimen of diet, medication, and exercise. Frequently monitoring blood glucose levels and controlling these are beneficial in avoiding long-term complications.

The American Diabetes Association recognizes HbA1C testing as a standard in medical care of diabetes. This is a test that measures glycosylated hemoglobin in the blood and is a good indicator of diabetes management.

Glycosylated hemoglobin is formed when the hemoglobin component of the blood is exposed to high glucose levels. Once the hemoglobin is glycosylated, it remains that way for the duration of the red blood cells' 2- to 3-month life. A high level of glycosylated hemoglobin indicates that the blood glucose levels of the individual have been high during the previous 2 to 3 months.

The higher the HbA1C, the greater the risk of developing complications such as eye disease, kidney disease, nerve damage, heart disease, and stroke. This is especially true if the HbA1C level remains high for long periods of time.

The closer the HbA1C is to normal, the lower the risk for complications. A normal HbA1C is 5% or less. Results above 7% indicate that diabetes is poorly controlled. Managing blood glucose levels and bringing the HbA1C level down decrease the risk of long-term complications. Testing is recommended every 3 to 6 months.

■ *PREVENTION.* Type 1 diabetes has a hereditary etiology and cannot be prevented. Research has demonstrated that people at risk for type 2 diabetes can prevent or delay developing type 2 diabetes by losing weight and exercising.

GESTATIONAL DIABETES

■ *DESCRIPTION.* Gestational diabetes is a type of diabetes that occurs only during pregnancy. It is usually short-lived, with blood sugar levels returning to normal soon after delivery.

■ *ETIOLOGY.* During pregnancy, the placenta produces estrogen and progesterone to maintain pregnancy. These hormones make the body cells more resistant to insulin. The mother's pancreas usually produces more insulin to overcome this resistance. As the placenta grows, more hormones are produced, placing more demand on the pancreas. If the pancreas reaches a point at which it cannot produce enough insulin to meet the need, less glucose moves into the body cells, and blood glucose levels rise. The developing fetus is also affected by the hyperglycemia and is usually overweight at birth.

■ *SYMPTOMS.* The condition can present the same symptoms as DM or be asymptomatic.

■ *DIAGNOSIS.* This type of diabetes is usually discovered with routine urine testing during prenatal visits. Further testing may include a 2- or 3-hour postprandial test. This test is a measurement of blood glucose levels at 2 or 3 hours after the individual has eaten. Normally, the blood sugar level will be down to normal in 2 to 3 hours after a meal. It is important to discover this condition and treat it because, otherwise, it can lead to fetal or neonatal mortality.

■ *TREATMENT.* Gestational diabetes is treated, like DM, with exercise, dietary control of carbohydrate intake, and medications. Injectable insulin might be needed to control blood sugar levels. Oral hypoglycemic medications are contraindicated because these pass across the placenta and can lead to fetal birth defects or hypoglycemia. Gestational diabetes usually disappears after delivery. If this condition does not disappear after delivery, the affected individual will need to continue diabetic management. Women affected with gestational diabetes are often affected later in life by adult-onset diabetes.

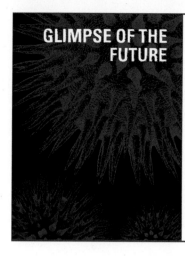

GLIMPSE OF THE FUTURE

A Link between Statins and Diabetes

A link has been found between statins (medications used to lower cholesterol) and diabetes in older women. Some studies have found that women who have been on statin drugs for several years have an increased risk for developing type 2 diabetes. This does not mean individuals who have high cholesterol should not be taking these medications. However, health care providers should monitor these women for early signs of diabetes. It is not understood why the statins increase the risk of diabetes, but all drugs have some side effects. In the future, researchers will try to determine why this occurs and what can be done to prevent increasing the patient's risk for diabetes when taking statins.

Source: Szabo (2012).

COMPLEMENTARY AND ALTERNATIVE THERAPY

Reduce the Risk of Diabetes: Drink Black Tea

New research has reported that individuals who drink black tea may be reducing their risk of developing diabetes. The research determined that it takes at least three cups of black tea ingested daily for this effect. The polysaccharides in black tea have glucose-inhibiting action and, thus, slow the absorption of glucose. The study also reported that black tea reduced the risk of heart attack. Black tea contains antioxidants and theanine, which help prevent blood clotting and also lower blood pressure.

Source: The Global Diabetes Community (2012).

■ **PREVENTION.** There is no absolute prevention, but those who observe a healthy lifestyle and a normal weight at conception are at less risk of developing the condition.

HYPOGLYCEMIA

■ **DESCRIPTION.** Hypoglycemia (HIGH-poh-gly-SEE-me-ah; hypo = decreased, glyc = glucose, emia = blood) is an abnormally low blood sugar. Hypoglycemia occurs whenever the blood glucose level drops below 60 mg/dl, although individuals can become symptomatic at different blood glucose levels. Some individuals tolerate unusually low blood glucose levels, whereas others do not.

■ **ETIOLOGY.** Some common causes of hypoglycemia are fasting, skipping meals, and excessive exercise. Hypoglycemia is also caused by administration of too much insulin, as previously discussed. Other causes of hypoglycemia include pancreatic adenoma, gastrointestinal disorders, and some hereditary disorders.

■ **SYMPTOMS.** Symptoms are the same as previously discussed for diabetes and include light-headedness, diaphoresis, and trembling. If untreated, symptoms can progress to include mental confusion and coma. Most individuals have had an episode of hypoglycemia at one time or another.

■ **DIAGNOSIS.** Physical examination to observe symptoms and blood glucose testing aid in the diagnosis. Blood testing may include a 5-hour glucose tolerance test (GTT). This test is performed in the same manner as the 3-hour test with an additional two hourly blood draws. A blood glucose level of less than 70 mg/dl at the time of symptoms and relief after eating confirm the diagnosis.

■ **TREATMENT.** Treatment of hypoglycemia is dependent on cause. Diabetics should carry glucose tablets or candy to take at the first sign of hypoglycemia. Acute hypoglycemia needs immediate emergency treatment with intravenous glucose administration.

PREVENTION. Preventive measures include eating a well-balanced diet, eating small meals often, keeping snacks available, avoiding sugary foods on an empty stomach, avoiding drinking alcohol on an empty stomach, keeping body weight at a healthy level, not smoking, and maintaining an exercise program.

Reproductive Gland Diseases

Sexual development can be affected by the release of androgens from the adrenal cortex, as previously discussed; by the pituitary; and by the sex organ (**gonad**). The male gonad is the testis, and the female gonad is the ovary. Gonads function as endocrine glands in the production of hormones, and the pituitary controls the function of the gonads by releasing gonadotropin. Gonadotropin stimulates the testes to produce the male hormone, testosterone, and the ovaries to produce the female hormone, estrogen. Dysfunction of the pituitary or the gonad can lead to endocrine disorders.

HYPERGONADISM

DESCRIPTION. Hypergonadism is the condition of increased hormone production before puberty, which produces precocious sexual development in both sexes.

ETIOLOGY. Causes of hypergonadism include unknown causes, testicular tumors, and pituitary tumors. Hypergonadism in females is primarily due to idiopathic causes. Uncommon causes include ovarian and adrenal tumors.

SYMPTOMS. In the male, onset of puberty usually occurs around age 13; with hypergonadism, this development occurs before age 10.

Signs of precocious sexual development in the male include:

- The growth of a beard and pubic hair
- Enlargement of the penis and testes
- Spermatogenesis, rendering the individual fertile
- Rapid growth of muscle and bone, leading to early uniting of the epiphyses and a premature halt of long bone growth

In the female, onset of puberty usually occurs around age 10; with hypergonadism, this development occurs before age 8. Signs of precocious sexual development in the female include:

- Onset of menarche
- Appearance of pubic and underarm hair

- Breast enlargement
- Ovarian development, rendering the individual fertile and making pregnancy possible

DIAGNOSIS. Diagnosis of hypergonadism is confirmed by positive clinical history and blood testing for evidence of elevated sex hormones.

TREATMENT. Treatment for both sexes involves removal or radiation of tumors and administration of hormones to suppress or counteract the sex hormone.

PREVENTION. There is no known prevention for hypergonadism.

HYPOGONADISM

DESCRIPTION. Hypogonadism is the condition of decreased sex hormone production by the age of normal puberty.

ETIOLOGY. In the male, causes of hypogonadism include dysfunctional testes, undescended testes, or loss of the testes due to castration. Testes also might fail to develop due to a pituitary disorder, resulting in the lack of gonadotropin. In the female, causes of hypogonadism include missing or dysfunctional ovaries.

SYMPTOMS. Loss of the male gonads before puberty causes eunuchism, or the lack of development of sex characteristics, because male characteristics are brought about by testosterone. Castration in the adult male will lead to a decrease in libido, but masculinity is maintained.

Without estrogen, female sex characteristics do not develop. Female children become abnormally tall because the long bones do not fuse normally without estrogen.

DIAGNOSIS. Hormone testing for males includes testosterone, thyroid level, and sperm count. For females, hormone testing of estrogen, FSH, LH, prolactin, thyroid, and anemia aid in diagnosis. If pituitary disease is suspected, an MRI or CT scan of the brain might be needed.

TREATMENT. Administration of testosterone is quite effective in treating hypogonadism in the male, and administration of estrogen is quite effective in treating hypogonadism in the female.

PREVENTION. Most cases cannot be prevented, but maintaining a healthy body weight and lifestyle might aid in prevention.

TRAUMA

Head injury can lead to multiple-organ dysfunction if the pituitary is involved. Hypersecretion and hyposecretion can occur with injury to any of the individual organs. Organ destruction and failure can be life-threatening when the pituitary, pancreas, and adrenal glands are all involved.

RARE DISEASES

Most previously discussed diseases of the endocrine system are relatively uncommon, with the exception of thyroid problems and DM. Other extremely rare endocrine disorders can be found in children or young adults, however. Cancer of most of the glands of the endocrine system is also somewhat rare, although the thyroid, ovaries, and testes are the most common sites for cancer development.

EFFECTS OF AGING ON THE SYSTEM

As the individual ages, changes occur in the endocrine glands. Decreases in the secretions from the glands alter the body's ability to respond to stressors, diseases, and other changes that occur from aging. The older adult is at high risk for hypoglycemic reactions and excessive fluid loss due to reduced levels of glucocorticoids and aldosterone. Digestive and metabolism problems are common due to reduced secretions of pancreatic and thyroid hormones. The secretions from the gonads are reduced, resulting in changes in secondary sex characteristics. Because glucose tolerance lessens with age, the serum glucose levels tend to be higher in the older adult. DM is common in the older population but usually can be regulated by dietary adjustments. With all the other changes that occur during the aging process, diabetes becomes a very serious condition, adversely affecting many systems.

SUMMARY

The endocrine system is a complex system of many glands located throughout the body. Each of the glands has a unique function and delivers its hormones into the bloodstream. The hormones help the body's growth, regulation, and metabolism. Overproduction or underproduction of any one gland can cause dysfunction in other systems. If the gland malfunctions in childhood, the result is a different disorder than if the gland malfunctions in adulthood.

The most common endocrine disorder overall is DM. Although, historically, type 2 diabetes was most commonly found in middle-aged or older adults, it is now frequently diagnosed in younger populations and is related to the increasing rate of obesity in the population. The older adult with an endocrine disorder is at risk for other systemic problems. Secretions from the endocrine glands decrease slowly with age.

REVIEW QUESTIONS

Short Answer

1. What are the functions of the endocrine system?

2. Which signs and symptoms are associated with common endocrine system disorders?

3. Which diagnostic tests are most commonly used to determine the type and cause of endocrine system disorders?

Multiple Choice

4. Which of the following is not an endocrine gland?

a. Pituitary

b. Adrenal

c. Liver

d. Ovaries

5. What function does the somatotropin hormone perform?

a. Promotes absorption of calcium in the bones

b. Stimulates the thyroid to produce its hormones

c. Stimulates growth

d. Promotes development of sex characteristics

6. Acromegaly is defined as which of the following?

a. An overgrowth of the long bones of the body

b. An abnormal decrease in the activity of the pituitary gland

c. A tumor located in the anterior pituitary

d. A chronic disorder characterized by large feet, hands, and facial bones

7. Cretinism is defined as which of the following?

a. Congenital hypothyroidism

b. Congenital hypopituitarism

c. Severe chronic lack of growth hormone

d. An impaired growth of all body parts

8. Hypoadrenalism is also known as which of the following disorders?

a. Acromegaly

b. Myxedema

c. Cushing's syndrome

d. Addison's disease

9. In type 1 DM, the individual needs replacement of which of the following?

a. Steroids

b. Antidiuretic hormone

c. Insulin

d. Estrogen

10. The individual affected by type 2 DM can usually control the disorder by:

a. Insulin injections

b. Diet and oral medications

c. Replacement hormones

d. Steroid therapy

Matching

11. Match the hormone in the left column with its gland in the right column. Some glands may be used more than once.

_____ ACTH

_____ T$_3$

_____ Oxytocin

_____ Mineralocorticoids

_____ Melatonin

_____ Estrogen

_____ Insulin

_____ Norepinephrine

_____ ADH

_____ Calcitonin

a. Anterior pituitary

b. Posterior pituitary

c. Pineal

d. Thyroid

e. Adrenals

f. Testes or ovaries

g. Pancreatic islets

CASE STUDIES

■ Ms. Jenson is a young woman who routinely uses a variety of herbal products to treat and prevent diseases. She knows there is a strong history of type 2 diabetes in her family and has read on the Internet about drinking black tea to prevent diabetes. She asks you whether you think that would work for her. What should you tell her? Do you think it is a good option for her? What has the research shown about black tea as a preventive treatment for diabetes? Where could she find evidence-based information about this?

■ Mrs. Webb is 78 years old and has been hospitalized frequently for repeated respiratory infections. Until the past 2 years, she has been relatively healthy. She has not been diagnosed with any serious chronic diseases but does have some osteoporosis. Based on your knowledge of the aging process and the endocrine system changes, what might be contributing to the development of these repeated respiratory infections? What can she do to decrease her risk and improve her immunity to infections?

Study Tools

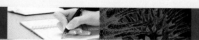

Workbook

Complete Chapter 14

Online Resources

PowerPoint® presentations

Animation

BIBLIOGRAPHY

American Diabetes Association. (2012). Assessing risk for diabetes. *www.diabetes.org* (accessed February 2012).

Botrugno, I., Lovisetto, F., Cobianchi, L., Zonta, S., Klersy, C., Vailati, A., & Jemos, V. (2011). Incidental carcinoma in multinodular goiter: Risk factors. *American Surgeon 77*(11), 1553–1558.

Bronstein, M. D., Paraiba, D. B., & Jallad, R. S. (2011). Management of pituitary tumors in pregnancy. *Nature Reviews Endocrinology 7*(5), 301–310.

Burke, L. E., & Wang, J. (2011). Treatment strategies for overweight and obesity. *Journal of Nursing Scholarship 43*(4), 368–375.

Centers for Disease Control and Prevention (CDC). (2012). Adolescents and school health: Childhood obesity facts. *www.cdc.gov* (accessed August 2012).

Clarke, J. L. (2012). Seeking patient-centered solutions to a national epidemic. *Population Health Management 14*(Suppl), S3–S16.

Crawford, A., & Harris, H. (2011). Balancing act: Hypomagnesemia & hypermagnesemia. *Nursing 41*(10), 52–55.

Crawford, A., & Harris, H. (2012). Balancing act: Calcium & phosphorus. *Nursing 42*(1), 36–43.

Funnell, M. M. (2011). Diabetes under control. The National Diabetes Education Program. *American Journal of Nursing 111*(12), 65–67.

Horowitz, S. (2011). Medicinal mushrooms: Research support for modern applications of traditional uses. *Alternative & Complementary Therapies 17*(6), 323–329.

Hughes, L. (2012). Think "SAFE": Four crucial elements for diabetes education. *Nursing 42*(1), 58–61.

Losa, M., Picozzi, P., Redaelli, M., Laurenzi, A., & Mortini, P. (2010). Pituitary radiotherapy for Cushing's disease. *Neuroendocrinology 92*, 107–110.

Marquess, J. G. (2011). Managing special populations among patients with type 2 diabetes mellitus. *Pharmacotherapy 31*(12), 65S–72S.

Messick, B. H., Casmus, R. J., & Comadoll, J. L. (2010). Hyperthyroidism in a foot ball player. *Athletic Therapy Today 15*(3), 26–28.

Mosher, M. C. (2011). Amiodarone-induced hypothyroidism and other adverse effects. *Dimensions of Critical Care Nursing 30*(2), 87–93.

News you can use. (2011). *Alternative & Complementary Therapies 17*(6), 229–301.

Płoski, R., Szymański, K., & Bednarczuk, T. (2011). The genetic basis of Graves' disease. *Current Genomics 12*(8), 542–563.

Propylthiouracil/thiamazole. (2010). *Reactions Weekly* (1289), 35.

Shehzad, A., Ha, T., Subhan, F., & Lee, Y. (2011). New mechanisms and the anti-inflammatory role of curcumin in obesity and the obesity-related metabolic diseases. *European Journal of Nutrition 50*(3), 151–161.

Shields, L. E., Balko, M., & Hunsaker J. C. III. (2012). Sudden and unexpected death from pituitary tumor apoplexy. *Journal of Forensic Sciences 57*(1), 262–266.

Smart, M. (2011). Oncology update. *Oncology Nursing Forum 38*(4), 485–486.

Szabo, L. (2012). Study links statins to higher diabetes in older women. *USA Today* online. *www.usatoday.com* (accessed January 2012).

The Global Diabetes Community. (2012). Three cups of black tea each day could help reduce risk of diabetes. *www.diabetes.co.uk* (accessed January 2012).

Tritos, N. A., Biller, B. K., & Swearingen, B. (2011). Management of Cushing disease. *Nature Reviews Endocrinology 7*(5), 279–290.

Trojan-Rodrigues, M. M., Alves, T. S., Soares, G. G., & Ritter, M. R. (2012). Plants used as antidiabetics in popular medicine in Rio Grande do Sul, southern Brazil. *Journal of Ethnopharmacology 139*(1), 155–163.

Turns, M. (2011). Chairside assessment of peripheral arterial disease in diabetes patients. *British Journal of Community Nursing* Suppl, S24–S33.

Turns, M. (2011). The diabetic foot: An overview of assessment and complications. *British Journal of Nursing* Suppl, S19–S25.

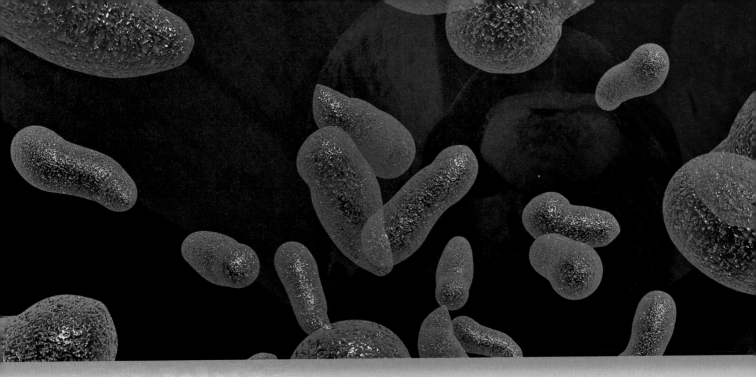

OUTLINE

- **Anatomy and Physiology**
  The Central Nervous System
  The Peripheral Nervous System

- **Common Signs and Symptoms**

- **Diagnostic Tests**

- **Common Diseases of the Nervous System**
  Infectious Diseases
  Vascular Disorders
  Functional Disorders
  Dementias
  Sleep Disorders
  Tumors

- **Trauma**
  Concussions and Contusions
  Skull Fractures
  Epidural and Subdural Hematomas
  Spinal Cord Injury: Quadriplegia and Paraplegia

- **Rare Diseases**
  Amyotrophic Lateral Sclerosis
  Guillain–Barré Syndrome
  Huntington's Disease
  Multiple Sclerosis

- **Effects of Aging on the System**

- **Summary**

- **Review Questions**

- **Case Studies**

- **Bibliography**

KEY TERMS

Amnesia (p. 347)
Aura (p. 340)
Carotid endarterectomy (p. 338)
Cauterization (p. 350)
Cephalalgia (p. 339)
Chorea (p. 353)
Convulsion (p. 340)
Decompress (p. 351)
Dysphagia (p. 337)
Dysphasia (p. 337)
Epidural (p. 349)
Grand mal (p. 341)

Hemiparesis (p. 337)
Hydrophobia (p. 335)
Hypothermia (p. 351)
Intractable (p. 339)
Nuchal rigidity (p. 333)
Paraplegia (p. 351)
Paresthesia (p. 353)
Petit mal (p. 341)
Quadriplegia (p. 351)
Seizure (p. 340)
Spinal stenosis (p. 339)
Status epilepticus (p. 341)
Subdural (p. 349)

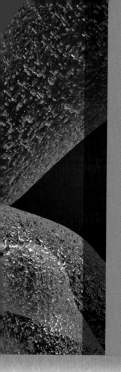

15

Nervous System Diseases and Disorders

LEARNING OBJECTIVES

Upon completion of the chapter, the learner should be able to:

1. Define the terminology common to the nervous system and the disorders of the system.

2. Discuss the basic anatomy and physiology of the nervous system.

3. Identify the important signs and symptoms associated with common nervous system disorders.

4. Describe the common diagnostics used to determine the type and cause of nervous system disorders.

5. Identify common disorders of the nervous system.

6. Describe the typical course and management of the common nervous system disorders.

7. Describe the effects of aging on the nervous system and the common disorders associated with aging of the system.

OVERVIEW

The nervous system is a complex network that provides communication from the brain to the rest of the body and from the body back to the brain. It facilitates the individual's ability to reason, interact with other individuals, understand complex ideas, and respond both intellectually and physically. Disorders of the system can affect any or all other normal functioning in the individual. Because brain and spinal cord injury often causes irreversible damage, the individual with a nervous system disorder can become a victim of severe, permanent, neurologic deficits. ■

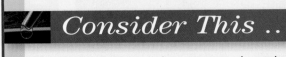

Consider This ...

The brain stops growing at approximately age 18.

◼◼◼ ANATOMY AND PHYSIOLOGY

The nervous system is composed of the brain, spinal cord, and nerves (Figure 15–1). It is divided into the central nervous system (CNS) and the peripheral nervous system (PNS). The CNS includes the brain and the spinal cord. The PNS includes the autonomic nervous system (ANS), the cranial nerves, and the spinal nerves. The CNS communicates with organs and other body systems through the PNS.

The Central Nervous System

The brain is a complex structure located within the protective covering of the skull. It is divided into the cerebrum, cerebellum, and brain stem. The cerebrum is divided into two hemispheres that can be further subdivided into lobes. Each of these lobes has a specialized function (Figure 15–2). The basal ganglia, called the gray matter, are located deep in the hemispheres. Another part of the cerebrum is called the diencephalon. This is where the hypothalamus and thalamus are located. They are active in controlling the body's sleep–wake pattern and are involved in the actions of the hypophysis (pituitary) gland. (See Chapter 14, "Endocrine System Diseases and Disorders," for more information.)

The cerebellum, important in coordination and fine motor movements, is located in the lower back part of the brain.

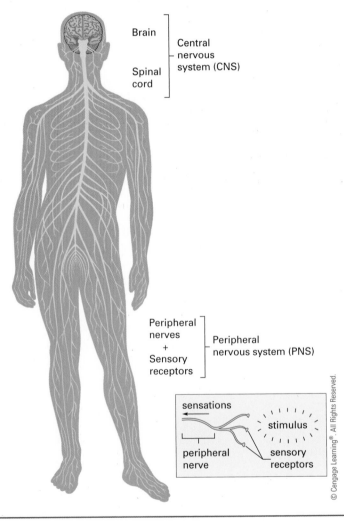

FIGURE 15–1 The nervous system.

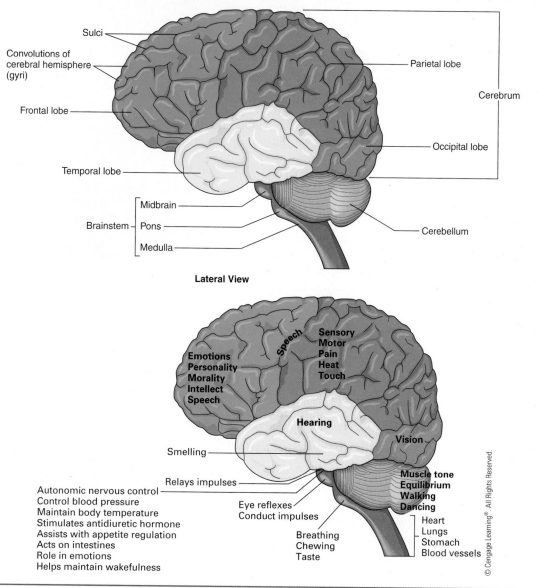

Lateral View

Sulci

Convolutions of cerebral hemisphere (gyri)

Frontal lobe

Temporal lobe

Brainstem — Midbrain, Pons, Medulla

Parietal lobe

Cerebrum

Occipital lobe

Cerebellum

Emotions
Personality
Morality
Intellect
Speech

Speech

Sensory
Motor
Pain
Heat
Touch

Hearing

Vision

Smelling

Relays impulses

Autonomic nervous control
Control blood pressure
Maintain body temperature
Stimulates antidiuretic hormone
Assists with appetite regulation
Acts on intestines
Role in emotions
Helps maintain wakefulness

Eye reflexes
Conduct impulses

Breathing
Chewing
Taste

Muscle tone
Equilibrium
Walking
Dancing

Heart
Lungs
Stomach
Blood vessels

FIGURE 15–2 The cerebral lobes and their specialized functions.

The brain stem makes up the last part of the brain. It is subdivided into the midbrain, pons, and medulla; contains some nerves; and is responsible for transmitting impulses that control respiration, swallowing, wakefulness, and other activities.

The spinal cord is a continuous structure running through the vertebral column from the medulla to the tailbone. The spinal cord is composed of both white and gray matter. It has ascending and descending pathways that transmit impulses. Sensory impulses (pain, temperature, and touch) travel from the spinal

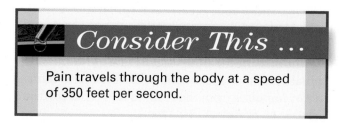

Consider This ...

The brain holds five times as much information as the Encyclopedia Britannica, or the equivalent of 1,000 computer terabytes.

Consider This ...

Pain travels through the body at a speed of 350 feet per second.

TABLE 15–1   **The Cranial Nerves**

Cranial Nerve	Function
I. Olfactory	Smell
II. Optic	Sight
III. Oculomotor	Movement of the eyeball, pupil, and eyelid
IV. Trochlear	Movement of the eyeball
V. Trigeminal	Chewing; pain, temperature, and touch of face and mouth
VI. Abducens	Movement of the eyeball
VII. Facial	Movement of the face and secretion of saliva; taste
VIII. Auditory	Hearing and balance
IX. Glossopharyngeal	Swallowing and secretion of saliva; taste and sensation in the mouth and pharynx
X. Vagus	Sensation and movement in the pharynx, larynx, thorax, and gastrointestinal system
XI. Accessory	Movement of the head and shoulders
XII. Hypoglossal	Movement of the tongue

cord to the brain. Motor impulses (for movement of muscles) travel from the brain to the spinal cord.

The meninges are membranes that cover the brain and spinal cord. The meninges are divided into three layers: the dura mater (outer cover), the arachnoid (middle layer), and the pia mater (inner layer). They provide both protection and support for the system.

The Peripheral Nervous System

The ANS controls the functions of the body's organs and innervates smooth muscle and cardiac muscle. It is divided into the parasympathetic and sympathetic systems. The parasympathetic system controls the changes in the body needed to relax and restore function, such as returning blood pressure to normal after it has increased in response to some need. The sympathetic system controls the changes in the body needed to respond to stressors, such as increasing the heart rate or blood pressure—the fight-or-flight response.

Twelve pairs of cranial nerves control sensation and movement in the area of the head and neck (Table 15–1). Thirty-one pairs of spinal nerves are divided into 8 cervical, 12 thoracic, 5 lumbar, 5 sacral, and 1 coccygeal. Each spinal nerve innervates designated areas, called dermatomes, of the skin (Figure 15–3). Each of the spinal nerves sends sensory impulses from the body organs and surfaces to the spinal cord for transmission to the brain and returns motor impulses from the brain to the spinal cord and then to the muscles.

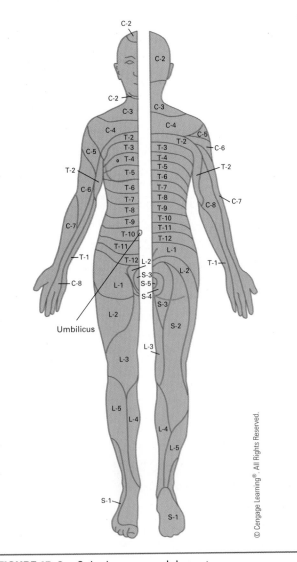

FIGURE 15–3   Spinal nerves and dermatomes.

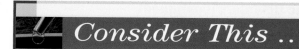

Consider This ...

Twenty-five percent of the brain is used to control the eyes.

COMMON SIGNS AND SYMPTOMS

Common signs and symptoms of nervous system disorders include headache, nausea, vomiting, weakness, mood swings, and fever. Symptoms specific to the nervous system include the following:

- Disturbance in motor function (or ability to move), including:
  1. Stiffness in the neck, back, or extremities
  2. Inability to move any part of the body
  3. Seizures or convulsions
  4. Paralysis

- Disturbance in sensory function (or ability to sense or feel), including:
  1. Visual difficulties
  2. Inability to speak
  3. Paralysis

- Alteration in mental alertness or cognitive function, including:
  1. Extreme or prolonged drowsiness
  2. Stupor, unconsciousness, or coma
  3. Amnesia or extreme forgetfulness

DIAGNOSTIC TESTS

A neurologic examination includes testing motor, sensory, and mental function. This examination is often performed on any individual presenting with an injury to the head, neck, or spinal column or exhibiting neurologic symptoms. Motor testing includes checking reflexes, gait, and posture. Sensory testing includes checking the ability to feel, using pinprick or application of heat, cold, or vibration. Ability to see and smell also can be part of sensory testing. Testing of mental or cognitive function includes asking simple questions related to name, occupation, and location. Further testing might include simple math problems or questions about current events.

The most important laboratory test in a neurologic examination is the analysis of cerebrospinal fluid (CSF). The fluid is examined under a microscope to determine the presence of bacteria, leukocytes, red blood cells, neoplastic cells, and other microorganisms. To obtain this fluid, a lumbar puncture must be performed, a procedure that consists of positioning the

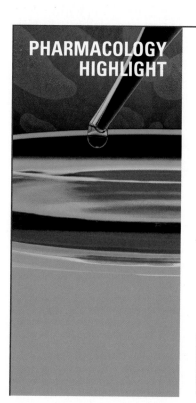

PHARMACOLOGY HIGHLIGHT

Common Drugs for Neurologic Disorders

CATEGORY	EXAMPLES OF MEDICATIONS
Anticonvulsants Drugs used to treat convulsive disorders	
Aldehydes	paraldehyde
Barbiturates	phenobarbital or barbexaclone
Benzodiazepines	clonazepam, diazepam, or lorazepam
Carbamates	felbamate
Carbozamides	carbamazepine or eslicarbazepine
Fatty acids	progabide or tiagabine
Fructose based	topiramate
GABAs	gabapentin or pregabalin
Hydantoins	phenytoin, mephenytoin, or fosphenytoin
Triazines	lamotrigine
Ureas	pheneturide or phenacemide
Others	beclamide, primidone, sultiame, or mesuximide
Antibiotics Drugs used to prevent or stop bacterial infections	ampicillin, amoxicillin, ciprofloxacin, doxycycline, erythromycin, penicillin, or tetracycline

(continued)

Common Drugs for Neurologic Disorders (continued)

CATEGORY	EXAMPLES OF MEDICATIONS
Anticoagulants Drugs used to prevent clotting	tissue plasminogen activator, warfarin, heparin, or dabigatran
Antipyretics/Analgesics Drugs used to reduce fever and pain	acetaminophen, aspirin, ibuprofen, or naproxen
Anti-inflammatories Drugs used to reduce inflammation	
Steroids	hydrocortisone, beclomethasone, or amcinonide
Nonsteroidal	acetaminophen, aspirin, or ibuprofen
Antidementias Drugs used to treat dementia disorders by maintaining mental function or controlling moods or behaviors	
Cholinesterase inhibitors	donepezil, galantamine, or rivastigmine
Antipsychotics	risperidone or olanzapine
Antidepressants	amitriptyline, amoxapine, doxepin, imipramine, or sertraline
Others	memantine or tacrine

affected individual on his or her side in a knee–chest position to widen the vertebral disk space, inserting a spinal needle into the meningeal space around the spinal cord, and withdrawing CSF. During the procedure, a special manometer might be connected to the spinal needle so intracranial pressure (ICP) can be measured.

Because the skull is a rigid structure, any increase in the size of the brain tissue by swelling, tumor, infection, or hematoma will cause an increase in ICP. If pressure becomes too high, the brain will herniate or move downward through the foramen magnum, the only opening available. When this occurs, coma and rapid death can occur because this places pressure on vital centers in the brain stem.

Radiologic examinations include X-rays of the skull and vertebral column for fractures and other abnormalities. A myelogram, or picture of the spinal cord, might be used for diagnosis of a tumor, nerve root compression, herniated nucleus pulposus (HNP), or herniated disk. Angiograms can help determine vessel occlusion and hematomas in individuals exhibiting symptoms of cerebrovascular accident or stroke.

Electroencephalography (EEG) measures electrical brain activity. A damaged area of the brain might exhibit abnormal electrical activity as might occur with cerebrovascular accident and epilepsy. EEG is also used to determine brain death.

Computerized tomography (CT) and magnetic resonance imaging (MRI) scanning are both valuable tools to assess the anatomy of the brain and spinal cord.

COMMON DISEASES OF THE NERVOUS SYSTEM

The diseases of the nervous system can range from mild to severe, depending on the particular condition. Age-related factors can influence the severity of the disease, but many nervous system disorders can affect the individual at any age.

Infectious Diseases

Infections of the nervous system are more common in the young but can be found in older adults as well. Early diagnosis and treatment are essential to reduce the permanent neurologic deficits that can result from the infection.

ENCEPHALITIS

■ **DESCRIPTION.** Encephalitis is an inflammation of the brain tissue.

■ **ETIOLOGY.** Encephalitis is caused by a variety of microorganisms, including bacteria and viruses, or as a complication of measles, chicken pox, or mumps. Such viruses can be spread also by mosquitoes and carried from animal to human or from human to human.

■ **SYMPTOMS.** Symptoms include headache, elevated temperature, and a stiff neck and back but can progress to lethargy, mental confusion, and even coma.

■ **DIAGNOSIS.** Encephalitis is usually diagnosed by finding the causative agent in spinal fluid obtained by lumbar puncture.

■ **TREATMENT.** Treatment is supportive. Antiviral medication might be effective in some types of encephalitis, but prognosis is guarded because some forms of encephalitis have a high mortality rate. Severe encephalitis can leave the individual with permanent neurologic impairment.

■ **PREVENTION.** Prevention is related to avoiding transmission of the disease by mosquitoes. Activities include avoiding outdoor activity when mosquitoes are active—usually near or after dark—wearing protective clothing with long sleeves and long pants, and using repellents that contain DEET.

Consider This ...

The female mosquito is the only one that bites. The male mosquito feeds on flower nectar, but the female needs blood proteins in order to produce fertile eggs. The piercing bite mixed with the mosquito saliva creates the stinging skin irritation associated with a mosquito bite.

MENINGITIS

■ **DESCRIPTION.** Meningitis is inflammation of the meninges, the covering of the brain and spinal cord.

■ **ETIOLOGY.** Meningitis can be caused by anything that causes an inflammatory response, including bacteria, viruses, fungi, and toxins such as lead and arsenic. Some forms of meningitis are more contagious and more lethal than other forms of the disease. The

most common cause of meningitis is bacterial invasion by *Neisseria meningitides*. Bacteria and viruses usually reach the meninges after invading and infecting other parts of the body such as the middle ear, sinuses, and upper respiratory tract; or they can be carried to the meninges in the blood, as in septicemia.

■ **SYMPTOMS.** Symptoms of meningitis often include a sudden onset of high fever, severe headache, photophobia (fear of light), and a stiffness in the neck that resists bending the neck forward or sideways (**nuchal rigidity**). As the disease progresses, drowsiness, stupor, seizures, and coma might occur.

■ **DIAGNOSIS.** Diagnosis is usually confirmed by finding the causative agent in the spinal fluid obtained by lumbar puncture.

■ **TREATMENT.** Antibiotic treatment of bacterial meningitis is usually quite effective. Other treatments include antipyretics; anticonvulsive medications; and a quiet, dark environment. If untreated, meningitis can be fatal, especially in infants, children, and older individuals. It can cause permanent neurologic damage in children, leading to hearing loss, learning and developmental challenges, and epilepsy. Good hand washing practices can help prevent the spread of the disease.

■ **PREVENTION.** Good hand washing helps reduce exposure to infectious organisms. Avoiding those who are infected is also a preventive activity.

POLIOMYELITIS

■ **DESCRIPTION.** Poliomyelitis, or polio, is a viral infection affecting the brain and spinal cord. Polio was a major crippling and life-threatening disease affecting children prior to the development of a vaccine in the 1950s. Immunization programs since that time have virtually eliminated the disease in the United States.

■ **ETIOLOGY.** The poliomyelitis virus enters the body through the mouth and nose. It crosses the gastrointestinal tract into the blood and then travels to the brain and spinal cord. The virus is spread by oropharyngeal secretions and by infected feces.

■ **SYMPTOMS.** Symptoms of polio include muscle weakness, neck stiffness, and nausea and vomiting. As the disease progresses, muscles atrophy and deteriorate. Muscles of the arms, legs, and respiratory system can become paralyzed.

■ **DIAGNOSIS.** Diagnosis is made by clinical examination and confirmed by culturing the virus from the throat, feces, or spinal fluid.

■ **TREATMENT.** Treatment is supportive and includes analgesics and bed rest during the acute phase. Long-term physical therapy and limb braces might be needed. If the respiratory system is involved, mechanical ventilation might be necessary.

Ten to forty years after the initial polio attack, many survivors experience postpolio syndrome (PPS), characterized by further weakening of muscles that were previously affected by the polio infection. Symptoms can include joint pain, fatigue, and increasing skeletal deformities such as scoliosis. The problems caused by PPS usually mirror the severity of the original polio attack. If the original attack was not severe, the PPS condition is usually not bad. PPS tends to affect females more often than it does males. This is not an infectious condition, and it is rarely life-threatening.

■ **PREVENTION.** The most effective prevention is with polio vaccine.

TETANUS

■ **DESCRIPTION.** Tetanus is a highly fatal infection of nerve tissue.

■ **ETIOLOGY.** Tetanus disease is caused by the *Clostridium tetani* bacterium. The effects of the toxin produced by this bacterium on the CNS lead to voluntary or skeletal muscle contraction.

■ **SYMPTOMS.** The first symptom is typically a stiffness of the jaw, commonly called lockjaw, and is due to strong jaw muscle contractions. This disease affects both the musculoskeletal system and the nervous system.

More detailed information about tetanus is found in Chapter 6, "Musculoskeletal System Diseases and Disorders."

RABIES

■ **DESCRIPTION.** Rabies is an often fatal encephalomyelitis.

■ **ETIOLOGY.** Rabies is caused by a virus and primarily affects animals such as dogs, cats, foxes, raccoons, squirrels, and skunks but can be transmitted to humans through a bite by an infected animal. Like tetanus, this virus travels slowly to the spinal cord and brain, so the location of the bite is significant.

HEALTHY HIGHLIGHT

Polio Vaccine Precautions

There are three distinct polioviruses, designated as types 1, 2, and 3. Dr. Jonas Salk developed an injectable vaccine against only one form of polio, so that vaccine is called a monovalent vaccine. It used dead virus to stimulate the production of antibodies against polio. Dr. Albert Sabin later developed an oral vaccine (trivalent oral polio vaccine [TOPV]) against all three forms of the virus; that vaccine is, therefore, called a trivalent vaccine and is a live vaccine using weakened virus to stimulate antibody production.

Immunosuppressed individuals must follow precautions with polio vaccines. Immunosuppressed individuals include those who are:

■ Affected with chronic disease.
■ Taking chemotherapy.
■ Receiving radiation treatments.
■ Taking immunosuppressive medications for organ transplants.
■ On long-term steroid treatment.

Precautions for immunosuppressed individuals include the following:

■ Do not take the live trivalent vaccine because this can lead to contracting polio.
■ Do not change diapers or come in contact with feces of children recently treated with TOPV.
■ Do not come in contact with nasal secretions or vomitus of children recently treated with TOPV.

HEALTHY HIGHLIGHT

CDC Recommends Tdap for All Ages

The Centers for Disease Control and Prevention (CDC) now recommends the Tdap (tetanus, diphtheria, and acellular pertussis) shot be given to adults age 65 and older. Previously, the recommendation was for older adults only if they had close contact with infants under age 1 and if they had not been vaccinated with Tdap before. Pertussis cases have been increasing during the last 30 years and peaked in 2010. About 700 of these cases involved older adults. There are two Tdap vaccines on the market, but only one (Boostrix®) is approved by the Food and Drug Administration for older adults.

Source: Lowes (2012).

Incubation time is from 1 to 3 months. Shorter incubation times are related to the position of the bite, making bites to the face and neck more serious than those to the extremities.

■ **SYMPTOMS.** Symptoms of rabies include fever, pain, paralysis, convulsions, and rage. In animals, a change in temperament is often noticed. Wild animals can become friendly, and family pets can become aggressive. Another classic symptom is spasm and paralysis of the muscles of swallowing. The sight of water or attempting to drink water causes throat spasms, leading to **hydrophobia** (hydro = water, phobia = fear). Inability to swallow also causes a drooling of frothy saliva, an identifying symptom in animals.

■ **DIAGNOSIS.** Diagnosis is based on a history and physical exam, observing for symptoms of muscle spasms, stiffness, and pain. Laboratory tests are not helpful with diagnosis.

■ **TREATMENT.** Treatment of rabies includes immediate washing of the area with soap and water, followed by medical attention. A series of antirabies injections must be given before the virus has had time to reach the brain. Any animal bite needs to be investigated immediately. The biting animal should be confined and placed under observation for symptoms of rabies, and viral cultures should be obtained. If the animal cannot be captured and must be killed, care should be taken not to destroy the head because the brain must be examined for presence of disease. If the animal cannot be found, the injured individual will need to take the series of injections immediately.

There is no cure for rabies. Treatment is palliative and includes strong muscle relaxants to reduce convulsions. Untreated cases end with severe convulsions

and respiratory arrest. Death usually occurs within 2 to 5 days after onset of symptoms.

■ **PREVENTION.** Prevention of rabies begins with vaccination of family pets and education of children in recognizing and avoiding animals with rabid symptoms.

SHINGLES

■ **DESCRIPTION.** Shingles is an acute viral disease. It is fairly common in the elderly, with approximately 50% of people over age 80 having an episode of shingles.

■ **ETIOLOGY.** Shingles is caused by herpes zoster, the same virus that causes chicken pox. The only difference between chicken pox and shingles is the level of the affected individual's immunity. Chicken pox usually appears in children with little or no immunity, and shingles occurs in adults with limited immunity. It is thought that herpes zoster virus is a chicken pox virus that has been dormant, usually for years, after recovery from chicken pox. This virus tends to flare up or become active during periods of stress or immunosuppression caused by other disease processes, trauma, and aging.

■ **SYMPTOMS.** Shingles is characterized by an itching, painful, red rash, and small vesicles or blisters that follow the course of a sensory nerve (Figure 15–4). The resulting neuritis or inflammation of the nerve results in a stabbing, sharp pain that usually is more severe at night. Symptoms can last from 10 days to several weeks. The pattern of rash and blisters usually appears on the body trunk and runs toward the midline but also can appear on the face, causing severe conjunctivitis.

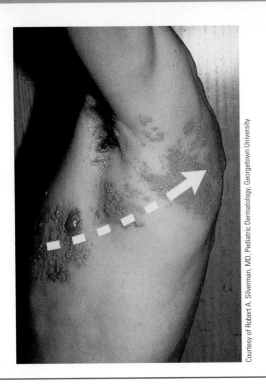

FIGURE 15–4   Shingles: vesicles follow a nerve pathway.

A more rare form of shingles is Zoster san herpes, or shingles without the typical rash. Pain may run more front to back and is often mistaken for a heart attack.

■ **DIAGNOSIS.** Diagnosis is made on the basis of the appearance of lesions. A viral culture or blood test for the herpes virus can be performed to confirm the diagnosis.

■ **TREATMENT.** There is no cure for shingles. Treatment is symptomatic and involves administration of antiviral medication (acyclovir, valacyclovir, famciclovir), analgesics (acetaminophen, aspirin, ibuprofen, and opioids, like codeine, for severe pain), topical antibiotics applied to prevent infections of the open blisters, and antipruritics (medications to reduce itching).

■ **PREVENTION.** Zostavax®, a vaccine to prevent shingles, has been available for individuals over age 60 since it was licensed by the Food and Drug Administration (FDA) in 2006. The vaccine is not a treatment for shingles.

Vascular Disorders

Vascular disorders of the nervous system can be quite severe, causing long-term debility. Some vascular disorders can be prevented or reduced in severity by lifestyle changes.

CEREBROVASCULAR ACCIDENT (CVA)

■ **DESCRIPTION.** CVA is commonly called a stroke. It is a major cause of death in people over 50 years of age.

> ## Consider This ...
>
> On average, someone in the United States has a stroke every 40 seconds and someone dies from a stroke every 3 minutes.

■ **ETIOLOGY.** CVA is due to poor blood supply to the brain. A common causative factor is arteriosclerosis. A CVA is to the brain what a heart attack is to the heart—lack of blood flow to the brain causes brain tissue death. The three common causes of poor blood supply or lack of blood flow are:

Cerebral thrombus a clot in a brain artery and the most common cause of vessel occlusion. Thrombus formation usually occurs in an area where the vessel is narrowed by arteriosclerosis. Symptoms usually appear gradually until blood flow is inadequate.

Cerebral embolism usually due to a small piece of a thrombus or arterial plaque breaking loose and traveling in the artery until it wedges and occludes the vessel. Symptoms usually appear quite suddenly.

Cerebral hemorrhage the rupture of an artery, filling the surrounding brain tissue with blood. Cerebral hemorrhage is usually due to hypertension and arteriosclerosis (see "Arteriosclerosis and Atherosclerosis" in Chapter 8, "Cardiovascular System Diseases and Disorders"), which cause the vessel to tear and hemorrhage. Another cause of cerebral hemorrhage is a weakened artery due to an aneurysm. Symptoms are very sudden with hemorrhage.

■ **SYMPTOMS.** When an area of the brain loses blood supply, the individual suddenly loses consciousness and can die or have permanent neurologic disability. About one-third of individuals with a CVA die. Some survive without functional disability, and others might have mild, moderate, or severe disability. The symptoms of CVA are numerous, depending on the area of the brain affected and the severity of the occlusion or hemorrhage. Common symptoms include **dysphasia** (dis-FAY-zee-ah; dys = difficulty, phasia = speaking), **dysphagia** (dis-FAY-jee-ah; dys = difficulty, phagia = swallowing), **hemiparesis** (HEM-ee-par-EE-sis; hemi = one half, paresis = paralysis), confusion, and poor coordination (Figure 15–5).

■ *DIAGNOSIS.* Diagnosis of CVA is made and confirmed by physical examination, EEG, and CT or MRI scan. One indicator of the location of brain damage is shown by the pattern of hemiparesis, if present. Hemiparesis affecting the left side is indicative of right-sided brain injury, whereas hemiparesis affecting the right side is indicative of left-sided brain injury. Symptoms of right- and left-sided brain damage vary to some degree (Figure 15–6).

■ *TREATMENT.* Treatment of CVA depends on the severity of the stroke and the symptoms. Anticoagulant

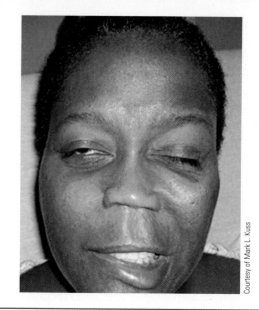

FIGURE 15–5 CVA: facial features.

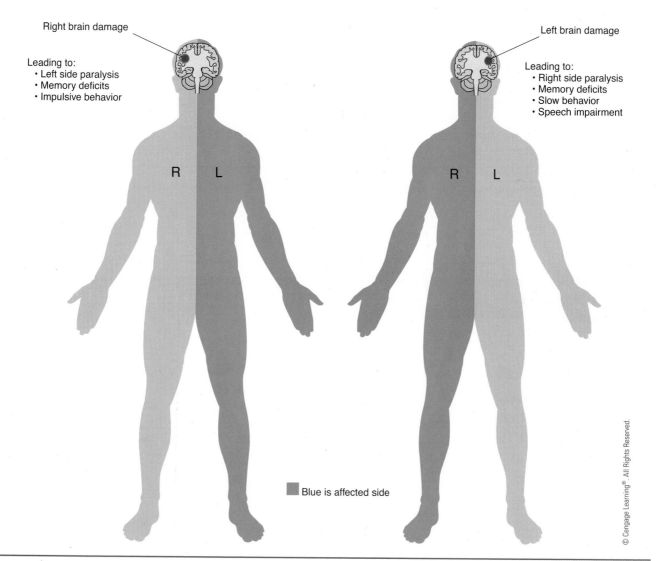

Right brain damage

Leading to:
• Left side paralysis
• Memory deficits
• Impulsive behavior

Left brain damage

Leading to:
• Right side paralysis
• Memory deficits
• Slow behavior
• Speech impairment

Blue is affected side

FIGURE 15–6 Symptoms of right and left CVA vary to some degree.

and hypertensive medications can be given to control the formation of clots and to lower blood pressure. For those individuals with physical disability, a rehabilitation program, including the needed services of physical therapy and speech therapy, must be set up early and continued until the individual has gained maximum potential.

■ **PREVENTION.** Prevention of stroke is directed toward avoiding risk factors that include:

1. Smoking
2. High-fat diet
3. Obesity
4. Lack of exercise

These factors also play a role in arteriosclerosis, a main cause of CVA.

Early detection and treatment of occluded arteries can aid in prevention of some types of CVA. Carotid artery screening involves a physician auscultating the carotid arteries and listening for vessel narrowing. As blood rushes through a narrowed vessel, a rushing sound called a bruit (BREW-ee) can be heard. Ultrasound imaging can also be performed to determine the condition of the vessel. Surgical intervention to open the vessel might prevent CVA and includes removal of plaque in the carotid arteries to improve blood flow and reduce the risk of a thrombus. This surgical procedure is called a **carotid endarterectomy**.

TRANSIENT ISCHEMIC ATTACK (TIA)

■ **DESCRIPTION.** TIAs are sudden, mild mini-strokes.

■ **ETIOLOGY.** TIAs are due to insufficient blood supply to the brain. They can serve as a warning of an impending stroke and are often due to artery narrowing by arteriosclerotic plaque.

■ **SYMPTOMS.** Symptoms, like those of CVA, depend on the area of the brain that is affected. Some common symptoms are weakness of an arm, leg, or both; dizziness; slurred speech; and a mild loss of consciousness. Total loss of consciousness usually does not occur. Symptoms usually subside within a few minutes to an hour.

■ **DIAGNOSIS.** Symptoms can be completely resolved by the time medical advice is sought. The diagnosis is made on the medical history and physical examination including a neurologic exam. Blood pressure is also checked for hypertension. A stethoscope may be placed over neck veins (auscultation) to determine blood flow irregularities. Arteriograms can locate suspected vessel blockage or occlusion. A CT scan of the head might also be part of the diagnostic testing.

■ **TREATMENT.** Arteriograms showing blocked blood flow can be followed up with surgery to open vessels or bypass blockage. Carotid endarterectomy is one of the more common surgeries to correct blood flow for TIA.

COMPLEMENTARY AND ALTERNATIVE THERAPY

Too Many Supplements Could Be Harmful, but Not Always

Many individuals today are taking mega-doses of vitamins for a variety of reasons. Some believe it gives them more energy, and others believe it might cure their disorders. However, a group of doctors and researchers warn the consumer that taking these large doses of vitamins might actually be harmful to their health. They state that large amounts of vitamin D and calcium are unnecessary and large amounts of vitamin E could increase a person's risk of hemorrhagic stroke by 22%. However, they also note that it might reduce the risk of ischemic stroke by 10%. B complex vitamins have been shown to help maintain cognitive function. Perhaps the best warning to the consumer is to use these products wisely, be aware of side effects, read the labels, and communicate with a primary care provider about taking supplements.

Source: Challem (2011).

■ **PREVENTION.** Quitting smoking is the best preventive measure. Knowing risk factors and living a healthy lifestyle are also helpful preventive measures.

Functional Disorders

Functional disorders of the nervous system include degenerative disk disease, headache, epilepsy, and Bell's palsy. These conditions, although varying in severity, are some of the most common problems of the system. The cause of the disorder might be found, but in many cases, it is unknown. Treatment of structural disorders is directed toward the relief of symptoms and assisting the individual in maintaining maximum function in activities of daily living.

DEGENERATIVE DISK DISEASE

■ **DESCRIPTION.** Degenerative disk disease is actually a degeneration, or wearing away, of the intervertebral disk of the musculoskeletal system, but the results so severely affect the neurologic system that it will be considered in this chapter.

■ **ETIOLOGY.** The wearing away of the disk between the vertebrae of the back allows the vertebrae to bump or rub against each other. As these vertebrae move closer together, the opening for the spine and nerve roots becomes smaller, causing pressure on the nerves. The condition of narrowing of nerve root openings in the spinal column is called **spinal stenosis** (stenosis = narrowing).

■ **SYMPTOMS.** Common symptoms include difficulty walking and radiating pain in the back and in one or both legs. This pain often follows the nerve path and can be **intractable** (difficult to stop or control). Degenerative disk disease usually affects older individuals but can be related to trauma or congenital defects in younger individuals.

■ **DIAGNOSIS.** Diagnosis is made on the basis of clinical history, X-ray, myelography, CT, or MRI.

■ **TREATMENT.** Treatment initially involves resting the back and legs. A back brace might be beneficial. Long-term treatment involves analgesics, anti-inflammatory medications, and exercise to ease the pain. A laminectomy, surgery to remove part of the vertebrae and widen the nerve root opening, can be the treatment of choice. In severe cases, surgery to fuse the vertebrae and free the nerve root can be performed. Often, older individuals affected with degenerative disk disease and spinal stenoses are not medically stable enough to endure surgery.

■ **PREVENTION.** Since degenerative disk disease primarily affects the elderly due to the aging process, many cases cannot be prevented. Moderate exercise, especially daily walking programs, and good nutrition can help slow or stop painful symptoms.

HEADACHE

■ **DESCRIPTION.** Headache, or **cephalalgia** (SEF-ah-LAL-jee-ah; cephal = head, algia = pain), is one of the most common disorders of humans. It is usually a symptom of another disease rather than a disorder in and of itself. Disorders that typically have headaches as a symptom can include sinusitis, meningitis, encephalitis, hypertension, anemia, constipation, premenstrual tension, and tumors, to name only a few. Most headaches are not related to disease but are basically caused by two mechanisms:

■ Tension on the facial, neck, and scalp muscles

■ Vascular changes in arterial size (dilation or constriction) of the vessels inside the head

■ **ETIOLOGY.** Many factors produce headaches, including allergies, stress, noise, toxic fumes, lack of sleep, and alcohol consumption.

■ **SYMPTOMS.** Headaches can be acute or chronic and can affect different areas of the head. The pain can range from mild to unbearable and incapacitating; it can be constant or intermittent and might be described as pressure, throbbing, or stabbing. Interestingly, brain tissue does not contain sensory nerves, so the sense of pain must come from the pain receptors in the meninges, facial tissue, or scalp. Some of the more common types of headaches include:

Tension headache caused by stress, strain, and tension on the facial, neck, and scalp muscles. Pain is typically in the occipital area.

Cluster headache can be caused by stress, emotional trauma, or unknown reasons. These headaches occur at night after falling asleep. The pain is generally a severe, throbbing pain behind the nose and one eye. The skin in this area becomes reddened, and the nose and eye water. The pain generally subsides after 1 or 2 hours but might recur several times during the night.

Post–lumbar puncture headache a severe headache affecting up to 40% of individuals, following a lumbar puncture. It is thought to be due to leakage of spinal fluid through the needle puncture site. This type of headache is often prevented by positioning the individual flat in bed without a pillow for 2 or 3 hours following this procedure.

Migraine headache a severe, incapacitating headache commonly accompanied by nausea, vomiting, and visual disturbances. Individuals affected by migraines can experience a visual **aura**, a sensation that precedes the event, including flashing light, dim vision, or photophobia. This type of headache can begin in adolescence and diminish in intensity and frequency with age. Migraine headaches occur twice as often in women than in men. The cause is still unknown, although they tend to run in families, suggesting some type of inheritance pattern. Some foods that trigger migraines are chocolate, wine, and cheese. It is also thought that these are vascular headaches caused by altered arterial blood flow.

■ *DIAGNOSIS.* Diagnosis of the cause of headache depends on individual history and physical examination. Testing can include X-ray, EEG, and MRI and CT scans.

■ *TREATMENT.* Headache treatment depends on the cause, severity, and frequency of occurrence. Often, lifestyle changes, such as improvements in diet, sleep, and exercise, help. Pain medications may be over the counter, such as acetaminophen (Tylenol®) or ibuprofen. Prescription pain medication and antinausea medications might also be needed.

■ *PREVENTION.* Diet and lifestyle changes and stress reduction are measures that can help prevent headaches. Severe headaches might require prescription medication.

EPILEPSY

■ *DESCRIPTION.* Epilepsy is a chronic disease of the brain, characterized by intermittent episodes of abnormal electrical activity in the brain, activity that might be compared to an arrhythmia of the heart.

■ *ETIOLOGY.* The cause of epilepsy can be due to brain tumors, neurologic disease, or scar tissue in the brain due to trauma or stroke. More commonly, the cause cannot be determined during the individual's life or even on autopsy.

■ *SYMPTOMS.* The most noted symptom of epilepsy is a convulsive seizure. A **convulsion** is an abnormal muscle contraction. A **seizure** is actually a sudden attack, but it is commonly used to indicate a convulsive seizure. Not all seizures are characterized by convulsions, and not all convulsions are due to epilepsy. Convulsions can occur in a nonepileptic individual due to conditions such as excessive temperature (hyperpyrexia), hypoglycemia, hypocalcemia, and drug or alcohol toxicity.

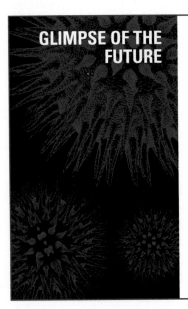

GLIMPSE OF THE FUTURE

High-Vitamin Diets = Better Test Scores?

Your diet could affect your scores on thinking tests according to recent research. Diets high in vitamins B, C, D, and E and omega-3 fatty acids and low in trans-fats may be good for brain health. Studies have shown that these vitamins are the most supportive of healthy brain aging. The studies were done on older adults who did not have other common diseases of their age group such as diabetes or high blood pressure. The participants were given thinking tests, and their scores were compared with laboratory tests analyzing their nutrient levels. The studies found that diets high in vitamins and omega-3 fatty acids were good for brain health. A diet high in trans fats was determined to be most unfavorable for brain health. Further research needs to determine how much of an individual's declining mental ability is related to diet and how much to other factors such as environment or other diseases. What will future research tell us about our diet and health?

Source: Doheny (2011).

The most common types of seizures are:

- **Petit mal** These seizures are also called absence seizures and commonly occur in children; they are often outgrown during puberty, but they can last a lifetime. These seizures consist of a brief change in the level of consciousness without convulsions. The involved individual might show symptoms of blank staring, blinking, and twitching of the eyes or mouth, or all these. The individual might remain seated or standing with loss of awareness of surroundings. Often, the seated individual appears to have only a loss of attention or absentmindedness. Episodes often last only a few seconds but can occur multiple times during the day.

- **Grand mal** These seizures are the type most often thought of as epilepsy. They are characterized by convulsions, loss of consciousness, urinary and fecal incontinence, and tongue biting. Epileptic individuals often perceive an aura with grand mal seizures, allowing time to lie down or call for support. Auras can include tingling of the fingers, ringing in the ears, and visual disturbances. Grand mal seizures often begin with a crying out as the contraction of the respiratory muscles forces exhalation, followed by generalized rhythmic contractions of the skeletal muscles of the body, arms, and legs. Contractions can last 1 to 2 minutes, but consciousness will return more slowly. The involved individual is often weak, drowsy, and confused and has no memory of the seizure event.

- **Status epilepticus** is a life-threatening event, a state of continued convulsive seizure with no recovery of consciousness. This is a medical emergency because treatment is needed to prevent cerebral anoxia and possible death.

■ *DIAGNOSIS.* Diagnosis of epilepsy is made on the basis of EEG, CT, and cerebral angiograms. EEG can reveal altered brain activity; CT can indicate alteration in brain structure, including tumors; and cerebral angiograms can reveal alteration in blood flow. Blood tests can be performed to indicate disorders of hypoglycemia and drug or alcohol toxicity.

■ *TREATMENT.* Anticonvulsive medications are the treatment of choice for epilepsy. Close monitoring and adjustment of medications are needed to get the best effect. Medications are effective in preventing or reducing seizures 80% of the time. Education and emotional support of the affected individual and family members are necessary because this disease is often feared due to lack of education. The goal for epileptic individuals should be maintenance of a normal lifestyle.

■ *PREVENTION.* Because the cause of epilepsy in many cases is not clear, it is not possible to prevent it. In the case of epilepsy brought on by head injury,

HEALTHY HIGHLIGHT

First Aid for Seizures

A seizure is a sign of a malfunction of some part of the brain's electrical system. Most seizures in individuals diagnosed with epilepsy are not emergencies, but they could be in others. It is always wise to call for assistance (medical personnel) when unsure.

In the event of a seizure, complete the following steps:

- Look for a medical ID.
- Loosen tight clothing.
- Protect the individual from harm or nearby hazards.
- Protect the head by placing a cushion or padding under it.
- Do not attempt to place a tongue blade, any hard object, or your fingers in the individual's mouth.
- Turn the individual to a side-lying position.
- Avoid tightly restraining the individual.
- Stay with the individual until other assistive personnel arrive.
- Reassure the individual and offer assistance as consciousness returns.

prevention measures include wearing a seat belt in the car and a helmet when riding a motorcycle, ATV, bike, or horse or while skating or skiing.

BELL'S PALSY

■ **DESCRIPTION.** Bell's palsy is a disease affecting the facial nerve (seventh cranial nerve), causing unilateral (one-sided) paralysis of the face. It commonly occurs in individuals 20 to 60 years of age. Bell's palsy can affect either side of the face, and both genders are affected equally. There appears to be an increased risk for pregnant women and those with an upper respiratory infection, influenza, and diabetes.

■ **ETIOLOGY.** This disease is idiopathic, but possible causes include autoimmune problems and viral disease.

■ **SYMPTOMS.** Symptoms include a drooping weakness of the eye and mouth, with inability to close the affected eye and drooling of saliva. The affected individual is unable to whistle or smile and has a distorted facial appearance (Figure 15–7).

■ **DIAGNOSIS.** Diagnosis is made on the basis of clinical history and symptoms. An electromyography can be completed to measure voluntary muscle movement and determine the extent of nerve weakness. An MRI scan is helpful also.

■ **TREATMENT.** Treatment includes analgesics and anti-inflammatory medications. If the individual is unable to close the affected eye, protection of the eye with a patch and artificial tear medication might be needed. Warm, moist heat, electrical nerve

stimulation, and massage can be prescribed to prevent facial muscle atrophy. Prognosis for Bell's palsy is good, with most cases resolving spontaneously in 2 to 8 weeks. Plastic surgery might be prescribed to correct the facial deformities caused by chronic disease.

■ **PREVENTION.** There are no known preventive measures.

PARKINSON'S DISEASE

■ **DESCRIPTION.** Parkinson's disease is a slow, progressive brain degeneration, usually developing in individuals in their late 50s and 60s. Parkinson's affects men more often than it does women.

■ **ETIOLOGY.** The cause is unknown, but individuals with Parkinson's have been found to have a deficiency of the neurotransmitter dopamine in the brain.

■ **SYMPTOMS.** Classic symptoms include the following:

- Rigidity and immobility of the hands and a very slow speech pattern

- A fine tremor in the hands described as a pill-rolling motion of the fingers

- An expressionless facial appearance with a fixed stare and infrequent blinking called Parkinson's facies (fay-SHEEZ)

- An abnormal bent-forward posture that includes a bowed head and flexed arms (Figure 15–8)

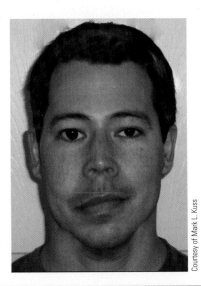

Courtesy of Mark L. Kuss

| **FIGURE 15–7**   Facial appearance of Bell's palsy.

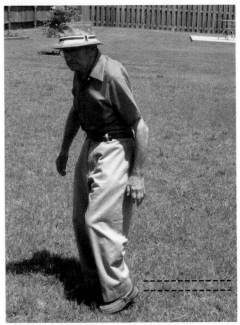

Courtesy of Larry J. Butler

| **FIGURE 15–8**   Classic posture in Parkinson's disease.

COMPLEMENTARY AND ALTERNATIVE THERAPY

Chinese Herbs for Parkinson's Disease Treatment

Mixtures of herbs have long been the basis of Chinese medicine. Western medicine did not give much credence to these treatments in the past, but new studies have shown many of them to be effective for a variety of illnesses. Parkinson's disease symptoms have been treated by the Chinese for centuries with the herb *gou teng* or with a combination of herbs. Recent research found that patients with Parkinson's disease who took a combination of herbs, which included *gou teng*, were able to sleep well and had more understandable speech patterns. A new drug being tested for Parkinsonism treatment has serious side effects, whereas *gou teng* seems to have no ill effects on the user. Other combinations of herbs are still being tested.

Source: Zukerman (2011).

- A peculiar gait of short, fast-running steps due to the abnormal posture that makes the individual tend to stumble forward, leading to frequent falls

■ **DIAGNOSIS.** Diagnosis is usually easy to make after a thorough history and physical exam. Criteria for Parkinson's disease are bradykinesia and at least one of the following: muscle rigidity, resting tremor, and/or postural instability.

■ **TREATMENT.** Treatment of Parkinson's is symptomatic. Dopamine replacement medications can be used; they do not stop the progression of the disease, but they might help with symptoms. Psychological support and physical therapy for muscle soreness are also helpful.

■ **PREVENTION.** There is no known prevention for Parkinson's disease.

Dementias

Dementia (dee-MEN-she-ah) is a loss of mental ability due to the loss of neurons or brain cells caused in several ways. One of the most common dementias is senile (old) dementia and is related to degeneration of cells with aging. The most common cause of senile dementia is Alzheimer's disease. Therefore, Alzheimer's and senile dementia are often used synonymously, but in reality, an individual can have senile dementia without Alzheimer's. Vascular dementia also can be considered a form of senile dementia because it tends to occur in older individuals.

ALZHEIMER'S DISEASE

■ **DESCRIPTION.** Alzheimer's (ALTZ-high-merz) disease is a form of dementia characterized by the

---

HEALTHY HIGHLIGHT

Not All Hand Tremors Are Caused by Parkinson's Disease

Not all hand tremors are due to Parkinson's disease. The most common tremor type is called "essential" tremor. This type of tremor most often affects the hands, but can affect the voice, legs, and head. Essential tremor is often inherited or of unknown cause. This tremor usually occurs when an individual holds a posture such as holding a fork or holding the arms outstretched. It usually does not occur at rest. β-blocker and anticonvulsant medications may be of some help if the tremors worsen to the point of making day-to-day tasks difficult to perform.

Short-lived "physiologic" tremors may occur due to stress, anxiety, low blood sugar, thyroid problems, or withdrawal from caffeine or alcohol. The cause and treatment of physiologic tremors should be addressed by a physician.

Source: Mayo Clinic (2012).

death of neurons and replacement of these neurons by microscopic plaques. It is the most common cause of dementia among older people. The disease usually affects individuals 70 years of age and older. The number of cases increases with age, with an estimated 50% of individuals over age 85 affected.

■ *ETIOLOGY.* The cause of Alzheimer's disease is unknown, but factors being considered are heredity, viral infection, autoimmunity, and aluminum toxicity. Research also shows a higher rate of Alzheimer's in individuals with a history of head trauma.

■ *SYMPTOMS.* Symptoms of the disease begin with mild mental impairment characterized by loss of short-term memory, inability to concentrate, and slight changes in personality. As the disease progresses, the affected individual struggles with communication skills, uses meaningless words, and cannot form sentences. Increased forgetfulness and difficulties in communication lead to irritability and agitation. In the final stages, which can take 5 to 10 years to develop, the affected individual's mental and physical capabilities are severely affected. The affected individual becomes restless, disoriented, incontinent, hostile, and combative and is totally dependent on a caregiver. Death is usually due to a secondary cause such as infection.

■ *DIAGNOSIS.* Diagnosis cannot be positively made except from autopsy. Initially, a diagnosis can be made on the basis of symptoms after ruling out other brain diseases. In the final stage of the disease, CT or MRI scans might reveal the characteristic brain atrophy and microscopic plaques.

■ *TREATMENT.* Treatment is supportive because there is no known cure for Alzheimer's disease. As the individual's capabilities decline, care is focused on safety and maintaining adequate nutrition, hydration, and personal hygiene. Mobility and mental capabilities are supported for as long as possible. Emotional support of family members and caregivers is of primary concern.

■ *PREVENTION.* According to the Alzheimer's Research and Prevention Foundation, there is some proof that preventive measures should include avoiding a diet high in trans-fat and saturated fat, especially red meats. Other prevention activities include taking high-potency multiple vitamins and minerals that include folic acid, vitamin E, and at least 2,000 mg of vitamin C.

VASCULAR DEMENTIA

■ *DESCRIPTION.* Vascular dementia is caused by atrophy and death of brain cells due to decreased blood flow.

■ *ETIOLOGY.* Atherosclerotic plaque is the common cause of decreased blood flow and is common with aging.

■ *SYMPTOMS.* Because the atherosclerotic plaques develop slowly, so do symptoms, which progress so slowly that they often go unnoticed by family members until they become quite severe. Symptoms include changes in memory, personality, and judgment. Irritability, depression, and sleeplessness also can occur. Personal hygiene is lacking and is often the sign that alerts family members to the condition. The affected individual can become disoriented and lost in familiar surroundings.

■ *DIAGNOSIS.* Diagnosis is made on the basis of a history and physical and blood flow testing. Arteriograms of the carotid and cerebral arteries will reveal narrowing of vessels, stenosis, and arteriosclerotic plaques.

■ *TREATMENT.* Treatment is aimed at increasing blood flow to the brain. If the cerebral arteries are involved or narrowed, medications may help improve blood flow. Carotid artery plaques can be surgically cleaned by a carotid endarterectomy (END-ar-ter-ECK-toh-me; endo = inside, arter = artery, ectomy = excision of). Prognosis depends on the effectiveness of treatment and the amount of brain cell death. If treatment is not possible or effective, or if a large amount of brain tissue has been lost, the affected individual will become progressively more demented and might need institutionalization for care.

■ *PREVENTION.* The best preventive measures are to quit smoking, lead a healthy lifestyle, and control hypertension.

HEAD TRAUMA DEMENTIA

■ *DESCRIPTION.* Head trauma can damage any part of the brain. This term fails to capture all the symptoms and long-term disabilities that can be related to such trauma. Males experience head injuries more often than females, with the most injuries occurring in those age 14 to 24 years. Very young children commonly have the worst outcomes.

■ **ETIOLOGY.** Head trauma dementia is due to death of brain cells related to head trauma. One type is Boxer's dementia, caused by repeated blows to the head as in the sport of boxing. Other types of trauma can be those sustained in accidents, especially motor vehicle accidents, and sports-related activities. The death of brain cells can be caused by the injury itself or by edema and increased ICP, which decreases or halts blood flow to brain cells, leading to cell death.

■ **SYMPTOMS.** Symptoms of head trauma dementia include a prolonged or permanent decrease in mental intellect, cognitive function, or both. The affected individual might be unable to perform activities that were easily completed prior to the injury. There are often symptoms of loss of the ability to reason, remember, and show appropriate emotions and behaviors following such injury. Changes in personality are not uncommon. Chronic psychological trauma can bring about major life changes, mania, major depression, and post-traumatic stress and anxiety disorders.

■ **DIAGNOSIS.** Diagnosis is made on the basis of history, cranial X-rays, and MRI and CT scans.

■ **TREATMENT.** Treatment is aimed at correcting the damage if possible, preventing further damage, and maintaining the existing healthy tissue. Dead brain cells cannot be replaced, so damage is permanent. Therapy and rehabilitation are needed to regain as much function as possible. Individuals suffering severe head trauma might need institutionalization for long-term care.

■ **PREVENTION.** Head injury is often easy to prevent with proper use of protective equipment. Preventive activities include:

- Wearing seat belts in automobiles.

- Wearing a helmet when riding bikes, ATVs, and skateboards.

- Wearing work-related safety equipment along with hard hats when needed.

- For elderly individuals, altering the surroundings by removing rugs or furniture that might slide easily and cause falls.

SUBSTANCE-INDUCED DEMENTIA

■ **DESCRIPTION.** This type of dementia is often cured because the cause of the dementia is curable. In some cases of substance abuse dementia, the individual might not have dementia at all but, rather, suffer from severe depression.

■ **ETIOLOGY.** Substance-induced dementia is due to brain cell death caused by toxicity from drugs and toxins. This type of dementia can be caused by repeated exposure to, or use or abuse of, certain substances. Commonly, those substances include alcohol, cocaine, heroin, lead, mercury, and fumes of paints, paint thinners, and insecticides, to name only a few. Brain cell death often persists long after the exposure to the substance ends.

■ **SYMPTOMS.** Symptoms of mental impairment and decreased cognitive ability can be permanent and often worsen over a period of time.

■ **DIAGNOSIS.** Substance abuse dementia is usually difficult to diagnose. A history and physical exam along with family and caregiver history of the individual's symptoms and history are helpful. A mental health exam is often needed.

■ **TREATMENT.** Once properly diagnosed, treating the dementia is usually a matter of removing the toxin (drugs, alcohol, fumes, or insecticides). Depending on the degree of dementia, removing the toxin might not restore normal function.

■ **PREVENTION.** Avoiding the toxin prevents this type of dementia.

Sleep Disorders

Sleep may be described as a necessary state of unconsciousness. It is thought that sleep is a period of time during which the body is actively restoring and repairing itself because an increased amount of growth hormone is released during sleep. Sleep also provides a time of recuperation of mental activities. It is believed that there is an increase in metabolic rate in the brain during sleep that allows it to be more alert and efficient during waking hours.

Sleep deprivation of just one night can lead to changes in personality, lack of muscle coordination, and decreased coping ability. There is a great variability in sleep requirements among individuals and different ages: infants need 16 to 20 hours of sleep every 24 hours. The need for sleep decreases into adulthood, with adults generally requiring between 6 and 9 hours of sleep and older adults requiring even less sleep. Sleep disorders can be due to a variety of causes and can be tested by polysomnography, a procedure measuring a variety of physical variables related to sleep.

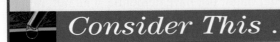
INSOMNIA

■ **DESCRIPTION.** Insomnia is the most common sleep disorder in the United States, with about one-third of the adult population experiencing it at some time. Insomnia is the perception or feeling of inadequate or poor sleep, the inability to fall or stay asleep, or waking up too early in the morning. The affected individual arises physically and mentally tired, irritable, and anxious. Insomnia is more common in females and occurs increasingly with age.

■ **ETIOLOGY.** The cause of insomnia can be related to stress, pain, fear, depression, and cardiovascular or thyroid disorders. Drugs such as caffeine, alcohol, nicotine, and bronchodilators also can cause insomnia. Eventually, the fear of being unable to fall asleep can become a cause.

■ **SYMPTOMS.** The symptom is sleeplessness, often leading to fatigue and irritability. The diagnostic definition of insomnia is sleeplessness for more than 1 month that is interfering with the individual's social or work habits.

■ **DIAGNOSIS.** Diagnosis is determined by taking a careful account of an individual's sleep history. Referral to a sleep lab might help if a breathing disorder is suspected.

■ **TREATMENT.** Treatment consists of identifying and removing the cause(s). One can develop a sleep routine with a scheduled bedtime and awakening time, and counseling might be needed to assist the individual in managing or reducing stress and anxiety. The affected individual is encouraged not to worry about when and how much he or she sleeps and to take naps and sleep as they can rather than build up anxiety about sleeping at night. The total amount of sleep in 24 hours is more important than the sleeping schedule.

■ **PREVENTION.** Prevention centers on living a healthy lifestyle, balancing rest, exercise, and recreation with stress management and healthy diet.

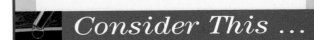
SLEEP APNEA

■ **DESCRIPTION.** Sleep apnea (AP-nee-ah; a = without, pnea = breathing) is a sleep disorder characterized by periods of apnea or breathlessness.

■ **ETIOLOGY.** This condition occurs more frequently in men and might be related to obesity, hypertension, and airway obstruction. Alcohol ingestion and smoking also can be causative factors.

■ **SYMPTOMS.** The diagnostic definition of sleep apnea is more than five periods of apnea lasting for at least 10 seconds each per hour of sleep. These breathless periods are followed by sudden gasps or snorts for air. Other symptoms can include (1) excessive daytime sleepiness to the point of falling asleep during driving, at work, or in the middle of a conversation; (2) extreme snoring that might not awaken the affected individual but easily awakens family members; and (3) personality changes, depression, and impotence. Sleep apnea can be divided into three categories:

- Obstructive apnea, caused by nasal obstruction
- Central apnea, caused by a disorder in the brain's respiratory control center
- Mixed apnea, a combination of both obstructive and central apnea

■ **DIAGNOSIS.** Diagnosis is confirmed by monitoring the affected individual during sleep for apnea and low blood oxygen levels.

■ **TREATMENT.** Treatment is based on cause. Obstructive types and mixed types are treated with weight-loss therapy and, if needed, surgery to correct nasal obstruction. Individuals affected by obstructive apnea also might benefit from oxygen administration, oral appliances, adjustable airway pressure devices, and continuous positive airway pressure (CPAP) devices during sleep. Central apnea is more difficult to control and might be treated with medications to stimulate breathing.

■ *PREVENTION.* Most cases of sleep apnea can be prevented by maintaining a healthy weight, avoiding alcohol, not smoking, and avoiding environmental smoke.

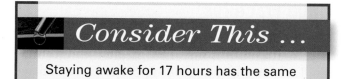

Consider This ...

Staying awake for 17 hours has the same effect on your body as drinking two glasses of wine.

Tumors

Tumors may be classified as benign and malignant. (See Chapter 3, "Neoplasms.") Benign tumors of the brain often become malignant if surgical removal is not possible. The growth of benign tumors in the confined space of the skull places pressure on the brain tissue and blood vessels, leading to loss of function and death of normal tissue. Tumors can occur in any area of the brain and at any age, although many are fairly age-specific or commonly occur in a particular age group. Gliomas and meningiomas are most common in adults.

BRAIN TUMOR

■ *DESCRIPTION.* Brain tumors may be classified as primary or secondary. Primary tumors start in the brain tissue, whereas secondary tumors occur in other areas and metastasize to the brain. Brain tumors in children are commonly primary tumors. Secondary tumors are not called brain tumors; they are named after the organ of origin. In other words, breast tumor that metastasizes to the brain is still called breast cancer with metastasis to the brain. Common sites of secondary tumors that metastasize to the brain include breast and lung.

■ *ETIOLOGY.* The cause of primary tumors is unknown.

■ *SYMPTOMS.* Symptoms are varied, depending on the area involved, and include headache, vomiting, seizures, mood and personality changes, visual disturbances, and loss of memory.

■ *DIAGNOSIS.* Diagnosis is made on the basis of clinical history, symptoms, X-ray examinations, CT and MRI scans, and biopsy. A biopsy is the most definitive study to determine the type of tumor and the best study to assist with treatment and prognosis. Further studies might be needed to determine the primary location of metastatic brain tumors.

■ *TREATMENT.* Treatment can include surgery, radiation, and chemotherapy. Treatment and prognosis depend on the type and location of the tumor.

■ *PREVENTION.* Reducing or avoiding exposure to radiation, certain medications, and head trauma can benefit prevention.

■ TRAUMA

Injuries to the brain, neck, and spinal cord are a main cause of disability and death. Trauma to the head can cause edema, increased ICP, hemorrhage, and infection, resulting in brain damage. Injury to the neck and spinal cord can lead to temporary or permanent paralysis.

Concussions and Contusions

■ *DESCRIPTION.* A concussion is the less serious of the two conditions and does not involve injury to the brain. A contusion, however, is a physical bruising of the brain tissue. Brain contusions are often accompanied by skull fractures.

■ *ETIOLOGY.* A blow to the head caused by an object, fall, or other trauma such as an automobile accident can cause a concussion or contusion.

■ *SYMPTOMS.* Both concussions and contusions cause a disruption of normal electrical activity in the brain, which, in turn, causes immediate unconsciousness, often described as being knocked out. This state of unconsciousness can last from a few seconds to several hours, and the affected individual often awakens with **amnesia**, or loss of memory. Other symptoms are headache, blurred vision, and irritability. The individual might suddenly draw up the knees and begin vomiting.

The physical bruising of a contusion can lead to the development of a hematoma, increased ICP, and permanent brain damage. If the bruised tissue is in the area of the impact, it is referred to as a coup (COO) lesion. Coup lesions often occur with direct injury such as is incurred from a direct blow to the head. If the injury occurs on the opposite side of the brain, it is called a contracoup (CON-tra-coo) lesion, which often occurs when the head is in motion and is stopped suddenly, causing a rebound effect to the opposite side (Figure 15–9), as is often found in automobile accidents. Contracoup injuries are commonly accompanied by a coup injury at the point of impact.

■ **DIAGNOSIS.** Diagnosis of both conditions is made on the basis of a history of the injury, neurologic examination, cranial X-ray, and CT or MRI scans.

■ **TREATMENT.** Treatment of a concussion consists of bed rest in a quiet area under direct observation. The individual should be awakened every 2 to 4 hours and observed for changes in consciousness, eye pupil size, mood, and behavior. An individual suffering with a contusion should be hospitalized for continuous monitoring. Analgesic, sedative, and stimulant medications should not be given to individuals with head injuries because these medications can mask symptoms and make assessment difficult.

■ **PREVENTION.** Head injury prevention includes activities such as wearing a seat belt in an automobile, wearing helmets with recreational activity, and preventing falls by removing clutter and slippery rugs.

Media Link

View an animation on contracoup injuries on the Online Resources.

Skull Fractures

■ **DESCRIPTION.** A skull fracture is a break in a cranial (skull) bone. The greatest danger of a skull fracture is the resulting brain tissue damage (Figure 15–10). Bony fragments can cut into the brain tissue, severing a vessel and causing a hematoma. Brain damage from a fracture can be temporary or permanent.

■ **ETIOLOGY.** A fracture can occur with head injuries from falls, a severe blow to the head, automobile accidents, or sports injuries.

■ **SYMPTOMS.** The position of the fracture will cause a variety of symptoms. For instance, a fracture near the base of the skull might injure the respiratory center of the brain, causing the individual to stop breathing. Fractures in other areas can

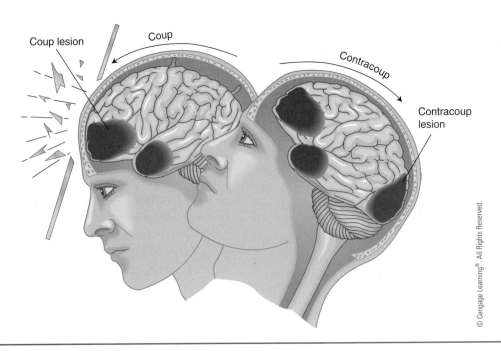

FIGURE 15–9   Coup and contracoup lesions.

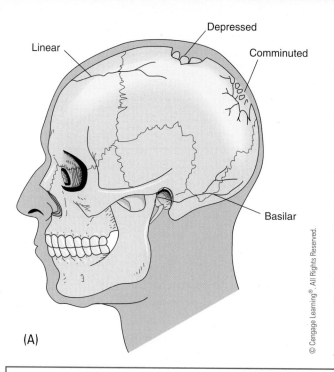

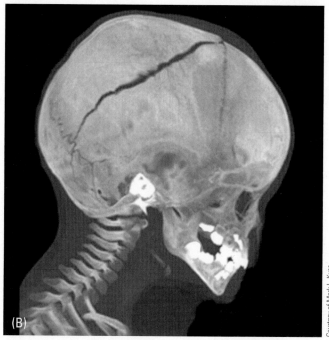

FIGURE 15–10 (A) Common sites and types of skull fractures. (B) Skull fracture (X-ray).

lead to hemiparesis and seizures. Another potential problem is infection of the brain tissue through the fracture site.

■ *DIAGNOSIS.* Diagnosis is made on the basis of clinical history, physical examination, cranial X-rays, and CT scan.

■ *TREATMENT.* Treatment depends on the type and position of the fracture. A craniotomy (cranio = skull, otomy = incision) might be performed to relieve ICP due to swelling. Surgical repair of the fracture might be performed if the fractured bone is pressing on the brain tissue. Protective headgear might be needed until the fracture site is healed.

■ *PREVENTION.* Preventive actions include practicing safety measures and avoiding risky activities to prevent head injury.

Epidural and Subdural Hematomas

■ *DESCRIPTION.* An epidural hematoma is a collection of blood between the skull and dura mater, the thin membrane that covers the brain. Epidural hematomas occur more often in young adult males. A subdural hematoma is a collection of blood between the outer (dura mater) layer and the middle (arachnoid) layer. Subdural hematomas occur twice as often as epidural hematomas.

■ *ETIOLOGY.* A blow to the head, such as might be obtained in a fight or accident, is the common cause of an **epidural** (EP-ih-DER-al); epi = above, dural = dura, outer meninges) hematoma. Blood vessels are ruptured and hemorrhage or seep blood between the bony skull and the first, or outer, meninges, the dura mater (Figure 15–11). Blood usually collects rapidly over a period of hours, pushing the dura away from the inner bony skull.

A **subdural** (SUB-DOO-ral) hematoma is usually the result of the head hitting a stationary object, as is often seen with falls, characterized by striking the head on the floor or a solid object. Subdural hematomas are characterized by blood collecting between the outer (dura mater) layer and the middle (arachnoid) layer. Subdural hematomas generally develop more slowly over a period of days.

■ *SYMPTOMS.* Symptoms of an epidural hematoma occur within a few hours after injury and can include headache, dilated pupils, nausea, vomiting, and dizziness. As the hematoma grows, the individual might lose consciousness and develop an increase in ICP.

Symptoms of a subdural hematoma are due to increased ICP. Symptoms might include hemiparesis, nausea, vomiting, dizziness, convulsions, and loss of consciousness.

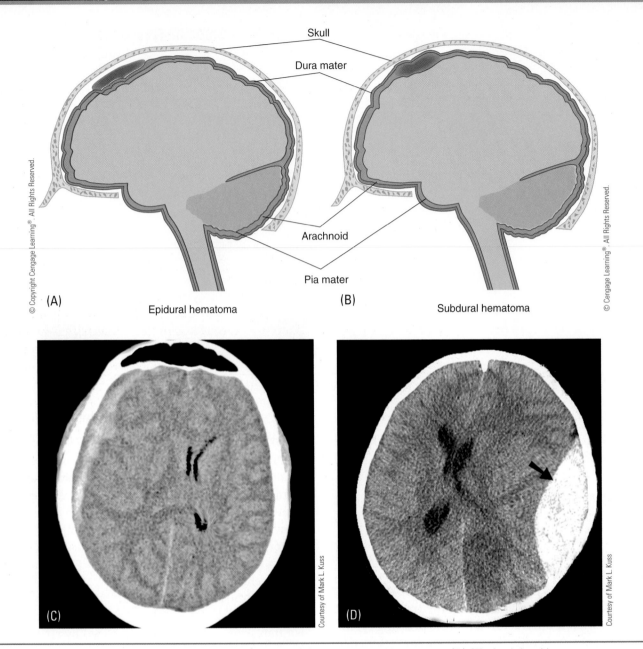

Skull

Dura mater

Arachnoid

Pia mater

(A)

Epidural hematoma

(B)

Subdural hematoma

© Copyright Cengage Learning®. All Rights Reserved.

© Cengage Learning®. All Rights Reserved.

Courtesy of Mark L. Kuss

(C)

(D)

Courtesy of Mark L. Kuss

FIGURE 15–11 (A) Epidural and (B) Subdural hematomas. (C) CT of epidural hematoma. (D) CT of subdural hematoma.

■ *DIAGNOSIS.* Diagnosis of a cerebral hematoma is made on the basis of clinical history, cranial X-ray, or CT or MRI scan. Hematomas, generally, are accompanied by a skull fracture.

■ *TREATMENT.* Treatment of epidural and subdural hematomas is aimed at decreasing ICP. Pressure can be relieved by a special craniotomy called burr holes to drain the blood and **cauterization** (KAW-ter-eye-ZAY-shun; electrical burning of tissue) to stop the bleeding. If ICP is treated promptly, prognosis is good. Untreated, increased ICP can be fatal.

■ *PREVENTION.* Preventive actions include activities to prevent head injury.

Spinal Cord Injury: Quadriplegia and Paraplegia

■ *DESCRIPTION.* The spinal cord is protected by the bony vertebral column. When this column is fractured or injured, the spinal cord also can suffer injury. The spinal cord can be injured at any level, but the mobility of the neck causes this area to be the most vulnerable. The site of the injury, the type of trauma, and the degree of injury will all play a role in determining whether paralysis will occur and whether it will be temporary or permanent. Paralysis of the lower part of the body including both legs is called paraplegia. If the body and both arms and both legs are affected, it is called quadriplegia.

■ *ETIOLOGY.* The leading cause of spinal cord injury is automobile accidents. Other causes are gunshot and knife wounds, falls, and recreational and sports injuries.

■ *SYMPTOMS.* Injury to the spinal cord can result in varying degrees of loss of movement and feeling below the area of injury. If the damage to the spinal cord is severe, there is little or no hope of regaining movement and feeling. Paralysis, initially, results in the inability to move the extremities; but with time, reflex functions might return, leading to spastic movements. Refer to Figure 15–12 while reading the following material for a better understanding of spinal cord injuries and preventive measures.

Injury to the neck is common in automobile accidents and sports accidents. Automobile accidents commonly lead to injury in the form of whiplash.

Injury to the highest level of the cervical spine (C1–C3) is usually fatal. Injuries to the cervical spine or neck area (C1–C4) can lead to **quadriplegia** (KWAD-rih-PLEE-jee-ah; quadri = four, plegia = paralysis). Quadriplegia is the loss of movement and feeling in the trunk and all four extremities with the accompanying loss of bowel, bladder, and sexual function. Other life-threatening symptoms include hypotension, **hypothermia** (hypo = low, thermia = heat or temperature), bradycardia, and respiratory problems. In some cases, respirations must be permanently assisted with mechanical ventilation. Injury to the lower cervical spine (C5–C7) can lead to varying degrees of paralysis of the arms and shoulders.

Injury to the thoracic or lumbar section of the spinal cord can lead to **paraplegia** (PAR-ah-PLEE-jee-ah; para = beyond or two like parts, plegia = paralysis), a loss of movement and feeling in the trunk and both legs. Loss of bladder, bowel, and sexual function is common. Paraplegia is often the result of a fall or an injury resulting in compression to the lower spine.

■ *DIAGNOSIS.* Diagnosis is made on the basis of history of the injury and physical examination along with X-rays, CT scan, MRI, and myelography.

■ *TREATMENT.* Treatment of suspected spinal cord injury victims includes seeking emergency medical treatment immediately and not moving the victim unless the surroundings are unsafe or life-threatening as in the case of fire or flood. The head and neck should be moved only in life-threatening situations such as choking or respiratory arrest. Movement at

this time should be very cautious. Emergency medical treatment is aimed at maintaining the position of the spine by limiting movement with use of special collars and backboards. The head, neck, and spine are stabilized prior to transporting in an emergency vehicle.

Hospitalization includes diagnosis and treatment of the injury, including medications, emergency surgery, and, often, immobilization with traction or traction-like devices. Much of the early treatment is aimed at preventing further spinal cord injury.

Further treatment can include surgery to realign and stabilize the bony spinal column and **decompress**, or release, pressure on the spinal cord. Early and intensive rehabilitation is necessary for the best prognosis. Generally, the earlier the treatment is begun, the better the prognosis.

During treatment, medical attention must also focus on preventing problems that arise from immobilization, including muscle wasting, contractures, decubitus (commonly called bed sores), blood clots, and urinary tract infections.

Long-term care includes rehabilitation and supportive treatment, which might include medications, electric wheelchair, computer devices, and ventilator support.

■ *PREVENTION.* Preventive actions include activities to prevent spinal cord injury as shown in Figure 15–12.

Media Link

View an animation on spinal cord injuries on the Online Resources.

RARE DISEASES

Although some of the disorders discussed in this section are familiar to the public due to their exposure in the media and to intensive solicitations for research, they are actually rare diseases of the nervous system, considering all the various disorders that affect this system.

Amyotrophic Lateral Sclerosis

Amyotrophic lateral sclerosis (ALS), also known as Lou Gehrig's disease, is a destructive disease of the motor, or movement, neurons. The cause of ALS is unknown, although genetic and viral-immune factors have been suggested.

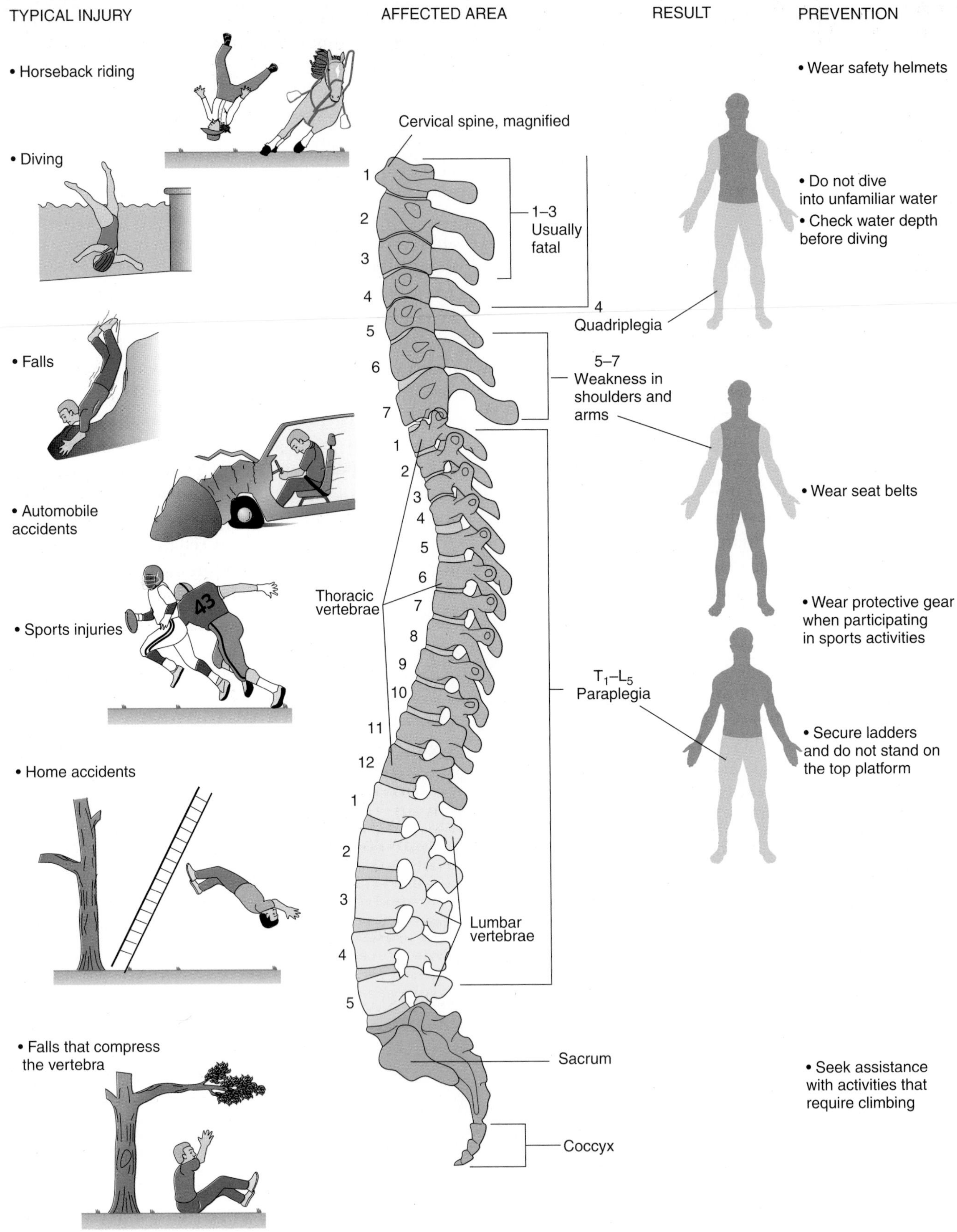

TYPICAL INJURY	AFFECTED AREA	RESULT	PREVENTION

- Horseback riding

- Diving

Cervical spine, magnified

1
2
3
4

1–3
Usually
fatal

4
Quadriplegia

- Wear safety helmets

- Do not dive
into unfamiliar water
- Check water depth
before diving

- Falls

5
6
7

5–7
Weakness in
shoulders and
arms

- Automobile
accidents

- Sports injuries

Thoracic
vertebrae

1
2
3
4
5
6
7
8
9
10
11
12

T_1–L_5
Paraplegia

- Wear seat belts

- Wear protective gear
when participating
in sports activities

- Home accidents

1
2
3
4
5

Lumbar
vertebrae

- Secure ladders
and do not stand on
the top platform

- Falls that compress
the vertebra

Sacrum

Coccyx

- Seek assistance
with activities that
require climbing

FIGURE 15–12 Spinal cord injuries.

ALS is characterized by atrophy of the muscles, leading to a progressive loss of movement of the hands, arms, and legs. As the disease progresses, loss of muscle function in the face and chest area leads to difficulty talking, chewing, swallowing, and breathing. Eventually, the loss of motor function causes quadriplegia.

One distinguishing factor of ALS is that there is not a loss of sensory neurons. The individual can feel the extremities, but movement is impaired. Mental function is unaffected, so the affected individual is aware of the condition and can take an active role in planning care. ALS usually affects men twice as often as it affects women, with onset of the disease after age 50.

Treatment is supportive because there is no cure for ALS. Management of respiratory complications is vital because most individuals affected with ALS die of respiratory failure. ALS is eventually fatal, with death usually occurring 4 to 6 years after onset. In some cases, affected individuals have remained active for 10 to 20 years after onset.

Guillain–Barré Syndrome

Guillain–Barré syndrome is an acute, progressive disease affecting the spinal nerves. The cause of this disease is unknown, but it is suggested to be an autoimmune disorder because the symptoms usually begin 10 to 21 days after a febrile illness such as a respiratory infection or gastroenteritis.

Early symptoms include nausea, fever, and malaise. Within 24 to 72 hours, **paresthesia** (PAR-es-THEE-see-ah; abnormal sensation, burning, tingling, or numbness), muscle weakness, and paralysis usually begin. These symptoms generally begin in the legs and move upward but can also start in the face and arms and move downward.

Guillain–Barré syndrome becomes life-threatening if respiratory muscles are involved. Symptoms can progress for several days to some weeks. When progression ceases, recovery begins and can require 3 to 12 months. Treatment is supportive. Recovery is usually complete.

Huntington's Disease

Huntington's disease, also known as Huntington's chorea, is an inherited disease. It is a dominant gene disorder affecting 50% of all children in families in which one parent has Huntington's. This disorder does not appear until middle age, so children are often grown before the parent shows symptoms.

Symptoms of Huntington's consist of a progressive degeneration of the brain, characterized by loss of muscle control and **chorea**, a constant, jerky, uncontrollable movement. The disease also leads to mental deterioration with symptoms of personality change, moody behavior, and loss of memory. Over a period of years, dementia (total mental incapacitation) occurs.

There is no cure for Huntington's disease. Treatment is supportive and protective with institutionalization often necessary to provide the needed care. Genetic counseling is needed in families with this inheritance pattern.

Multiple Sclerosis

Multiple sclerosis (MS) is a disease that causes demyelination of the nerves of the CNS. Myelin, remember, acts as an insulator around nerves, much like the insulation around an electric cord. Demyelination allows information to leak from the nerve pathway, leading to poor or absent nerve transmission.

The cause of MS is not clear. It is thought that a genetic predisposition plays some part because it is 15 times more likely to occur in first-degree relatives of affected persons. It is also believed that the immune system and viral infection play a part.

Symptoms caused by demyelinating lesions are muscle weakness, lack of coordination, paresthesia, speech difficulty, loss of bladder function, and visual disturbance, especially diplopia (double vision). Symptoms are varied, depending on the location of the lesions, making diagnosis difficult.

MS usually affects young adults between the ages of 20 and 40 years. It is characterized by periods of remission and exacerbation, usually over a period of several years.

Physical therapy and muscle relaxants can be helpful to maintain muscle tone and reduce spastic movement. The severity of the disease varies from individual to individual, but generally speaking, most affected individuals live a normal life span.

EFFECTS OF AGING ON THE SYSTEM

The effects of aging on the nervous system are some of the most noticeable to the older adult. With aging, there is a decrease in nervous system activity in the brain and spinal cord due to a loss of neurons and shrinkage of the hypothalamus. Research has shown that continued active use of the brain decreases this process to some extent, but some changes still occur. With these changes in the brain and spinal cord come many changes in the individual's functioning, for instance, a loss in short-term memory but not in long-term memory. There is also a slower general reaction time. The older person also might have difficulty completing fine motor skills. General touch perception is somewhat diminished, too, so the individual might have difficulty distinguishing temperature changes and pain stimuli.

Vision ability is one of the first changes the individual often notices. There is a loss of visual acuity and a decrease in peripheral vision. Some individuals also become intolerant of very bright light and have difficulty adapting to changes in light from dark to bright. Some hearing loss is a subtle process that occurs at different levels in individuals. Taste sensation also can diminish over time.

Sleep patterns are usually affected in the aging process. Generally, the older adult does not sleep as well at night but makes up for this deficit by taking short naps throughout the day or in the early evening.

SUMMARY

The nervous system is a highly complex system responsible for the individual's ability to reason, interact with other individuals, understand complex ideas, and respond both intellectually and physically. Disorders of the system usually result in symptoms involving many other systems.

Injuries to the brain, neck, and spinal cord are a main cause of disability and death nationwide. Permanent neurologic deficits are common in brain and spinal cord injuries.

Changes in the nervous system with aging result in some of the most commonly seen symptoms; losses in the senses are the most noticeable problems. Changes in vision and hearing are some of the earliest symptoms realized by the middle-aged individual. Alzheimer's disease is one of the most common disorders of the nervous system diagnosed today.

REVIEW QUESTIONS

Short Answer

1. What are the functions of the nervous system?

2. Which signs and symptoms are associated with common nervous system disorders?

3. Which diagnostic tests are most commonly used to determine the type and cause of nervous system disorders?

Matching

4. Match the disorders listed in the left column with the correct description in the right column:

_____ Encephalitis   a. Inflammation of the covering of the brain and spinal cord

_____ Tetanus   b. A disorder affecting the seventh cranial nerve

_____ Meningitis   c. Disruption in the electrical activity of the brain, causing unconsciousness

_____ TIA   d. Blood collection between the dura mater and arachnoid layer of the brain

_____ Cephalalgia   e. Physical bruising of the brain

_____ Concussion   f. Infection of nerve tissue

_____ Contusion   g. Disease characterized by the demyelination of nerves of the CNS

_____ Subdural hematoma   h. Inflammation of brain tissue

_____ Alzheimer's disease   i. Headache

_____ ALS   j. A neurodegenerative disease characterized by cognitive dysfunction

_____ MS   k. Destructive disease of the motor neurons

_____ Bell's palsy   l. Mild stroke

CASE STUDIES

■ Mr. Speed is a 57-year-old gentleman who has been recently diagnosed with Alzheimer's disease. He is in the early stage of the disease at this point. Mrs. Speed is quite concerned about the progression of the disease, whether Mr. Speed can still be employed, if he can be left alone for several hours at a time, and what medications he will be required to take. How would you respond to her concerns? Is there other information that would be helpful to the Speeds? Where can they find more information about Alzheimer's disease?

■ Mrs. Simpson, age 56, comes to the clinic for her yearly routine physical examination. She asks you about receiving the vaccine for shingles that she heard about on television. She thought she should get it because her sister had shingles a year ago. Mrs. Simpson stated that her sister really suffered with the disease, and she does not want to have that same experience. What can you tell her about the vaccine? Is she a candidate for Zostavax®? Who should receive the vaccine? Where can she find more information about this vaccine?

Study Tools

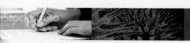

Workbook

    Complete Chapter 15

Online Resources

    PowerPoint® presentations

    Animation

BIBLIOGRAPHY

Ashton, J., Baker, S. N., & Weant, K. A. (2011). When snakes bite: The management of North American Crotalinae snake envenomation. *Advanced Emergency Nursing Journal 33*(1), 15–22.

Cahill, J. E., & Armstrong, T. S. (2011). Caring for an adult with a malignant primary brain tumor. *Nursing 41*(6), 28–34.

Carney, P. R., Myers, S., & Geyer, J. D. (2011). Seizure prediction: Methods. *Epilepsy & Behavior 22*, S94–S101.

Challem, J. (2011). Medical journal watch: Context and applications. *Alternative & Complementary Therapies 17*(1), 57–61.

Cilia, R., & Eimeren, T. (2011). Impulse control disorders in Parkinson's disease: Seeking a roadmap toward a better understanding. *Brain Structure & Function 216*(4), 289–299.

Clinical digest. Brain tumor risk persists for many years after epilepsy. (2011). *Nursing Standard 25*(40), 16–17.

Do antidepressants work in the damaged brain? (2011). *Harvard Health Letter 37*(1), 6–7.

Doheny, K. (2011). Diet patterns linked with brain health: People with diets high in vitamins B, C, D, E and omega-3s had less brain shrinkage, higher scores on thinking tests. WebMD Health News. *www.webmd.com* (accessed December 2011).

Emery, V. (2011). Alzheimer disease: Are we intervening too late? *Journal of Neural Transmission 118*(9), 1361–1378.

Galimberti, D., & Scarpini, E. (2012). Progress in Alzheimer's disease. *Journal of Neurology 259*(2), 201–211.

Gialanella, B., Bertolinelli, M., Lissi, M., & Prometti, P. (2011). Predicting outcome after stroke: The role of aphasia. *Disability & Rehabilitation 33*(2), 122–129.

Hallett, M. (2012). Parkinson's disease tremor: Pathophysiology. *Parkinsonism & Related Disorders 18*(Suppl.), S85–S86.

Ibarretxe-Bilbao, N., Junque, C., Marti, M. J., & Tolosa, E. (2011). Cerebral basis of visual hallucinations in Parkinson's disease: Structural and functional MRI studies. *Journal of the Neurological Sciences 310*(1/2), 79–81.

Japan Cholesterol and Diabetes Mellitus Investigation Group. (2011). Age, gender, insulin and blood glucose control status alter the risk of ischemic heart disease and stroke among elderly diabetic patients. *Cardiovascular Diabetology 10*(1), 86–97.

Laredo, L., Vargas, E., Blasco, A., Aguilar, M., Moreno, A., & Portolés, A. (2011). Risk of cerebrovascular accident associated with use of antipsychotics: Population-based case-control study. *Journal of the American Geriatrics Society 59*(7), 1182–1187.

Lowes, R. (2012). All ages should get Tdap shots, says CDC panel. Medscape Medical News. *www.medscape.com* (accessed February 2012).

Margrove, K. L., Thapar, A. K., Mensah, S. A., & Kerr, M. P. (2011). Help-seeking and treatment preferences for depression in epilepsy. *Epilepsy & Behavior 22*(4), 740–744.

Mayo Clinic. (2012). Hand tremors. Mayo Clinic Newsletter, July. *www.HealthLetter.MayoClinic.com* (accessed July 2012).

Mount, H. R., & Schlaudecker, J. D. (2011). A stroke—or something else? *Journal of Family Practice 60*(9), 513–516.

Natale, G., Pasquali, L., Paparelli, A., & Fornai, F. (2011). Parallel manifestations of neuropathologies in the enteric and central nervous systems. *Neurogastroenterology & Motility 23*(12), 1056–1065.

Nuttall, A. (2010). Learning zone: Assessment meningitis. *Nursing Standard 24*(48), 59.

Pandey, P., Singh, M., & Gambhir, I. S. (2011). Alzheimer's disease: A threat to mankind. *Journal of Stress Physiology & Biochemistry 7*(4), 15–30.

Paul, S., Wellesley, A., & O'Callaghan, C. (2011). Meningococcal disease in children: Case studies and discussion. *Emergency Nurse 19*(4), 24–29.

Perucca, P., Hesdorffer, D. C., & Gilliam, F. G. (2011). Response to first antiepileptic drug trial predicts health outcome in epilepsy. *Epilepsia (Series 4) 52*(12), 2209–2215.

Philip, A., & Thakur, R. (2011). Post-herpetic neuralgia. *Journal of Palliative Medicine 14*(6), 765–773.

Raymond, L. A., André, V. M., Cepeda, C., Gladding, C. M., Milnerwood, A. J., & Levine, M. S. (2011). Pathophysiology of Huntington's disease: Time-dependent alterations in synaptic and receptor function. *Neuroscience 198*, 252–273.

Rozen, T. (2011). Juvenile myoclonic epilepsy presenting as a new daily persistent-like headache. *Journal of Headache & Pain 12*(6), 645–647.

Unger Lithner, C., Hedberg, M. M., & Nordberg, A. (2011). Transgenic mice as a model for Alzheimer's disease. *Current Alzheimer Research 8*(8), 818–831.

Whisenant, M. (2011). Informal caregiving in patients with brain tumors. *Oncology Nursing Forum 38*(5), E373–E381.

Williams, I. I., Leen, C. C., & Barton, S. S. (2011). 6 Herpes viruses. *HIV Medicine 12*(S2), 61–69.

Wreghitt, T. (2011). Medicolegal aspects of the mismanagement of patients with herpesvirus infections. *Clinical Risk 17*(2), 62–64.

Zukerman, W. (2011). Chinese medicine to treat Parkinson's. *New Scientist 210*(2818), 14.

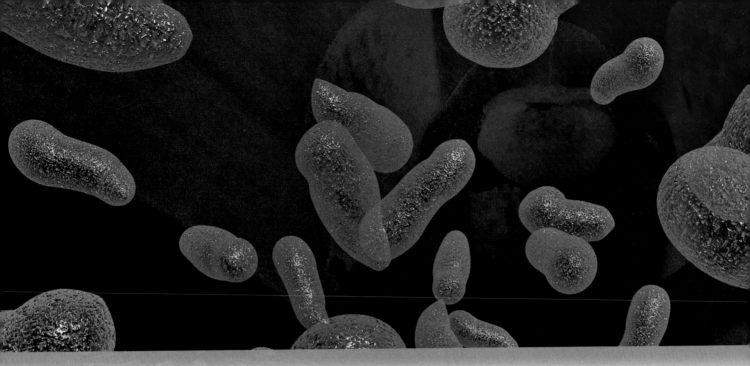

OUTLINE

KEY TERMS

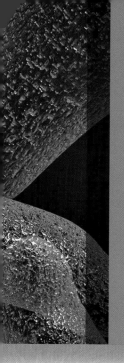

16

Eye and Ear Diseases and Disorders

LEARNING OBJECTIVES

Upon completion of the chapter, the learner should be able to:

1. Define the terminology common to the eye and ear.

2. Discuss the basic anatomy and physiology of the eye and ear.

3. Identify the important signs and symptoms associated with common eye and ear disorders.

4. Describe the common diagnostics used to determine the type and cause of eye and ear disorders.

5. Identify common disorders of the eye and ear.

6. Describe the typical course and management of the common eye and ear disorders.

7. Describe the effects of aging on the eye and ear and the common disorders associated with aging of these organs.

OVERVIEW

The eyes and ears are the major sensory organs of the body. They are extremely important to most individuals to maintain quality of life and ease of functioning. However, although sensory deficits affect many people adversely, a high-quality lifestyle is still possible after sensory losses. Individuals with visual and hearing impairment learn to function extremely well in activities of daily living. Disorders of the sensory organs are frequently the result of other system problems. Early detection of vision or hearing impairment can prevent permanent loss of these senses. ■

ANATOMY AND PHYSIOLOGY

The eye and ear are sensory organs that perform highly complex functions in the individual. They each are unique in their structure and function.

Eye

The eyeball is the sensory organ of sight located in the bony orbit of the skull. It is about 1 inch in diameter and consists of extraocular and intraocular structures (Figure 16–1). The extraocular structures include the following:

- Muscles that hold the eyeball in place and facilitate movement of the eyeball
  - Superior and inferior rectus—move eye up and down
  - Medial and lateral rectus—move eye toward the nose and toward the temple
  - Superior and inferior oblique—move the eye to the right and left vertically
- Cranial nerves that innervate the eye and its structures
  - Optic (II)
  - Oculomotor (III)
  - Trochlear (IV)
  - Trigeminal (V)
  - Abducens (VI)
  - Facial (VII)
- Eyelids that cover the anterior portion of the eyeball, regulate light entering the eye, protect the eye, and lubricate the eye
- Conjunctivae (clear transparent membranes) to protect the eye from foreign objects
- Lacrimal glands (tear glands) to clean and moisten the eye

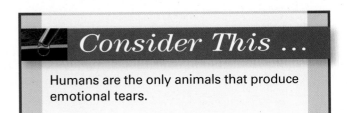

Consider This ...

Humans are the only animals that produce emotional tears.

The intraocular structures consist of some parts of the eye that are visible externally and some parts visible only through an ophthalmoscope. The intraocular structures include the following:

- Sclera—white area covering the outside of the eye except over the pupil and iris
- Cornea—clear tissue covering the pupil and iris
- Iris—round disk of smooth and radial muscles giving the eye its color

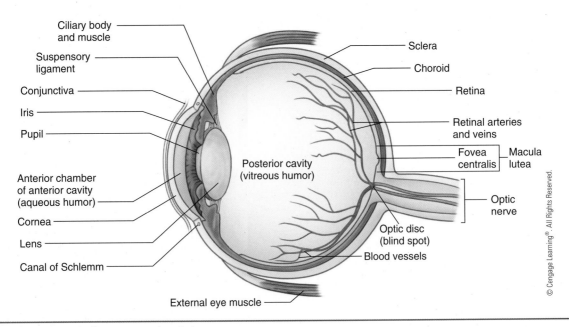

FIGURE 16–1 The eyeball: cross-sectional view.

- Pupil—round opening in the iris that changes size as the iris reacts to light and dark
- Anterior chamber—space between the cornea and iris/pupil that is filled with clear fluid called aqueous humor
- Posterior chamber—space between the iris and lens that is filled with aqueous humor
- Lens—clear fibers enclosed in a membrane that refract and focus light to the retina
- Posterior cavity—the space in the posterior two-thirds of the eyeball, filled with a thick, gelatinous material called vitreous humor
- Posterior sclera—white opaque layer covering the posterior part of the eyeball
- Choroid layer—the layer containing blood vessels between the sclera and retina
- Retina—the inner layer of the posterior part of the eye that receives the light rays (visual stimuli)

The mechanism of vision occurs after impulses leave the retinae and travel through the optic nerves to the brain. At the optic chiasm, the nerve fibers cross and continue to the thalamus. These fibers synapse with other neurons that send the impulses to the right and left visual area of the occipital lobe of the brain. Because the tracts cross at the optic chiasm, the stimuli coming from the right visual fields are translated in the visual area of the left occipital area, and the stimuli coming from the left visual fields are translated in the visual area of the right occipital lobe (Figure 16–2).

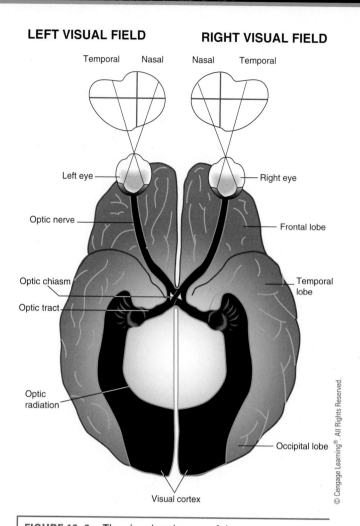

FIGURE 16–2 The visual pathways of the eye.

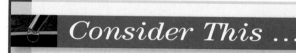

If an individual becomes blind in one eye, they lose about 20% of their vision but 100% of their depth perception.

Media Link

View an animation about the structures of the eye on the Online Resources.

Ear

The structures of hearing and equilibrium are divided into the external ear, the middle ear, and the inner ear (Figure 16–3). The external ear includes the pinna (auricle) and the external auditory canal. The pinna is mostly cartilaginous tissue with a small amount of adipose tissue in the earlobe. The external auditory canal is about 1 inch long and contains hair and wax (**cerumen**, se-ROO-men) producing glands. The external ear and middle ear are separated by the tympanic membrane (eardrum).

The middle ear, also called the tympanic cavity, is a small space containing three bones: the malleus (hammer), incus (anvil), and stapes (stirrup). Next to the stapes is the oval window that leads to the inner ear.

The inner ear is the most sophisticated part of the ear and is responsible for both hearing and equilibrium (balance). It consists of a fluid-filled space

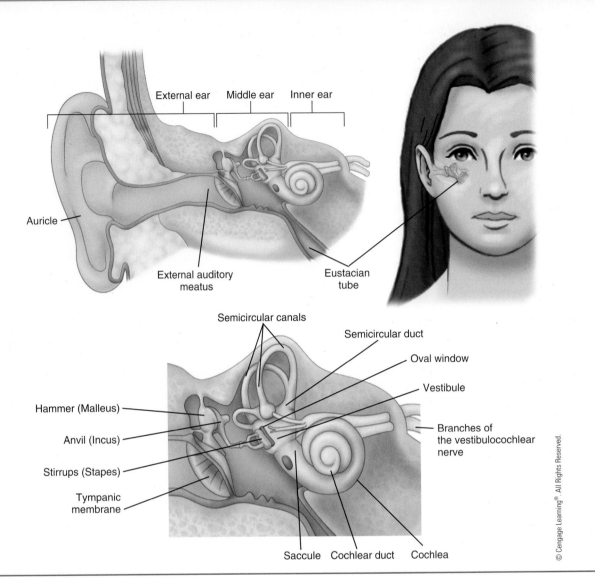

FIGURE 16–3 The ear.

housing the vestibule, the semicircular canals, the round window, and the cochlea. The structures in the vestibule maintain equilibrium during movement of the head. The semicircular canals assist the body in adjusting to changes in direction, and the movement of fluid in this area can cause symptoms of dizziness. The cochlea is the organ of hearing.

The outer ear (pinna) picks up sound waves sent through the external auditory canal to the tympanic membrane. The membrane vibrates in reaction to the sound waves striking it. These vibrations pass through the three tiny middle ear bones, through the oval window, and into the fluid in the cochlea. Receptor cells respond and transfer the sounds into electrical impulses that travel to the brain through the acoustic nerve. The receiving area of the brain for auditory impulses is in the temporal lobe.

Media Link

View an animation about the structures of the ear on the Online Resources.

▓▓ COMMON SIGNS AND SYMPTOMS

Common signs and symptoms of eye disease that need medical attention include:

- Pain or burning in or around the eye
- Decreased visual acuity or ability to see

- Any visual disorder such as seeing flashes of light
- Eye redness

Common signs and symptoms of ear disease that need medical attention include:

- Otalgia (oh-TAL-gee-ah; oto = ear, algia = pain; ear pain)
- Deafness
- Vertigo (VER-tih-go; dizziness)
- Tinnitus (tin-EYE-tus; ringing in the ears)

DIAGNOSTIC TESTS

Diagnostic Tests of the Eye

An **ophthalmoscope** (aft-THAL-moh-skope; ophthalm = eye, scope = instrument used to look) is the instrument used for a basic examination of the eye. During an ophthalmoscopy (ophthalm = eye, oscopy = procedure to look), the fundus, or interior aspect of the eye, is examined. The retina, vessels, and optic disk of the eye can be visualized easily.

Visual acuity is measured by the use of a Snellen chart (Figure 16–4). The chart contains lines of letters in varying sizes with predetermined numbers at the end of each line. The predetermined numbers indicate the distance from which an individual with normal vision can see that particular line of letters. Normal vision is expressed as 20/20 and is considered normal vision for an individual viewing a particular line of the chart from 20 feet away.

For testing, the individual is positioned 20 feet from the chart, or this distance can be simulated with reflective mirrors. During the testing, one eye is covered, allowing measurement of each eye separately. The smallest line of letters the individual can read is noted, and the predetermined numbers at the end of that line are recorded in a fraction. The first number, 20, expresses the fact that the individual is tested from 20 feet, and the second number expresses the distance from which an individual with normal vision could view those same images. For example, 20/220 means that the tested individual can see at 20 feet what most people can see at 220 feet.

Diagnostic testing includes tonometry, slit-lamp examination, and retinal angiography. **Tonometry** (toh-NOM-eh-tree; tono = tone or pressure, metry = measurement) measures the pressure inside the eye

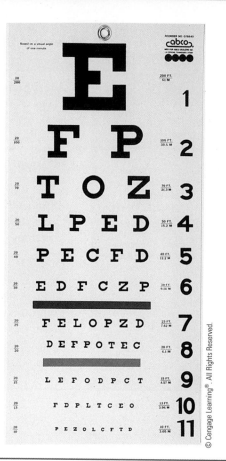

FIGURE 16–4 The Snellen chart.

and is therefore useful in determining the presence of glaucoma. A slit-lamp examination uses a microscope to magnify the surface of the eye by directing a beam of light, narrowed to a slit, at the cornea. Instilling fluorescein dye in the eye prior to the examination can improve visualization of eye disorders. A slit-lamp examination is helpful in determining corneal abrasions, keratitis, and cataracts. **Angiography** (AN-jee-OG-rah-fee; angio = vessel, graphy = procedure to record) is used to discover vessel disease and problems with blood flow to the eye. For this test, fluorescein dye is injected into a vein, usually in the arm, and after the dye fills the vessels of the eye, X-rays show the vessels. Vascular disorders such as those caused by diabetic retinopathy can be visualized.

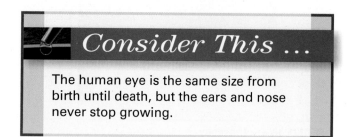

Consider This ...

The human eye is the same size from birth until death, but the ears and nose never stop growing.

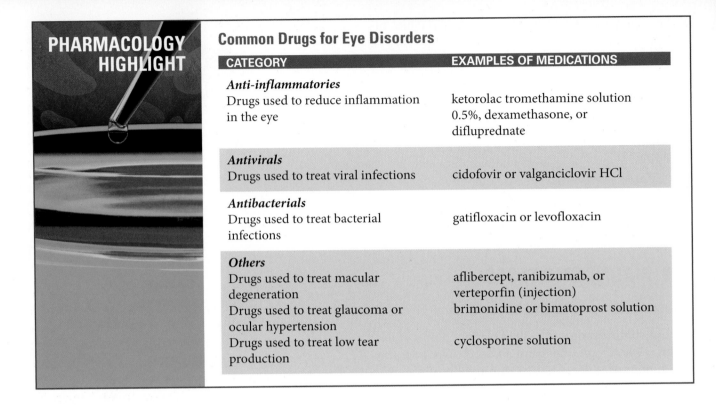

PHARMACOLOGY HIGHLIGHT

Common Drugs for Eye Disorders

CATEGORY	EXAMPLES OF MEDICATIONS
Anti-inflammatories Drugs used to reduce inflammation in the eye	ketorolac tromethamine solution 0.5%, dexamethasone, or difluprednate
Antivirals Drugs used to treat viral infections	cidofovir or valganciclovir HCl
Antibacterials Drugs used to treat bacterial infections	gatifloxacin or levofloxacin
Others Drugs used to treat macular degeneration	aflibercept, ranibizumab, or verteporfin (injection)
Drugs used to treat glaucoma or ocular hypertension	brimonidine or bimatoprost solution
Drugs used to treat low tear production	cyclosporine solution

Diagnostic Tests of the Ear

An **otoscope** (OH-toh-skope; oto = ear, scope = instrument to look) is the instrument used to examine the ear. During an otoscopy (oto = ear, scopy = procedure to look), or otoscopic examination (Figure 16–5), the external canal and tympanic membrane can be visualized easily. Otitis externa and a ruptured tympanic membrane can be diagnosed using the otoscope.

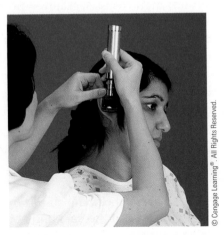

FIGURE 16–5 Otoscopy.

The basic test for hearing is called **audiometry** (AW-dee-OM-eh-tree; audio = sound, metry = measure). During the test, sound is delivered in varying levels, or decibels, through a headset to each ear separately. The greater the amount of sound needed for the individual to hear or recognize it, the greater the amount of deafness or hearing loss.

COMMON DISEASES OF THE EYE

The most common problem of the eyes is a decrease in visual acuity, the ability to see clearly. The most common cause of poor visual acuity is refractive errors. Other common problems include those related to inflammation or infection, which usually affects the outer eye because of its contact with the environment. Other eye disorders are clouding of the lens (cataract), increased inner eye pressure (glaucoma), altered eye movement (nystagmus, strabismus), degenerative disorders (such as macular degeneration), secondary disease (diabetic retinopathy), and hereditary disorders (color blindness).

PHARMACOLOGY HIGHLIGHT

Common Drugs for Ear Disorders

CATEGORY	EXAMPLES OF MEDICATIONS
Antibiotics Drugs used to treat ear infections	azithromycin, amoxicillin, or cefdinir
Analgesics Drugs used to treat pain in the ear	acetaminophen, naproxen, or codeine
Others Drugs used to help remove excessive ear wax	antipyrine-benzocaine otic

Consider This ...

The pupil of the eye gets approximately 45% larger when an individual looks at something or someone they find pleasing.

Refractive Errors

■ **DESCRIPTION.** Refractive errors are those caused by the eye's inability to focus images correctly on the retina. Approximately one-third of the population is affected by refractive errors.

■ **ETIOLOGY.** The cause of refractive errors is unknown, although some run in families, suggesting an inheritance pattern. Although these disorders affect individuals of all ages, incidence increases with age. There are four common types of refractive errors:

■ Myopia (my-OH-pee-ah) is commonly called near-sightedness or shortsightedness. Individuals with myopia can see nearby objects but have difficulty seeing distant objects. Light entering the eye of a myopic individual falls short of the retina due to the eyeball being abnormally long from front to back (Figure 16–6). Myopia can be treated with prescriptive lenses, radial keratotomy (RK), automated lamellar keratoplasty (ALK), laser-assisted in-situ keratomileusis (LASIK), and implantable contact lenses (ICL) surgery (as described in the section titled, "Treatment").

■ Hyperopia (HIGH-per-OH-pee-ah) is commonly called farsightedness. Individuals with hyperopia can see objects that are far away but have difficulty seeing close objects. Light entering the eye of a hyperoptic individual falls too far past the retina due to the eyeball being abnormally short from front to back (see Figure 16–6). Hyperopia can be treated with prescriptive lenses, conductive keratoplasty (CK), ALK, laser epithelial keratomileusis (H-LASEK), and thermal keratoplasty.

■ Presbyopia (PRES-bee-OH-pee-ah; presby = old age) is hyperopia that is age-related. It is not due to the shape of the eyeball but, rather, is related to the inability of the aging lens to focus light rays properly. When the eye focuses on a distant object, the muscles of the eye pull the lens into a flatter shape. As the eye focuses on nearby objects, the muscles relax, allowing the lens to return to a more spherical shape. In presbyopia, the lens does not return to the normal shape, causing light rays to fall beyond the retina (see Figure 16–6). Presbyopia usually affects individuals age 40 or older and can be corrected with reading glasses, bifocals, CK, and monovision LASIK.

■ Astigmatism (ah-STIG-mah-tizm) is an irregularity in the surface of the cornea, causing light rays to spread over the retina rather than focus properly on part of the retina (see Figure 16–6). This refractive error can lead to blurred or fuzzy vision, often described as seeing halos around objects. Astigmatism can be treated with prescriptive lenses or LASIK.

■ **SYMPTOMS.** Common symptoms of refractive errors include squinting, blurred vision, headaches, and rubbing of eyes.

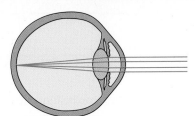

Normal eye
Light rays focus on the retina

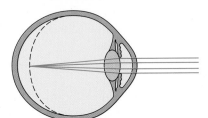

Myopia (nearsightedness)
Light rays focus in front
of the retina

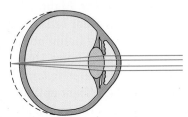

Hyperopia (farsightedness)
Light rays focus beyond
the retina

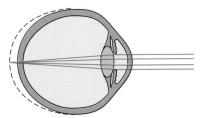

Presbyopia
Light rays focus
behind the retina

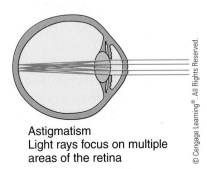

Astigmatism
Light rays focus on multiple
areas of the retina

FIGURE 16–6 Normal eye vision, myopia, hyperopia, presbyopia, and astigmatism.

■ **DIAGNOSIS.** Tests for visual acuity include an ophthalmoscopic examination to look inside the eye and the individual reading a Snellen chart.

■ **TREATMENT.** Refractive errors are commonly corrected with prescriptive eyeglasses or contact lenses. Surgical treatments include the following:

■ **Radial keratotomy (RK)** (KER-ah-TOT-oh-me; kerato = cornea, otomy = incision) is a procedure to correct myopia. Incisions are made in a radial fashion in the cornea to flatten the cornea, shortening the length of the eyeball and correcting the refractive error (Figure 16–7). RK is still performed and even recommended for certain eye cases, but it is quickly being replaced by laser procedures.

■ **Automated lamellar keratoplasty (ALK)** is a surgery using a device called a microkeratome to separate and remove a thin disc of cornea. The thickness of the disc removed determines the change in the refractive error.

■ **Laser-assisted in-situ keratomileusis (LASIK)** is the newest form of RK and is rapidly becoming the procedure of choice. This process uses a precisely controlled, intense beam of ultraviolet laser light to vaporize selected cells and flatten the curvature of

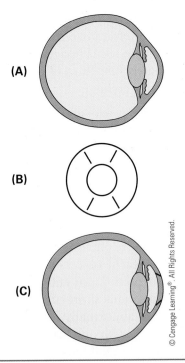

(A)

(B)

(C)

FIGURE 16–7 Radial keratotomy. (A) Cross-section of the eye prior to surgery. (B) Small incisions are made in the cornea from the middle outward. (C) This causes the cornea to become flatter, thereby improving vision.

the cornea. With this procedure, the tissue around and underneath the tissue that is removed is not affected.

- **Implantable contact lenses (ICL)** permanently implant contact lenses into the eye. An advantage of ICL over surgeries that flatten the cornea is that overcorrection or undercorrection can be remedied by replacing the contact lens with the correct prescription.

- **Conductive keratoplasty (CK)** surgery uses mild heat from radio waves to shrink connective tissue (collagen) around the edge of the cornea. This circular pattern acts like a belt that tightens around the cornea, causing it to bulge or steepen the center of the cornea, thus lengthening the too-short eyeball.

- **Laser epithelial keratomileusis (H-LASEK)** surgery loosens the surface area of the cornea and pushes it to the side; a laser reshapes the inner layer of the cornea, and then the outer surface is replaced.

- **Thermal keratoplasty (TK)** uses heat to change the shape of the cornea by shrinking collagen fibers.

- **Monovision** surgery adjusts or fits one eye to see at a distance, leaving the other eye unadjusted for seeing close up, such as is needed for reading. (Normally, the eyes work equally to look at an object, a process called binocular vision.) The monovision idea is easy to achieve also with contact lenses in that one lens can be left out, allowing one eye to be corrected while the other is not.

LASIK surgeons are capable of producing monovision in presbyopic patients by purposefully adjusting one eye to see nearsighted. This technique does not work in all cases because some individuals cannot become accustomed to monovision. Monovision can affect depth perception and should be avoided by individuals such as airplane pilots, professional drivers, and some athletes.

■ **PREVENTION.** There are no preventive measures for refractive errors.

Consider This ...

Individuals with poor eyesight are often found to have a higher IQ.

Inflammation and Infection

Inflammation of the eye and related structures is commonly caused by infectious microorganisms. Internal infections, or infection affecting the inside of the eye, are rare and are usually related to trauma; more common are inflammations or infections of the surface of the eye and its related structures. Eye infections are commonly caused by viruses and bacteria and can be secondary to allergies, trauma, and upper respiratory infections. Microorganisms can reach the eye from the individual's hands and contaminated washcloths and towels. Good hand washing and cleanliness are preventive measures.

CONJUNCTIVITIS

■ **DESCRIPTION.** Conjunctivitis is an inflammation of the conjunctiva, the pink membrane lining the inner eyelids (Figure 16–8).

■ **ETIOLOGY.** Conjunctivitis can be caused by excessive exposure to wind, sun, heat, and cold. The eyelids become red and swollen.

■ **SYMPTOMS.** Affected individuals might complain of excessive tearing, itching, burning, and pain. An acute, contagious bacterial infection of the conjunctiva is called pinkeye, which can become epidemic among school-aged children.

■ **DIAGNOSIS.** Diagnosis is usually simple because of obvious symptoms and is confirmed by a medical history and physical examination of the eye. If infection is a consideration, a swab of eye drainage can be obtained for a bacterial culture and sensitivity test.

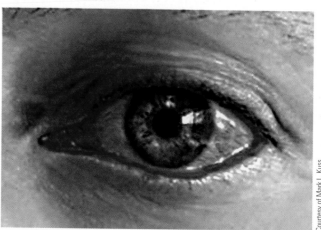

Courtesy of Mark L. Kuss

FIGURE 16–8 Conjunctivitis.

■ **TREATMENT.** Treatment includes warm compresses, anti-inflammatory medications, and analgesics to relieve pain. If a culture identifies a microorganism, antibiotic ointment or drops might be needed.

■ **PREVENTION.** Good hygiene measures, including frequent hand washing, using protective eye wear, avoiding allergens such as dust and pollen, and using a clean tissue to remove drainage in the eye, can prevent most cases.

BLEPHARITIS

■ **DESCRIPTION.** Blepharitis is inflammation of the edge of the eyelid, including the eyelash follicles and glands (Figure 16–9).

■ **ETIOLOGY.** Blepharitis can be caused by bacterial infection and allergic reaction to smoke, dust, or chemicals. Seborrhea, a disorder of the sebaceous gland, or oil-secreting gland, also can cause blepharitis.

■ **SYMPTOMS.** Affected individuals might complain of itching and burning and a feeling of something in the eye. The eyelids appear red, swollen, and crusted.

■ **DIAGNOSIS.** A routine examination of the eye with a slit-lamp microscope is usually all that is needed for diagnosis.

■ **TREATMENT.** Treatment is directed toward removal of the cause and can include antibiotics, allergy medication, or treatment for seborrhea.

■ **PREVENTION.** Good eyelid hygiene and a regular cleaning routine usually control blepharitis. Eyelid hygiene includes frequent hand and face washing, warm water soaks on the eyelids, and eyelid and eyelash cleansing with warm water and baby shampoo. Good eyelid hygiene is very important upon awakening due to the secretions that accumulate on the eyelids during sleep.

KERATITIS

■ **DESCRIPTION.** Keratitis is inflammation of the cornea, usually unilateral, affecting only one eye.

■ **ETIOLOGY.** A frequent cause of keratitis is infection by herpes simplex virus secondary to an upper respiratory infection involving cold sores (herpes simplex). Allergies and contact lenses can also lead to this condition.

■ **SYMPTOMS.** Symptoms include pain, **photophobia** (photo = light, phobia = fear), and excessive tearing.

■ **DIAGNOSIS.** A slit-lamp examination of the surface of the cornea will confirm the diagnosis.

■ **TREATMENT.** Treatment can include antibiotic ointment or drops to treat or prevent infection, analgesics for pain, and an eye patch to treat photophobia.

■ **PREVENTION.** Preventing trauma and avoiding unnecessary touching and rubbing of the eye help prevent keratitis.

STYE (HORDEOLUM)

■ **DESCRIPTION.** A stye, or hordeolum (hor-DEE-oh-lum), is an inflammatory infection of a sebaceous (oil-secreting) gland of the eyelid (Figure 16–10) at the base of a hair follicle or eyelash.

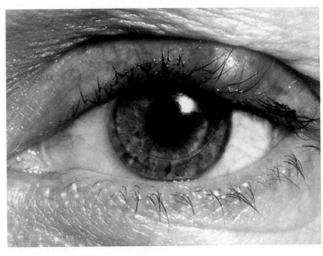

FIGURE 16–10 Stye (hordeolum).

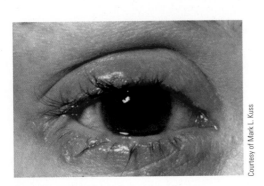

FIGURE 16–9 Blepharitis.

ETIOLOGY. Most styes are caused by *Staphylococcus* bacteria and are often seen in blepharitis. They are also found more frequently in individuals who have diabetes and seborrhea.

SYMPTOMS. A tender, painful, red bump, often resembling a pimple, is located at the base of an eyelash or inside the eyelid. Often there is swelling or edema along the entire lid. Purulent drainage can come from the eyelash line or on the conjunctival surface of the eye.

DIAGNOSIS. Diagnosis is made on the basis of examination of the eye and presence of symptoms.

TREATMENT. Warm compresses may relieve pain, help localize the infection, and promote drainage. Styes usually form a soft spot, open, and drain and heal without further treatment. In some cases, styes may need to be incised to promote drainage and healing. In chronic conditions, **topical** (placed on the skin) antibiotic or systemic (taken by mouth or injection) antibiotics may be needed.

PREVENTION. Good eyelid and eye hygiene are preventive measures.

Cataract

DESCRIPTION. A cataract is a clouding of the lens of the eye (Figure 16–11).

ETIOLOGY. Cataracts develop from a change in metabolism and nutrition within the lens, most commonly from aging. Approximately 60% of all individuals 70 years of age or older will have clouding of a lens. Cataracts also can be caused by trauma, birth defects, and other diseases such as diabetes mellitus. Cataracts usually develop very slowly in one or both eyes.

SYMPTOMS. The main symptom is a decrease in visual acuity or a complaint about not being able to see clearly. Other symptoms include blurred vision, glare, and a decrease in color perception. In advanced cases, the cataract can be seen through the pupil, giving the pupil a white, cloudy appearance.

DIAGNOSIS. Diagnosis is confirmed by slit-lamp examination.

TREATMENT. Cataracts are commonly treated with surgery, which involves removing the cloudy lens and replacing it with a clear artificial lens (Figure 16–12). This surgery, commonly called cataract extraction with placement of intraocular lens, is routinely performed as outpatient surgery. Postoperative prognosis is usually good.

PREVENTION. There are no known preventive measures but those who smoke, have diabetes, or have exposure to UV light are more likely to develop cataracts.

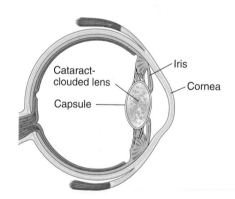

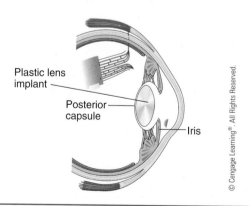

FIGURE 16–12 Cataract extraction with placement of intraocular lens.

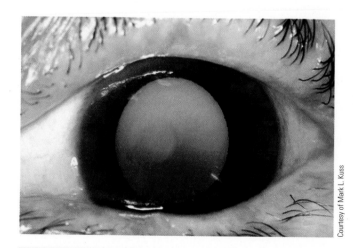

FIGURE 16–11 Cataract.

Glaucoma

■ **DESCRIPTION.** Glaucoma is a common condition characterized by excessive pressure inside the eye from the fluid inside the eye, known as aqueous humor, which is produced constantly by blood. It circulates through the eye and is reabsorbed into the bloodstream.

■ **ETIOLOGY.** Excessive pressure inside the eye occurs if too much fluid is produced or does not drain properly. There are several forms of glaucoma, including open angle and closed angle glaucoma.

■ **SYMPTOMS.** Generally speaking, glaucoma progresses slowly, might or might not be symptomatic, and rarely affects individuals under age 40. Increased pressure inside the eye for a continued period of time can lead to damage of the optic nerve and blindness, and permanent damage is often done before symptoms occur. For this reason, intraocular pressure should be checked on an annual basis.

■ **DIAGNOSIS.** Diagnosis is made on the basis of an ophthalmic examination and tonometry revealing an increase in intraocular pressure.

■ **TREATMENT.** Early treatment is essential to prevent permanent blindness. Depending on the form of glaucoma, treatment can include use of eye drops or surgery. Both are directed toward either reducing the amount of aqueous humor produced or improving the drainage.

■ **PREVENTION.** Regular eye examination with monitoring of eye pressure to discover glaucoma before any damage is done is the best preventive measure.

Nystagmus

■ **DESCRIPTION.** Nystagmus (nis-TAG-mus) is a constant, involuntary movement of the eyes that might be unnoticed by the affected individual. Movement can be vertical, horizontal, circular, or a combination of these. One or both eyes might be affected.

■ **ETIOLOGY.** Nystagmus might be the result of brain tumors, disease, alcohol abuse, or congenital defects. Diseases that cause nystagmus include Ménière's disease and multiple sclerosis.

■ **SYMPTOMS.** Abnormal eye movement as described.

■ **DIAGNOSIS.** It is usually easy to diagnosis nystagmus but difficult to diagnose the cause. Computerized tomography (CT) scan, magnetic resonance imaging (MRI), myelogram, angiography, and spinal tap might be needed to confirm the cause of the condition.

■ **TREATMENT.** Treatment is directed toward correction of the underlying cause. Congenital nystagmus is often untreatable and permanent.

■ **PREVENTION.** Prevention is aimed at curing or preventing the cause.

Strabismus

■ **DESCRIPTION.** Strabismus (strah-BIZ-mus) is a disorder in which the eyes fail to look in the same direction at the same time (Figure 16–13). Strabismus is often incorrectly referred to as lazy eye and as crossed eye or cockeye.

COMPLEMENTARY AND ALTERNATIVE THERAPY

Antioxidants for Eye Strain

Research has shown that carotenoid antioxidants increase blood flow and reduce eye irritation and inflammation often associated with sitting for long hours in front of a computer screen or other digital device. Eye strain and fatigue associated with this activity is now called computer vision syndrome and is becoming more common among all ages. Healthy doses of vitamins have long been touted to be good for eye problem prevention. Since it has been shown that these antioxidants have a positive effect on the syndrome, a new vitamin formula specifically targeting eye strain and eye fatigue has been developed by one company.

Source: EyeScience Launches Eye Strain Formula (2011).

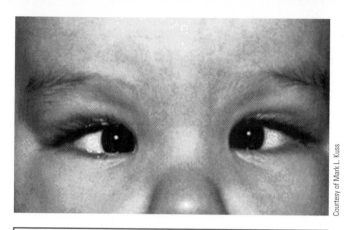

Courtesy of Mark L. Kuss

FIGURE 16–13 Strabismus.

■ **ETIOLOGY.** Strabismus is the result of muscle weakness in one or both eyes. The affected eye can deviate upward or downward, but more commonly, it looks inward (convergent strabismus) or outward (divergent strabismus). Strabismus commonly occurs in children and requires early intervention to prevent **amblyopia** (AM-blee-OH-pee-ah), a decrease in the vision of the affected eye due to a lack of visual stimuli.

■ **SYMPTOMS.** The primary symptoms of strabismus are **diplopia** (dih-PLOH-pee-ah), or double vision, and altered eye movement.

■ **DIAGNOSIS.** A cover test is helpful in diagnosis. This involves covering each of the eyes while the individual is looking at an object. The straight eye will continue to look at the object when the opposite eye is covered. When the straight eye is covered, the strabismic eye will shift or straighten to fixate on the object.

■ **TREATMENT.** Treatment often consists of covering the normal eye in an effort to force the affected eye to function. Eye exercises and corrective lenses also can be ordered. The earlier the treatment is begun, the better. If correction is not made by the age of 6 or 7, the visual impairment can be permanent. Surgical intervention might be needed to correct strabismus.

■ **PREVENTION.** Strabismus cannot be prevented, but complications can be prevented with early detection and proper treatment.

Macular Degeneration

■ **DESCRIPTION.** Macular degeneration is a degeneration of the macular area of the retina, which is important in seeing fine detail.

■ **ETIOLOGY.** The cause of this degeneration can be due to the effects of drugs, but the most common cause is aging. Risk factors include farsightedness, light eye color, and cigarette smoking. This disease is the leading cause of visual impairment in individuals 50 years of age and older.

■ **SYMPTOMS.** The primary symptom is a loss of central vision. Peripheral vision and color perception are unaffected. The disease generally develops slowly and painlessly, and both eyes are usually affected. As the disease progresses, reading and activities that require fine, detailed vision become impossible. There can be a complete loss of central vision, but generally, blindness does not occur.

■ **DIAGNOSIS.** Diagnosis is made on the basis of fluorescein angiography and routine examination.

■ **TREATMENT.** Vision might be improved in some cases by laser surgery or by taking antioxidant vitamins. There are also several new drugs on the market to treat age-related macular degeneration, and the Food and Drug Administration recently approved an implantable miniature telescope.

■ **PREVENTION.** Since the most common cause is due to aging, this condition cannot always be prevented. Some activities aid prevention and include smoking cessation, eating foods high in antioxidants, eating fish regularly, wearing sunglasses that block ultraviolet light, managing other diseases such as cardiovascular disease and hypertension, and getting regular eye exams.

Diabetic Retinopathy

■ **DESCRIPTION.** Diabetic retinopathy (RET-ih-NOP-ah-thee; retino = retina, opathy = disease) is a complication of diabetes and the leading cause of blindness in the United States. This condition can happen to any individual with type 1 or type 2 diabetes. The longer the individual has diabetes, the more likely is the development of diabetic retinopathy.

■ **ETIOLOGY.** Diabetes mellitus causes vascular changes in the retina that lead to a decrease in visual acuity. These changes include capillary aneurysms (also called microaneurysms), microhemorrhages, venous dilation, and new vessel growth (Figure 16–14). The affected vessels tend to bleed easily into the retina and produce scarring.

HEALTHY HIGHLIGHT

Foods to Help Dry Eyes

Dry eye syndrome (DES) can be helped by using artificial tears but also by eating a healthy diet. Studies have shown that people with DES often have low levels of omega-3 fatty acids in their food choices. Some of the foods that contain these include walnuts, flaxseeds, beans, fish, olive oil, and winter squash. Other supplements that help DES are the antioxidant vitamins C and E, agents that can be naturally found in vegetables, fruits, and plants. Antioxidants are also synthesized in the body and are essential to the immune system. They can be found in vegetables, fruits, legumes, and whole-grain foods.

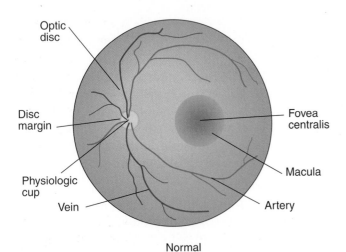

Normal

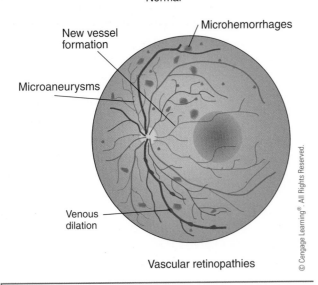

Vascular retinopathies

FIGURE 16–14 Vascular changes caused by diabetic retinopathy.

■ **SYMPTOMS.** Retinal scarring decreases visual acuity and can ultimately cause permanent blindness. These vascular changes tend to occur in both eyes and are more extensive in uncontrolled diabetes or in individuals whose blood sugar is not controlled. Diabetic retinopathy can be asymptomatic in the early stages, but as the disease progresses, symptoms include blurred vision, poor night vision, floating spots in the visual field, and vision loss.

■ **DIAGNOSIS.** This condition is best diagnosed with a dilated-eye exam to allow the physician to see abnormal blood vessels, blood or fatty deposits in the retina, retinal detachment, and damage to the nerve tissue, all symptoms of diabetic retinopathy.

■ **TREATMENT.** Laser photocoagulation treatment is usually effective, but the condition tends to recur and might need repeated treatment.

■ **PREVENTION.** Prevention is directed toward controlling blood sugar levels to reduce the retinopathy. Other preventive methods include monitoring and controlling blood pressure and cholesterol levels, not smoking, reducing stress, and getting regular eye examinations.

Color Blindness or Color Vision Deficiency

■ **DESCRIPTION.** Normal ability to see colors diminishes with age due to the progressive yellowing of the lens. Colors become less intense, and the colors of green and blue often become more difficult to distinguish. Difficulty in distinguishing colors also can occur in young individuals affected with color vision deficiency (CVD).

■ **ETIOLOGY.** Color blindness also commonly occurs as an inherited, X-linked disorder that affects approximately 1 in 10 males. It is rarely seen in females.

■ *SYMPTOMS.* There are three main kinds of color vision defects. Red–green color vision defects are the most common, occur more often in men, and affect the ability to distinguish between red and green. The other major types are blue–yellow defects and complete absence of color vision.

■ *DIAGNOSIS.* CVD can be diagnosed using color plates or charts. A common plate is the Ishihara color plate shown in Figure 16–15.

■ *TREATMENT.* There is no known treatment or cure for color blindness. Interestingly, affected individuals might be sought to perform military duties that include the discovery of camouflage. Color-blind individuals might exhibit an uncanny ability to see through camouflage, especially that using shades of green.

■ *PREVENTION.* There are no preventive measures.

■ COMMON DISEASES OF THE EAR

The common diseases of the ear include infections and conditions of decreased hearing or total hearing loss. Gradual hearing loss can be due to a primary ear disorder, such as an infection, or secondary to a disease or injury.

Infection

The ear and related bony structures are commonly subject to infection. The middle ear is connected to the nasopharynx by way of the Eustachian tube, making it easily accessible to bacteria that cause throat and respiratory infections. The external ear is open to the external environment, allowing infection from air and water. The bony mastoid process connects with the middle ear and is subject to infections affecting

the middle ear. Ear infections are more common in infants and children.

Consider This ...

Wearing head phones for an hour increases the bacteria in an individual's ear by 700 times.

OTITIS MEDIA

■ *DESCRIPTION.* Otitis media is inflammation in the middle ear. It usually affects infants and young children and is commonly called middle-ear infection, but it might not necessarily be an infection. The middle ear is normally filled with air, but when this area fills with fluid, inflammation occurs. For this reason, otitis media is classified by the type of fluid that fills the ear. Fluid types are:

Serous

■ *ETIOLOGY.* The fluid is clear and can be due to a Eustachian tube obstruction, allergy, or change in middle-ear pressure. Middle-ear pressure commonly occurs with air flight. Any of these situations may allow clear serous fluid to accumulate in the middle ear. This fluid accumulation causes inflammation of the middle ear but without infection.

■ *SYMPTOMS.* Symptoms are usually mild and include a feeling of fullness in the ear and conductive hearing loss.

Suppurative

■ *ETIOLOGY.* The fluid is pus due to a bacterial infection in the middle ear. The **suppurative** (SUP-you-RAY-tiv; formation of pus) form of otitis media is often due to bacteria entering the middle ear, usually from the Eustachian tube during an upper respiratory infection. Blowing the nose forcefully often drives respiratory bacteria through the Eustachian tube into the middle ear. Swimming in contaminated water can be another cause of suppurative infection.

■ *SYMPTOMS.* Symptoms include varying degrees of **otalgia** (oh-TAL-gee-ah; ot = ear, algia = pain),

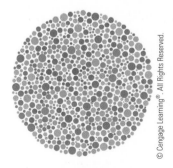

FIGURE 16–15 Ishirara color test plate. The numeral "74" should be clearly visible to viewers with normal color vision.

nausea, vomiting, fever, chills, **vertigo** (VER-tih-go; dizziness), and conductive hearing loss.

The structure and position of the Eustachian tube is an important factor with either type of otitis media. If the Eustachian tube is narrower, shorter, more horizontally placed than normal, or all three of these conditions, the individual is more prone to otitis media. Infants and young children normally have narrower and more horizontally placed Eustachian tubes, thus predisposing them to otitis media. As the child grows, the tube becomes more vertical, which explains why children often outgrow ear infections.

■ **DIAGNOSIS.** Diagnosis is made on the basis of otoscopy revealing a bulging tympanic membrane or eardrum (Figure 16–16). The normally pearly colored tympanic membrane is red and swollen. If the tympanic membrane is ruptured, a culture of the fluid can be performed; otherwise, cultures are not obtainable. An elevated white blood cell count is also indicative of infection.

■ **TREATMENT.** Treatment for both types of otitis media includes analgesics for pain and decongestants to promote drainage. Suppurative otitis media requires antibiotic therapy.

Chronic otitis media, both forms, might need surgical removal of fluid by **myringotomy** (MIR-in-GOT-oh-me; myringo = eardrum, tomy = incision into) to prevent rupture of the tympanic membrane, permanent hearing loss, and possible mastoiditis. To prevent further accumulation of fluid and to relieve pressure, **tympanostomy** (TIM-pan-OSS-toh-me; tympano = eardrum, ostomy = new opening) tubes, commonly called pediatric ear (PE) tubes, can be placed through the tympanic membrane during a

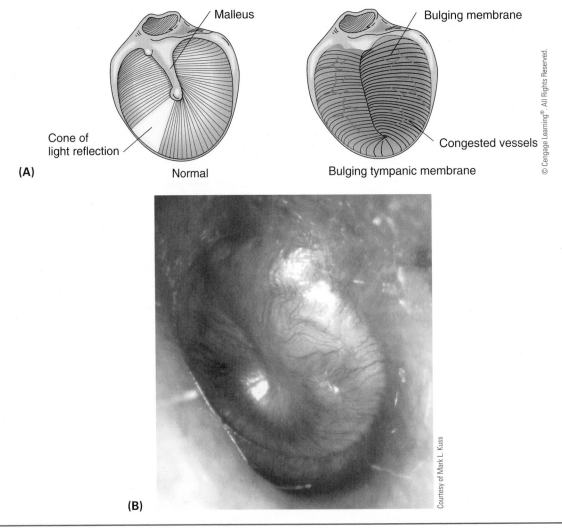

FIGURE 16–16 (A) Bulging tympanic membrane indicative of otitis media. (B) Bulging tympanic membrane.

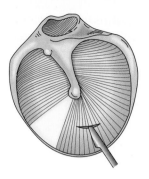
Tympanic membrane incision

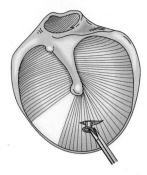
Tube placement

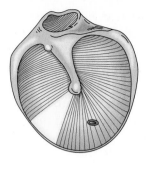
Tympanoplasty completed

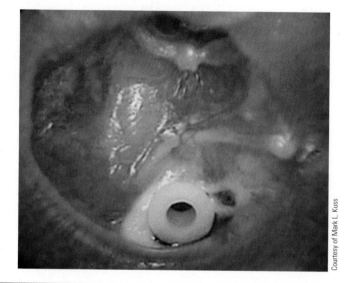

FIGURE 16–17   Tympanoplasty.

procedure called a **tympanoplasty** (TIM-pah-no-PLAS-tee; tympano = eardrum, plasty = surgical repair) (Figure 16–17). Tubes commonly fall out after several months but can be removed after 6 months to a year. Prognosis for both types of otitis media is good if given prompt treatment. Chronic untreated otitis media, however, can lead to severe ear damage and permanent hearing loss. Prevention of complications is directed toward prevention and prompt treatment of upper respiratory infections and otitis media.

■ **PREVENTION.** Avoiding bottle feeding, smoking environments, and group child care are all preventive measures. Babies who are breast-fed, cared for in their homes, and kept in nonsmoking environments have fewer bouts of otitis media.

OTITIS EXTERNA

■ **DESCRIPTION.** Otitis externa, also called swimmer's ear or external otitis, is an inflammation of the external ear canal.

■ **ETIOLOGY.** This disease commonly affects swimmers who spend many hours in the water. Other causes include trauma to the ear canal, such as can occur when attempting to scratch or clean the ear canal, and when swimming in contaminated water. The condition often is due to bacterial or fungal infection. Wearing headphones also creates a favorable environment for the growth of microorganisms.

■ **SYMPTOMS.** Symptoms of otitis externa include an inflamed ear canal with extreme pain, fever, **pruritus** (proo-RYE-tus; itching), and hearing loss. The ear also might drain clear or **purulent** (PYOU-roo-lent; containing pus) fluid.

■ **DIAGNOSIS.** Diagnosis is made on the basis of an otologic examination. If an infection is suspected, a culture and sensitivity test might be needed.

■ **TREATMENT.** Treatment includes keeping the ear canal clean and dry and giving analgesics for pain and antibiotics if an infection is detected.

■ **PREVENTION.** Prevention includes wearing earplugs while showering or swimming to keep the external canal clean and dry. Decreasing the amount of time headphones are worn and keeping foreign objects out of the ears also can be helpful. Otitis externa tends to be a recurring disease that can eventually become chronic and cause hearing loss.

MASTOIDITIS

■ **DESCRIPTION.** Mastoiditis (MAS-toy-DYE-tis) is inflammation of the mastoid bone or process. This bone is porous or honeycombed in appearance and located behind the ear (Figure 16–18). This condition commonly affects children and is usually the result of a middle-ear infection. Prior to antibiotics, this was a leading cause of death in children. With current diagnosis and treatment regimens, it is less common and rarely dangerous.

■ **ETIOLOGY.** Acute mastoiditis is usually the result of a middle-ear infection commonly caused by *Streptococcus*.

■ **SYMPTOMS.** Symptoms include **tinnitus** (tin-EYE-tus; ringing in the ears), otalgia (oh-TAL-gee-ah; ot = ear, algia = pain), fever, and headache. The mastoid also can become swollen and painful, and ear drainage can be present.

■ **DIAGNOSIS.** Diagnosis is made on the basis of examination and otoscopy (OH-TOS-koh-pee; oto = ear, scopy = procedure to look into), X-ray of the mastoid bone, CT scan, and bacterial cultures.

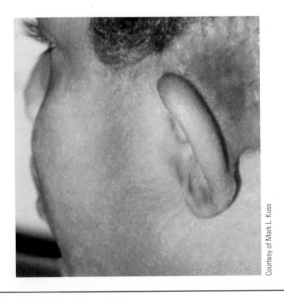

Courtesy of Mark L. Kuss

FIGURE 16–18 Mastoiditis.

■ **TREATMENT.** Mastoiditis generally responds to antibiotic therapy. Severe or chronic mastoiditis might need surgical treatment with a **mastoidectomy** (MAS-toy-DECK-toh-me; mastoid = shaped like a nipple; referring to mastoid process; ectomy = removal or excision) to prevent complications and preserve hearing.

■ **PREVENTION.** Prompt and thorough treatment of ear infections reduces the risk of developing mastoiditis.

Deafness

Deafness, or loss of hearing, is a common disease affecting millions of Americans. There are multiple reasons for deafness, but most causes fall into two basic categories: conductive and sensory. Conductive deafness is caused by external or middle-ear disorders that decrease or stop conduction of sound to the inner ear. Conductive disorders include impacted cerumen, otosclerosis, and a ruptured tympanic membrane. Sensory deafness is the result of cochlear or auditory nerve damage that impairs the ability of sound to be carried to the brain. Sensory deafness is often related to damaging noise levels and ototoxic medications.

IMPACTED CERUMEN

■ **DEFINITION.** Cerumen is the soft, yellow-brown secretion produced by the external ear, commonly called ear wax.

■ **ETIOLOGY.** Impacted cerumen is a common cause of conductive hearing loss. If cerumen accumulates and becomes impacted (pressed firmly) in the ear canal, it can cause tinnitus and temporary deafness. An abnormal amount of cerumen can build up in the ear due to skin dryness, excessive hair in the ear, or a narrow ear canal. Another cause of buildup is due to excessive dust in the ear, which occurs among construction workers, farmers, and cabinetmakers, to name a few.

■ **SYMPTOMS.** The common symptom is a partial loss of hearing. Itching, tinnitus, and pain can also be symptoms.

■ **DIAGNOSIS.** An otologic examination will confirm the diagnosis.

■ **TREATMENT.** Cerumen is normally washed out of the ear during routine showering and shampooing. Impacted cerumen is often removed with ear

HEALTHY HIGHLIGHT

**Removing
Impacted
Cerumen**

Impacted cerumen should be softened and removed gently in the following manner.

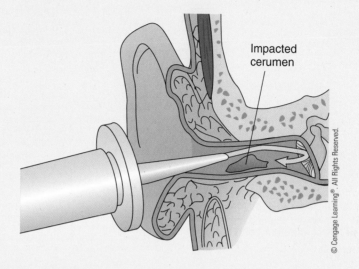

Impacted cerumen

1. Warm mineral oil or glycerin by holding it between the hands or placing the bottle in a cup of warm water.
2. Check the temperature to ensure that it is not too hot. It should be lukewarm.
3. Drop two or three drops of oil in the ear canal.
4. Gently irrigate the ear canal by using a bulb syringe filled with lukewarm water.
5. Aim the water flow toward the top of the ear canal, not toward the eardrum.
6. Continue to irrigate until the impacted cerumen is removed. This can take 10 to 15 minutes.
7. Repeat steps 1–6 until the impacted cerumen is removed.

---

irrigations. This condition tends to recur, so routine examination should be performed.

■ **PREVENTION.** Placing two to three drops of mineral oil into the ear once a week, allowing it to remain for 3 to 4 minutes, and then rinsing it out with warm water is a preventive method.

OTOSCLEROSIS

■ **DESCRIPTION.** Otosclerosis (OH-toh-skleh-ROH-sis; oto = ear, scler = hardening, osis = condition) is a condition characterized by bony fixation of the small bones of the middle ear. This fixation prevents the bones from conducting vibrations from the eardrum to the inner ear, causing a conductive hearing loss. Otosclerosis occurs more commonly in females than in males; it usually affects females under the age of 35 and can be aggravated by pregnancy.

■ **ETIOLOGY.** The cause of otosclerosis is unknown, but there is evidence of familial tendency, suggesting a hereditary cause.

■ **SYMPTOMS.** The primary symptom is slow hearing loss that continues to worsen.

■ **DIAGNOSIS.** Diagnosis is made on the basis of physical examination, audiogram, and otoscopy.

■ **TREATMENT.** A common treatment for otosclerosis is a **stapedectomy** (STAY-peh-DECK-toh-me; stape = stapes, ectomy = removal or excision of). A stapedectomy involves removal of the stapes bone in the middle ear and replacement with a **prosthesis** (pros-THEE-sis; an artificial part) (Figure 16–19).

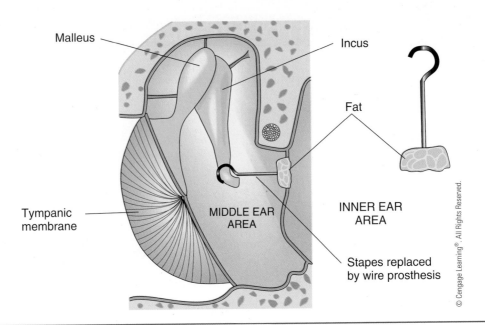

Malleus

Incus

Fat

Tympanic
membrane

MIDDLE EAR
AREA

INNER EAR
AREA

Stapes replaced
by wire prosthesis

FIGURE 16–19   Stapedectomy with wire prosthesis.

Hearing is generally improved soon after surgery. If a stapedectomy is not an option for the affected individual, a hearing aid might improve hearing.

■ **PREVENTION.** Otosclerosis cannot be prevented.

SENSORINEURAL DEAFNESS

■ **DESCRIPTION.** Sensorineural deafness is a type of sensory deafness due to damage to the cochlea or the auditory nerve.

■ **ETIOLOGY.** There are many causes of this condition; some are congenital, or inherited, whereas others are acquired. Acquired causes are more common and include stroke, tumors, certain medications, infections, diseases, and trauma. The most common trauma is due to exposure to loud noise. Occupational noise, including that from heavy machinery, jackhammers, and airplane engines, can lead to deafness. Teenagers and young adults are at high risk due to the popularity of playing loud music, especially while using personal ear buds, and attending music concerts that use large amplifiers.

■ **SYMPTOMS.** The primary symptom is a gradual loss of hearing.

■ **DIAGNOSIS.** Diagnosis is made on the basis of audiometry.

■ **TREATMENT.** Sensorineural deafness caused by cochlear or auditory nerve damage is often permanent. Treatment is limited to use of hearing aids or cochlear implants.

A hearing aid is a tiny microphone, amplifier, and speaker in one device. It fits in the external ear and increases volume to the internal ear.

A cochlear implant is an electronic device that is implanted behind the ear. It directly stimulates the auditory nerve fibers to increase hearing.

■ **PREVENTION.** Prevention is aimed at avoiding the cause if possible. Reducing the amount of noise and protecting the ears by using protective earphones and earplugs are beneficial.

PRESBYCUSIS

■ **DESCRIPTION.** Presbycusis (PRES-beh-KOO-sis; presby = old age, cusis = hearing) is a progressive sensory hearing loss related to aging.

■ **ETIOLOGY.** The cause of presbycusis is from degenerative changes in the organs of hearing.

■ **SYMPTOMS.** Onset of symptoms is gradual and usually begins after age 50. Initially, there is a loss of hearing of high tones, but as hearing loss progresses, lower tones become difficult to hear as well. In affected individuals, the speech of others might seem mumbled or slurred, and conversations might be difficult to hear, especially against background noise.

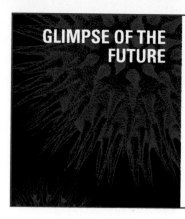

Cochlear Implants Improve Quality of Life

Placement of bilateral cochlear implants has improved the quality of life of those receiving them according to a recent study. Children with deafness who had these implants have reported a significant improvement in quality of life especially on the disease-related questionnaires. The researchers administered three types of quality-of-life questionnaires to the participants. Perhaps in the future, as greater numbers of children receive cochlear implants, there will be even more significant improvements in the lives of these individuals.

Source: Doctors Lounge (2012).

■ **DIAGNOSIS.** Diagnosis is made after physical examination and medical history to rule out other causes of hearing loss. An audiogram confirms the diagnosis.

■ **TREATMENT.** Use of a hearing aid can be helpful initially, but as the hearing declines, aids might become less useful.

■ **PREVENTION.** Much of the hearing loss caused by trauma and noise can be prevented. Avoiding activities with damaging noise levels and wearing ear muffs or ear plugs to protect the ears are helpful preventive measures.

Motion Sickness

■ **DESCRIPTION.** Motion sickness is the nauseated feeling some individuals experience when traveling by automobile, boat, or airplane.

■ **ETIOLOGY.** The cause of motion sickness is abnormal movement of the organs of balance—the semicircular canals—that are located in the inner ear. These semicircular canals are accustomed to traveling in a horizontal plane, but movement in a vertical plane, as in a boat or bumpy airplane ride, produces an abnormal sensation in these organs, leading to motion sickness. Watching motion on a widescreen picture also can cause motion sickness, even though the individual is not actually moving.

■ **SYMPTOMS.** Symptoms of motion sickness include varying degrees of nausea, vomiting, diaphoresis, and vertigo. Fortunately, motion sickness usually subsides when movement stops.

■ **DIAGNOSIS.** A history and description of symptoms are usually adequate to diagnose this condition. Laboratory testing is usually not needed.

■ **TREATMENT.** Antihistamine medications are generally used to treat and prevent this condition. These medications appear to work by calming the stimulation of the inner ear. Meclizine (Antivert®, Dramamine II®) can treat symptoms. Motion sickness can also be relieved or reduced by lying down and closing the eyes.

■ **PREVENTION.** Meclizine is also helpful in prevention of motion sickness if taken at least 1 hour prior to travel.

Scopolamine is the most commonly prescribed preventive medication. It is available in a skin patch (Transderm Scop®) that is applied behind the ear; the medication is then slowly absorbed into the skin. To be most effective, this patch should be placed at least 4 hours in advance of the motion activity. Effects of the patch last up to 3 days.

Promethazine, dimenhydrinate, and cyclizine are all preventive medications when taken prior to the motion activity.

Other considerations that might decrease the effect or prevent the occurrence of motion sickness include:

- Avoiding heavy meals prior to a trip.
- Finding a seat in the most stable area of the boat or plane.
- During automobile rides, making frequent stops for short walks in the fresh air.
- Not reading while traveling.
- Avoiding stuffy areas, especially those with odors such as cigarette smoke.
- Trying to stay cool with plenty of fresh air when possible.
- Avoiding too much heat.

TRAUMA

Corneal Abrasion

■ **DESCRIPTION.** The cornea, the transparent outer layer of the eye, is subject to trauma because of its position.

■ **ETIOLOGY.** Corneal abrasions can be caused by:

■ Trapping a foreign object such as sand or sawdust between the eyelid and the cornea.

■ Contact lenses that do not fit properly, are dirty or scratched, or are worn for too long a time period.

■ Accidentally poking a finger in the eye.

■ Extreme light, as with welding.

■ **SYMPTOMS.** Symptoms are often delayed, occurring 12 to 18 hours after the trauma, and include severe pain, tearing, and photophobia.

■ **DIAGNOSIS.** Diagnosis is made on the basis of history and visual examination. Abrasions can be stained easily with fluorescein and viewed with a slit lamp.

■ **TREATMENT.** Treatment includes removal of the foreign body and administration of antibiotic ointment or drops to prevent infection. Analgesic medications for pain might be prescribed. A pressure dressing can be applied to the eye to keep the eyelid from moving against the cornea and to reduce the pain of photophobia. Interestingly, the pain caused by corneal abrasion comes from the inside of the eyelid rubbing over the abrasion on the cornea. The cornea does not have sensory nerves.

■ **PREVENTION.** Abrasions can often be avoided by use of protective eyewear.

Retinal Detachment

■ **DESCRIPTION.** This is a disorder of the eye in which the retina peels away from the underlying tissue. Detachment usually starts in a small area but can quickly lead to detachment of the entire retina. If this occurs, blindness can occur. Retinal detachment is a medical emergency.

■ **ETIOLOGY.** Retinal detachment often occurs with trauma, diabetes, and other retinopathies that cause an opening or hole in the retinal layer. This opening allows fluid from the vitreous humor to leak between

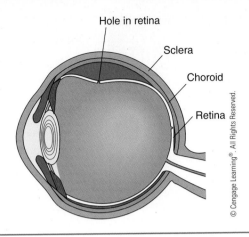

FIGURE 16–20 Retinal detachment.

the retina and choroid layer. The fluid lifts or floats the retina away from the choroid (Figure 16–20).

■ **SYMPTOMS.** Because the retina has no sensory nerves, this condition is painless. The individual experiences loss of vision in the affected area with symptoms of blurred vision, flashes of light, and floating spots. As more of the retina detaches, the symptoms become more pronounced.

■ **DIAGNOSIS.** Ophthalmoscopic examination will readily show the detachment.

■ **TREATMENT.** Surgery is the usual treatment to seal the opening and reattach the retina to the choroid layer. This can be done using laser technology. The retina usually regains function unless extreme detachment has occurred.

■ **PREVENTION.** Most cases cannot be prevented, although prompt treatment of the cause, when known, does reduce risk. Some eye injuries cause damage to the retina that leads to detachment. Prevention of these injuries by wearing safety glasses, sports glasses, or goggles also reduces risk.

Ruptured Tympanic Membrane

■ **DESCRIPTION.** A ruptured tympanic membrane, also called perforated eardrum, is a tear or hole in the tympanic membrane (Figure 16–21). This thin membrane separates the ear canal from the middle ear and vibrates when sound waves strike it, starting the process of hearing.

■ **ETIOLOGY.** The most common causes include severe middle-ear infection or trauma from inserting something, such as a pencil, into the ear canal.

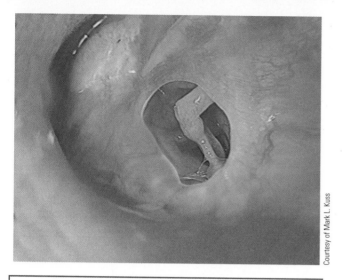

Courtesy of Mark L. Kuss

FIGURE 16–21   Ruptured tympanic membrane.

■ **SYMPTOMS.** Symptoms include pain, partial loss of hearing, and usually bloody or purulent drainage. The main risk of a ruptured membrane is from infection.

■ **DIAGNOSIS.** Diagnosis can be confirmed by otoscopy.

■ **TREATMENT.** Treatment can include antibiotics to prevent infection and surgical patching of the membrane with a tissue graft. Minimal hearing loss is associated with a ruptured tympanic membrane.

■ **PREVENTION.** Getting prompt and thorough treatment for middle-ear infection and keeping the ears free of foreign objects are preventive measures.

■ RARE DISEASES

Retinoblastoma

Retinoblastoma is a malignant tumor of the eye. It occurs during infancy and childhood and tends to be hereditary. Often, both eyes are affected. Retinoblastomas grow as intraocular masses that fill the eye and can extend into the optic nerve. The mass is usually recognized by a white light reflex seen at the pupil (cat's eye). Untreated retinoblastoma is fatal. With treatment, 90% of affected children survive. Treatment includes **enucleation** (removal of the eyeball), radiation, and chemotherapy.

Ménière's Disease

Ménière's disease usually affects individuals between the ages of 40 and 60. The cause is unknown, although predisposing factors appear to include middle-ear infections and head trauma. Ménière's disease is a chronic disease of the inner ear characterized by tinnitus, vertigo, progressive hearing loss, and a feeling of fullness in the ear.

Acute attacks can last from a few hours to several days with symptoms of nausea, vomiting, diaphoresis, and vertigo. Treatment for acute attacks includes medications to control nausea and vomiting. A low-salt diet, diuretics, antihistamines, and cessation of smoking are usually effective for long-term treatment. Surgery can be performed if the disease does not respond to treatment, but a major complication of surgery is permanent deafness.

COMPLEMENTARY AND ALTERNATIVE THERAPY

Eat Fish for Healthy Eyes

To protect eyes through the aging process, new research results show that eating more fish high in omega-3 fatty acids is a good prevention strategy. Age-related macular degeneration (AMD) is a frequent cause of blindness in older adults. This research found that participants who ate fish high in omega-3 fatty acids were 42% less likely to develop AMD than those who only ate fish once per month. The study also found that participants with high levels of vitamin D in their system were 59% less likely to develop AMD. However, this was only true for women under age 75. Other nutrition studies have shown similar results. Researchers now feel confident recommending that older adults eat more fish.

Source: New Clues to Dietary Defenses against Vision Loss with Aging (2011).

EFFECTS OF AGING ON THE SYSTEM

The effects of aging on the sensory organs are significant. Changes in vision begin in middle age and progress through the older adult years. The change is obvious in most people, beginning with the inability to read small print or to see well in low light. These changes affect the older adult's ability to function well in society and often cause social isolation and dependence on others.

Vision changes begin around age 40 and continue through the life span. Inability to focus on near objects, diminishing color perception, some sensitivity to light, and decreased visual acuity are all normal physiologic changes that occur during the aging process. Although the changes vary among individuals, most persons have about a 20/70 visual acuity by age 65. Glaucoma and cataracts are common problems of older adults, reducing even further their ability to see. In the diabetic older person, retinopathy is a very common problem that often eventually leads to blindness. Arcus senilis is an opaque, grayish ring at the periphery of the cornea that frequently occurs in an older person. It results from fatty granule deposits in, or hyaline degeneration of, the lamellae and cells of the cornea (Figure 16–22). Age-related macular degeneration (AMD) is the leading cause of severe vision loss and blindness in the older adult. Vision exams for older adults should include screening for this problem. Since more individuals are living into their 80s and 90s, AMD will continue to be a significant problem for older adults in the future. Early treatment is important.

Hearing changes in the older adult affect the ability to perceive what is heard and might affect behavior, personality, and attitudes. Many hearing problems can be corrected but, because of financial constraints or social concerns, are not attended to. The inability

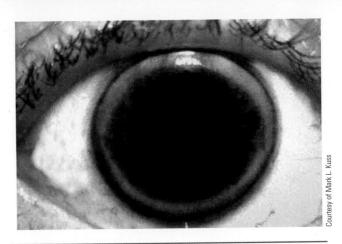

FIGURE 16–22   Arcus senilis.

to hear often affects the individual's ability to communicate and interferes with one's social life and independence. In some instances, speaking in a clear, concise manner to someone with such hearing loss is more beneficial than raising one's voice.

As the individual ages, the tympanic membrane becomes thinner and less flexible, reducing the conduction of sound. This is a conductive hearing loss associated with aging. If there has been damage to the eighth cranial nerve, the individual has a sensorineural loss. If both types of hearing loss are present, it is called a mixed hearing loss.

The slow but gradual loss of hearing, called presbycusis, affects more men than women and is due to degenerative changes in neurons, the bones of the middle ear, and the cochlea. High-pitched sounds become the most difficult to hear at first, but gradual loss of low-pitched sounds also occurs eventually.

Other hearing conditions apparent in the older adult include otosclerosis, tinnitus, and Ménière's disease. Although some of these can begin in younger life, they are most commonly detected in later years.

SUMMARY

The sensory organs of the body are often regarded as the most important to the individual to maintain quality of life. Visual and hearing impairments are often correctable, especially if diagnosed early in the degenerative period. Other system diseases such as diabetes often affect the sensory organs and can destroy their ability to function. Some of the most common disorders of the eyes include myopia, presbyopia, hyperopia, diabetic retinopathy, cataracts, and glaucoma. The most common diseases of the ear include tinnitus, otitis media, conduction loss, otosclerosis, and Ménière's disease. In the older adult, sensory organ disorders are common. Some losses of vision and hearing occur naturally through the aging process. Other losses of vision are a result of other system diseases. Diagnosis and treatment of vision and hearing losses should be implemented early to prevent some of the complications of sensory dysfunction.

REVIEW QUESTIONS

Short Answer

1. What are some of the most common problems affecting the eyes?

2. What are some of the most common problems affecting the ears?

3. What diagnostic tests are used to diagnose or evaluate eye disorders?

4. What diagnostic tests are used to diagnose or evaluate ear disorders?

Fill in the Blanks

5. _____ is the chronic inflammation of the eyelid.

6. The lay term for _____ is pinkeye.

7. Extreme sensitivity to light is called _____.

8. Another term for nearsightedness is _____.

9. Farsightedness is also called _____.

10. A common eye disorder that occurs with aging is called _____.

11. The main symptom of a cataract is the gradual _____ of vision.

12. In _____, aqueous humor is produced faster than it can be drained.

13. Sudden flashes or spots before the eyes can be a sign of _____.

14. Flushing the eye with large amounts of water is the best immediate treatment for a _____ of the eye.

15. The cranial nerves that control the muscles of eye movement include _____, _____, and _____.

16. Within the ear, the organ of hearing is the _____.

17. The major symptom of ear disorders is _____.

18. Buzzing or ringing in the ear(s) is called _____.

19. Pediatric ear tubes can be placed through the tympanic membrane during a procedure called _____.

20. _____ is also commonly called swimmer's ear.

21. The most common cause of a progressive hearing loss is _____.

22. The surgical treatment for progressive otosclerosis is a _____.

23. Vertigo is the common complaint of an individual with _____.

24. The slow but gradual loss of hearing common in the older adult is called _____.

25. Chronic otitis media can result in perforation of the _____.

CASE STUDIES

■ Ms. Tesar is a 52-year-old woman who has been doing intricate needlework for years. She has exhibited her work in many fairs and received awards for her unique original patterns. While having lunch with her one day, she confides that she is having difficulty seeing the eye of the needle while trying to thread it. She is also having some difficulty drawing the minute details of the patterns. She has noticed, however, that she can see a little better if she holds the needle out away from her while threading it rather than holding it close, as she was used to doing. Having just completed a unit on vision and hearing disorders in your Human Disease course, you think you can explain what is probably occurring with Ms. Tesar's eyesight. What would you tell her about this problem? How would you explain the natural changes that occur with aging? Would you recommend she make an appointment to have her eyes checked?

■ Suzie Lindquist is a friend who has suffered from motion sickness for several years. What medications might help her? What other suggestions could you could give her to decrease the frequency of her motion sickness problems?

Study Tools

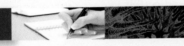

Workbook

Complete Chapter 16

Online Resources

PowerPoint® presentations

Animation

BIBLIOGRAPHY

Abelson, M. B., Ciolino, J., & Tobey, C. (2012). Treating the problem: Fungal keratitis. *Review of Optometry January 15*, 2–13.

Audiology in brief. (2011). *ASHA Leader 16*(14), 5.

Bernardes, T., & Bonfioli, A. (2010). Blepharitis. *Seminars in Ophthalmology 25*(3), 79–83.

Bilkhu, P. S., Wolffsohn, J. S., & Naroo, S. A. (2012). A review of non-pharmacological and pharmacological management of seasonal and perennial allergic conjunctivitis. *Contact Lens & Anterior Eye 35*(1), 9–16.

Campbell, K. M., & Le Prell, C. G. (2011). Potential therapeutic agents. *Seminars in Hearing 32*(3), 281–296.

Carruthers, J. (2010). Is eye care a sinking ship or a rising tide? *Eye Care Review 4*(3), 30–31.

Charters, L. (2011). Evaluate tear film before surgery. *Ophthalmology Times 36*(16), 19.

Doctors Lounge. (2012). Sequential bilateral cochlear implantation ups life quality. *www.doctorslounge.com* (accessed February 2012).

EyeScience launches eye strain formula. (2011). *Review of Optometry 148*(9), 129.

Fong, D. S., & Poon, K. T. (2012). Recent statin use and cataract surgery. *American Journal of Ophthalmology 153*(2), 222–228.

Hampson, C. (2011). Listen up. *Working Mother 35*(1), 25.

Honaker, J. (2011). Hearing loss as a result of common and rare medical conditions: Clinical findings, management options, and prevention strategies. *Seminars in Hearing 32*(4), 297–298.

How and when to use eyedrops. (2010). *Consumer Reports on Health 22*(5), 6.

Kirchner, D. B., Evenson, E., Dobie, R. A., Rabinowitz, P., Crawford, J., Kopke, R., & Hudson, T. W. (2012). Occupational noise-induced hearing loss. *Journal of Occupational & Environmental Medicine 54*(1), 106–108.

Layman, W., & Zuo, J. (2012). An unheard benefit of Cialis. *Nature Medicine 18*(2), 206–207.

Loftus, P. (2012). New drug approved to treat glaucoma. *Wall Street Journal - Eastern Edition*, February 14, D2.

Meinke, D. K., & Morata, T. C. (2012). Awarding and promoting excellence in hearing loss prevention. *International Journal of Audiology 51*(Suppl.), S63–S70.

Mohan, R. R., Tovey, J. C. K., Sharma, A., & Tandon, A. (2012). Gene therapy in the cornea: 2005–present. *Progress in Retinal & Eye Research* (1), 43–64.

New clues to dietary defenses against vision loss with aging. (2011). *Tufts University Health & Nutrition Letter 29*(5), 8.

Patel, P. B., Shastri, D. H., Shelat, P. K., & Shukla, A. K. (2010). Ophthalmic drug delivery system: Challenges and approaches. *Systematic Reviews in Pharmacy 1*(2), 113–120.

Salim, S. (2012). Education key for glaucoma care. *Ophthalmology Times 37*(2), 25.

Skarzynski, H., Lorens, A., Matusiak, M., Porowski, M., Skarzynski, P. H., & James, C. J. (2012). Partial deafness treatment with the nucleus straight research array cochlear implant. *Audiology & Neuro-Otology 17*(2), 82–91.

Tseng, S. G. (2012). Tissue aids glaucoma surgery. *Ophthalmology Times 37*(2), 20.

Twamley, K., Evans, J., & Wormald, R. (2011). Why involve consumers in eye health research? *Eye 25*(8), 969–970.

Understanding amblyopia. (2011). *Review of Optometry May 15*, 49A.

Watkinson, S., & Scott, E. (2010). Care of patients undergoing intra-vitreal therapy. *Nursing Standard 24*(25), 42–47.

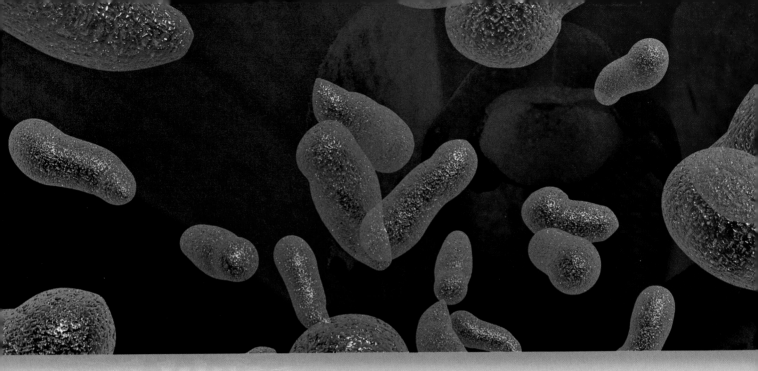

OUTLINE

KEY TERMS

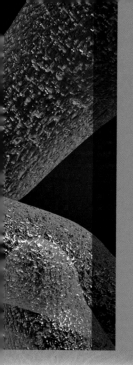

17

Reproductive System Diseases and Disorders

LEARNING OBJECTIVES

Upon completion of the chapter, the learner should be able to:

1. Define the terminology common to the reproductive system and the disorders of the system.

2. Discuss the basic anatomy and physiology of the reproductive system.

3. Identify the important signs and symptoms associated with common reproductive system disorders.

4. Describe the common diagnostics used to determine the type and cause of reproductive system disorders.

5. Identify common disorders of the reproductive system.

6. Describe the typical course and management of the common reproductive system disorders.

7. Describe the effects of aging on the reproductive system and the common disorders associated with aging of the system.

OVERVIEW

The reproductive system is a complex system of structures with a variety of physiologic functions. Some parts of the reproductive system are endocrine glands (ovaries and testes) with purpose throughout a person's lifetime, whereas other parts are strictly involved in procreation for a specific time during the individual's life span. Disorders of the system are common at all ages and can range from mild to severe, especially if not diagnosed early in the development of the disorder. Changes in the system during the aging process have both physiologic and psychosocial implications. ■

ANATOMY AND PHYSIOLOGY

The reproductive system is quite different between the male and female. Although the anatomy and physiologic features have a few commonalities, there are enough differences to discuss them separately.

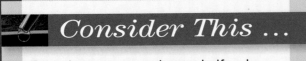

Consider This ...

Every human spent about a half an hour as a single cell—as a fertilized ovum.

Female Anatomy and Physiology

The female reproductive system consists of external structures that include the vulva, labia majora, labia minora, clitoris, vestibule, hymen, vaginal orifice, and vestibular glands. Internal structures include the ovaries, fallopian tubes, uterus, cervix, and vagina (Figure 17–1). The ovaries secrete the female sex hormones, estrogen and progesterone, and produce ova, the reproductive cells, within the Graafian follicles (microscopic sacs). After a follicle releases an ovum, it develops into a corpus luteum, created by the luteinizing hormone from the pituitary gland. The corpus luteum secretes estrogen and progesterone. The fallopian tubes are ducts that carry the ova (eggs) from the ovaries to the uterus.

The uterus is a pear-shaped muscular structure lying above the bladder in the pelvis. It measures only about 2 inches by 3 inches in the nonpregnant state. The lower part of the uterus is called the cervix (neck); the inner layer of the uterus is the endometrium. During menstruation, part of this layer is sloughed off and passed through the vagina and vaginal orifice. The vagina is the structure that receives the penis during intercourse and becomes the birth canal during delivery of the fetus.

The hormones secreted by the ovaries are estrogens and progesterone. Secretion occurs in response to the effects of the follicle-stimulating hormone (FSH) and the luteinizing hormone (LH) produced by the anterior pituitary gland. Estrogen affects the development of secondary sex characteristics (characteristics occurring at puberty), changes in the endometrium, and growth of the uterus and vagina. Progesterone affects the development of the endometrium, assists in the development of the placenta, causes enlargement of the breasts during pregnancy, prevents ova from being produced during pregnancy, and assists in the development of cells in the mammary glands.

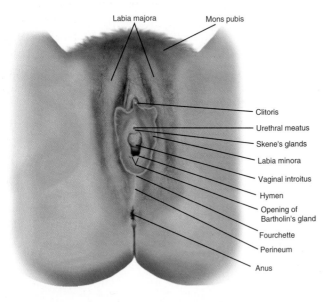

External genitalia.

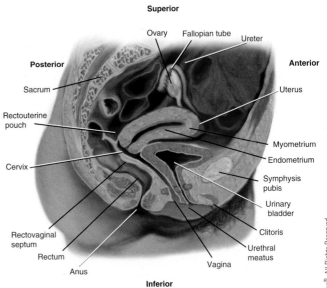

Cross-section of internal structures.

FIGURE 17–1 The female reproductive system.

The menstrual cycle is the process of secretion of hormones, the preparation of the endometrium for the implantation of the fertilized egg, and, if the egg is not implanted, the sloughing of the layer with bleeding from torn capillaries. The cycle runs for about 28 days but varies among individuals. The start of the menstrual flow is the first day of the cycle and usually lasts about 4 to 5 days. After that, estrogen is secreted until the Graafian follicle matures and ruptures, about halfway through the cycle. Progesterone is then secreted by the corpus luteum. As the corpus luteum ages, progesterone levels decline. Declining progesterone levels cause menses and the beginning of the next cycle. Pregnancy will sustain progesterone levels, maintaining the endometrium. The menstrual cycle can begin (menarche) in females as young as 10 years of age but typically begins at age 11 or 12. The cessation of the cycle is called menopause, which usually occurs between ages 40 and 50 but also varies with the individual.

The female breasts are located between the second and seventh ribs over the pectoralis major muscle of the chest. They are usually almost symmetrical and might be small or very large, depending on the individual's structure, body weight, and other factors. Endocrine secretions during menstruation and pregnancy affect the breast size and composition. The breasts show little sign of development until puberty, when, over a 2- to 3-year period, the breasts change from the flattened preadolescent stage to full breast maturity. As the female enters menopause, the breasts begin to atrophy and become more relaxed with a reduction in size.

The female breasts consist of three types of tissue: glandular, fibrous, and adipose (fat). The structure of the breast includes the nipple, areola, lactiferous ducts, lobules lined with milk-producing glands called acini, and fibrous dividers (septa). The breast also contains a network of lymph glands that drains the lymph and returns it to the circulatory system.

Media Link

View an animation on the male reproductive system on the Online Resources.

Male Anatomy and Physiology

The male reproductive system includes the external organs, scrotum and penis, and the internal organs, testes, epididymis, vas deferens, urethra, seminal vesicles, bulbourethral glands, and the prostate (Figure 17–2). The penis houses the urethra, a tube that carries urine from the bladder and semen from the ejaculatory duct. At the tip of the penis is the prepuce (foreskin). The penis is composed of erectile tissue and arteries that dilate during sexual arousal, causing the penis to become erect for the purpose of intercourse. The scrotum is a sac that hangs below the penis and holds the testes. The testes secrete testosterone (the male sex hormone) and produce sperm (the reproductive cells). Testosterone is responsible for the changes occurring during puberty and secondary sex characteristics in the male.

The epididymis is the duct leading from each testis to the vas deferens, the excretory duct. The vas deferens from each testis extends up into the abdomen, where it connects to create the ejaculatory duct that opens into the urethra. The seminal vesicles sit behind the bladder near the neck. They secrete fluid that is part of the thick, white secretion called semen. The prostate gland and bulbourethral glands also secrete fluid that becomes part of the semen.

Consider This ...

An average sperm can swim about 8 inches per hour.

Consider This ...

The largest cell in the human body is the female egg, while the smallest is the male sperm.

Media Link

View an animation on the female reproductive system on the Online Resources.

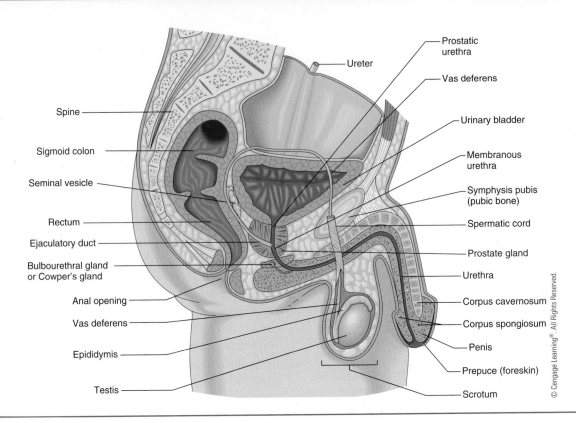

FIGURE 17–2   The male reproductive system.

Labels (clockwise / by region):
- Spine
- Sigmoid colon
- Seminal vesicle
- Rectum
- Ejaculatory duct
- Bulbourethral gland or Cowper's gland
- Anal opening
- Vas deferens
- Epididymis
- Testis
- Ureter
- Prostatic urethra
- Vas deferens
- Urinary bladder
- Membranous urethra
- Symphysis pubis (pubic bone)
- Spermatic cord
- Prostate gland
- Urethra
- Corpus cavernosum
- Corpus spongiosum
- Penis
- Prepuce (foreskin)
- Scrotum

COMMON SIGNS AND SYMPTOMS

Common signs and symptoms of female reproductive system diseases and disorders include:

- Abdominal and pelvic pain
- Fever and malaise
- Abnormal vaginal drainage
- Burning, itching, or both of the genitals
- Pain during sexual intercourse
- Any change in breast tissue
- Abnormal discharge from the nipple

Common signs and symptoms of male reproductive system diseases and disorders include:

- Urinary disorders, including frequency, dysuria, nocturia, and incontinence
- Pain in the pelvis, groin, or reproductive organs
- Lesions on the external genitalia
- Swelling or abnormal enlargement of the reproductive organs
- Abnormal penile drainage
- Burning, itching, or both of the genitals

DIAGNOSTIC TESTS

Physical examination of the female reproductive system to aid in diagnosis of diseases begins with a pelvic examination that includes inspection of the external genitalia, visual examination of the vagina and cervix through a speculum or instrument used to spread and hold the vaginal wall in an open position (Figure 17–3), and palpation of female internal organs by **bimanual examination**. A bimanual (two-handed) examination is so named because the physician places one hand on the abdomen and inserts fingers of the other hand into the vagina to feel the female organs between the two hands. A bimanual rectal examination allows palpation of the posterior aspect of the uterus and the rectum.

The most common test of the female reproductive system is the Papanicolaou (Pap smear) of the cervix (see Figure 17–3). Pap smears are **cytologic** (sigh-toe-LAWG-ic; cyto = cell, logic = study) examinations to

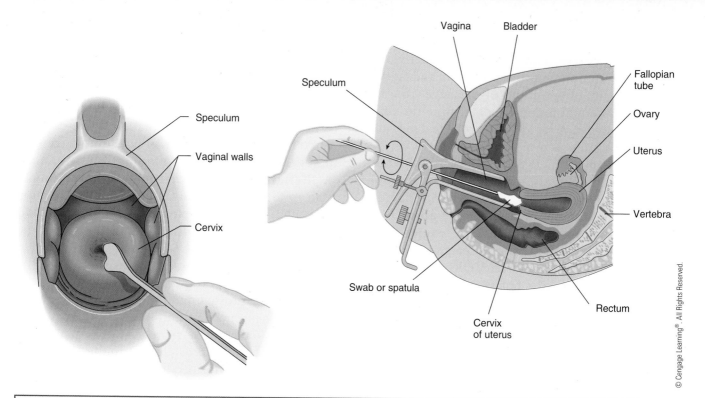

FIGURE 17–3 Use of a speculum and obtaining a Pap smear.

discover cervical cancer. If an abnormal Pap smear is obtained, follow-up can involve a cervical biopsy that entails taking a small piece of tissue from the cervix for microscopic examination. A special type of biopsy, called a cone biopsy, refers to taking a cone-shaped piece of cervical tissue including the cervical os and endocervical lining. The diagnosis of endometrial cancer is best discovered by obtaining tissue for biopsy during a **dilatation and curettage** (KYOU-reh-TAHZH) (D&C). This procedure involves a light surgical sedative, dilation of the cervix (dilatation), and scraping (curettage) of the uterine endometrial tissue. D&C is also commonly performed for abnormal uterine bleeding and following a spontaneous abortion.

A **laparoscopy** (LAP-ah-ROS-ko-pee; laparo = abdomen, scopy = scope procedure), or looking inside the abdominal cavity with a lighted scope (Figure 17–4), is commonly used to view the female organs for abnormalities, diagnose endometriosis, and perform a tubal ligation. To determine the size, position, and patency of the uterus and fallopian tubes, a **hysterosalpingogram** (hystero = uterus, salpingo = fallopian tubes, gram = picture), or X-ray, of these organs can be obtained. During a hysterosalpingogram, a small tube is passed

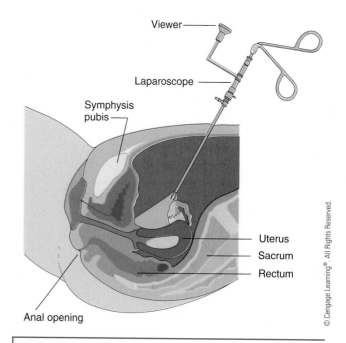

FIGURE 17–4 Laparoscopy.

through the cervix and a radiopaque dye is injected. As the dye fills the uterus and fallopian tubes and spills into the abdominal cavity, X-rays are taken to show patency, or openness, of the tubes.

This procedure is commonly done as part of infertility testing.

Laboratory tests to determine reproductive diseases include microscopic examination and culture and sensitivity of secretions or drainage from the vagina and genital lesions to determine the presence of infection. A rapid DNA probe test may also be used. This test is sensitive to the DNA of specific microorganisms. Blood tests to measure hormone levels, including estrogen and progesterone, are also common. Other blood testing includes the **florescent treponemal antibody absorption test (FTA-ABS)** and **rapid plasma reagin (RPR)** test, and the Venereal Disease Research Laboratory (VDRL) test for syphilis. The VDRL is the oldest of the tests for syphilis but is still used in some cases.

Mammography (mam-OG-rah-fee; mammo = breast, ography = procedure to take a picture) is an X-ray or radiologic examination of breast tissue (Figure 17–5) to determine the presence of cysts or tumors. Digital mammography is a newer technique that takes an electronic image of the breast and stores it in a computer for the radiologist to view. If an abnormal mass is discovered during mammography, further diagnostic techniques include fine-needle aspiration and incisional biopsy.

Ultrasound can be performed on the pelvis to determine the presence of tumors and pregnancy and to visualize pelvic organ position and size. Benign breast cysts can be differentiated from solid tumors by ultrasonography.

Physical examination of the male reproductive system includes visual examination of the external genitalia for tumors, lesions, or penile drainage. The testes are palpated to determine presence of tumors. A **digital rectal examination** allows the physician to feel the prostate (Figure 17–6) for abnormal enlargement (hypertrophy or hyperplasia) and tumors.

A **cystoscopy** (sis-TOS-koh-pee; cysto = bladder, scopy = scope procedure) is performed to view the urethra and bladder with a lighted scope to evaluate the size of the prostate and the degree of obstruction the gland is placing on the urethra.

Biopsy of the male reproductive organs commonly involves the prostate and the testicle. Both procedures are performed to determine malignancy. To obtain a prostatic biopsy, a fine needle is guided through the rectum and into the prostate. A testicular biopsy involves the use of local anesthetic and a fine needle to withdraw a small piece of tissue. Testicular biopsy also can be used to evaluate sperm production.

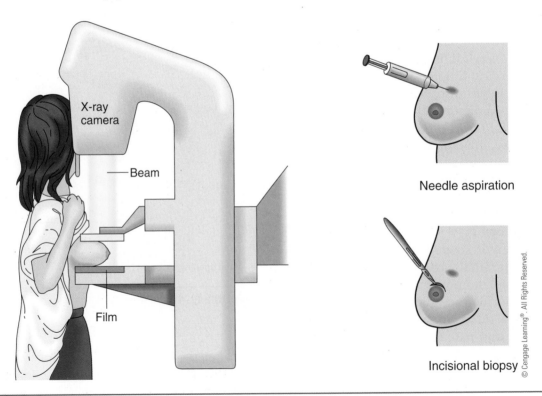

X-ray camera

Beam

Film

Needle aspiration

Incisional biopsy

FIGURE 17–5 Mammography, needle aspiration, and incisional biopsy.

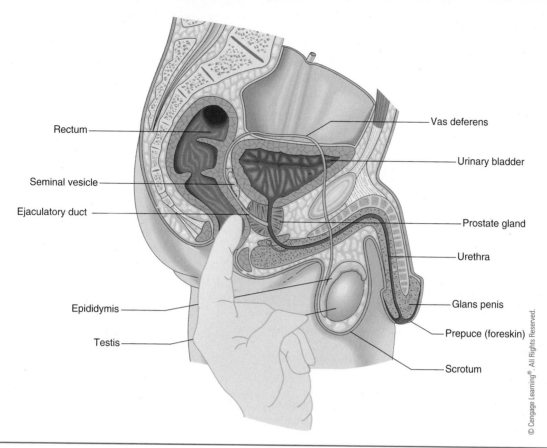

Rectum

Seminal vesicle

Ejaculatory duct

Epididymis

Testis

Vas deferens

Urinary bladder

Prostate gland

Urethra

Glans penis

Prepuce (foreskin)

Scrotum

FIGURE 17–6   Digital rectal examination.

Laboratory tests used in the determination of diseases of the male reproductive system include cultures and sensitivities of penile drainage, lesions, and urine to determine the presence of infection. DNA probe test may also be used. A blood test called a prostate-specific antigen (PSA) is helpful in the detection of prostate cancer. PSA levels also assist in determining effectiveness of prostate cancer treatment. Urine estrogen levels can assist in the diagnosis of testicular cancers.

Specific laboratory tests used for infertility testing include microscopic examination of semen to perform a sperm count, to check sperm viability or ability to survive, and to look for abnormally shaped sperm. Blood tests for the hormones testosterone and LH are also used.

COMMON DISEASES OF THE REPRODUCTIVE SYSTEM

Common diseases of the reproductive system involve those affecting both sexes, including the pregnant female. These diseases are divided into female reproductive system diseases, diseases of the breast, disorders of pregnancy, male reproductive system diseases, sexually transmitted diseases (STDs), and sexual dysfunction.

Female Reproductive System Diseases

The female reproductive system is affected by numerous diseases and disorders caused by inflammation, infection, tumors, cysts, and hormonal imbalances. Diseases can range from mild to life-threatening. Common symptoms include pain and abnormalities in the menstrual cycle.

MENSTRUAL ABNORMALITIES

■ **DESCRIPTION.** Menstrual abnormalities are a common problem in the ovulating female.

■ **ETIOLOGY.** Causes of menstrual abnormalities vary, as does treatment. Common abnormalities include premenstrual syndrome, amenorrhea,

PHARMACOLOGY HIGHLIGHT

Common Drugs for Female Reproductive Disorders

CATEGORY	EXAMPLES OF MEDICATIONS
Antibiotics Drugs used to prevent or stop bacterial infections	ampicillin, amoxicillin, ciprofloxacin, doxycycline, erythromycin, penicillin, or tetracycline
Hormones Drugs to reduce the symptoms of menopause	estrogen
Antineoplastics Drugs used to treat cancer	
Alkylating agents	chlorambucil, cyclophosphamide, or lomustine
Antimetabolites	5-flourauracil, mercaptopurine, or methotrexate
Antitumor antibiotics	mitomycin or streptozocin
Hormones/antihormones	estrogens, androgens, flutamide, or tamoxifen
Other substances	vincristine, L-asparaginase, paclitaxel, carboplatin, cisplatin, or etoposide
Antipyretics/Analgesics Drugs used to reduce fever and pain	acetaminophen, aspirin, ibuprofen, or naproxen

PHARMACOLOGY HIGHLIGHT

Common Drugs for Male Reproductive Disorders

CATEGORY	EXAMPLES OF MEDICATIONS
Antibiotics Drugs used to prevent or stop bacterial infections	ampicillin, amoxicillin, ciprofloxacin, doxycycline, erythromycin, penicillin, or tetracycline
Antineoplastics Drugs used to treat cancer	
Alkylating agents	chlorambucil, cyclophosphamide, or lomustine
Antimetabolites	5-flourauracil, mercaptopurine, or methotrexate
Antitumor antibiotics	mitomycin or streptozocin
Hormones/antihormones	estrogens or androgens
Other substances	vincristine, L-asparaginase, paclitaxel, carboplatin, cisplatin, or etoposide
Antipyretics/Analgesics Drugs used to reduce fever and pain	acetaminophen, aspirin, ibuprofen, or naproxen
Hormones Drugs used to treat prostate cancer or other male reproductive disorders	estrogen or testosterone

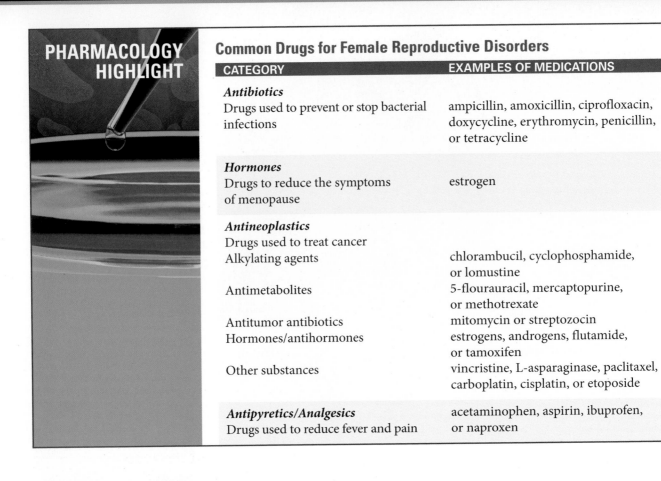

HEALTHY HIGHLIGHT

Coffee and Tea for Women's Health?

A recent study on women's health found that coffee drinkers had less depression than those who did not drink coffee. However, decaf coffee did not improve depression, nor did tea. Coffee also contains some antioxidants that might help prevent blood clots and can help control the blood sugar level. Tea also contains antioxidants that help keep blood vessels healthy and, thus, reduce the risk of heart attack or stroke. In addition, tea contains estrogen-like factors that might help improve bone density. Low bone density is a problem for women, especially older women, and leads to osteoporosis. Caution is recommended for women who drink too much caffeine. Overdoing it might cause anxiety, tremors, or palpitations. Coffee usually contains about twice as much caffeine per cup as tea.

Source: Coffee or Tea: Which for Thee? (2011).

---

dysmenorrhea, menorrhagia, and metrorrhagia. A short description of these disorders follows.

PREMENSTRUAL SYNDROME

■ **DESCRIPTION.** Premenstrual syndrome, commonly called PMS, is a group of symptoms occurring prior to the onset of menses.

■ **ETIOLOGY.** The cause of PMS is uncertain, but research has shown an increase in PMS with rapid hormonal changes in estrogen levels that occur during the menstrual cycle. Other causes might be related to vitamin deficiencies and psychological disturbances. In the past, PMS was thought to be entirely due to emotional factors and stress, but it is now known to have a true physical cause.

■ **SYMPTOMS.** Symptoms of PMS usually begin mid-cycle with ovulation and increase in severity until a few hours after the onset of menses. PMS symptoms can affect virtually every system of the body and include headache, nausea, and back and joint pain. An increase in water retention can cause edema, bloating, weight gain, and breast tenderness and engorgement. Psychological symptoms can include irritability, mood swings, depression, and sleep disturbances. Symptoms of PMS vary significantly from one individual to another. It is unknown why some females have severe, disabling PMS, whereas others are virtually unaffected.

■ **DIAGNOSIS.** Diagnosis is difficult because the cause of this disorder is not clearly understood. A thorough history and physical examination might help determine the correlation of the onset of symptoms in relation to the menstrual cycle. Thyroid testing and tests for dysmenorrhea and endometriosis aid in ruling out other causes. Because depression is common, some women might undergo psychological testing to rule out psychiatric disorders and confirm that the depression is related to PMS.

■ **TREATMENT.** Due to the variation in symptoms, treatment must be individualized because affected individuals have differing symptoms and respond differently to treatment. Dietary changes might be helpful and include avoidance of caffeine, chocolate, nicotine, sugar, salt, and alcohol. Developing a regular exercise program of brisk walking or swimming can be beneficial. Medications might be helpful and include diuretics, analgesics, and progesterone.

■ **PREVENTION.** PMS cannot be prevented, but certain activities can reduce the symptoms. These activities include quitting smoking, limiting caffeine, taking daily calcium (1,200 mg) and vitamin B_6 (50 mg), exercising, eating a balanced diet, and reducing stress.

AMENORRHEA

■ **DESCRIPTION.** Amenorrhea (ah-MEN-oh-REE-ah; a = without, menorrhea = menstruation) is the absence of menstrual periods. Primary amenorrhea is defined as not having menses by age 18. This can be caused by hormonal disorders, malformation or absence of female organs, pregnancy, or anorexia. Secondary amenorrhea is the absence of menses for 6 months or more in a female who has had regular cycles.

■ **ETIOLOGY.** Causes include hormonal imbalance, emotional upset, depression, malnutrition, excessive fitness training, ovarian tumor, and pregnancy.

■ **DIAGNOSIS.** Diagnosis is made on the basis of a physical examination and hormonal blood and urine studies.

■ **TREATMENT.** Treatment depends on cause. If no abnormalities are present, hormone administration will usually begin the menstrual cycle in primary amenorrhea.

■ **PREVENTION.** Preventive measures include adequate nutrition, exercise, and stress reduction.

DYSMENORRHEA

■ **DESCRIPTION.** Dysmenorrhea (DIS-men-oh-REE-ah; dys = difficult, menorrhea = menses) is painful or difficult menses, one of the most common gynecologic disorders.

■ **ETIOLOGY.** Causes of dysmenorrhea include pelvic infections, cervical stenosis, endometriosis, and unknown causes.

■ **SYMPTOMS.** Symptoms include dull to severe cramping pain in the pelvic area and low-back pain. Pain also might radiate into the upper back, thighs, and genitalia. Pain associated with cervical stenosis and endometriosis often occurs in females prior to childbearing and is often relieved after the birth of a child. Prognosis is good if the cause can be found and treated.

■ **TREATMENT.** Oral contraceptives can be effective in reducing dysmenorrhea because they regulate and decrease menstrual flow. Nonsteroidal anti-inflammatory medications are helpful in reducing inflammation and pain. Application of a heating pad to the pelvic area also might be helpful.

MENORRHAGIA

■ **DESCRIPTION.** Menorrhagia (MEN-oh-RAY-jee-ah; meno = menses, orrhagia = bursting forth, abnormal, excessive) is excessive or prolonged menstrual flow.

■ **ETIOLOGY.** Cause can be due to uterine tumors, pelvic inflammatory disease (PID), and hormone imbalances.

■ **TREATMENT.** Treatment is related to cause and can include surgery to remove tumors, antibiotics to treat PID, and hormone therapy for hormone imbalances.

METRORRHAGIA

■ **DESCRIPTION.** Metrorrhagia (MET-roh-RAY-jee-ah; metro = uterus, orrhagia = bursting forth, abnormal, excessive) is abnormal bleeding between menstrual periods.

■ **ETIOLOGY.** The cause is commonly due to hormonal imbalance, leading to an abnormal thickening and shedding of the endometrial tissue.

■ **TREATMENT.** Treatment can be a D&C, returning the endometrium to normal and ending metrorrhagia.

MENOPAUSE

■ **DESCRIPTION.** Menopause is the natural halting of menstruation.

■ **ETIOLOGY.** Menopause is not a disease but rather a normal physical change related to aging, but many women consider menopause a disorder because they commonly have physical and psychological symptoms. Menopause usually takes place between the ages of 40 and 50 years. As a female ages, the ovaries produce less estrogen, causing cessation of ovulation and menstruation. This process can be surgically induced by removal of both ovaries (bilateral oophorectomy).

■ **SYMPTOMS.** Common physical symptoms of menopause include hot flashes, night sweats, and vaginal dryness. Some women also experience psychological symptoms of depression, sleep disorders, and decreased libido (sex drive). Hormonal changes brought about by menopause increase a woman's risk of cardiac disease and osteoporosis.

■ **DIAGNOSIS.** The blood testing for presence of FSH aids in diagnosis of menopause.

■ **TREATMENT.** Menopausal hormone therapy (MHT) has been the treatment of choice for more than 60 years for prevention of hot flashes and vaginal dryness in menopausal women. In the mid-1980s, estrogen also was approved as preventive treatment of heart disease and osteoporosis.

In 2002, a federally funded Women's Health Initiative (WHI) prematurely halted a hormone study, finding that hormone therapy not only did not protect against heart disease but actually led to a slight increase in risk of heart attacks, breast cancer, strokes, and blood clots. The results of this study led to a drastic and immediate decline in the use of MHT. Since the WHI study, expert panels of scientist have found that the overall conclusions of the WHI study do not apply to most menopausal women starting MHT. The study group actually started MHT several years after onset of menopause, and the average age of the women in the study was 63, more than 10 years older than the average age of most menopausal women. Most women begin menopause around age 53 and start MHT shortly thereafter. This study did not look at that group of women.

More current research has found that women who are less than 60 years old do not appear to be at an increased risk for heart disease. This research also found that the benefits of MHT do outweigh the risk in most cases, especially for the relief of symptoms related to low estrogen levels. Other studies have shown that lower doses of estrogen than were given in the WHI research not only reduce symptoms but also assist in maintaining bone density.

Since 2002, there has been much confusion about the safety of MHT. While many questions remain unanswered, there are several treatment considerations that most clinicians do agree upon.

First, decisions about MHT should be made, like most treatments, on an individual basis by the individual and her physician. Treatment options, the individual's medical and family history, and the potential risk should all be discussed and carefully considered.

The dosage and delivery method should also be individualized to meet the individual's particular needs. The National Cancer Institute has determined that MHT should be given for the shortest time and in the lowest dose needed to control menopausal symptoms.

Other resources on menopausal hormone therapy include:

- National Institutes of Health, Menopausal Hormone Therapy Information: www.nih.gov/PHTindex.htm
- The National Library of Medicine, MedlinePlus: www.medlineplus.gov

■ **PREVENTION.** There are no preventive measures.

VAGINITIS

■ **DESCRIPTION.** Vaginitis (VAJ-ih-NIGH-tis) is inflammation of the vagina.

■ **ETIOLOGY.** Vaginitis is a very common disease caused by a variety of microorganisms including bacteria and yeast. It is not dangerous but is irritating and uncomfortable and often leads to a bladder infection.

■ **SYMPTOMS.** Symptoms of vaginitis are burning, itching, and swelling of the vagina and external genitalia. A white cottage cheese–appearing discharge is common with *Candida* vaginitis.

■ **DIAGNOSIS.** Basic diagnosis is made by review of symptoms, testing the pH level of vaginal fluid, and microscopic (wet prep) examination. More sensitive testing includes culture, antigen detection, and DNA probe test.

■ **TREATMENT.** The key to proper treatment of vaginitis is to determine the correct cause of the infection. Yeast infections that occur more often than four times a year need physician treatment. Abstaining from sexual intercourse until the condition has healed is recommended primarily to decrease the risk of reinfection.

■ **PREVENTION.** Preventive activities include keeping the vaginal area clean and dry; wearing cotton underwear to help absorb moisture; always wiping genital area front to back; avoiding excessive douching; avoiding deodorized tampons; eating yogurt, especially if taking antibiotics; removing and replacing tampons as directed; and decreasing intake of sweets and alcohol. The most common types of vaginitis include the following.

CANDIDA VAGINITIS

■ **DESCRIPTION.** *Candida* vaginitis is a type of fungus or yeast vaginitis that normally cohabits with *Lactobacillus* bacteria in the vagina, maintaining vaginal normal flora. (See Chapter 4, "Inflammation and Infection," for more details on normal flora.)

■ **ETIOLOGY.** If the balance between the *Candida* and the *Lactobacillus* is disturbed, the affected individual develops a *Candida* vaginitis, the most common type of vaginitis, commonly called a yeast infection (Figure 17–7). To maintain normal healthy vaginal flora, sufficient estrogen must be produced to enhance the growth of lactobacilli, a beneficial, normal flora bacterium. Lactobacilli aid in the production of lactic acid, causing a lower vaginal pH of 4 or 4.5. This acid environment is also a deterrent to the growth of harmful microorganisms.

Use of tampons, diaphragms, condoms, spermicides, vaginal douche, and deodorant sprays can

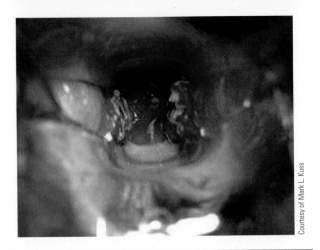

Courtesy of Mark L. Kuss

FIGURE 17–7 Candida vaginitis: view through speculum.

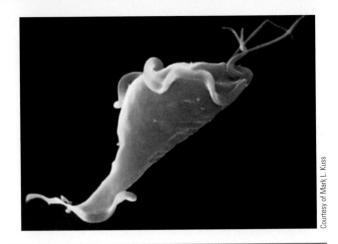

Courtesy of Mark L. Kuss

FIGURE 17–8 Trichomonas vaginalis protozoan.

easily upset the normal flora of the vagina and lead to vaginitis. Antibiotic use commonly kills lactobacilli and can lead to severe vaginitis. *Candida* infection is usually not spread by sexual transmission except in severe cases.

■ ***TREATMENT.*** Home remedies include douching with 1 teaspoon of vinegar in 1 gallon of water and eating yogurt or adding the yogurt in the douche to restore the normal flora. Over-the-counter, vaginal antifungal ointments and tablets such as clotrimazole (Gyne-Lotrimin®, Femcare®) and miconazole are beneficial in most cases. Oral antifungal medications such as fluconazole (Diflucan®) might be needed for more severe cases.

TRICHOMONAS VAGINITIS

■ ***ETIOLOGY.*** *Trichomonas* (TRICK-oh-MOH-nas) vaginitis is caused by the protozoan parasite *Trichomonas vaginalis*. This parasite is commonly transmitted during sexual intercourse (Figure 17–8).

■ ***TREATMENT.*** Both sexual partners must be treated with an oral antiparasitic medication to eradicate the infection.

ATROPHIC VAGINITIS

■ ***ETIOLOGY.*** Atrophic vaginitis commonly occurs after menopause and is caused by a decrease in secretion of estrogen, which is needed to maintain the vaginal lining. Without an adequate supply, the lining becomes more susceptible to infection.

■ ***DIAGNOSIS.*** Diagnosis is usually confirmed by microscopic examination of vaginal secretions, revealing the presence of the infecting organism.

■ ***TREATMENT.*** Treatment often includes estrogen therapy and the use of adequate lubrication during sexual intercourse to prevent injury to the vaginal lining.

OTHER FEMALE REPRODUCTIVE SYSTEM DISEASES AND DISORDERS

ENDOMETRIOSIS

■ ***DESCRIPTION.*** Endometriosis (EN-doh-ME-tree-OH-sis; endo = inside, metri = uterus, osis = condition of) is the abnormal growth of endometrial tissue outside the uterus. Endometrial tissue might flow retrograde during menses and escape into the abdominopelvic cavity through the fallopian tubes or, even worse, escape into the blood supply and be carried to sites all over the body.

■ ***ETIOLOGY.*** The cause of retrograde flow is unknown, but use of tampons might be a causative factor. For this reason, the use of tampons is discouraged. Common sites of endometrial implantation include the ovaries, fallopian tubes, abdominal wall, and intestine. Other sites of implantation include the urinary bladder, the diaphragm, nerves and ligaments of the back, and the vulva, to name only a few (Figure 17–9).

This endometrial tissue continues to act under the influence of hormones, thickening and bleeding with menstrual cycles, causing irritation and inflammation of normal tissue surrounding the implanted endometrial tissue, and thus causing the development of a special blood-filled cyst (chocolate cyst), scar tissue, and adhesions.

■ ***SYMPTOMS.*** This bleeding of endometrial tissue in the abdominopelvic cavity and other **ectopic**

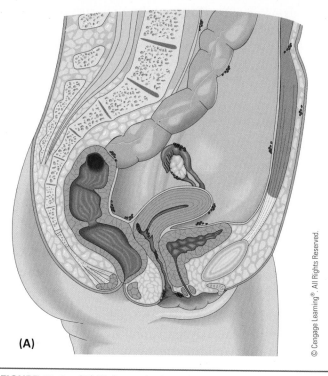

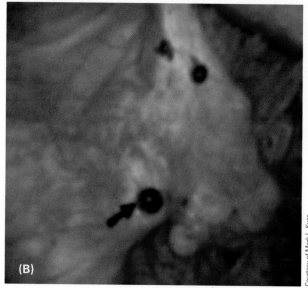

(A)

(B)

FIGURE 17–9   (A) Endometriosis—common sites of endometrial implants. (B) Endometriosis—internal abdominal wall implant.

(eck-TOP-ick, out of normal place) areas causes **dysmenorrhea** (DIS-men-oh-REE-ah; dys = painful, menorrhea = menses), beginning a few days before menses and extending several days into the menstrual cycle. There might be a constant cramping pain in the low back, pelvis, and vagina. Affected individuals, usually females of childbearing age, also might experience heavy menses and **dyspareunia** (DIS-pah-ROO-nee-ah; painful sexual intercourse).

The primary complication of endometriosis is infertility. Other complications include ectopic pregnancy and spontaneous abortion.

■ **DIAGNOSIS.** Diagnosis is made on the basis of history and pelvic examination. A laparoscopy will confirm the diagnosis and allow visualization of the extent of the condition.

■ **TREATMENT.** Treatment depends on the affected individual's age and desire to have children. Young females wishing to have children should not delay childbearing. Treatment with various hormonal medications might be helpful in younger individuals. Pregnancy, nursing, and menopause will not cure the condition but do cause a remission in symptoms because the abnormal tissue shrinks when menstrual hormones are halted. In severe cases, a total hysterectomy, or **panhysterectomy**

(removal of ovaries, fallopian tubes, and uterus), might be indicated.

■ **PREVENTION.** Endometriosis cannot be prevented, primarily because the etiology is not well understood. Long-term birth control hormones might prevent the condition from worsening.

PELVIC INFLAMMATORY DISEASE

■ **DESCRIPTION.** PID is an inflammation of some or all of the pelvic reproductive organs. It can be mild to severe and might involve the cervix (**cervicitis**), the inner lining of the uterus (**endometritis**), fallopian tubes (**salpingitis**), and ovaries (**oophoritis**) (Figure 17–10).

■ **ETIOLOGY.** This inflammation is commonly due to infection by bacteria that ascend from the vagina and travel upward to the pelvic cavity. Bacteria can be introduced into the female reproductive system during childbirth, miscarriage, abortion, or other gynecologic procedures. The most common cause of PID is STD, including gonorrhea and chlamydia infection. Young, sexually active females and those who use intrauterine devices (IUDs) are most at risk of developing PID.

■ **SYMPTOMS.** Symptoms are typical of an infection and include fever, chills, pain in the pelvic area, and

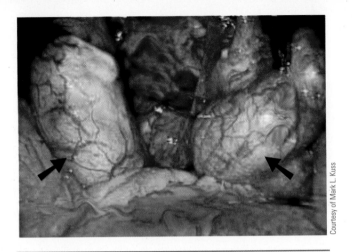

FIGURE 17–10 Pelvic inflammatory disease.

leukorrhea (LOO-koh-REE-ah; leuk = white, orrhea = flow or discharge), a white, usually foul-smelling vaginal discharge.

■ *DIAGNOSIS.* Diagnosis is made on the basis of a pelvic examination including a positive culture of vaginal discharge.

■ *TREATMENT.* Treatment includes antibiotic therapy, analgesics, and bed rest. Without proper treatment, the infection can lead to **septicemia** (SEP-tih-SEE-me-ah; septic = dirty or contaminated, emia = blood), or blood-borne, and life-threatening. Inflammation of the reproductive organs can lead to the development of scar tissue and adhesions that can cause the complications of infertility and ectopic pregnancy.

■ *PREVENTION.* PID can usually be prevented by practicing safe sex with proper use of condoms.

This will reduce but not eliminate risk of contracting STDs, the primary cause of the disease. Monogamous sexual relationships and abstinence also help prevent STDs.

OVARIAN CYST

■ *DESCRIPTION.* Ovarian cysts are commonly benign, fluid-filled sacs on or near the ovary (Figure 17–11).

■ *ETIOLOGY.* There are two types of cysts: physiologic—those caused by a normally functioning ovary—and neoplastic, an abnormal type not related to the function of the ovary. Physiologic cysts are the most common and can become very large (grapefruit size) before producing symptoms.

■ *SYMPTOMS.* Symptoms include low back pain, pelvic pain, and dyspareunia. Acute, extreme pain, nausea, and vomiting can occur if the ovary becomes twisted from the weight of the cyst.

■ *DIAGNOSIS.* Diagnosis is made on the basis of history, pelvic examination, and ultrasound.

■ *TREATMENT.* Treatment depends on the type and size of the cyst. Small physiologic cysts usually do not need treatment and often resolve spontaneously. Oral contraceptive medication can be given for several months to help resolve physiologic tumors of various sizes. Large cysts or those of questionable type are often viewed by laparoscopy, during which the cyst can be removed or drained. Determination should be made of the type of cyst because cancerous cysts need immediate treatment.

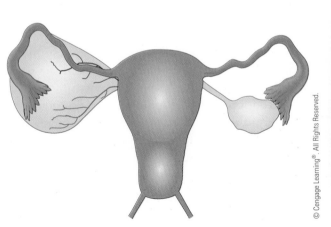

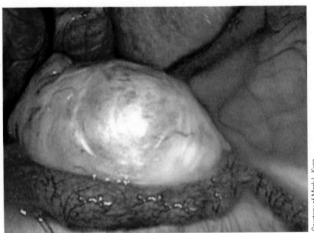

FIGURE 17–11 Ovarian cyst.

■ **PREVENTION.** Anything that prevents ovulation, such as birth control hormones, breast feeding, pregnancy, and menopause, reduces the risk of ovarian cysts.

FIBROID TUMOR

■ **DESCRIPTION.** Leiomyomas, commonly called fibroid tumors, are benign tumors of the smooth muscle of the uterus (Figure 17–12). They are the most common tumor of the female reproductive system, occurring in one out of five women over age 35.

■ **ETIOLOGY.** The cause of fibroid tumors is unknown, but it is known that these tumors are stimulated by estrogen and, thus, tend to occur during reproductive years and regress or calcify after menopause. They often appear in multiples and vary in size from small to quite large. Small fibroids are often asymptomatic.

■ **SYMPTOMS.** Symptoms include abnormal uterine bleeding, excessive menstrual bleeding, and pain.

■ **DIAGNOSIS.** Diagnosis is made on the basis of pelvic examination and ultrasound.

■ **TREATMENT.** Treatment depends on the individual's age and desire for childbearing. Fibroids can be removed surgically, but in older individuals, a hysterectomy is often the treatment of choice. A technology called high-intensity focused ultrasound (HIFU) that uses sound waves to destroy tumors can be used to treat the uterine fibroids.

■ **PREVENTION.** Fibroid tumors cannot be prevented. Estrogen therapy and oral contraceptives do increase risk of developing these tumors.

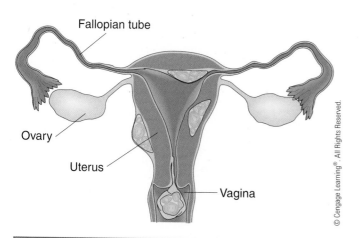

FIGURE 17–12   Fibroid tumors.

Fallopian tube

Ovary

Uterus

Vagina

TOXIC SHOCK SYNDROME

■ **DESCRIPTION.** Toxic shock syndrome (TSS) is a severe, life-threatening illness found almost exclusively in menstruating females using tampons.

■ **ETIOLOGY.** TSS is thought to be caused by *Staphylococcus aureus*, a normal flora bacterium of the skin that produces an increased amount of toxin when in contact with the synthetic fibers found in tampons.

■ **SYMPTOMS.** Symptoms include the sudden onset of high fever, vomiting, diarrhea, and a dropping blood pressure.

■ **DIAGNOSIS.** Diagnosis is made on the basis of history of tampon use and symptoms. Complete blood count (CBC), chest X-ray, and electrocardiogram (ECG) may be completed to rule out other serious conditions.

■ **TREATMENT.** Treatment includes intravenous fluids to counteract shock and antibiotics to treat the infection. Untreated or delayed treatment may be fatal.

■ **PREVENTION.** The best preventive measure is to avoid use of tampons. If this is not a good option, proper tampon usage helps reduce risk. Proper usage includes:

- Good hand washing to decrease the number of bacteria on the individual's hands prior to tampon insertion
- Avoiding superabsorbent tampons
- Changing the tampon every 2 to 3 hours

UTERINE PROLAPSE

■ **DESCRIPTION.** Uterine prolapse occurs when the uterus drops or protrudes downward into the vagina. There are varying degrees of prolapse (Figure 17–13).

■ **ETIOLOGY.** Prolapse is commonly due to aging and childbirth because these weaken the pelvic floor muscles.

■ **SYMPTOMS.** Symptoms include heaviness in the pelvic area; urinary stress, incontinence, or dysuria; and low back pain. With a complete prolapse, one can easily see the uterus bulging out of the vaginal opening (Figure 17–14). Although quite uncomfortable, this condition is not an emergency or even a health risk unless there is bleeding or an inability to urinate.

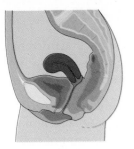
Normal uterus

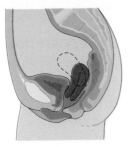
First-degree prolapse

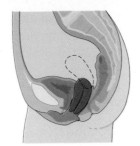
Second-degree prolapse

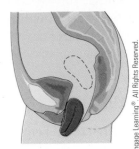
Third-degree prolapse

FIGURE 17–13 Uterine prolapse—varying degrees.

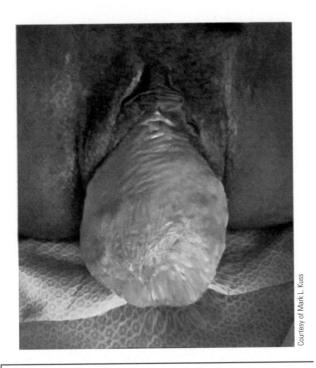

FIGURE 17–14 Uterine prolapse—complete.

■ *DIAGNOSIS.* Diagnosis is made on the basis of a pelvic examination.

■ *TREATMENT.* A hysterectomy is often the surgical treatment of choice, depending on the woman's age and desire to bear children.

■ *PREVENTION.* This condition might not be preventable. Preventive behavior includes not smoking, maintaining a healthy weight, exercising daily, performing Kegel exercises to strengthen pelvic floor muscles, and controlling coughing.

CYSTOCELE

■ *DESCRIPTION.* Cystocele (SIS-toh-seel; cysto = urinary bladder, cele = hernia) is the herniation, or protrusion, of the urinary bladder through the anterior vaginal wall (Figure 17–15).

■ *ETIOLOGY.* Cystocele is often due to weakening of or trauma to the pelvic muscles related to aging and childbirth.

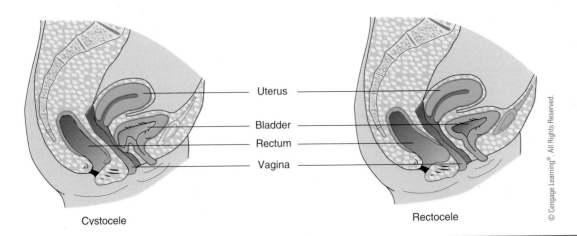

Uterus

Bladder

Rectum

Vagina

Cystocele

Rectocele

FIGURE 17–15 Cystocele and rectocele.

■ **SYMPTOMS.** Symptoms include pelvic pressure, urinary urgency, frequency, and incontinence.

■ **DIAGNOSIS.** Diagnosis is made on the basis of a pelvic examination.

■ **TREATMENT.** Treatment depends on the degree of herniation. Strengthening the pelvic floor muscles with exercise can be beneficial. The specific exercise (Kegel exercise) is performed by contracting the pelvic floor muscles (this group of muscles is tightened to cut off urine flow) and releasing the muscles several times a day. If the cystocele is large or exercise is ineffective, surgery (anterior colporrhaphy) might be necessary.

■ **PREVENTION.** Preventive activities include not smoking, controlling coughing, avoiding heavy lifting, maintaining a healthy weight, controlling constipation, and performing Kegel exercises.

RECTOCELE

■ **DESCRIPTION.** Rectocele is the herniation or protrusion of the rectum through the posterior vaginal wall (see Figure 17–15).

■ **ETIOLOGY.** Rectocele, like a cystocele, is due to trauma to this area during childbirth.

■ **SYMPTOMS.** Symptoms include discomfort, constipation, and fecal incontinence.

■ **DIAGNOSIS.** Diagnosis is made on the basis of a physical examination.

■ **TREATMENT.** Treatment commonly is surgical repair (posterior colpoplasty). Often, the affected individual needs both a cystocele repair and a rectocele repair, called an anterior–posterior, or A&P, repair.

■ **PREVENTION.** Preventive activities include not smoking, avoiding coughing, maintaining a healthy body weight, and performing Kegel exercises.

CERVICAL CANCER

■ **DESCRIPTION.** Cervical cancer is the fifth-leading cause of cancer-related death in females. This cancer usually begins with **carcinoma in situ**—neoplastic cells that sit on the basement membrane and have not invaded into deeper tissue. As the cancer progresses, ulceration and cervical bleeding occur (Figure 17–16).

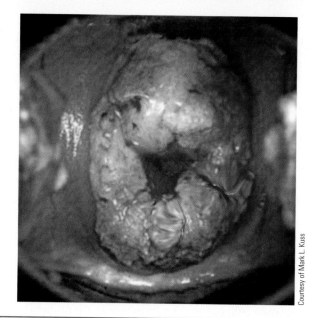

FIGURE 17–16 Cervical cancer.

Courtesy of Mark L. Kuss

■ **ETIOLOGY.** Infection with high-risk human papillomavirus (HPV) often causes changes to the cells of the cervix and is the major cause of cervical cancer. There are over 60 types of HPV. Some types cause warts on the hands and feet of children, whereas other types cause genital warts. Infection with HPV is also known to cause cancers of the oropharynx, vagina, vulva, penis, and anus.

HPV is generally acquired through sexual contact. Condoms cannot prevent the spread of HPV because it is found on all genital tissues of the infected individual. Males and females are usually asymptomatic with HPV infection. Discovery of HPV is usually made when cervical changes are found with a Pap smear. It is very difficult to trace exposure to the virus because it can lie dormant on the cervix for 20 years before it causes changes to the cells of the cervix.

Activities that increase risk of HPV infection include:

■ Beginning sexual intercourse at an early age. This activity generally results in an increase in the number of sex partners over the individual's lifetime.

■ Having multiple sexual partners. Studies show that approximately 40% of young, sexually active females carry HPV in their vaginas. Presumably, a similar percentage of males are infected.

One fact in support of these identified risk factors is that females who abstain from sexual intercourse throughout life do not get cervical cancer.

HPV infection does not cause cervical cancer in all females. Most women who have evidence of HPV on their cervix never get cervical cancer. Studies suggest that whether a female will develop cervical cancer depends on a variety of factors acting together with HPV infection. These factors include:

- **Decreased resistance to infection**.
- **Smoking** Women who smoke concentrate nicotine in their cervix, which harms the cells.
- **Sexual intercourse with males who smoke** Men also concentrate nicotine in their genital secretions and can bathe the cervix with these chemicals during intercourse.
- **Marriage to a male whose previous spouse was diagnosed with cervical cancer** Females married to men whose former spouse was diagnosed with cervical cancer are at greater risk of also developing cervical cancer.
- **Obesity**.
- **Excessive alcohol consumption**.

■ *SYMPTOMS.* Development of cervical cancer is usually slow, and symptoms of abnormal cervical bleeding are easily noticed, leading to early detection of this form of cancer.

■ *DIAGNOSIS.* Diagnosis of cervical cancer is made on the basis of a Pap smear.

■ *TREATMENT.* Treatment is usually surgical removal of the tumor. If metastasis has occurred, surgery is often followed by radiation therapy. If the tumor has spread into adjacent tissues, a complete hysterectomy might be performed. Untreated, the tumor becomes inoperable and fatal.

■ *PREVENTION.* Cervical cancer is one of the few preventable cancers. Regular Pap smear testing aids in identifying precancerous cells, allowing treatment prior to cancer development. Other activities to reduce risk include not smoking, limiting the number of sexual partners, using condoms, and following up on abnormal Pap tests.

The Food and Drug Administration (FDA) has now approved two HPV vaccines, Gardasil® and Cervarix®, for girls age 9 to 26. Gardasil® has also been approved for both girls and boys age 9 to 26 for prevention of genital warts caused by HPV.

These vaccines are given in three individual doses and are proven to be effective only if given *before* infection with HPV. It is also recommended that the vaccines be given before the individual becomes sexually active.

Neither of these vaccines has been proven to provide complete protection against all strains of HPV, nor will they prevent other sexually transmitted diseases. Approximately 30% of cervical cancers will not be prevented by these vaccines. In 2010, approximately 48% of age-eligible girls had received only one vaccine dose, whereas less than 2% of age-eligible boys had been vaccinated with one dose.

UTERINE CANCER

■ *DESCRIPTION.* Uterine cancer develops in the inner lining of the uterus, the endometrium, and spreads into the uterine wall (Figure 17–17). Uterine cancer also may be called endometrial cancer.

■ *ETIOLOGY.* This type of cancer usually occurs in postmenopausal females who have never had children. Increased risk factors include infertility, obesity, and prolonged estrogen stimulation as occurs with hormone replacement therapy.

■ *SYMPTOMS.* A symptom of uterine cancer is abnormal bleeding, which is quite noticeable in postmenopausal females and usually leads to early detection of this form of cancer.

■ *DIAGNOSIS.* Diagnosis is made on the basis of visual examination and endometrial biopsy.

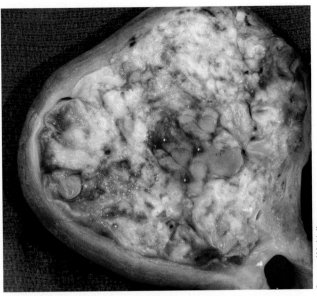

Courtesy of Mark L. Kuss

FIGURE 17–17 Uterine cancer.

■ **TREATMENT.** Treatment is very successful if the cancer is discovered in its early stages and includes surgical removal of the ovaries and uterus, combined with radiation therapy.

■ **PREVENTION.** Most cases are not preventable, but reducing risk factors is helpful. Risk reduction includes a history of taking oral contraceptives or birth control pills and taking hormone therapy with progestin after menopause. Other activities to reduce risk include not smoking and maintaining a healthy weight.

OVARIAN CANCER

■ **DESCRIPTION.** Ovarian cancer is quite common and often fatal (Figure 17–18).

■ **ETIOLOGY.** The cause of ovarian cancer is unknown, and the ovaries' position deep in the pelvis makes discovery of this tumor difficult. Often, extensive metastasis will occur before noticeable symptoms present.

■ **SYMPTOMS.** Symptoms include a feeling of pressure on the bladder, low abdominal or pelvic pain, and a general feeling of ill health.

■ **DIAGNOSIS.** Diagnosis is made on the basis of physical examination and visualization of the mass during an exploratory laparoscopy.

■ **TREATMENT.** Treatment depends on the stage of the cancer and often includes a complete hysterectomy,

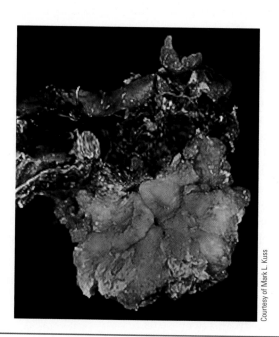

FIGURE 17–18   Ovarian cancer.

radiation, and chemotherapy. Prognosis is good with early detection, but as stated previously, this is not the usual case. If metastasis has occurred, this cancer can be fatal in 1 to 2 years. The only preventive measure is early detection through annual gynecologic exams.

■ **PREVENTION.** Activities that lower risk include a history of taking oral contraceptive (birth control pills), bearing at least one child, and breast feeding for at least 1 year. An interesting fact about preventive activities is that having a tubal ligation reduces risk more than having a hysterectomy. The reason for this is unknown.

Diseases of the Breast

Diseases of the breast are quite common, affecting one in eight women in the United States and ranging from mild to life-threatening. Breast self-examination and mammography are important methods of screening for cancer. Although women are most often affected with breast diseases, men also can be affected. Any change from normal in tissue shape or appearance in males or females should be called to the attention of a physician.

Consider This ...

Breast pain is the second most common breast symptom for which women seek medical attention, second only to finding a lump in the breast.

FIBROCYSTIC DISEASE

■ **DESCRIPTION.** Fibrocystic disease of the breast is the most common breast disorder of premenopausal females between the ages of 30 and 55.

■ **ETIOLOGY.** It is thought that the development of cysts is linked to estrogen levels.

■ **SYMPTOMS.** This disorder is characterized by:

■ An irregular, lumpy feeling in the breast, usually in the upper outer quadrant area of the breast.

■ Breast discomfort that is persistent or occurs on and off, typically peaking around the menstrual period and receding afterward.

- Breast often feeling heavy, full, and tender.
- A tendency to run in families.

Fibrocystic disease causes an increased risk of cancer approximately one-and-a-half times that of the normal population. Multiple cysts also make detection of neoplasm more difficult. For these reasons, affected females need to perform monthly breast self-examinations routinely and have yearly mammograms. Females with severe fibrocystic disease and at high risk of breast cancer might decide to have a **prophylactic** (preventive) mastectomy.

■ *DIAGNOSIS.* Diagnosis is made primarily by feeling, or palpation, of lumpy areas in the breast. Breasts that have many areas of fibrocystic disease can be difficult to palpate and to mammogram properly. In this case, breast ultrasound can be helpful. If there is a suspicious area, a needle or surgical biopsy can be performed to confirm diagnosis.

■ *TREATMENT.* Measures to decrease breast pain due to fibrocystic disease include elimination of caffeine in the diet, reduction of salt intake, the use of a mild diuretic the week prior to menstruation, and the use of mild analgesics. For severe cases, hormonal therapy with synthetic androgen might be helpful.

■ *PREVENTION.* This condition is often not preventable, but decreasing dietary fat and caffeine can be helpful. Several researchers have studied the correlation between wearing brassieres and fibrocystic lumps, with 90% of the women in one study finding improvement in symptoms when they stopped wearing their brassieres (Singer & Grismaijer, 1995).

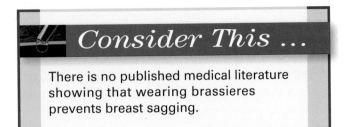

Consider This ...

There is no published medical literature showing that wearing brassieres prevents breast sagging.

MASTITIS

■ *DESCRIPTION.* Mastitis (mas-TYE-tis; mast = breast, itis = inflammation) is inflammation of the breast tissue and is a broad term covering a variety of diseases and disorders. The type of mastitis commonly thought of is **puerperal** (pyou-ER-pier-al; childbirth) mastitis (Figure 17–19).

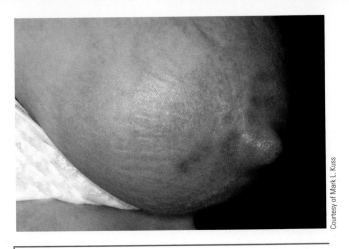

Courtesy of Mark L. Kuss

FIGURE 17–19   Mastitis.

■ *ETIOLOGY.* Puerperal mastitis occurs when bacteria from the nursing baby's mouth or mother's hands enter the breast tissue through the nipple and cause infection.

■ *SYMPTOMS.* Symptoms include redness, heat, swelling, pain, and, often, bloody discharge from the nipple.

■ *DIAGNOSIS.* Diagnosis is made on the basis of symptoms.

■ *TREATMENT.* Treatment includes antibiotics, application of heat, analgesics, and a firm support brassiere to decrease discomfort.

■ *PREVENTION.* Preventive measures include complete emptying of the breast when breast feeding. The baby should completely empty one breast before the other is offered.

BREAST CANCER

■ *DESCRIPTION.* Breast cancer is an adenocarcinoma (adeno = gland, carcinoma = cancer) of the breast ducts. It is the most common neoplasm affecting breast tissue and occurs in one out of eight females. It is second only to lung cancer as the leading cause of cancer-related deaths in females in the United States (Centers for Disease Control and Prevention & National Cancer Institute, 2010). Monthly breast self-examinations and routine mammograms are a must for early detection of breast cancer.

■ *ETIOLOGY.* The cause of breast cancer is unknown, but possible identified risk factors include:

- Age 40 and over
- Family member affected with breast cancer

- Onset of menses before age 13
- Menses continuing after age 50
- Nullipara (nuh-LIP-ah-rah; nulli = none or no, para = births)
- First child after age 30
- Obesity
- Chronic breast disease
- Brassiere wear time

■ **SYMPTOMS.** Symptoms of breast cancer include a nontender lump of varying size. These occur most often in the upper outer quadrant of the breast, near the axillary area. The lump might cause a dimpling of the skin, or the nipple might be retracted. Often, there are no visual symptoms.

■ **DIAGNOSIS.** Diagnosis is made on the basis of the presence of the lump, mammogram, and biopsy. A biopsy is the definitive test and can be performed by aspiration or surgery. Prognosis is good if the lump is found early. However, metastasis is common and usually affects the lungs, liver, brain, and bone. If metastasis has occurred, the prognosis can be poor.

■ **TREATMENT.** Treatment is usually surgical removal of the mass or the breast (**mastectomy**: mas-TECK-toh-me; mast = breast, ectomy = excision), followed by chemotherapy, radiation therapy, or both. Carcinoma spreads through the lymphatic system, so removal of the lymph nodes and lymph vessels is a common procedure. Several types of surgical procedures are performed for breast cancer, depending on the location, size, and metastasis of the tumor. Commonly, these types of surgery include:

- Lumpectomy, involving removal of the lump only.
- Simple or total mastectomy, involving removal of the breast and nipple.
- Modified radical mastectomy, involving removal of the breast, nipple, and lymph nodes.
- Radical mastectomy, involving removal of the breast, nipple, lymph nodes, and underlying chest (pectoral) muscles (Figure 17–20).

Mastectomy surgery not only causes an alteration in the physical image but also can lead to a variety of psychological disorders for a female. For this reason, many women decide to have reconstructive surgery (mammoplasty) performed along with the mastectomy in an effort to reduce the physical and psychological trauma. **Mammoplasty** (MAM-oh-PLAS-tee; mammo = breast, plasty = surgical repair or restructuring) involves reconstruction of the breast with plastic surgery and prosthetic breast implants or skin flaps.

Many new postmastectomy or postlumpectomy treatments are reducing the rate of recurrence of the disease. Depending on the type of breast cancer, medications that target the specific problem (such as hormone, protein receptor, or blood vessel problems) are having a positive impact on the disease.

■ **PREVENTION.** Preventive measures include reducing identified risk factors. Several researchers have supported the theory of a relationship between brassiere wear time and breast cancer.

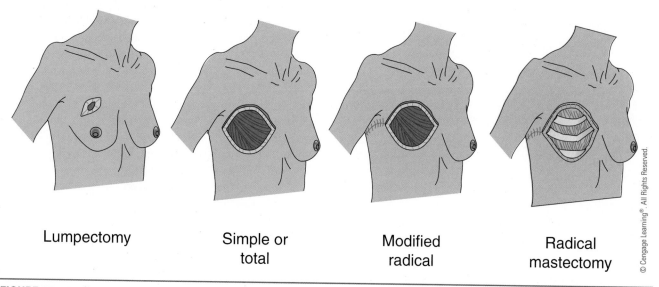

| Lumpectomy | Simple or total | Modified radical | Radical mastectomy |

FIGURE 17–20 Types of mastectomy.

Weightlifting after Breast Cancer Treatment

Women who participate in weightlifting exercises after breast cancer treatment might reduce their risk for developing lymphedema. New research has shown that weightlifting reduced the symptoms in women who have not yet developed lymphedema after breast cancer surgery. Lymphedema is one of the complications of breast cancer surgery and is a significant problem for women who develop it. Previous research demonstrated that weightlifting helped women who had already developed lymphedema, but now this research shows that it also helps prevent the development of lymphedema. Historically, it was not recommended that women lift anything over 5 pounds after breast cancer surgery. Based on this study and others, the recommendations for weightlifting restrictions after breast cancer surgery may change significantly. It seems it might be a good idea rather than something to avoid.

Source: Schmitz et al. (2010).

Researchers at Harvard School of Public Health published a medical journal article on breast cancer risk. Their research supported the fact that women who did not wear brassieres had a 60% lower rate of breast cancer than women who did wear brassieres. Explanations included that the tightness of the brassiere slows lymphatic flow. Lymph fluid helps dilute and wash away cellular toxins. A second explanation is that brassieres hold heat, thus increasing the temperature of breast tissues, a possible cause of increased cancer (Hiseh, 2009).

The book, *Dressed to Kill: The Link Between Breast Cancer and Bras*, reports results of a study of 4,600 women, half of whom had breast cancer and half who did not. The authors found that the more hours per day that a bra is worn, the higher is the rate of breast cancer, and women who did not wear a bra had a dramatically reduced rate of breast cancer.

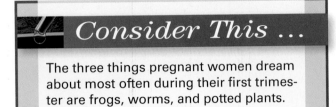

Consider This ...

The three things pregnant women dream about most often during their first trimester are frogs, worms, and potted plants.

Disorders of Pregnancy

Pregnancy is a normal condition of developing a fetus in the female body. However, disorders of pregnancy range from mild to life-threatening, sometimes risking the lives of the mother and the fetus. For this reason, the importance of prenatal care cannot be stressed enough.

ECTOPIC PREGNANCY

■ **DESCRIPTION.** Ectopic (eck-TOP-ick; displaced) pregnancy occurs when a fertilized ovum attaches to tissue outside the uterus, most commonly in the fallopian tubes.

■ **ETIOLOGY.** Strictures, adhesions, and scarring of the fallopian tubes due to PID, inflammation, infection, and structural defects can cause the tube to be narrowed, allowing microscopic-sized sperm to travel up the tube and fertilize the ovum, whereas the larger ovum is unable to travel down the tube and implant normally in the uterus. Other ectopic sites include the ovary, intestine, and outside wall of the uterus (Figure 17–21).

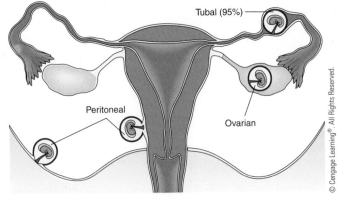

FIGURE 17–21 Sites of ectopic pregnancy.

■ **SYMPTOMS.** Symptoms of ectopic pregnancy include acute pelvic pain, vaginal bleeding, and a positive pregnancy test. If large blood vessels are ruptured, bleeding can be heavy, and the affected female might show symptoms of shock.

■ **DIAGNOSIS.** Diagnosis is made on the basis of symptoms, a pelvic examination, and ultrasound.

■ **TREATMENT.** Treatment is prompt surgery to terminate the pregnancy and decrease the possibility of shock, which can be life-threatening. Blood replacement also might be needed. If the female wants to bear children, every effort is made to preserve the affected ovary and tube.

■ **PREVENTION.** Two preventive measures are to not smoke and to practice safe sex. Those who smoke, or who have smoked in the past, are at higher risk of ectopic pregnancy. Practicing safe sex lowers the risk of STD, the most common cause of this condition.

SPONTANEOUS ABORTION (MISCARRIAGE)

■ **DESCRIPTION.** Spontaneous abortion is the natural termination of pregnancy before the fetus is able to live on its own. This type of abortion is commonly called miscarriage.

■ **ETIOLOGY.** The cause of spontaneous abortion is unknown. It is believed that it might be due to infection, drug use by the pregnant mother, abnormal fetal development, or an incompetent cervix (one that dilates prematurely). Approximately one in every six pregnancies ends with spontaneous abortion, and 75% of these occur in the first 12 weeks. The risk is higher during a woman's first pregnancy.

■ **SYMPTOMS.** Symptoms of miscarriage include vaginal bleeding, cramping, and pelvic pain, usually in the first trimester of pregnancy. If bleeding is severe, shock is of major concern.

■ **DIAGNOSIS.** Diagnosis is made on the basis of symptoms and pelvic ultrasound.

■ **TREATMENT.** Bed rest is the treatment of choice if bleeding is not severe. Bed rest is continued until spotting stops. If the individual is hemorrhaging and showing signs of shock, hospitalization might be needed to control hemorrhage and give blood replacement. After spontaneous abortion begins, its progression is difficult to stop. A surgical D&C can be performed to remove any tissue remaining in the uterus after the abortion.

■ **PREVENTION.** There is no way to prevent spontaneous abortion, but activities to reduce risk include not smoking, eating healthy foods, monitoring and controlling chronic diseases, and taking folic acid prior to becoming pregnant.

MORNING SICKNESS

■ **DESCRIPTION.** Morning sickness is the nausea and vomiting associated with pregnancy, usually occurring in the first trimester of pregnancy.

■ **ETIOLOGY.** The cause of morning sickness is unknown, but it is thought to be due to hormonal changes related to pregnancy. It is also believed that hunger might play some part in the cause.

■ **SYMPTOMS.** Morning sickness, as its name implies, usually occurs in the morning, but it also can occur later in the day. Approximately 50% of pregnant females experience varying degrees of morning sickness.

■ **DIAGNOSIS.** Morning sickness is diagnosed by symptoms in a pregnant female.

■ **TREATMENT.** Treatment is not necessary unless there is excessive vomiting, which can lead to dehydration and weight loss. This condition is then termed *hyperemesis gravidarum*. No antiemetic (anti = against, emetic = vomiting) medication has been approved by the FDA for morning sickness, and taking medications at this time in pregnancy can lead to fetal abnormalities.

■ **PREVENTION.** Morning sickness might not be preventable, but activities that might help reduce morning sickness include:

- Eating something light such as soda crackers before getting out of bed in the morning.
- Eating dry foods before drinking liquids.
- Eating several small meals during the day instead of three large ones.
- Avoiding fatty foods such as fried foods, butter, and margarine.
- Resting after meals.

HYPEREMESIS GRAVIDARUM

■ **DESCRIPTION.** Hyperemesis (hyper = excessive, emesis = vomiting) gravidarum is excessive vomiting during pregnancy.

■ **ETIOLOGY.** The cause is unknown but is thought to be due to an increased production of chorionic gonadotropin by the fetus. This thought is supported by the fact that hyperemesis gravidarum occurs more often in pregnancies with multiple fetuses.

■ **SYMPTOMS.** This condition can lead to dehydration, weight loss, and possible electrolyte imbalances in the mother and baby. The condition is not usually life threatening, but prompt medical attention is needed to preserve the health of the mother and baby.

■ **DIAGNOSIS.** Diagnosis is made on the basis of symptoms.

■ **TREATMENT.** Severe cases can be treated with intravenous fluids and by withholding all foods and oral fluids. Most cases subside by the second trimester of pregnancy.

■ **PREVENTION.** This condition cannot be prevented. Vomiting might be lessened by maintaining a healthy diet, eating dry foods, taking several small meals throughout the day, getting adequate sleep, reducing stress, and eating soda crackers before rising from bed in the morning.

TOXEMIA

■ **DESCRIPTION.** Toxemia is a condition usually appearing in the third trimester of pregnancy. The name of this condition is misleading because there is no toxin in the blood, but it was once thought that the fetus produced a toxin that led to toxemia.

■ **ETIOLOGY.** The cause of toxemia is unknown, but it does tend to occur more frequently in:

- Individuals with poor prenatal care.
- **Primigravid** (PRE-mih-GRAV-id; primi = first, gravid = pregnancy) females younger than 20 years of age and older than 30.
- Individuals with poor nutritional intake.
- Those who are hypertensive prior to becoming pregnant.
- **Multiparity** (mul-TIP-ah-rah-tee; multiple births), especially in individuals who have had five or more pregnancies.

■ **SYMPTOMS.** Toxemia is characterized by hypertension, sudden weight gain, proteinuria (protein = blood protein, uria = urine), and edema in the face, hands, and feet. It is also called **preeclampsia**

(PREE-ee-KLAMP-see-ah). The individual with toxemia is preeclamptic before convulsions occur. Toxemia or preeclampsia, if untreated or unresolved, can progress into **eclampsia** (eh-KLAMP-see-ah), a condition characterized by all the symptoms of toxemia or preeclampsia plus convulsions. Eclampsia can lead to abruptio placentae and become life-threatening to the mother and baby.

■ **DIAGNOSIS.** Diagnosis is made on the basis of symptoms.

■ **TREATMENT.** Treatment includes frequent monitoring of blood pressure, weight, and urine protein as part of prenatal care. If symptoms of toxemia occur, a low-salt diet and antihypertensive medications might be recommended. If toxemia becomes severe, hospitalization in a quiet environment with frequent monitoring and administration of antihypertensive medications is the usual therapy to prevent convulsions. Prognosis is good because delivery of the baby or termination of the pregnancy resolves the problem.

■ **PREVENTION.** This condition is not preventable, but good prenatal care and good nutrition greatly reduce the risk of toxemia.

ABRUPTIO PLACENTAE

■ **DESCRIPTION.** Abruptio placentae is the sudden separation of the placenta from the uterus prior to or during labor (Figure 17–22).

■ **ETIOLOGY.** Often, the cause is unknown, but convulsions, trauma, multiple births, and chronic hypertension are known causes.

■ **SYMPTOMS.** The degree of separation determines the symptoms. A partial separation during labor might be asymptomatic, whereas a complete separation prior to labor can be life-threatening to the mother and baby. Symptoms of a complete separation can include severe abdominal pain with large amounts of vaginal bleeding (hemorrhage), shock, a decrease in fetal heart tones, and a decrease in fetal activity. Complete separations are a medical emergency because these can lead to maternal death from hemorrhage and death of the baby from a lack of oxygen and nutrition.

■ **DIAGNOSIS.** Diagnosis is usually made on the basis of clinical history because there is not time for other testing.

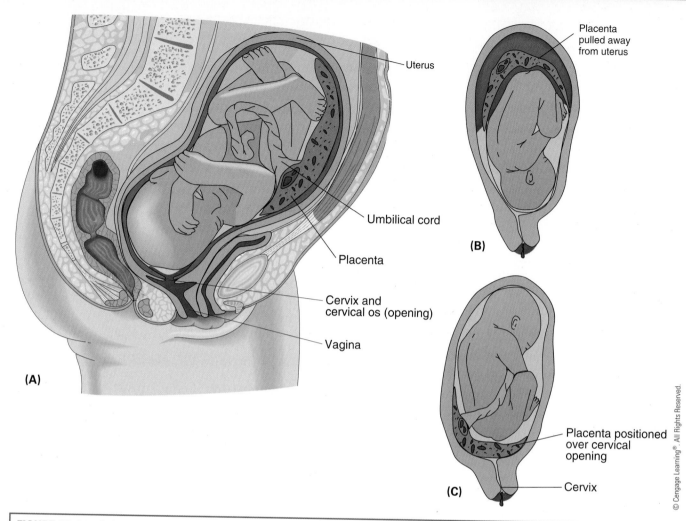

Uterus

Placenta pulled away from uterus

Umbilical cord

Placenta

(B)

Cervix and cervical os (opening)

Vagina

(A)

Placenta positioned over cervical opening

Cervix

(C)

FIGURE 17–22   (A) Normal uterine pregnancy, (B) abruptio placentae, and (C) placenta previa.

■ **TREATMENT.** Treatment is prompt delivery, either vaginally or by surgical cesarean section (C-section). Blood replacement also might be needed.

■ **PREVENTION.** Abruptio placentae is often not preventable. Controlling risk factors such as not smoking, preventing maternal trauma such as that caused by domestic violence, and avoiding substance abuse are all helpful in reducing risks.

PLACENTA PREVIA

■ **DESCRIPTION.** Placenta previa is the abnormal positioning of the placenta in the lower uterus, often near or over the cervical os or opening (see Figure 17–22). If the placenta is totally over the os, it is a complete placenta previa; partial covering is a partial placenta previa.

■ **ETIOLOGY.** The cause of this condition is unknown. Some risk factors include multiparity, maternal age over 35, and previous uterine surgery.

■ **SYMPTOMS.** The affected individual has symptoms of painless, bright red vaginal bleeding during the third trimester of pregnancy. Vital signs can indicate shock if the bleeding is severe. Placenta previa can be life-threatening to the mother due to hemorrhaging and to the baby due to anoxia.

■ **DIAGNOSIS.** Diagnosis is made by pelvic ultrasound.

■ **TREATMENT.** Vaginal delivery might be possible if the mother is asymptomatic or if bleeding is not severe. Severe maternal bleeding or fetal anoxia is reason to perform an emergency C-section.

COMPLEMENTARY AND ALTERNATIVE THERAPY

Saw Palmetto for Prostate Problems

Saw palmetto is the extract from a fruit called *Serenoa repens*. It has been used in folk and alternative medicine for years as a treatment for prostate problems, especially benign prostatic hyperplasia (BPH). Recent studies by the National Center for Complementary and Alternative Medicine have found that it does not relieve the symptoms of enlarged prostate. In fact, it was reported that saw palmetto is no more effective than a placebo for BPH. The study recommended that individuals do not use herbal treatments for prostate problems.

Source: Stewart (2012).

■ **PREVENTION.** Because the cause is unknown, prevention is not possible.

Male Reproductive System Diseases

The most common diseases affecting the male reproductive system include infection and diseases affecting the prostate. The positional relationship of the male urinary bladder and the prostate causes the male to experience urinary symptoms when the prostate is affected with disease.

PROSTATITIS

■ **DESCRIPTION.** Prostatitis (PROS-tah-TYE-tis; prost = prostate, itis = inflammation) is inflammation of the prostate gland. This condition is more common in men over 50 years of age.

■ **ETIOLOGY.** Cause can be unknown or the result of a urinary tract infection or infection by STDs.

■ **SYMPTOMS.** Symptoms include **dysuria** (dis-YOU-ree-ah; dys = painful, uria = urine), **pyuria** (pye-YOU-ree-ah; py = pus, uria = urine), fever, and low back pain.

■ **DIAGNOSIS.** Diagnosis is made on the basis of a urinalysis, urine culture, and digital rectal examination.

■ **TREATMENT.** Treatment depends on cause but often includes antibiotic therapy with penicillin. Warm sitz baths, increased fluid intake, and analgesics also can be prescribed. Prognosis is good because prostatitis usually responds well to treatment.

■ **PREVENTION.** Preventive activities include not smoking, drinking plenty of fluids, seeking early treatment for urinary symptoms, and practicing good hygiene by keeping the penis clean. This takes extra effort in an uncircumcised male.

BENIGN PROSTATIC HYPERPLASIA

■ **DESCRIPTION.** Benign prostatic hyperplasia (BPH) is also called benign prostatic hypertrophy, the enlargement of the prostate due to normal cells overgrowing and enlarging (Figure 17–23). BPH is common in men over the age of 60. Approximately 50% of males over age 65 have some degree of prostate enlargement.

■ **ETIOLOGY.** The cause of BPH is unknown, but it is thought to be due to hormonal changes, including alterations in testosterone, estrogen, and androgen levels associated with aging.

■ **SYMPTOMS.** The enlargement of the prostate places pressure on the bladder and prostatic urethra, causing urinary obstruction and a variety of urinary symptoms. The primary symptoms of BPH are **nocturia** (nock-TOO-ree-ah; noct = night, uria = urine), or frequently getting up at night to void; inability to start urination; a weak urinary stream; and inability to empty the bladder. The inability to empty the bladder often causes the excess urine to fill the ureters, leading to hydroureter, hydronephrosis, and frequent urinary tract infections.

■ **DIAGNOSIS.** Diagnosis is made on the basis of symptoms and digital rectal examination revealing an enlarged prostate.

■ **TREATMENT.** Treatment is symptomatic and might include prostatic massage, sitz baths, and catheterizations. Regular sexual intercourse can be helpful in reducing prostatic congestion. Surgery to resect or

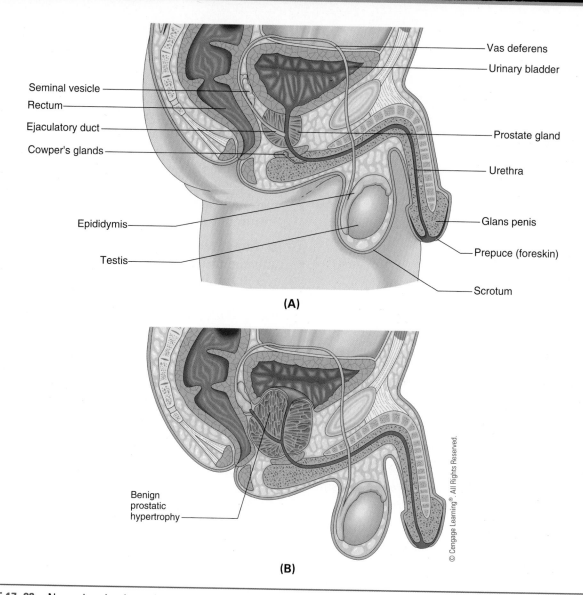

Seminal vesicle

Rectum

Ejaculatory duct

Cowper's glands

Epididymis

Testis

Vas deferens

Urinary bladder

Prostate gland

Urethra

Glans penis

Prepuce (foreskin)

Scrotum

(A)

Benign prostatic hypertrophy

© Cengage Learning®. All Rights Reserved.

(B)

FIGURE 17–23 Normal and enlarged prostate. (A) Normal. (B) Benign prostatic hypertrophy or hyperplasia (enlarged).

decrease the size of the prostate is one common treatment. This procedure is called a transurethral (trans = through, urethral = urethra) resection of the prostate (TURP). This procedure is performed, as the name indicates, through the urethra. No surgical incision is needed. During a TURP, the surgeon uses a cystoscope to chisel away the excess prostate tissue causing the urinary obstruction (Figure 17–24).

■ **PREVENTION.** There are no known preventive measures for BPH. An annual prostate exam is recommended for males after age 40. Some people believe that regular ejaculation will help prevent prostate enlargement, but there is no scientific proof of this belief.

PROSTATIC CARCINOMA

■ **DESCRIPTION.** Prostatic carcinoma is a neoplasm of the prostate gland that commonly affects men after age 50. It is the second most common cause of cancer-related death in men; lung cancer is first.

■ **ETIOLOGY.** The cause of this cancer is unknown, although some believe that testosterone levels are involved. A puzzling fact with this theory is the great racial inequity in incidence of prostatic cancer. Caucasian men are affected with prostatic cancer 10 times more often than Asian men. This fact leads to the belief that environmental and lifestyle factors are involved. Diets high in fat are also

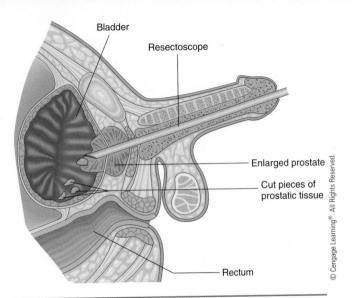

Bladder

Resectoscope

Enlarged prostate

Cut pieces of prostatic tissue

Rectum

FIGURE 17–24 Transurethral resection of prostate (TURP).

believed to be associated with an increase in prostate cancer. It is known that incidence does increase with age.

This adenocarcinoma grows in the outer layer of the prostate and often does not cause symptoms until it has metastasized. Common sites of metastasis include the bones of the spine and pelvis.

■ **SYMPTOMS.** Symptoms, when present, are similar to BPH as the urethra becomes obstructed.

■ **DIAGNOSIS.** Digital rectal examination will reveal a hard, abnormal mass. A blood test measuring PSA will be elevated with prostatic cancer. A serum PSA test result of 2.0 to 5.5 might be within the normal range, depending on the patient's age. Biopsy is the definitive test.

■ **TREATMENT.** Treatment depends on the age and physical condition of the affected individual and the degree of metastasis. If the tumor has not metastasized, complete removal and cure can be accomplished with a prostatectomy. If metastasis has occurred, treatment might involve hormone therapy to slow the growth of the neoplasm. Hormone therapy might include:

■ Administration of estrogen to counteract testosterone.

■ Surgical **orchiectomy** (OR-kee-ECK-toh-me; orchi = testicle, ectomy = removal), removal of the testicles to halt testosterone production.

■ A combination of both treatments.

Much controversy exists over the benefits of hormone therapy. Many urologists do not believe an orchiectomy improves the survival rate of the affected individual. Chemotherapy and radiation treatments also might be beneficial treatments. The prognosis of prostatic carcinoma varies, depending on the age of the affected individual and the degree of spread. If the individual is older than 60 years of age, he will probably outlive the cancer and die of some other disease process. Younger individuals and those with extensive metastasis do not have as positive a prognosis. Overall, 50% to 75% of affected individuals live 5 years or more.

■ **PREVENTION.** There are no preventive measures, although getting an annual prostate examination is recommended for early detection.

EPIDIDYMITIS

■ **DESCRIPTION.** Epididymitis (EP-ih-did-ih-MY-tis; epididym = epididymis, itis = inflammation) is inflammation of the epididymis.

■ **ETIOLOGY.** Common causes include prostatitis, urinary tract infection, mumps, and STDs such as chlamydia, syphilis, and gonorrhea. Epididymitis is one of the most common diseases of the male reproductive tract and usually affects only one epididymis (unilateral).

■ **SYMPTOMS.** Symptoms include a swollen, hard, and painful epididymis, often accompanied by severe scrotal pain and swelling. Scrotal discomfort makes walking difficult, and the affected individual might walk straddle-legged to protect the scrotum.

■ **DIAGNOSIS.** Diagnosis is made on the basis of symptoms, urinalysis, and urine culture.

■ **TREATMENT.** Prompt, appropriate antibiotic therapy is usually very effective. A delay in treatment can lead to complications of scarring and **sterility** (inability to impregnate a female, related to sperm quality or quantity). Other treatment includes bed rest, analgesics, use of a scrotal support, and avoidance of alcohol, spicy foods, and sexual stimulation.

■ **PREVENTION.** Prevention is aimed at cause and includes sexual abstinence, or use of condoms during sexual intercourse to decrease the risk of infection with STDs, and prompt treatment of causative infections.

ORCHITIS

■ **DESCRIPTION.** Orchitis (or-KYE-tis; orch = testis, itis = inflammation) is inflammation of one or both

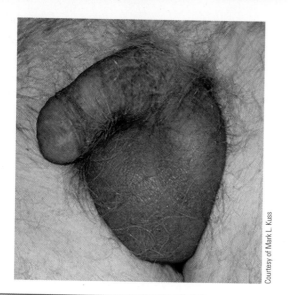

Courtesy of Mark L. Kuss

FIGURE 17–25 Orchitis.

testes, usually due to bacterial or viral infection or trauma (Figure 17–25).

■ *ETIOLOGY.* Viral mumps is the most common cause of orchitis in the adult male. Commonly, orchitis occurs in conjunction with or as a complication of epididymitis.

■ *SYMPTOMS.* Symptoms include swelling, pain and tenderness of one or both testes, fever, and malaise.

■ *DIAGNOSIS.* Diagnosis is made on the basis of symptoms, blood testing, and urinalysis.

■ *TREATMENT.* Treatment depends on cause. If the cause is bacterial, antibiotic therapy is usually effective. Orchitis caused by mumps is treated symptomatically and includes bed rest and analgesic and antipyretic medications. A scrotal support might be helpful. Prognosis is good, although atrophy of the involved testicle does occur 50% of the time. If both testes are involved, sterility can occur.

■ *PREVENTION.* Prevention is aimed at causative factors and includes mumps vaccination and prevention of infection from STDs.

TESTICULAR TUMORS

■ *DESCRIPTION.* Testicular tumors commonly affect young males aged 20 to 35 and are the most common type of cancer for this age group. Testicular tumors rarely occur in males over age 40.

■ *ETIOLOGY.* The cause of this cancer is unknown, but predisposing factors include individuals who

have been affected by **cryptorchidism** (krip-TOR-kih-dizm; crypt = hidden, orchid = testicle, ism = condition), or undescended testicle, and an inguinal hernia as a child. Cryptorchidism increases the risk of developing testicular tumor by 10-fold (American Cancer Society, 2008).

■ *SYMPTOMS.* The primary symptom of a testicular tumor is a painless mass felt in the testicle.

■ *DIAGNOSIS.* Diagnosis is made on the basis of palpation of a testicular mass with confirmation by biopsy.

■ *TREATMENT.* Treatment commonly includes surgery (orchiectomy), followed by chemotherapy and radiation. Because there is no direct lymphatic connection between the testes, testicular tumors do not usually spread from one testicle to the other. Surgical removal of the affected testis is often the treatment of choice. This procedure leaves the unaffected testis, and the male is not rendered sterile or **impotent** (inability to achieve or maintain a penile erection).

Metastatic testicular cancers can be treated with radical surgery involving removal of both testes and adjacent lymph nodes. This surgery might or might not affect impotency, but it will cause sterility. Males wishing to father children might elect to bank sperm prior to surgery so they can father children at a later date by artificial insemination. If discovered early, prognosis of testicular tumor is good, with an approximately 90% cure rate. If metastasis has occurred, the prognosis is poor.

■ *PREVENTION.* There are no preventive measures for testicular cancer because most of the risk factors are unavoidable, such as age, race, and conditions occurring at birth. The best method of controlling spread of the disease is to discover the tumors prior to metastasis; the American Cancer Society (ACS) recommends a testicular exam as part of a routine annual checkup.

CRYPTORCHIDISM

■ *DESCRIPTION.* Cryptorchidism is a condition commonly referred to as an undescended testicle. As the unborn male fetus develops, the testes appear first in the abdominal cavity. As the fetus grows and develops, the testes should move downward through the inguinal canal and into the scrotum.

■ *ETIOLOGY.* If this process does not occur properly, the testes might become lodged in any position in

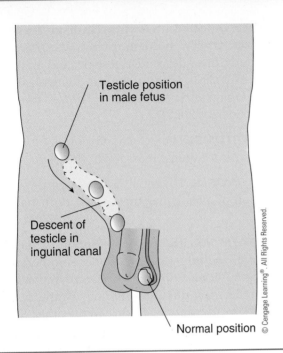

Testicle position
in male fetus

Descent of
testicle in
inguinal canal

Normal position

© Cengage Learning®. All Rights Reserved.

FIGURE 17–26   Cryptorchidism—pathway and common sites of hidden testis.

the abdominal cavity (Figure 17–26). Premature birth is a common cause of cryptorchidism and is usually time limited. The failure of both testes to descend is uncommon.

■ *SYMPTOMS.* Primary symptom is an undescended testis.

■ *DIAGNOSIS.* Diagnosis is made on the basis of physical examination noting an undescended testis.

■ *TREATMENT.* If a testis remains undescended into childhood, surgical intervention is necessary to move and secure the testis in the scrotum. This surgery is usually performed during infancy or prior to the age of 5. If the testis is left in the abdominal cavity, it will not function properly, but this will not affect potency or sterility because one testis can maintain adequate male hormone levels. If both testes are undescended, the male will be sterile. Men who have an undescended testicle at birth are at increased risk of developing testicular cancer in both testes.

■ *PREVENTION.* There is no way to prevent this condition because the cause is still unknown.

Sexually Transmitted Diseases

STDs, formerly called venereal diseases, include a group of many diseases that are spread by intimate or sexual contact. The spread of STD is at an epidemic level in the United States. These infections are transmitted from one person to another by contact with infected skin, blood, semen, and vaginal secretions during vaginal, anal, and oral sex.

Treatment of STDs commonly consists of identifying sex partners and treating the infected individuals concurrently to avoid reinfection, or a ping-pong effect, of passing the infection back and forth between involved individuals. Follow-up testing is needed after treatment to ensure that the disease has been eradicated in all infected individuals.

Prevention of STDs is best achieved by avoiding intimate contact with infected individuals. Other precautions include use of a condom during sexual intercourse, avoiding multiple sex partners, avoiding sex with someone with an unknown sexual history, and avoiding the use of alcohol that can impair judgment concerning a sexual encounter.

ACQUIRED IMMUNODEFICIENCY SYNDROME

Acquired immunodeficiency syndrome (AIDS) is a blood-borne infection commonly transmitted sexually. AIDS is the most dreaded disease of modern society and has reached global epidemic proportion. Prevention is imperative and must include health and AIDS education. For more details about AIDS, see Chapter 5, "Immune System Diseases and Disorders."

HEPATITIS

Hepatitis B and C can be spread by sexual intercourse and are, therefore, considered STDs. For more information, see Chapter 12, "Liver, Gallbladder, and Pancreatic Diseases and Disorders."

GENITAL HERPES

■ *DESCRIPTION.* Genital herpes is an extremely painful, recurring viral infection characterized by multiple, blister-like lesions (Figure 17–27). The incidence of genital herpes in the United States is increasing at a frightening rate, with one in every six individuals currently infected (Centers for Disease Control and Prevention, 2012).

■ *ETIOLOGY.* Genital herpes is caused by herpes simplex virus (HSV) type 2. (Herpes viruses are discussed in detail in Chapter 18, "Integumentary System Diseases and Disorders.") This is a highly contagious virus transmitted by intimate contact between

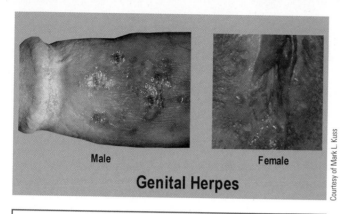

Male   Female

Genital Herpes

Courtesy of Mark L. Kuss

FIGURE 17–27 Genital herpes.

two mucous membrane surfaces. HSV-2 is commonly spread by sexual intercourse but can be spread also to the lips by oral–genital exposure or by self-infection with the hands by touching an infected area and then touching the lips, genitals, or eyes. Extreme care should be taken to avoid infection of the mucous membranes of the eyes.

Herpes disease cannot be cured. The virus remains dormant in the tissues until activated by stress or lowered immunity. Sunlight, fever, emotional stress, and menses are common activators of the herpes virus.

■ *SYMPTOMS.* When activated, the virus produces blisters that enlarge, rupture, and ulcerate. The lesions are extremely painful, especially during sexual intercourse. Severe itching and painful urination (dysuria) are common. Genital herpes infection in the male commonly produces blisters on the glans penis, the shaft of the penis, scrotum, and inner thighs.

Lesions in the female commonly appear on the vulva, vagina, inner thighs, and rectal area. Childbirth in a female with active herpes infection is fatal to the infant 50% of the time. If the infant survives, major neurologic and ophthalmic complications usually occur. For this reason, delivery by C-section is performed in mothers with active genital herpes.

Herpes lesions generally last between 1 and 3 weeks but can recur weekly, monthly, or yearly.

■ *DIAGNOSIS.* Diagnosis is made on the basis of the presence of characteristic lesions and a positive viral culture of active lesions.

■ *TREATMENT.* Treatment is symptomatic and involves antiviral medications to reduce symptoms. Sitz baths, ice therapy, analgesics, and keeping the lesions clean and dry can help with the discomfort. Females with genital herpes should have Pap smears

every 6 months because they are eight times more likely to develop cervical cancer.

■ *PREVENTION.* Avoid intimate contact with infected individuals.

GONORRHEA

■ *DESCRIPTION.* Gonorrhea, also known as clap, is one of the most common STDs in the United States. It is a highly contagious STD.

■ *ETIOLOGY.* Gonorrhea is caused by the *Neisseria gonorrhoeae* bacterium. The transmission of gonorrhea is often difficult to control because the infected individual, either male or female, might be asymptomatic. In this case, the infected individual is a carrier of the infection and might unknowingly spread the infection.

Infants born to mothers with gonorrhea run the risk of developing gonorrheal eye infection, which can lead to blindness. To prevent infant blindness, it is a common practice, and is state law in some instances, to treat all newborns' eyes with a prophylactic antibiotic or silver nitrate drops at birth.

■ *SYMPTOMS.* This bacterial infection causes inflammation of mucous membranes of the genital and urinary systems in both males and females. In males, symptoms include urethritis with purulent discharge from the penis, dysuria, and urinary frequency. Females commonly show signs of cervicitis with purulent vaginal discharge, dysuria, urinary frequency, genital itching, and a burning pain.

■ *DIAGNOSIS.* Diagnosis of gonorrhea may be made on the basis of a culture of secretions or using a DNA probe test.

■ *TREATMENT.* Treatment with antibiotics, including penicillin, tetracycline, and ceftriaxone, is usually effective. Untreated gonorrhea can lead to life-threatening, systemic infections such as meningitis and endocarditis. Arthritis and sterility are also common in both the untreated male and female.

■ *PREVENTION.* Avoid intimate contact with infected individuals.

SYPHILIS

■ *DESCRIPTION.* Syphilis is a serious STD. If untreated, it has a much worse outcome than gonorrhea because it can become a chronic, life-threatening disease.

HEALTHY HIGHLIGHT

Preventing Sexually Transmitted Infections: Practice Safe Sex

Preventing a sexually transmitted infection (STI) is easier than treating the infection once it occurs.

- Talk with your partner about STIs before beginning a sexual relationship. Find out whether he or she is at risk for an STI. Remember that it is quite possible to be infected with an STI without knowing it. Some STIs, such as human immunodeficiency virus (HIV), can take up to 6 months before they can be detected in the blood. Ask your partner:

  1. How many sex partners has he or she had?
  2. What high-risk behaviors does he or she have?
  3. Has he or she ever had an STI?
  4. Was it treated and cured?
  5. If the STI is not curable, what is the best way to protect yourself?

- Always be responsible:

  - Avoid sexual contact or activity if you have symptoms of an STI or are being treated for an STI.
  - Avoid sexual contact or activity with anyone who has symptoms of an STI or who may have been exposed to an STI.
  - Remember some STIs can also be spread through oral-to-genital or genital-to-anal sexual contact.
  - Don't have more than one sex partner at a time.
  - Abstain from sexual intercourse to prevent any exposure to STIs.

- Use condoms.

Source: WebMD (2012).

ETIOLOGY. Syphilis is caused by the *Treponema pallidum* bacterium (Figure 17–28). It is spread by sexual or intimate contact with contagious lesions. As soon as exposure occurs, these bacteria rapidly penetrate the skin or mucous membrane and gain access to the vascular system, producing a systemic infection.

SYMPTOMS. Syphilis progresses through three distinct stages with characteristic signs and symptoms. The stages are primary, secondary, and tertiary.

PRIMARY

SYMPTOMS. This stage is marked by the appearance of a painless, highly contagious lesion called a **chancre** (SHANG-ker) (Figure 17–29) that occurs at the site of bacterial entry and usually appears several weeks after contact. It can vary in appearance from pimple-like to an ulcerated sore. In the male, the chancre usually appears on the head of the penis.

In the female, the chancre commonly appears on the vulva, although it can be hidden inside the vaginal cavity and, thus, go unnoticed. The chancre can appear also at other sites in both sexes, including on the lips, fingers, anus, and tongue. Even without treatment, the chancre commonly disappears in 10 to 30 days, often leading to the false conclusion that the disease is cured. Lymphadenopathy, or sore swollen lymph nodes, is common.

TREATMENT. The disease is highly contagious during this stage but is easily cured with antibiotic therapy.

SECONDARY

DESCRIPTION. After the chancre heals, a period of rest occurs that can last from 6 weeks to 1 year.

SYMPTOMS. During this time, the bacteria rest and then rapidly grow and multiply, causing the characteristic

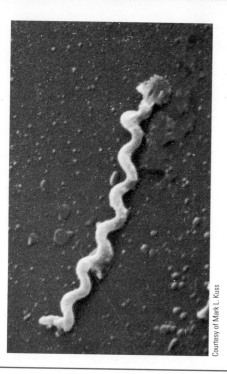

FIGURE 17–28   *Treponema pallidum.*

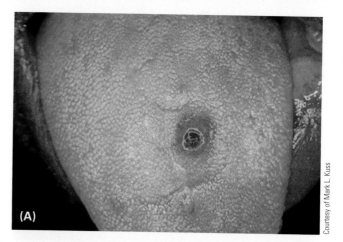

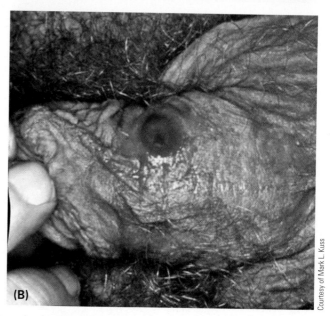

FIGURE 17–29   Syphilis chancre. (A) Chancre—tongue. (B) Chancre—penis.

rash of secondary syphilis (Figure 17–30). This rash can appear in any area of the body such as on the palms, the soles of the feet, and in the mouth, or it can spread over the entire body. The rash does not itch and might be erroneously diagnosed as mumps, chicken pox, or ringworm. The individual is highly contagious during this stage. If mouth sores are present, kissing can spread the disease.

■ *TREATMENT.* During this stage, it can be easily diagnosed based on a blood test and easily treated with antibiotics.

The primary and secondary stages are often combined and called early syphilis.

TERTIARY (LATE OR LATENT)

■ *DESCRIPTION.* If secondary syphilis is untreated, the bacterial organisms withdraw into single or multiple sites in the body and become dormant. The length of this dormant time ranges from 1 to 20 years. During this time, the infected individual can be unaware of the infection. Blood testing even might show negative results. The disease at this time is less contagious to others but is dangerous for the infected individual.

■ *SYMPTOMS.* Bacteria invade organs throughout the body, producing a characteristic soft gummy

lesion called **gumma** (GUM-mah) (Figure 17–31). Symptoms vary, depending on the organs attacked. Common problems include aortic aneurysm, heart failure, mental disorders, insanity, deafness, blindness, paralysis, and death.

■ *TREATMENT.* Tertiary syphilis can be cured with antibiotic treatment, but the effects of the lesions are irreversible.

Syphilis in pregnant females can cause spontaneous abortion or death of the infant. Infants that survive commonly have numerous defects, including physical and mental deformities, blindness, and deafness. Pregnant females should be tested for syphilis early because syphilis can be cured with antibiotic

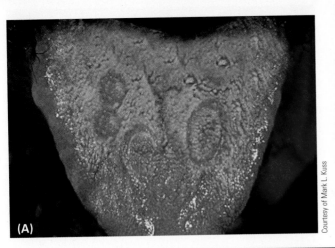

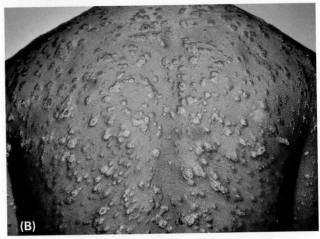

FIGURE 17–30 Syphilis rash—secondary. (A) Syphilis rash—tongue. (B) Syphilis rash—back.

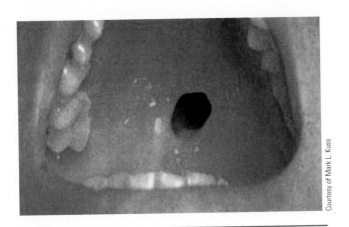

FIGURE 17–31 Tertiary—gumma.

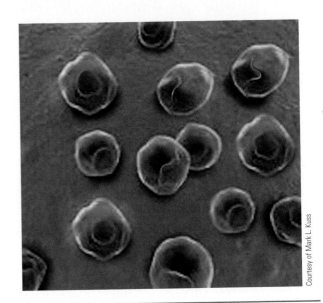

FIGURE 17–32 Chlamydia trachomatis bacteria.

treatment during the first 5 months of pregnancy, thus preventing infection in the unborn child.

■ *DIAGNOSIS.* Diagnosis is made on the basis of blood tests, VDRL, and RPR.

■ *PREVENTION.* Avoid intimate contact with infected individuals.

CHLAMYDIA INFECTION

■ *DESCRIPTION.* Chlamydia infection is very common in the United States and is one of the most damaging of the STDs. It is often called the silent STD because infected individuals can be asymptomatic until dangerous complications occur. Chlamydia infection is the leading cause of PID and is a major cause of female infertility.

■ *ETIOLOGY.* Chlamydia infection is due to the *Chlamydia trachomatis* bacterium (Figure 17–32).

■ *SYMPTOMS.* Males with chlamydia infection are usually symptomatic with drainage from the penis, burning and itching with urination due to urethritis, and epididymitis. Symptomatic females experience vaginal drainage with burning and itching of the genital area. Abdominal pain and dyspareunia can be indicative of PID.

■ *DIAGNOSIS.* Diagnosis is made on the basis of cytologic (microscopic examination of cells) examination for the bacteria, culture, and DNA probe test.

■ *TREATMENT.* Treatment with antibiotic therapy is effective. Prognosis is good if treatment occurs prior to the onset of complications. Untreated males can suffer with severe epididymitis, causing sterility.

■ **PREVENTION.** Avoid intimate contact with infected individuals.

TRICHOMONIASIS

■ **DESCRIPTION.** Trichomoniasis is a fairly common STD, affecting approximately 10% of all sexually active individuals.

■ **ETIOLOGY.** Trichomoniasis is caused by a protozoan, *Trichomonas vaginalis*.

■ **SYMPTOMS.** Most infected individuals are asymptomatic, resulting in extensive spread of the infection. If symptoms occur in the male, they commonly include urethritis, epididymitis, and prostatitis. Infected females, when symptomatic, have itching and burning of the genital area and a green, frothy vaginal drainage.

■ **DIAGNOSIS.** Diagnosis is made on the basis of microscopic examination of vaginal or penile secretions revealing the presence of the causative organism.

■ **TREATMENT.** Treatment with an antiparasitic medication is usually very effective.

■ **PREVENTION.** Avoid intimate contact with infected individuals.

GENITAL WARTS

■ **DESCRIPTION.** Genital warts, or venereal warts, are one of the most common types of STDs. As the names suggests, these warts affect the warm, moist tissues of the genital area.

■ **ETIOLOGY.** Genital warts are due to infection with HPV (Figure 17–33). Mode of transmission is usually through sexual contact, but autoinoculation, or self-inoculation, is also possible. These viral lesions

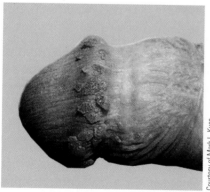
Courtesy of Mark L. Kuss

FIGURE 17–33 Genital warts.

commonly appear 1 to 6 months after exposure to an infected individual.

■ **SYMPTOMS.** Warts can be asymptomatic or cause tenderness in the affected area. The amount of discomfort is related to the size, location, and number of warts present. Size of genital warts might be very small, about the size of a ballpoint pen tip, or they might multiply into large clusters as wide as 3 or 4 inches in diameter. They can appear as small, flesh-colored bumps or have a stacked-up, cauliflower-like appearance.

In the male, warts are usually located on the head of the penis but also can be found along the penile shaft and around the anus. In the female, these lesions commonly appear around the vaginal opening and can spread to the perianal area.

Pregnancy tends to cause the warts to grow more rapidly and even reach a point of occluding the vaginal canal, thus making a C-section necessary. Cervical cancer is also more common in females with genital warts.

■ **DIAGNOSIS.** Diagnosis is made on the basis of visualization of the warts and biopsy to rule out carcinoma.

■ **TREATMENT.** Treatment is commonly surgical or chemical removal of the infected tissue. Surgical removal does not mean cure because recurrence of genital warts is common.

■ **PREVENTION.** Avoid intimate contact with infected individuals.

Sexual Dysfunction

A brief description of the most common sexual dysfunctions is provided in this section. Sexual dysfunction, whether due to physical or psychological conditions, can limit the ability of the individual to reproduce and to develop a close, nurturing sexual relationship with a significant other.

The human sexual cycle progresses through stages of arousal, sexual intercourse, and climax and ends with feelings of pleasure and relaxation. Any disorder that interrupts this cycle can be considered a sexual dysfunction.

Diagnosis of sexual dysfunction depends on general examination including a complete medical history, a sexual history including details of the dysfunction, a physical examination, and laboratory testing as indicated.

Psychological disorders leading to sexual dysfunction might need treatment by psychological counselors. Success in counseling often depends on both partners participating and maintaining a patient and sensitive attitude toward each other.

DYSPAREUNIA

■ **DESCRIPTION.** Dyspareunia is a condition of experiencing pain or discomfort with sexual intercourse. It can affect both males and females, although it is more common in women. Dyspareunia is not considered a disease but, rather, a symptom of a psychological or physical disorder.

■ **ETIOLOGY.** Dyspareunia for both sexes can be related to physical or psychological conditions. In females, common physical conditions causing dyspareunia include an intact hymen, vaginal deformity, insufficient lubrication, sensitivity to spermicide, presence of an STD, bladder infection, pelvic inflammatory disease, and endometriosis.

In the male, common physical conditions causing dyspareunia include penile deformity, presence of an STD, **phimosis** (figh-MOH-sis), or an abnormally tight foreskin (Figure 17–34), prostatitis, and epididymitis.

Psychological conditions in both sexes that might lead to dyspareunia include a history of past sexual abuse, anxiety, guilt, and fear of pregnancy.

■ **SYMPTOMS.** The pain can be mild or severe and appear in the pelvis, genitals, or low back. Females might feel pain specifically in the clitoris, labia, or vagina.

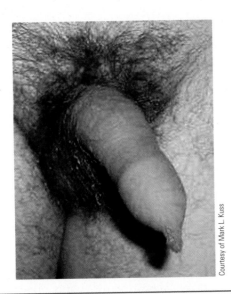

Courtesy of Mark L. Kuss

FIGURE 17–34 Phimosis.

■ **DIAGNOSIS.** Diagnosis is made on the basis of general examination including a description of the type of pain and the time of occurrence.

■ **TREATMENT.** Treatment depends on cause and can include instructions on extended foreplay, use of lubricating jelly, and manual stretching of the vaginal opening prior to intercourse. Infections need to be treated appropriately. Surgery might be needed to correct deformities, remove tumors, and treat endometriosis. Psychological conditions might need to be addressed with counseling.

■ **PREVENTION.** Some dyspareunia, like that caused by sexual trauma or abuse, is not preventable. Activities that reduce risk for the female include avoiding vaginal yeast infections, STDs, bladder infections, and sex on days near menstruation due to increased tenderness.

FEMALE AROUSAL–ORGASMIC DYSFUNCTION

■ **DESCRIPTION.** Female arousal–orgasmic dysfunction, also called *frigidity*, is the lack of sexual desire or responsiveness in a female.

■ **ETIOLOGY.** Frigidity is seldom caused by physical conditions, but neurologic disturbances such as those experienced with diabetes mellitus and multiple sclerosis can produce this condition. More commonly, frigidity is due to psychological conditions, including stress, depression, fatigue, past sexual abuse, guilt, and anxiety.

■ **SYMPTOMS.** Common signs include the inability to produce and maintain adequate vaginal lubrication and vasocongestive response indicative of sexual arousal. The primary symptom is an inability to reach orgasm.

■ **DIAGNOSIS.** Diagnosis is based on the history or complaint of an inability to reach orgasm.

■ **TREATMENT.** A physical examination to rule out physical disorders or disease is the first step in treatment. Psychological disorders might require the couple to visit a qualified specialist in sex therapy to identify and treat the cause.

■ **PREVENTION.** Education on healthy sex attitudes and sexual stimulation techniques will minimize problems. Couples who are able to communicate feelings and sexual needs effectively to one another are most likely to prevent this disorder.

IMPOTENCE

■ *DESCRIPTION.* Impotence, more recently called erectile dysfunction (ED), is the inability of the male to achieve or maintain an erection sufficient to complete sexual intercourse. Impotence does not affect fertility or the ability to produce offspring. It is a common disorder, affecting approximately half of all men over 40 years of age.

Interestingly, recent research has shown that ED might be the first indicator of cardiovascular disease, making it a helpful early warning for impending heart attacks, stroke, and death. There is a strong relationship between ED and high cholesterol, high blood pressure, and angina.

■ *ETIOLOGY.* ED is primarily caused by vascular insufficiency in the penis. Common causes are physical problems caused by endocrine disorders affecting testosterone levels; drug and alcohol abuse; neurologic disorders; spinal cord injury; urologic disorders; extensive pelvic surgery such as radical prostatectomy; diabetes mellitus; arteriosclerosis, which reduces blood flow; and certain medications such as diuretics, antihypertensives, and vasodilators.

Impotence is also caused by psychological factors, but these are not as common as physical problems. Psychological factors include depression, stress, guilt, sexual anxiety, sexual trauma, and disagreeable relationships.

■ *SYMPTOMS.* The only symptom is the inability of the male to achieve or maintain an erection sufficient to complete sexual intercourse.

■ *DIAGNOSIS.* Diagnosis is made on the basis of a medical history, sexual history, and physical examination including review of medications and laboratory testing.

■ *TREATMENT.* Treatment is based on diagnosis and might be as simple as a change in medications. Or treatment may be more involved and include psychological counseling and behavior modification. Systemically untreatable physical disorders can be treated with implantation of an inflatable penile implant. Erections also can be achieved artificially by use of external vacuum devices and injections into the penis with vasodilator medications.

■ *PREVENTION.* In some cases, ED is not preventable. However, preventive activities are those that control cardiovascular disease and diabetes, including not smoking, eating a healthy diet, maintaining a healthy body weight, and exercising.

PREMATURE EJACULATION

■ *DESCRIPTION.* Premature ejaculation, also known as rapid ejaculation or rapid climax, is expulsion of seminal fluid during foreplay, prior to complete erection or immediately after the beginning of sexual intercourse. Some researchers define premature ejaculation with time limits such as within 2 minutes of penetration, whereas others do not use time and simply state that premature ejaculation occurs any time a lack of control interferes with emotional and sexual well-being of both partners. This disorder is the most common sexual problem in males, especially in young males.

■ *ETIOLOGY.* The cause of this disorder is usually psychological rather than physical in nature. Common psychological causes include, but are not limited to, guilt, anxiety, and negative feelings or dislike for the sexual partner. Physical causes are rare but can include neurologic disorders, prostatitis, and urethritis.

■ *SYMPTOMS.* The only symptom is premature ejaculation.

■ *DIAGNOSIS.* Diagnosis is made on the basis of a medical history, sexual history, and a physical examination. Clinicians will consider factors that might lead to premature ejaculation such as duration of excitement, age of client, and frequency of sexual activity. Although the client's complaint of premature ejaculation might not meet all definitions, many clinicians diagnose premature ejaculation based on the client's feeling that the lack of control interferes with emotional and sexual well-being.

■ *TREATMENT.* Treatment is based on the diagnosis and can include sex therapy and instruction for both partners in techniques that help delay ejaculation. Control of male stimulation is important during lovemaking to allow the female time to reach orgasm and allow penetration into the vagina before ejaculation occurs. It is important for both partners to understand that this condition is reversible with treatment. In some cases, various medications might help slow arousal and thus delay ejaculation.

■ *PREVENTION.* Premature ejaculation can be prevented by masturbating and achieving orgasm several hours prior to intercourse.

INFERTILITY

■ **DESCRIPTION.** Infertility is the inability of a couple to achieve pregnancy after 1 year of unprotected sexual intercourse.

■ **ETIOLOGY.** Infertility can be due to male or female disorders or a combination of both. It was once thought that female disorders were the primary cause of infertility, but currently, male, female, and combination disorders are fairly equal in occurrence. Approximately 1 in 10 couples experiences difficulty with infertility. Of that group, it is estimated that half will eventually be able to have a child. Common causes of infertility in the female include:

- Presence of STD
- Hormonal disorders
- Abnormality of reproductive organs
- Endometriosis
- Scarring from PID or blockage of fallopian tubes
- Development of vaginal antibodies that kill sperm

   Common causes of infertility in the male include:

- Presence of STD
- Chronic genitourinary infection or blockage of the tract
- Structural abnormalities
- Hormone imbalances

■ **DIAGNOSIS.** Diagnostic testing for the female can include a complete medical and gynecologic history and examination. Hormone levels are determined by blood testing. Ovary function and ovulation can be evaluated by recording daily basal body temperatures. The structure of the uterus and patency (openness) of the fallopian tubes can be determined by a hysterosalpingogram. Endometriosis and other pelvic conditions can be assessed by visualization during a laparoscopy.

   Diagnostic testing for the male can include a complete medical history and physical examination with semen analysis. Blood testing for endocrine or hormone imbalances can be beneficial. A urinalysis might assist in determination of the presence of infection.

■ **TREATMENT.** Treatment is based on cause with the common goal of achieving pregnancy. Treatment can include surgery to correct anatomical abnormalities or remove blockages or medication therapy to correct endocrine or hormone imbalances and treat infection. Fertility drugs, artificial insemination with husband sperm (AIH), artificial insemination with donor semen (AID), and in vitro fertilization (IVF) can be beneficial in complicated cases.

■ **PREVENTION.** Many cases of infertility cannot be prevented. The following activities, however, might improve the chance of pregnancy:

- Do not smoke. Smoking reduces sperm count and increases miscarriage.
- Do not drink. Alcohol is toxic to sperm, disrupts hormone balances, and increases risk of miscarriage.
- Eat a healthy diet. Females should increase folic acid intake through dietary selection or supplements.
- Avoid excessive exercise. Excessive exercise can cause low sperm counts in men due to increased heat around the testicles and can lead to menstrual disorders in the female.
- Check with your physician to ensure that any medications, including herbal remedies, are not affecting fertility.
- Avoid STDs. These diseases can damage the reproductive system and cause infertility.
- Maintain proper body weight to reduce the possibility of hormone imbalance.

■ TRAUMA

Rape

Rape is sexual intercourse (vaginal or anal) without consent or against the will of the involved individual. Victims of rape can be any age and of either sex, but it is primarily an act violating females. The crime of rape occurs at an alarming rate, but many cases are unreported because the victim often feels embarrassed, ashamed, and guilty. Rape is a crime of violence more than of sexual passion. An acquaintance, date, spouse, or an unknown individual can carry out rape. Recent publicity has been devoted to date-rape drugs or medication that is placed in a drink and renders the individual unconscious to the point of becoming an easy victim.

   Signs and symptoms of rape can include, but are not limited to, torn clothing, disheveled appearance, bruises, and lacerations around the mouth, breasts, genitals, and rectum. Semen might be found on the inner thighs, in the vaginal cavity, and around the genital and rectal area if the victim has not bathed, showered, or douched after the act.

Diagnosis is made on the basis of history and physical examination. Special attention should be given to the emotional condition of the victim. Emergency guidelines are aimed at protecting the victim against disease and pregnancy and collecting legal evidence if the victim decides to press charges against the perpetrator. Gathering of criminal evidence is best if the individual has not bathed, showered, or douched, although, often, because the victim feels dirty and violated, these cleansing activities are performed immediately and prior to reporting the crime.

Sex crime evidence gathering can involve collecting samples of clothing, hair, scrapings from under fingernails, pubic hair, and semen, and taking pictures of areas of trauma. Sexual assault nurse examiners (SANEs) are often called in to collect the evidence and counsel the victim. These nurses have been educated and certified in the forensic specialty of sexual assault.

Recovery from rape is difficult. Crisis intervention counselors are needed, and follow-up is very important. Individuals involved with the victim need to be nonjudgmental, affirm that the individual is a victim, and assure the individual that this act of violence was not deserved.

RARE DISEASES

Vaginal Cancer

Vaginal cancer is a rare form of cancer that occurs in the daughters of mothers who used the synthetic hormone diethylstilbestrol (DES) to prevent spontaneous abortion. Symptoms include leukorrhea and bloody vaginal drainage. Diagnosis is made on the basis of a Pap smear and biopsy. Treatment usually consists of surgery, chemotherapy, and radiation.

Puerperal Sepsis

Puerperal (pyou-ER-pier-al; after childbirth) sepsis is an infection of the endometrium, usually with *Streptococcus* bacteria, following childbirth. Other names for puerperal sepsis include puerperal fever and childbed fever. In the 1800s, the cause and spread of this infection were unknown, and it was common for puerperal sepsis to sweep through maternity wards and kill most of the new mothers.

Symptoms of puerperal sepsis include chills, fever, and abdominal and pelvic pain. The modern use of aseptic technique has made this infection uncommon

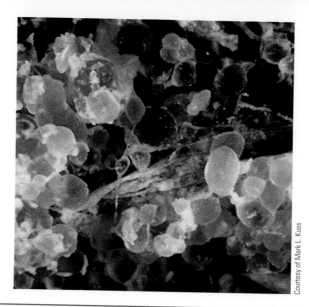

FIGURE 17–35   Hydatidiform mole.

in most of the world except for special instances when asepsis is not properly carried out. Without prompt and effective antibiotic treatment, this condition is often fatal.

Hydatidiform Mole

Hydatidiform mole is the formation of grape-like cysts in the uterus that fill the uterus and give indications of pregnancy (Figure 17–35). There is no fetus, although human chorionic gonadotropin levels get abnormally high. The cause of hydatidiform mole may be a genetic abnormality.

Toward the end of the third month, the affected individual might have symptoms of bright red vaginal bleeding, nausea, and vomiting. Diagnosis is made on the basis of symptoms and no fetal heart tones. Treatment is a surgical D&C to remove the abnormal tissue. Because individuals affected with hydatidiform mole are at higher risk for a certain type of carcinoma (choriocarcinoma), the individual should have frequent follow-up examinations.

EFFECTS OF AGING ON THE SYSTEM

As the female ages, changes in the reproductive system might seem more distinct than in the male. The pubic hair becomes thin and gray, and the external structures become less elastic and appear more wrinkled and sagging. The internal organs shrink in size, vaginal secretions diminish, and there is less elasticity of the vagina. Although sexual stimulation is still important, as in the male, it can take increased stimulation and the aid of a vaginal lubricant to enhance sexual intercourse. Using vaginal hormone cream might be recommended to reduce the dryness and improve the mucosal tone of the vagina. Some cancers of the female reproductive system, such as cancer of the uterus and ovaries, are more common in the older adult. Women over age 65 should be screened regularly for these disorders.

As the female enters menopause, the breasts also begin to atrophy and become more relaxed with a reduction in size. Women over age 50 are at increased risk for breast cancer. They should have yearly clinical exams as well as a mammogram.

As the male ages, production of testosterone and the formation of sperm decreases. The size of the testes also can diminish, but the functional ability of the male for sexual intercourse and reproduction continues. There is some loss of elasticity of the penis and scrotum, causing them to appear more wrinkled and sagging, and some thinning and graying of the pubic hair. Although the male is still able to have an erection, sometimes it takes greater stimulation to achieve this. The ejaculation amount also might be diminished. The prostate slowly enlarges in most men, beginning around age 50. This prostatic hypertrophy can cause problems with urination. The prostate is also a common site for cancer development in the older male. Routine rectal examination of the prostate and laboratory levels of PSA should be completed by all adult males over age 50.

SUMMARY

The reproductive system is a highly complex, multifunction system. It has important physiologic functions but is also very important in social relationships between individuals. Both procreation and the relationship and intercourse aspects of the system can be altered when disorders develop in the system. Common disorders of the system in the female include infections, inflammation, infertility, fibrocystic disease, pregnancy abnormalities, STDs, and cancer. In the male, common disorders include infections, STDs, impotence, and cancer. Signs and symptoms of reproductive disorders in both sexes can include pain, discharge, lesions, and abnormal enlargement of tissue. Changes occurring in the system in the older adult often affect the individual's ability to perform sexual intercourse satisfactorily. Other changes include decrease in hormone secretion, loss of elasticity of tissues, diminished lubricating secretions, and increased risk for cancer development.

REVIEW QUESTIONS

Short Answer

1. What are some of the common reproductive system disorders in the:

   a. Female?

   b. Male?

2. What are the common signs and symptoms of reproductive system disorders in the:

   a. Female?

   b. Male?

True or False

3. T F   Endometriosis is an ectopic occurrence of endometrial tissue.

4. T F   A hernia of the bladder into the vagina is called a urethrocele.

5. T F   Vaginal infections are very uncommon.

6. T F   TSS is characterized by high fever.

7. T F   Intermittent painless bleeding is the most common symptom of cervical cancer.

8. T F   Leiomyoma is a metastatic tumor of the uterus.

9. T F   A Pap smear should be performed every 2 years on a female who is not high risk.

10. T F   PMS is probably caused by a hormone imbalance.

11. T F   Phimosis is a narrowed opening of the prepuce.

12. T F   Epididymitis is usually caused by an infection from the bladder.

13. T F   STDs are not common in the male reproductive system.

14. T F   The best preventive measure for testicular cancer is the monthly self-examination.

15. T F   One of the symptoms of BPH is urinary retention.

16. T F   An orchiectomy is the removal of the prostate gland.

17. T F   The PSA test is a screening test for cancer of the prostate.

18. T F   The testosterone hormone is secreted by the prostate gland.

19. T F   There is some loss of elasticity of the penis and scrotum during the aging process.

20. T F   Increased stimulation and the aid of a vaginal lubricant may be needed to enhance sexual intercourse between the older adult male and female.

CASE STUDIES

■   Charles Roberts is a 63-year-old man who has been having difficulty urinating. He states he often gets up twice a night to void and has some difficulty getting the stream started. Is this a problem? He is basically quite healthy and does not have a family physician. He asks for your advice about this. What should you tell Mr. Roberts? Are there other questions you should ask him before giving him any information? How could you explain the effects of aging to him? Should he make an appointment with a physician?

■   Janice Simmonds is a 53-year-old first-grade school teacher. At the present time, she is single but dates on a fairly regular basis. She has been an active person all of her life. Janice has played on a tennis team for 20 years and works out at the local athletic club. She considers herself to be in great shape for her age and has never been concerned about any possible health problems. Her past laboratory history includes an average routine cholesterol level, normal blood sugar, and normal blood pressure. Her mother is still living and well, but her aunt died at age 69 of breast cancer. Her father is also living and well. Janice does not consider herself at risk for any major health problems. Do you agree with her? Would you consider her at risk for breast cancer? If so, what risk factors can you identify? Is she also at risk for cervical cancer? What routine clinical examinations should she have based on her age and gender?

Study Tools

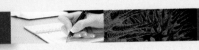

Workbook

Complete Chapter 17

Online Resources

PowerPoint® presentations

Animation

BIBLIOGRAPHY

American Cancer Society. (2008). Detailed guide: Testicular cancer. *www.cancer.org* (accessed March 2008).

Andersen, M., Sweet, E., Lowe, K. A., Standish, L. J., Drescher, C. W., & Goff, B. A. (2012). Involvement in decision-making about treatment and ovarian cancer survivor quality of life. *Gynecologic Oncology 124*(3), 465–470.

Annual report finds decrease in most cancer rates. (2011). *http://news.nurse.com* (accessed January 2011).

Ashizawa, K., Sugane, A., & Gunji, T. (1990). Breast from changes resulting from a certain brassiere. *Journal of Human Ergology (Tokyo) 19*(1), 53–62.

Avery Publishing Group. (1997). Fiji follow-up study supports "Dressed to Kill: The Link Between Breast Cancer and Bras." Avery News Release; October 31.

Breast cancer screening. (2011). *American Nurse 43*(6), 6–7.

Centers for Disease Control and Prevention. (2010). FDA licensure of bivalent human papillomavirus vaccine (HPV2, Cervarix) for use in females and updated HPV vaccination recommendations from the Advisory Committee on Immunization Practices (ACIP). *Morbidity and Mortality Weekly Report 59*(20), 626–629.

Centers for Disease Control and Prevention. (2011). Recommendations on the use of quadrivalent human papillomavirus vaccine in males—Advisory Committee on Immunization Practices (ACIP), 2011. *Morbidity and Mortality Weekly Report 60*(50), 1705–1708.

Centers for Disease Control and Prevention. (2012). Genital herpes: CDC fact sheet. *www.cdc.gov* (accessed September 2012).

Centers for Disease Control and Prevention & National Cancer Institute. (2010). United States cancer statistics: 1999–2007 incidence and mortality web-based report. *www.cdc.gov* (accessed September 2012).

Coffee or tea: Which for thee? (2012). *Consumer Reports on Health 24*(1), 6.

Diagnosed with prostate or breast cancer: Now what? (2010). *Consumer Reports on Health 22*(10), 1–5.

Drageset, S., Lindstrøm, T., Christine; Giske, T., & Underlid, K. (2011). Being in suspense: Women's experiences awaiting breast cancer surgery. *Journal of Advanced Nursing 67*(9), 1941–1951.

Eccles, D. M. (2011). Development of genetic testing for breast, ovarian and colorectal cancer predisposition: A step closer to targeted cancer prevention. *Current Drug Targets 12*(13), 1974–1982.

Forbat, L., White, I., Marshall-Lucette, S., & Kelly, D. Discussing the sexual consequences of treatment in radiotherapy and urology consultations with couples affected by prostate cancer. *BJU International 109*(1), 98–103.

"Free" prostate cancer screens can be costly. (2011). *Consumer Reports 76*(5), 12.

Garad, R., Burger, H., & Davison, S. (2011). Exploring the hormone replacement therapy debate. *Australian Nursing Journal 19*(5), 30–33.

Grover, S., Hill-Kayser, C. E., Vachani, C., Hampshire, M. K., DiLullo, G. A., & Metz, J. M. (2012). Patient reported late effects of gynecological cancer treatment. *Gynecologic Oncology 124*(3), 399–403.

Hiseh, C. C., & Trichopoulos, D. (1991). Breast size, handedness and breast cancer risk. *European Journal of Cancer 27*, 131–135.

Holloway, D. (2010). Nursing considerations in patients with vaginitis. *British Journal of Nursing (BJN) 19*(16), 1040–1046.

Johnston, J. J. (2011). Managing the menopause: Practical choices faced in primary care. *Climacteric, 14*(1), 8–12.

Johnston, S. B. (2011). Combating infection. Should males be vaccinated against HPV? *Nursing 41*(6), 62–63.

Kass-Wolff, J. H., & Fisher, J. E. (2011). Menopause and the hormone controversy: Clarification or confusion? *Nurse Practitioner 36*(7), 22–30.

Kazer, M. W., Bailey, D. E., Sanda, M., Colberg, J., & Kelly, W. K. (2011). An internet intervention for management of uncertainty during active surveillance for prostate cancer. *Oncology Nursing Forum 38*(5), 561–568.

Kuehn, B. M. (2011). Two doses of HPV vaccine may be sufficient. *JAMA: Journal of the American Medical Association 306*(15), 1643.

Larson, C. A. (2011). Evidence-based medicine: An analysis of prophylactic bilateral oophorectomy at time of hysterectomy for benign conditions. *Current Oncology 18*(1), 13–15.

Marroquin, J. (2011). To screen or not to screen: Ongoing debate in the early detection of prostate cancer. *Clinical Journal of Oncology Nursing 15*(1), 97–98.

Mcintyre, H. D., Oats, J. J. N., Zeck, W., Seshiah, V., & Hod, M. (2011). Matching diagnosis and management of diabetes in pregnancy to local priorities and resources: An international approach. *International Journal of Gynecology & Obstetrics Supplement 1*(115), S26–S29.

Menopause, prostate therapies rated. (2012). *Consumer Reports on Health 24*(2), 7.

Milman, N. (2012). Postpartum anemia II: Prevention and treatment. *Annals of Hematology, 91*(2), 143–154.

Most men don't need routine PSA tests. (2012). *Consumer Reports 77*(1), 13.

National Cancer Institute. (2012). Human papillomavirus (HPV) vaccines. *www.cancer.gov* (accessed September 2012).

National Heart, Lung, and Blood Institute. (2010). Women's Health Initiative (WHI). *www.nhlbi.nih.gov* (accessed September 2012).

National Institute on Aging. (2012). Hormones and menopause. *www.nia.nih.gov* (accessed August 2012).

New queries about PSA screenings. (2011). *Consumer Reports on Health 23*(6), 3.

Schmitz, K. H., Ahmed, R. L., Troxel, A. B., Cheville, A., Lewis-Grant, L., Smith, R., Bryan, C. J., Williams-Smith, C.T., & Chittams, J. (2010). Weight lifting for women at risk for breast cancer–related lymphedema. *JAMA, 304*(24), 2699–2705.

Singer, S. R., & Grismaijer S. (1995). *Dressed to Kill: The Link Between Breast Cancer and Bras.* New York: Avery Press, 1995.

Stewart, J. (2012). *Health Bulletin. Men's Health 27*(1), 36.

WebMD. (2012). Exposure to sexually transmitted diseases: prevention. *www.webmd.com* (accessed March 2012).

Wilson, K. M., Kasperzyk, J. L., Rider, J. R., Kenfield, S., van Dam, R. M., Stampfer, M. J., & Mucci, L. A. (2011). Coffee consumption and prostate cancer risk and progression in the health professionals follow-up study. *JNCI: Journal of the National Cancer Institute 103*(11), 876–884.

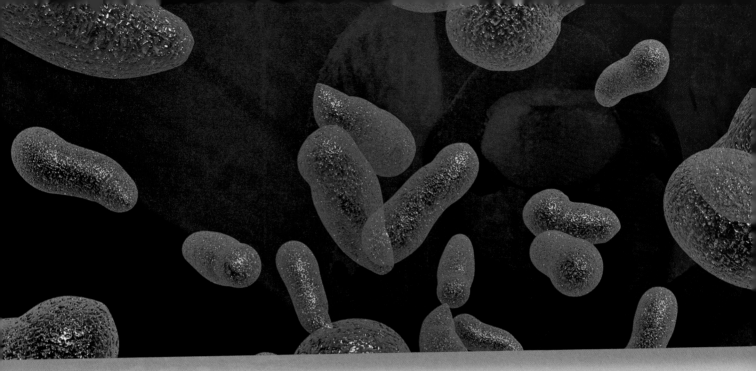

OUTLINE

- Anatomy and Physiology
- Common Signs and Symptoms
- Diagnostic Tests
- Common Diseases of the Integumentary System
  Infectious Diseases
  Metabolic Diseases
  Hypersensitivity or Immune Diseases
  Idiopathic Diseases
  Benign Tumors
  Premalignant and Malignant Tumors
  Abnormal Pigmented Lesions
  Diseases of the Nails
  Diseases of the Hair

- Trauma
  Mechanical Skin Injury
  Thermal Skin Injury
  Electrical Injury
  Radiation Injury
  Pressure Injury
  Insect and Spider Bites and Stings

- Rare Diseases
  Elephantiasis

- Effects of Aging on the System
- Summary
- Review Questions
- Case Studies
- Bibliography

KEY TERMS

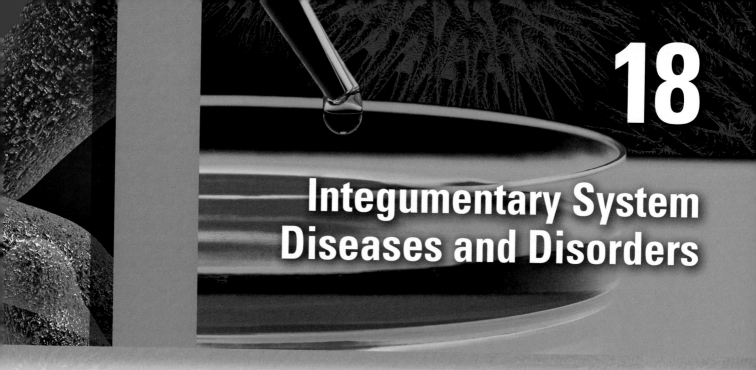

18

Integumentary System Diseases and Disorders

LEARNING OBJECTIVES

Upon completion of the chapter, the learner should be able to:

1. Define the terminology common to the integumentary system and the disorders of the system.

2. Discuss the basic anatomy and physiology of the integumentary system.

3. Identify the important signs and symptoms associated with common integumentary system disorders.

4. Describe the common diagnostics used to determine the type and cause of integumentary system disorders.

5. Identify common disorders of the integumentary system.

6. Describe the typical course and management of the common integumentary system disorders.

7. Describe the effects of aging on the integumentary system and the common disorders associated with aging of the system.

OVERVIEW

The integumentary system is composed of all the skin and its layers. The skin is also known as the largest organ of the body. It makes up about 15% of the total body weight. The skin is the first line of defense against disease. Many diseases of the integumentary system are the result of other body or system disorders. For instance, measles is a viral disease of the respiratory system, but it is characterized by the maculopapular rash seen on the skin. Skin disorders such as psoriasis are traumatic to the individual because of the obvious lesions and the effect it has on body image. Skin disorders range from mild to severe and acute to chronic. ■

ANATOMY AND PHYSIOLOGY

The skin is the largest organ of the body. It is a large, durable, and pliable organ and is the first line of protection for the body against invading organisms. The skin also provides a sense of touch, heat and cold, and pain and helps stabilize temperature and fluid and electrolyte balance. The skin is composed of two layers: the epidermis and the dermis, with a subcutaneous (hypodermis) level (Figure 18–1).

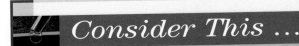

Consider This ...

The average person's skin weighs about 8 pounds and has the surface area of approximately 25 square feet.

The epidermis, or outer layer, is composed of five layers: the stratum corneum, stratum lucidum, stratum granulosum, stratum spinosum, and stratum basale. The cells of the epidermis are called stratified squamous epithelial cells. Most of these are keratinocytes; the others are melanocytes that produce melanin, the pigment that darkens the skin and gives it color. The dermis is the deeper layer, consisting of connective tissue and a variety of cell types. Blood vessels traverse the dermal layer to provide nutrients and oxygen, regulate heat, and remove waste products. Nerves also form a network in the dermis to provide the sensations of heat, cold, pain, and touch.

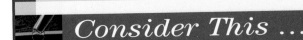

Consider This ...

There are approximately 45 miles of nerves in the skin of the average human.

The subcutaneous layer is composed of connective tissue containing fat cells and blood vessels and protects the body against cold. The amount of fat varies considerably with the individual.

Embedded in the dermis and extending to the epidermis are the sebaceous, apocrine, and eccrine sweat glands. The sebaceous glands produce oil called **sebum**. The apocrine sweat glands are located in the underarms (axillae), around the nipples of the breasts,

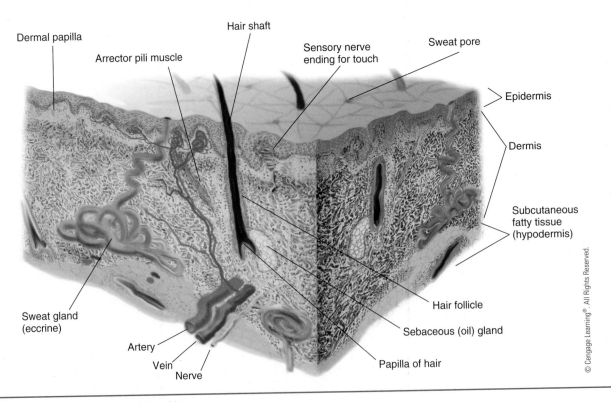

Dermal papilla · Arrector pili muscle · Hair shaft · Sensory nerve ending for touch · Sweat pore · Epidermis · Dermis · Subcutaneous fatty tissue (hypodermis) · Hair follicle · Sebaceous (oil) gland · Papilla of hair · Nerve · Vein · Artery · Sweat gland (eccrine)

FIGURE 18–1 The structures of the skin.

and around the umbilicus, anus, and genital areas. These glands are inactive until puberty and initiate their function with hormonal changes at that time. Their secretions are odorless, but bacteria that accumulate in these areas cause the smell referred to as body odor. Both the sebaceous glands and the apocrine glands secrete through the hair follicles. The eccrine sweat glands are found throughout the body surfaces and secrete through the skin pores to help the body regulate heat. Some electrolytes are also lost through these sweat glands.

The hair follicles are found in the dermal layer and extend through the epidermis. They grow in cycles, which vary with the individual, with an average growth of about 1 cm per month. Hair loss occurs continually but is not usually obvious until a large amount is lost and not replaced. Testosterone, the male hormone, influences hair growth, especially at puberty when hair begins to appear in the axillae and groin. It also triggers the male's baldness later in life. Generally, soft, tiny hairs cover most of the body, and terminal hairs (stiffer, longer, and often darker) are found on the scalp, axillae, groin, eyebrows, and eyelashes of both sexes and the face and trunk of males.

The nails are composed of **keratin** (epidermal cells in a tight web). Fingernails grow more rapidly than toenails, but they are composed of the same material. The thickness and growth rate of the nail varies with the individual. Health status, nutrition, and other factors can influence nail strength and growth.

Media Link

View an animation about skin on the Online Resources.

◼ COMMON SIGNS AND SYMPTOMS

Common signs and symptoms of integumentary diseases include the following:

- Skin **lesion** (LEE-zhun). A lesion is a very broad term meaning any discontinuity or abnormality of tissue. Lesions can be hard, soft, flat, raised, large, small, reddened, crusted, fluid-filled, or pus-filled, to name only a few characteristics (Figure 18–2).

- Pain.
- **Pruritus** (proo-RYE-tus) or itching.
- Edema (swelling).
- **Erythema** (ER-ih-THEE-mah) or skin redness.
- Inflammation.

Consider This …

Every half square inch of skin has approximately 10 hairs, 15 sebaceous glands, 100 sweat glands, and 32 feet of blood vessels.

◼ DIAGNOSTIC TESTS

There are numerous skin diseases; several have very characteristic lesions, leading to an easy diagnosis. However, many exhibit the same or similar types of lesions and symptoms, making diagnosis difficult. Biopsy might be used in diagnosing nodules and chronic lesions. Culture and sensitivity are effective in determining the presence of bacterial infections. Blood tests are helpful, especially if there is concern about a systemic infection or metabolic disorder. Diagnosis and identification of fungal and parasitic infections can be determined by using cultures and microscopic smear examinations.

Consider This …

Humans shed and regrow outer skin about once a month—approximately 1,000 new skins in a lifetime.

◼ COMMON DISEASES OF THE INTEGUMENTARY SYSTEM

The numerous diseases and disorders of the integumentary system often make diagnosis of skin disorders quite difficult because several diseases can be characterized by the same type or similar types of lesions. Common diseases include infections; metabolic, hypersensitivity, and idiopathic disorders; and tumors and can be categorized according to cause.

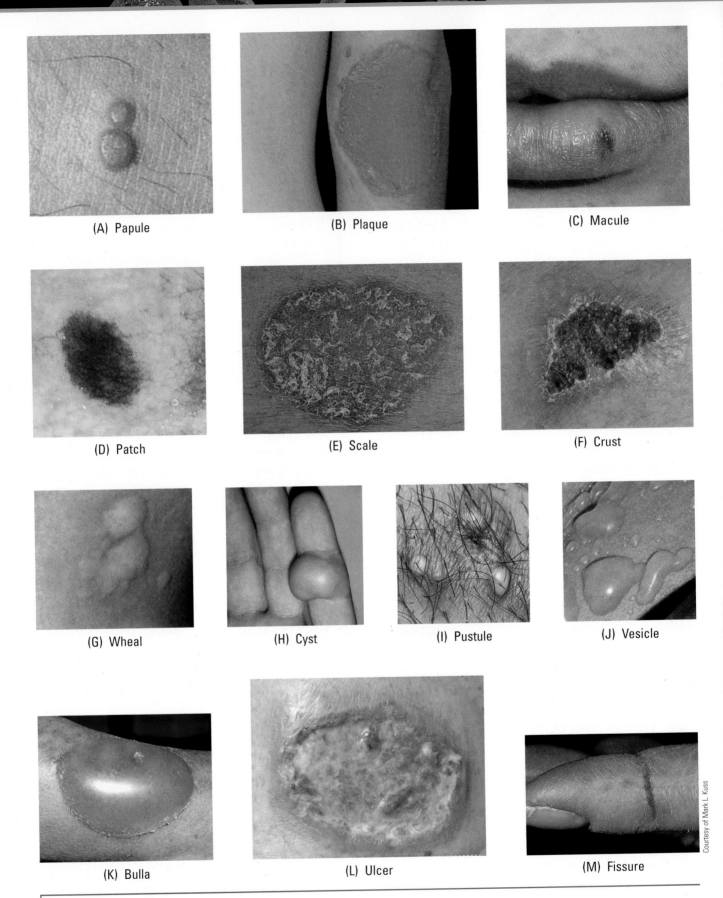

(A) Papule

(B) Plaque

(C) Macule

(D) Patch

(E) Scale

(F) Crust

(G) Wheal

(H) Cyst

(I) Pustule

(J) Vesicle

(K) Bulla

(L) Ulcer

(M) Fissure

Courtesy of Mark L. Kuss

FIGURE 18–2 Skin lesions.

PHARMACOLOGY HIGHLIGHT

Common Drugs for Integumentary Disorders

CATEGORY	EXAMPLES OF MEDICATIONS
Antibiotics Drugs used to treat skin infections	mupirocin, erythromycin, tetracycline, or clindamycin
Antifungals Drugs used to treat fungus infections	clotrimazole or ketoconazole
Antihistamines Drugs used to reduce the symptoms from allergies and contact dermatitis	carbinoxamine or levocabastine (prescription drugs), diphenhydramine or loratadine (over-the-counter drugs)
Anti-inflammatories Drugs used to reduce inflammation	hydrocortisone
Retinoids Drugs used to treat skin disorders like acne or psoriasis	acitretin, isotretinoin, or tazarotene
Biologics Drugs used to treat psoriasis	etanercept, calcipotriene, or salicylic acid
Anesthetics Drugs used to decrease pain in/on the skin	lidocaine or procaine
Parasiticides Drugs used to treat mites or lice	lindane or permethrin

Infectious Diseases

Skin infections are quite common and usually contagious, so care must be taken to prevent spread from one area of the body to another and from one person to another. Most infections are not serious unless systemic involvement occurs. Infections of the skin can be caused by viruses, bacteria, fungi, and parasites.

VIRAL DISEASES

Viral skin diseases can be acute or chronic. Acute viral diseases commonly affect children and usually resolve spontaneously, but many viral infections become lifelong with periods of remission and **exacerbation** (flaring up).

HERPES

■ **DESCRIPTION.** Herpes is a large family of viruses, including:

1. Cold sores and fever blisters (herpes simplex 1 or HSV-1).
2. Genital herpes (herpes simplex 2, HSV-2, or herpes genitalis).
3. Chicken pox (herpes varicella).

4. Shingles (herpes zoster).

5. Other, rarer herpes are ocular herpes, herpes simplex encephalitis, and neonatal herpes simplex. These cases can lead to blindness and high levels of morbidity and mortality, respectively.

Herpes simplex is very common and often appears on the mouth, nose, buttocks, and genitals. The herpes simplex viruses (HSV-1 and HSV-2) appear identical under a microscope, cause the same type of lesions, and, clinically, cannot be separated. Both can infect the mouth or genitals. Usually, HSV-1 appears above the waist and HSV-2 appears below the waist.

- **Herpes simplex type 1** Commonly called fever blisters and cold sores because febrile conditions and the common cold often bring about an exacerbation. The vesicles commonly appear around the lips and nose (Figure 18–3). Lesions appearing around the lips can be further identified as herpes labialis (labia = lip), and those occurring in conjunction with a fever can be further identified as herpes febrilis.

- **Herpes genitalis (herpes simplex type 2)** Commonly called genital herpes. This is a highly contagious disease and is spread by direct contact. Genital herpes can be a sexually transmitted disease, but transmission is not limited to sexual contact. Autoinoculation with the hands is also possible by touching the lips and then the genitals and vice versa. Herpes genitalis is discussed in detail in Chapter 17, "Reproductive System Diseases and Disorders."

- **Herpes varicella** Commonly called chicken pox. This is an acute, highly contagious childhood disease. Varicella is discussed in detail in Chapter 20, "Childhood Diseases and Disorders."

- **Herpes zoster** Commonly called shingles. The virus that causes chicken pox in children causes zoster in adults. It is characterized by painful lesions that follow the course of a spinal nerve. Zostavax® is the vaccine for shingles, but it is recommended only for adults over age 60. More detailed information can be found in Chapter 15, "Nervous System Diseases and Disorders."

■ **SYMPTOMS.** Herpes is characterized by inflammation of the skin and clusters of fluid-filled **vesicles** (VES-ih-kuls). The infection is painful, embarrassing, and often recurrent.

■ **DIAGNOSIS.** Diagnosis is made by observation of vesicles, positive viral culture, and blood testing for herpes antibodies.

■ **TREATMENT.** The virus is treatable but remains in the affected individual's body for life. Some type of balance between the host and the virus exists, with periods of viral remission and exacerbation. The virus exacerbates, or flares up, often during times of decreased immunity as occurs with stress. Valacyclovir, acyclovir, and famciclovir are approved to treat herpes genitalis but are also used for oral herpes. Penciclovir cream can also be prescribed for oral herpes.

■ **PREVENTION.** Prevention of simplex viruses includes avoiding skin-to-skin contact with anyone showing signs of infection. Use of a condom helps prevent herpes genitalis. Vaccination in children and those over 60 helps prevent varicella and zoster, respectively. In general, maintaining a healthy immune system by making healthy lifestyle choices helps reduce risk.

VERRUCAE (WARTS)

■ **DESCRIPTION.** Verrucae, or warts, a chronic skin condition, usually occur in multiples that can differ in size, shape, and appearance. They can appear at any age but more commonly affect children. The most common types are:

- **Common warts** Predominantly appear on the hands and fingers of children (Figure 18–4). These lesions are contagious and are spread by scratching and direct contact. Although unsightly, they are usually painless and harmless and often disappear spontaneously. Common warts occurring in adults

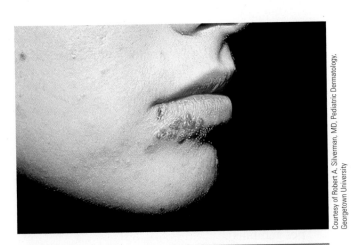

Courtesy of Robert A. Silverman, MD, Pediatric Dermatology, Georgetown University

FIGURE 18–3   Herpes simplex virus 1.

COMPLEMENTARY AND ALTERNATIVE THERAPY

Herb Treatment for Herpes

There are a variety of herbs used in the treatment of herpes. Herbs from the Lamiaceae family (mint group) are safe and effective for the treatment of herpes simplex virus. Research has shown that rosmanic, caffeic, and ferulic acids in herbs from the Lamiaceae family work by blocking the virus activity. These acids have antioxidant properties and are found in many products used in cooking, such as oregano, sage, lemon balm, rosemary, peppermint, apples, and artichokes, and are even in coffee.

Source: Yarnell et al. (2009).

should be called to the attention of a physician to ensure that they are not skin cancers.

- **Plantar warts** Appear on the sole of the foot. This wart usually grows inward, is smooth on the sole of the foot, and feels like a hard lump. Plantar warts contain small, clotted blood vessels that appear like dark splinters inside the wart and give it a cauliflower-like appearance (Figure 18–5). This wart commonly causes pain with walking; thus, surgical removal is often the treatment of choice.

- **Genital warts** A sexually transmitted disease. They are highly contagious and often need to be removed surgically. More detailed information can be found in Chapter 17.

■ *ETIOLOGY.* A verruca is caused by the papillomavirus affecting the keratin cells of the skin, causing cellular hypertrophy.

■ *SYMPTOMS.* The only symptom is a painless, often rough-surfaced skin lesion appearing on any surface of the body but primarily on the fingers and hands.

■ *TREATMENT.* Treatment depends on the location of the verruca. Warts on the finger and hands are commonly treated topically with over-the-counter medications. The best topical medications are those containing salicylic acid such as Trans-Ver-Sal, Sal-Acid Plaster, or Sal-Plant Gel. Genital and plantar warts are commonly removed surgically. Verrucae are often resistant to treatment, and recurrence is frequent.

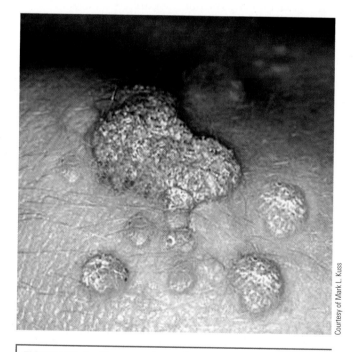

FIGURE 18–4 Verrucae (warts).

FIGURE 18–5 Plantar warts.

■ **PREVENTION.** The best prevention is to avoid skin-to-skin contact with those infected with verruca.

MEASLES

Measles is a highly contagious childhood disease that causes a characteristic maculopapular skin rash. For more information on measles, see Chapter 20.

BACTERIAL DISEASES

Bacterial skin infections are often highly contagious and affect individuals who are immunosuppressed or who practice poor personal hygiene. These skin infections are generally caused by normal flora bacteria and are treated effectively with antibiotics.

Consider This ...

The skin has its own ecosystem of microorganisms including yeast and bacteria that cannot be removed by any type of cleaning.

IMPETIGO

■ **DESCRIPTION.** Impetigo is a highly contagious skin disease. It is one of the most common skin infections of children and usually affects the face and hands.

■ **ETIOLOGY.** Impetigo is caused by *Streptococcus* and *Staphylococcus* bacteria.

■ **SYMPTOMS.** Impetigo is characterized by the appearance of vesicles and **pustules** (PUS-tyouls; small pus-filled lesions) that rupture, producing a yellow crust over the lesions (Figure 18–6). Impetigo occurs more readily in those with poor hygiene, anemia, and malnutrition.

■ **DIAGNOSIS.** Diagnosis is confirmed by symptoms and a positive bacterial culture of the infected lesion.

■ **TREATMENT.** Treatment includes washing and drying the affected area several times a day and applying antibiotic ointment. More serious conditions might also require oral antibiotics.

■ **PREVENTION.** Prevention is aimed at good personal hygiene, including frequent hand washing. Those with anemia and malnutrition need treatment to cure those conditions also.

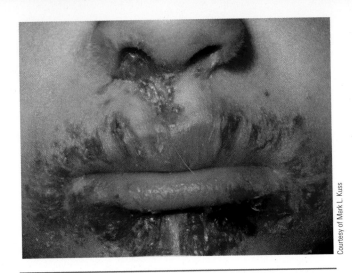

FIGURE 18–6   Impetigo.

FOLLICULITIS

■ **DESCRIPTION.** Folliculitis is inflammation and infection of the hair follicle and can occur anywhere on the skin.

■ **ETIOLOGY.** Folliculitis usually starts when hair follicles are damaged by shaving or friction from clothing. The damaged hair follicle then becomes infected with *Staphylococcus* bacteria.

■ **SYMPTOMS.** Common symptoms include rash, itching, and the formation of pimples or small pustules surrounding the hair (Figure 18–7) that can also

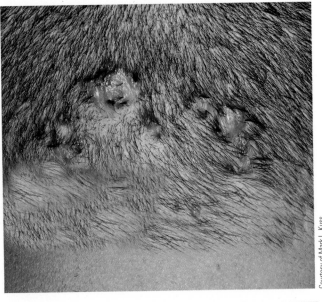

FIGURE 18–7   Folliculitis.

open, drain, and crust over. This condition commonly occurs in young men and affects the neck, groin, thighs, buttocks, beard, and scalp.

■ *DIAGNOSIS.* Diagnosis is based on physical examination of pustules and condition of the skin. Cultures can reveal bacterial or fungal infection.

■ *TREATMENT.* Warm, moist compresses help ease the pain and promote drainage of the pustules. Daily cleansing of the area with an antiseptic cleanser and application of antibiotic or antifungal creams for several weeks usually cure the condition. Severe or chronic cases might need additional treatment with oral antibiotics.

■ *PREVENTION.* Preventive measures include reducing friction from clothing, keeping skin clean and dry, avoiding bathing with dirty or contaminated washcloths, and avoiding shaving the area until the infection is healed.

ABSCESS, FURUNCLE, CARBUNCLE

■ *DESCRIPTION.* There are some differences in these lesions. An abscess is a localized collection of pus occurring in any tissue of the body, including the skin. Abscesses commonly occur around sites of trauma, embedded foreign material such as splinters, and hair follicles (Figure 18–8).

A small abscess occurring in the tissues of the skin is a furuncle, commonly called a boil. Furuncles generally

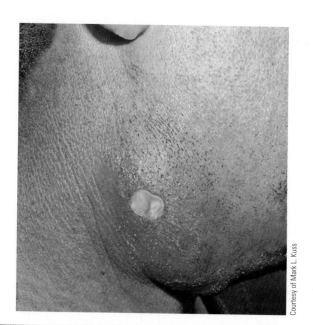

FIGURE 18–8 Abscess.

occur around a hair follicle and can develop during an acute case of folliculitis. Boils can develop in any hairy area of the body, with common sites including the skin of the neck, back, and buttocks.

Carbuncles are larger abscesses and involve several interconnected furuncles. These lesions arise in a cluster of hair follicles and have multiple drainage sites. Needless to say, carbuncles are much larger than furuncles and are less common.

■ *ETIOLOGY.* These lesions are commonly caused by the pyogenic, normal flora bacteria, *Staphylococcus*. Predisposing factors for these lesions include a lowered immunity due to the presence of other diseases and poor personal hygiene.

■ *SYMPTOMS.* Abscess, furuncle, and carbuncle are all characterized by inflammation, infection, and the formation of a capsule to wall off and prevent the spread of infection. All of these encapsulated lesions are extremely painful, usually develop a soft spot or come to a head, and need to be opened or surgically drained.

■ *DIAGNOSIS.* Diagnosis is based on history and physical examination of the lesion.

■ *TREATMENT.* Warm, moist compresses usually relieve pain and promote spontaneous drainage. If spontaneous opening and drainage do not occur, surgical opening and drainage might be necessary. Antibacterial or antifungal medications are usually prescribed to treat infection.

■ *PREVENTION.* Nothing can prevent these lesions, although using antibacterial soaps can help reduce bacterial count on the skin and thus aid in prevention.

Consider This ...

It is estimated that there are approximately 50 million individual bacteria on the surface of 1 square inch of skin.

CELLULITIS

■ *DESCRIPTION.* Cellulitis is a diffuse, or spreading, inflammation of the skin and subcutaneous tissue (Figure 18–9). It commonly appears on the lower legs but can affect any part of the body.

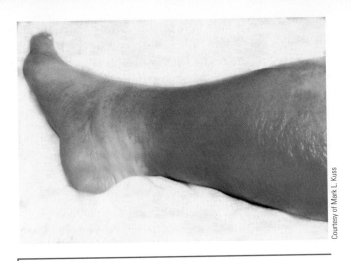

FIGURE 18–9   Cellulitis.

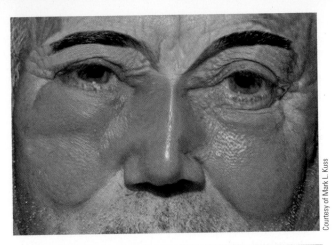

FIGURE 18–10   Erysipelas.

■ **ETIOLOGY.** Cellulitis is a bacterial infection commonly caused by *Streptococcus* and *Staphylococcus*. These bacteria are common bacteria of the skin (normal flora). Cellulitis often appears in open areas of the skin and can be the extension of a wound, **ulcer**, insect bite, blister, burn, or other skin infection.

■ **SYMPTOMS.** Cellulitis is characterized by pain, redness, swelling, warmth, and tenderness of the involved skin. Other symptoms might include headaches, fever, or chills. In advancing cases, red streaks can develop and travel from the affected area.

■ **DIAGNOSIS.** Medical history and physical examination of the involved area are helpful in diagnosis. If the leg is involved, an ultrasound can be performed to rule out deep vein thrombosis.

■ **TREATMENT.** Cellulitis is generally treated successfully with oral antibiotics. Analgesics for pain and resting the affected limb or affected area also can be part of the treatment plan. In extreme cases, intravenous antibiotics might be needed. Any cellulitis involving the face can be dangerous because this has the potential of spreading into the sinuses of the skull. If pain becomes severe, necrotizing fasciitis might have developed, which will require emergency surgical treatment.

■ **PREVENTION.** Good hand washing, proper cleansing, and care of open areas of the skin lower the risk of cellulitis. Deep, dirty, and open wounds need prompt medical treatment to prevent cellulitis.

ERYSIPELAS

■ **DESCRIPTION.** Erysipelas is an acute infection of the dermis that extends into underlying fat tissue.

It can affect the face, especially in children and older adults, but also affects the arms and legs (Figure 18–10).

■ **ETIOLOGY.** Most cases are due to *Streptococcus*, specifically group A *Streptococcus*. These bacteria can come from the skin or from the affected individual's throat or nasal passages and can enter the skin through any open area such as surgical incisions, ulcers, and minor trauma.

■ **SYMPTOMS.** Symptoms include fatigue, chills, fever, headaches, and vomiting. The infected skin develops a red, warm, hard, and painful rash showing a consistency similar to an orange peel. Swelling develops rapidly and exhibits sharply demarcated, raised edges.

■ **DIAGNOSIS.** A physical examination of the classic orange-peel rash and affected skin assists in diagnosis. Tests can determine that this skin condition is not herpes zoster or contact dermatitis.

■ **TREATMENT.** Antibiotics given orally or intravenously usually resolve the condition, but it often takes weeks for the skin to return to normal. In some cases, bacteria can infect the blood, leading to endocarditis and osteomyelitis.

■ **PREVENTION.** Prevention includes maintaining healthy skin, avoiding injuries to the skin, and promptly and completely treating streptococcal infections, including strep throat.

LYME DISEASE

■ **DESCRIPTION.** Lyme disease was first discovered in 1975 in the town of Lyme, Connecticut, for which it is named. It is more prevalent in the northeast and has become the most common tick-borne disease in the United States.

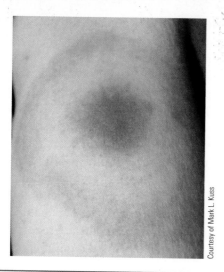

FIGURE 18–11 Lyme disease—bull's eye rash.

■ **ETIOLOGY.** Lyme disease is caused by the *Borrelia burgdorferi* bacterium and is transmitted to humans by the bite of an infected deer or blacklegged tick.

■ **SYMPTOMS.** The bacteria can affect any organ, causing a variety of symptoms and possibly delaying diagnosis. Symptoms can include flu-like symptoms, arthritis, malaise, chills, and fever. A characteristic bull's eye skin rash is a common sign (Figure 18–11). The bull's eye is a reddened circle with a lighter center and can appear days to weeks after the infected bite.

■ **DIAGNOSIS.** Lyme disease is diagnosed by a history confirming possible exposure to infected ticks and a physical examination revealing positive symptoms. Positive blood testing for antibodies confirms the diagnosis.

■ **TREATMENT.** Most cases can be treated successfully with a few weeks of antibiotics. If left untreated, the disease can cause arthritis and various neurologic and cardiovascular complications.

■ **PREVENTION.** Prevention of Lyme disease is aimed at preventing tick bites by using insect repellent; wearing long-sleeved shirts, long pants, and socks; and tucking the pants into the socks and boots when hiking or camping in grassy or wooded areas. Showering and inspecting the skin immediately after outside activities can also help prevent bites.

METHICILLIN-RESISTANT STAPHYLOCOCCUS AUREUS

■ **DESCRIPTION.** Methicillin-resistant *Staphylococcus aureus* (MRSA) is a strain of bacteria that is resistant to the antibiotics commonly used to treat

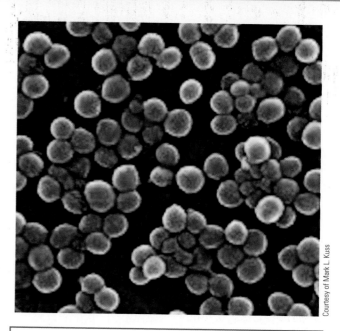

FIGURE 18–12 Staphylococcus aureus.

staphylococcal infections (Figure 18–12). This infection usually affects the elderly and those with other disease conditions and occurs in hospitals, nursing homes, and other health care settings and is known as health care–associated MRSA. More recently, MRSA is appearing in healthy people who might share personal items, such as athletes and students. These individuals are often in a community of people. In this case, MRSA is responsible for skin, tissue, and lung infections and is called community-associated MRSA.

Historically, MRSA has been a public health scare and superbug for about 7 years. In 2005, the Centers for Disease Control and Prevention (CDC) expressed concern that the number of MRSA deaths was increasing to the point that the number of MRSA deaths was higher than the number of deaths caused nationwide by acquired immunodeficiency syndrome (AIDS). In 2007, the CDC estimated that the number of MRSA infections in hospitals had doubled in only 6 years. These reports suggest a nationwide epidemic of MRSA. In 2010, encouraging results from the CDC showed that invasive (life-threatening) MRSA infections in health care settings had declined approximately 28% in 3 years from 2005 through 2008 (CDC, 2009).

■ **ETIOLOGY.** *S. aureus* is commonly found on the skin of individuals, is usually harmless, and does not cause illness. This presence of bacteria without illness is called being colonized. Individuals who are colonized with MRSA can easily pass these bacteria to others.

MRSA represents a group of bacteria that have developed a resistance to antibiotics, which is a natural survival method of bacteria. However, humans have helped build this resistance by excessive and unnecessary use of antibiotics. Many individuals insist on taking antibiotics for viral conditions such as flu and the common cold, even though it has been proven that these viruses are not affected by antibiotics. This overuse helps strengthen bacteria and build their resistance.

Even when antibiotics are used properly, they do not always kill every kind of bacterium. Those that survive become resistant to that antibiotic and many others. Because bacteria reproduce rapidly, they can build family resistance faster than new antibiotics can be developed. Staphylococcaceae is one of the families of bacteria that have built such a resistance that currently only a few drugs are effective to kill them.

Prescription medications are not the only sources of antibiotics that help build resistance. Antibiotics are often used in livestock. These antibiotics not only end up in meat products but eventually end up in groundwater supply from feedlot runoff.

■ **SYMPTOMS.** Symptoms of MRSA, like other staph bacteria, often start with small red bumps that resemble pimples or boils. These can quickly cause deep abscesses or become blood-borne. As a blood-borne infection, staph bacteria can invade all organs of the body, including bones, heart, and lungs. Symptoms of sepsis include a rash over most of the body along with fever, chills, headaches, joint pain, and shortness of breath. Sepsis with MRSA can be life-threatening, and infection requires immediate medical attention.

■ **DIAGNOSIS.** Diagnosis is determined by culture and drug sensitivity testing of wound and nasal secretions for MRSA.

■ **TREATMENT.** Current treatment of MRSA is with another, quite expensive antibiotic, vancomycin, which must be given intravenously. Even though it is currently effective, there are signs that some MRSA bacteria are building resistance to this medication also.

■ **PREVENTION.** Avoiding those with active infection is helpful along with maintaining a healthy lifestyle to keep natural immunity levels high. Other activities include frequent hand washing and carrying hand sanitizer for use when hand washing is not possible. Do not share personal items such as towels, clothing, combs, and eating utensils. Keep any open wounds covered and protected. Do not share or overuse antibiotics.

Prevention in health care facilities requires complete sanitation of all surface areas, fabrics, linens, and equipment in patient areas. Alcohol has been proven to be an effective sanitizer against MRSA. Therefore, many health care facilities have installed alcohol-based skin sanitizers in patient rooms, hallways, and utility rooms. Current best practices to prevent MRSA infection in health care settings include frequent hand washing by all staff, testing all patients upon admission for colonization with MRSA, placing all patients in isolation until culture results are reported as negative, and thorough cleansing regimens of patient rooms and common clinical areas.

FUNGAL DISEASES

Fungal infections are very common and usually affect the nails and hair. Pathogenic fungi are called dermatophytes, which often cause the skin to itch and crack, leaving it open to bacterial infections. Fungal infections are difficult to eradicate and can cause lifelong symptoms.

TINEA (RINGWORM)

■ **DESCRIPTION.** Tinea is a term used to identify any of a number of highly contagious fungal infections of the skin. They typically affect warm, moist areas of the body, feeding on perspiration and dead skin. Types of tinea include:

- **Tinea corporis** Affects the smooth skin of the arms, legs, and body. It is characterized by red, ring-shaped patches with pale centers and is commonly called ringworm, although no worm is involved. Tinea corporis is often spread from cats to humans and is common in children.

- **Tinea pedis** The most common form of tinea infection. It is typically called athlete's foot because it is a common condition in athletes. Tinea pedis is highly contagious and can be spread by direct contact with contaminated surfaces such as locker room floors, showers, and towels. Athlete's foot affects the spaces between the toes, causing intense itching and burning. The affected skin peels, leaving painful cracks or fissures (Figure 18–13). Untreated athlete's foot can spread to the entire foot. Wearing cotton socks, alternating shoes to allow complete drying, and wearing sandals help prevent and treat the fungus.

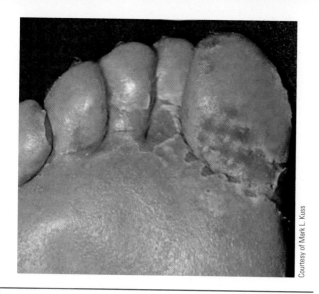

Courtesy of Mark L. Kuss

FIGURE 18–13   Tinea pedis.

- **Tinea cruris** Often occurs in conjunction with tinea pedis and is commonly called jock itch. It generally affects the scrotal and groin area of adult men. It tends to flare up during summer months and is aggravated by physical activity, tight-fitting jeans, and increased perspiration.

- **Tinea unguium** Involves the fingernail or toenail and is characterized by white patches in the nail. This tinea is difficult to treat because the fungus hides under the nail. Untreated, the fungus can destroy the entire nail, causing it to thicken, overgrow, turn white, and become brittle (Figure 18–14).

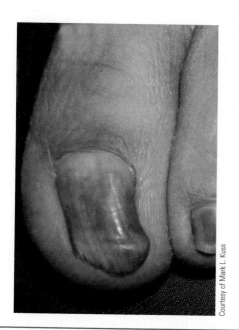

Courtesy of Mark L. Kuss

FIGURE 18–14   Tinea unguium.

- **Tinea capitis** Affects the scalp, causing areas of hair loss. This tinea occurs most often in children. (See Chapter 20 for more information.)

- **Tinea barbae** Affects bearded areas of the neck and face and, thus, is commonly called barber's itch. Shaving the affected area is helpful.

■ *ETIOLOGY.* Tinea is caused by a variety of fungi.

■ *SYMPTOMS.* Symptoms include itching, cracking, and weeping of the skin.

■ *DIAGNOSIS.* Diagnosis is made on the basis of clinical appearance and microscopic examination of skin scrapings, revealing the fungi.

■ *TREATMENT.* Treatment includes keeping the affected area clean and dry. Antifungal agents in liquid, cream, and powder forms are effective but must be used consistently over a long period of time to eradicate the fungus. Oral prescription medications might be needed and include ketoconazole (Nizoral®) and fluconazole (Diflucan®). Commonly, these fungal infections recur and become a chronic problem.

■ *PREVENTION.* Keeping the skin healthy, clean, and dry is the most helpful preventive measure. Other measures include avoiding tight-fitting clothing and avoiding areas where fungal infection might be prevalent such as community showers and hot tubs.

CANDIDIASIS

■ *DESCRIPTION.* Candidiasis (KAN-dih-DYE-ah-sis) is commonly called yeast infection or thrush (Figure 18–15). This fungal infection can be superficial or systemic and potentially life-threatening.

■ *ETIOLOGY. Candida* is a fungus that is normal flora of the skin, mouth, vagina, and intestines. It becomes an infection when some change in the body allows it to grow out of control. Taking antibiotics is a common cause of candidiasis. Antibiotics kill beneficial normal bacterial flora that help keep candidiasis under control.

Candidiasis also commonly affects individuals with chronic diseases such as diabetes mellitus, those who are on immunosuppressive medications, and those exposed to long-term water immersion such as dishwashers, bartenders, and waitresses.

■ *SYMPTOMS.* Symptoms of candidiasis differ, depending on the area affected. Infection in the mouth is called thrush and commonly occurs in infants. Symptoms include patches of white infection on the inner cheeks and tongue.

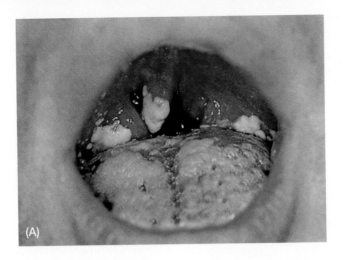

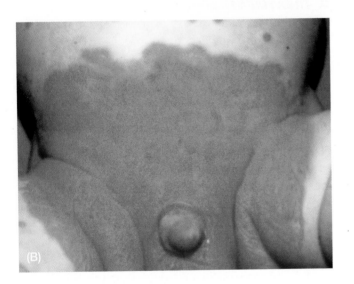

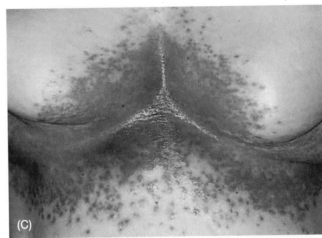

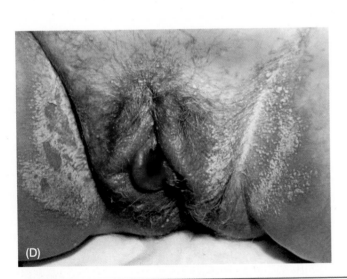

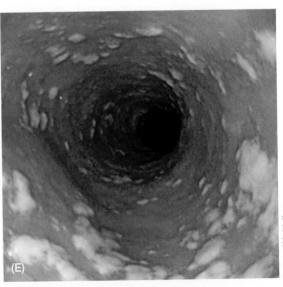

FIGURE 18–15   Candiasis. (A) Mouth—thrush. (B) Perineal area—diaper rash. (C) Skin—breast area. (D) Skin—vulva vaginitis. (E) Esophagus—view through endoscope.

Candidiasis infection on an infant's bottom is commonly called diaper rash and appears as a red, inflamed, and sometimes scaly rash.

Candidiasis also affects the fingernails and is called candidal onychomycosis. When it affects the area around the nail, is it paronychia. Infection between the fingers and toes often appears as itchy skin with blisters and pustules.

Candidiasis of the vagina causes vaginitis and is discussed in detail in Chapter 17.

■ **DIAGNOSIS.** Two primary methods for diagnosis include microscopic examination of the yeast and positive culture. A blood test and cultures might also be needed if the infection becomes blood-borne.

■ **TREATMENT.** Most *Candida* infections can be treated with over-the-counter or prescription antifungal medications. Topical creams, vaginal creams, and oral medications are available. More serious infections need long-term administration of intravenous antifungal medication. Even with a variety of antifungal medication available, fungal infections are often difficult to eradicate and can become chronic in some cases.

■ **PREVENTION.** Keeping skin clean, dry, and free from abrasions or cuts can help prevent skin *Candida* infections. Avoiding unnecessary antibiotics is also preventive.

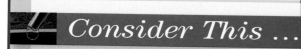

Consider This ...

The disease "ichthyosis" turns the skin scaly like a fish.

PARASITIC DISEASES

Parasites are organisms that feed on a host, sometimes a human. Human parasites affecting the skin are easily spread and cause intense itching. They commonly occur in crowded living conditions with inadequate bathing facilities. The two most common skin parasites are pediculosis (lice) and scabies.

PEDICULOSIS

■ **DESCRIPTION.** Pediculosis is an infestation of lice. Three types of lice commonly affect humans:

1. **Head lice** Commonly spread among school-aged children and their families (Figure 18–16). See Chapter 20 for more information.

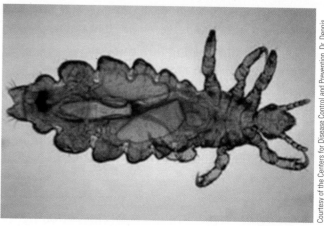

FIGURE 18–16 Head lice.

Courtesy of the Centers for Disease Control and Prevention, Dr. Dennis D. Juranek

2. **Body lice** Often occur in individuals with poor hygiene practices, such as transients and the homeless. Body lice can spread disease and were responsible for the spread of typhus during war times.

3. **Pubic lice** Spread by sexual contact with an affected individual and commonly called crabs. Pubic lice infect males and females and cause intense itching in the genital area. These lice also can spread to the eyelashes and eyebrows.

■ **ETIOLOGY.** Lice are easily spread by direct contact with an infected individual, or they can be carried by sharing combs, brushes, towels, clothing, or bed linens. Lice are not partial to any of the socioeconomic classes and, thus, affect anyone coming in contact with them.

■ **SYMPTOMS.** Lice can be seen in various areas, depending on the type of insect. Head lice are located on the scalp, crab lice in the pubic area, and body lice in the folds of the skin and on the clothing. Head lice lay their eggs (nits) on the hair shaft of the head. These lice are visible, as is the nit infestation in the hair. Lice crawl on the body and feed on human blood, causing severe itching.

■ **DIAGNOSIS.** Diagnosis is easily made by observation of lice on the body.

■ **TREATMENT.** Eradicating pediculosis is difficult. Treatment includes:

■ Bathing and shampooing with medicated shampoo. (Petroleum jelly can be applied to the eyelashes to kill lice.)

- Dry cleaning or washing all clothing and bed linens in hot water (140 degrees) for 20 minutes.
- Cleaning and treating furniture.

All lice on the body, clothing, bedding, and furniture must be killed to eradicate a lice infestation.

■ **PREVENTION.** Prevention includes avoiding contact with infested individuals and their clothing, bedding, and furniture.

SCABIES

■ **DESCRIPTION.** Scabies is an infestation by the itch mite.

■ **ETIOLOGY.** The mite responsible for scabies is *Sarcoptes scabiei*, a tiny (0.03–0.09 millimeter long), eight-legged parasite (in contrast to six-legged insects). The pregnant female mite burrows into the skin and lays her eggs in a short tunnel near the surface of the skin. The eggs hatch in 3 to 5 days; the mite matures on the surface of the skin in 2 to 3 weeks, then mates, and the cycle begins again.

Scabies mites can live off a host body for only 48 to 72 hours. Scabies is often transmitted throughout an entire household by skin-to-skin contact with an infected parent or child by hugging, holding, and sharing beds. Over a more extended period of time, relatives and close friends can also contact scabies. Sexual contact is the most common form of transmission among sexually active young people.

It is almost impossible to catch scabies by just touching or shaking hands with an infected individual. School settings, sports activities, and community shower rooms also do not provide the level of personal contact needed for transmission of the mites.

Mites cannot be picked up from animals, although cats and dogs do get mite infections. In dogs, scabies is called mange. Animal mites are different from scabies and do not infect humans but can produce a mild itch that goes away in a few days.

■ **SYMPTOMS.** The word *scabies* comes from a Latin word for scratch, the primary symptom for this condition. The action of the burrowing, along with movement of the mites within the skin, produces an intense itch that tends to be worse at night. Vesicles and pustules develop due to hypersensitivity to the bite, the mite's feces, and the presence of the ova.

Scabies are not visible with the naked eye but can be seen with a magnifying glass or microscope. The scabies burrow is visible and often appears as a

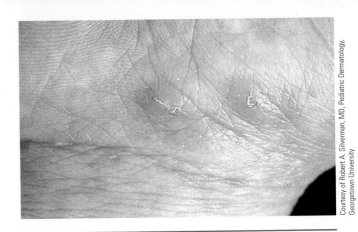

FIGURE 18–17   Scabies.

Courtesy of Robert A. Silverman, MD, Pediatric Dermatology, Georgetown University

slightly elevated, grayish white line. Common burrow sites are in the webs between the fingers and toes; in the folds of skin under the breast, armpits, and genital areas; on flexing surfaces of the wrist (Figure 18–17); along the belt line; and around underwear leg lines.

■ **DIAGNOSIS.** Diagnosis is made on the basis of microscopic skin examination revealing the presence of mites. Female mites can be viewed at the end of the burrowed tunnel and appear as a tiny black dot.

■ **TREATMENT.** Treatment includes application of lindane cream (Kwell®) to the entire body, leaving the cream on for 8 to 14 hours before showering or bathing. All infected individuals must be treated to prevent reinfection. Itching might persist for 3 to 4 weeks after successful treatment.

Cleaning and treating all personal items at the same time is recommended to prevent reinfection. Wash in hot water or dry clean all clothes, bedding, and towels. Treat furniture, carpets, and rugs. Place personal items that cannot be adequately cleaned, such as stuffed animals, brushes, gloves, hats, shoes, and pillows in plastic bags and freeze overnight or starve mites by placing items in zip-locked plastic bags and storing for a couple of weeks. Mites die after a week without food.

■ **PREVENTION.** Avoiding skin-to-skin contact with an infected individual is the best preventive measure.

Consider This ...

A large amount of dust in your home is actually dead skin cells.

Metabolic Diseases

Hyperactivity of the sebaceous gland causes several skin diseases. Inflammation and infection also can play a role in these diseases, although the primary cause is metabolic.

ACNE VULGARIS

■ **DESCRIPTION.** Acne is an inflammation of the sebaceous (oil-secreting) glands and hair follicles of the skin. It is characterized by the formation of **comedones** (KOM-eh-dones; a plugged skin pore; the open form of a comedone is a blackhead; the closed form is a whitehead) (Figure 18–18). Acne vulgaris is the most common form of acne and affects a large number, or crowd (vulgus = crowd), of individuals.

■ **ETIOLOGY.** The cause of acne is unknown, but it can be considered a metabolic disease because it occurs at puberty during increased production of sex hormones. An increase in these hormones, especially androgen, causes an increase in the size and activity of the sebaceous glands on the face, neck, chest, and back of males and females. Other factors contributing to the development of acne are heredity, food allergies, and endocrine disorders. Many misconceptions and misinformation exist concerning acne. It is not contagious nor due to lack of cleanliness, lack of sleep, or lack or excess of sexual release or masturbation. Acne vulgaris is not caused by venereal disease or consumption of chocolate, colas, or fried foods.

■ **SYMPTOMS.** Acne develops when sebaceous glands secrete excessive amounts of oil, or sebum, into a skin pore, eventually clogging the pore and causing the development of comedones. Sebaceous secretions at the opening of the pore can become oxidized and turn black, thus forming a blackhead. If bacteria enter the accumulated sebum and cause infection, the comedone becomes a whitehead or pimple. Acne can be mild to severe. Teens should be instructed to manage acne by:

- Cleansing the face and affected skin frequently with antibacterial soap to remove excess oil and bacteria.
- Avoiding the use of heavy makeup, which contributes to clogging the skin pores.
- Using over-the-counter acne creams or gels to help dry up excess oil.
- Avoiding tight-fitting clothing that traps heat.
- Showering often and especially after exercising or performing strenuous work.
- Avoiding the temptation to squeeze comedones because this can push the collected sebum farther into the skin pore, causing further inflammation and infection.

Comedones should be extracted gently, and pustules or pimples and cysts should be incised and drained.

■ **DIAGNOSIS.** Diagnosis is based on a history and physical examination of sebaceous lesions.

■ **TREATMENT.** Mild cases of acne are usually managed with proper cleansing and over-the-counter treatments. Severe cases need a treatment regimen prescribed by a dermatologist and often include cleansing with prescription medications, oral antibiotic therapy (tetracycline), steroids, and retinoic acid preparations or Retin-A®. Even with proper treatment, severe cases often result in permanent skin scarring. Symptoms of acne generally subside after puberty with or without treatment.

■ **PREVENTION.** Following treatment activities both treats and helps prevent acne.

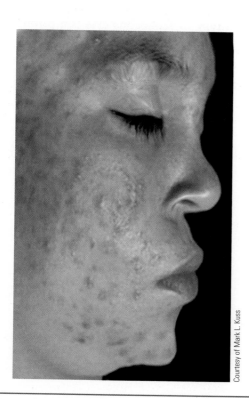

Courtesy of Mark L. Kuss

FIGURE 18–18   Acne vulgaris.

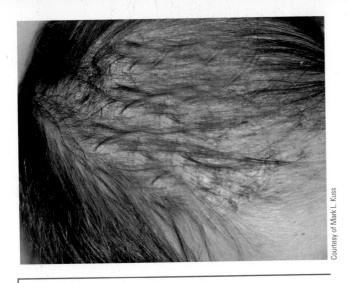

FIGURE 18–19   Seborrheic dermatitis.

SEBORRHEIC DERMATITIS

■ **DESCRIPTION.** Seborrheic dermatitis is a common type of dermatitis affecting the sebaceous, or oil-secreting, glands of the skin. It is not harmful or contagious but can be uncomfortable and unsightly. Seborrheic dermatitis affecting the scalp of infants is commonly called cradle cap (Figure 18–19) and usually clears by 12 months of age without treatment. Seborrheic dermatitis affecting the scalp of adults is called dandruff.

■ **ETIOLOGY.** The exact cause is unknown, although heredity and stress might be factors. This disease appears to run in families and appears more commonly in individuals who are obese; live with weather extremes; have other skin disorders such as acne; or have Parkinson's disease, stroke, head injury, and impaired immunity such as human immunodeficiency virus (HIV). Individuals recovering from stressful medical conditions such as myocardial infarction or who are confined for long periods of time in nursing homes are also more prone to this condition. The disease is characterized by an increase in the production of sebum, causing inflammation in the areas of the skin with the greatest number of glands. There is no cure for this disease.

■ **SYMPTOMS.** Seborrheic dermatitis affects the scalp, eyebrows, eyelashes, skin behind the ears (postauricular area), the sides of the nose, and the middle of the chest. Affected skin is usually reddened and covered with greasy-looking, yellowish scales. The eyebrows and eyelashes of an individual with seborrheic dermatitis show dry, dirty-white scales.

The affected nose area is generally reddened and itches. Mid-chest or sternal lesions are reddened and greasy-feeling. Itching might or might not be present.

■ **DIAGNOSIS.** The diagnosis is made based on physical examination of the location and appearance of the skin lesions.

■ **TREATMENT.** Treatment of the scalp involves use of over-the-counter medicated shampoo. If these are ineffective, a prescription-strength medicated shampoo might be necessary. Aggressive therapy includes the use of steroid lotion or creams.

Nonscalp areas often need to be cleaned and kept dry and treated often with antifungal or anti-itch medications. A prescription medication might be necessary if the disease is not manageable or if large areas of the body are involved.

■ **PREVENTION.** The severity of this condition can be lessened by controlling risk factors and treating appropriately.

SEBACEOUS CYST

■ **DESCRIPTION.** A sebaceous cyst is a closed sac of oily, cheese-like material located under the skin. This cyst can form anywhere on the body except in the palms of the hands and soles of the feet and commonly develops in the scalp, neck, and groin area. A special type of sebaceous cyst is a **pilonidal cyst**, which develops around a hair in the sacrococcygeal area (Figure 18–20).

■ **ETIOLOGY.** Sebaceous (seh-BAY-shus) cysts develop when a sebaceous gland becomes blocked and the

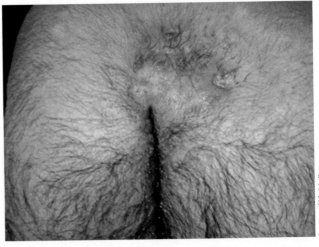

FIGURE 18–20   Pylonidal cyst.

sebum collects under the skin. They are often seen in individuals affected with acne, commonly result from a swollen hair follicle, and appear as slow-growing, painless lumps.

■ **SYMPTOMS.** The main symptom is the presence of the cyst. If it becomes infected, the skin will become red, warm, and tender over the area.

■ **DIAGNOSIS.** Diagnosis is made by physical examination of the cyst.

■ **TREATMENT.** No treatment is needed unless infection occurs. A warm, moist compress can be placed over the area to help relieve pain and promote drainage. Further treatment includes incising and draining the cyst, although it might tend to recur. Permanent treatment is surgical removal.

■ **PREVENTION.** There are no known measures that can prevent these cysts, but maintaining clean, healthy skin reduces the risk of occurrence.

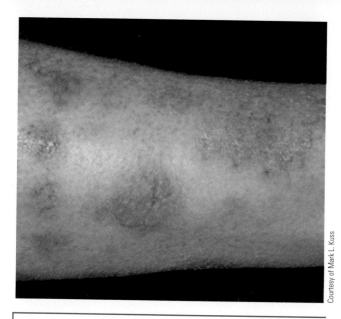

Courtesy of Mark L. Kuss

FIGURE 18–21 Eczema.

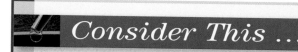

Consider This ...

Humans shed about 600,000 skin cells per hour—approximately 1.5 pounds per year—and by age 70 years, the average adult will have lost approximately 105 pounds.

Hypersensitivity or Immune Diseases

Hypersensitivity diseases are those caused by an immune reaction within the body. Frequently, the cause is unknown, and treatment is symptomatic.

ECZEMA

■ **DESCRIPTION.** Eczema (ECK-zeh-mah) is an inflammation of the skin or a type of dermatitis. It is not dangerous, not contagious, and often not curable.

■ **ETIOLOGY.** Eczema is also called atopic dermatitis because it tends to occur in atopic individuals—those with a genetic predisposition to allergies. Eczema is a common allergic reaction in children, often beginning in infancy and believed to be due to allergies to milk, orange juice, or some other foods. Eczema in infants often disappears when the offending food is discontinued. Factors that can cause eczema include

heredity, other diseases, allergies, and substances that irritate the skin.

■ **SYMPTOMS.** In adults, eczema often produces dry, leathery skin lesions characterized by itching, redness, vesicles, pustules, scales, and crust, appearing alone or in combination (Figure 18–21). Stress, humidity, and severe changes in temperature are a few of the identified factors causing an exacerbation or flare-up of the condition.

■ **DIAGNOSIS.** Diagnosis is made on the basis of clinical examination and history.

■ **TREATMENT.** Treatment is aimed at decreasing the occurrence and severity of the condition. Topical cortisone creams are often used along with antihistamines and sedatives to treat pruritus. Sunlight should be avoided, especially with light-sensitive eczema.

■ **PREVENTION.** Eczema is not preventable, but avoiding irritants reduces symptoms and exacerbation of the condition.

URTICARIA

■ **DESCRIPTION.** Commonly called hives or nettle rash, this is a vascular reaction of the skin.

■ **ETIOLOGY.** Urticaria is caused by contact with an external irritant such as insect bites, pollen, or plants. Urticaria also can be caused by internal irritants such as food, drugs, and contrast dye.

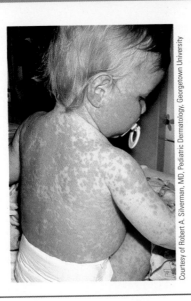

Courtesy of Robert A. Silverman, MD, Pediatric Dermatology, Georgetown University

FIGURE 18–22　Uriticaria.

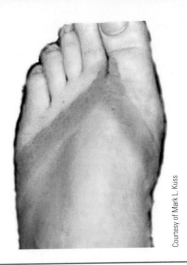

Courtesy of Mark L. Kuss

FIGURE 18–23　Contact dermatitis.

■ **SYMPTOMS.** Urticaria is characterized by slightly elevated lesions that are redder or paler than the surrounding skin and are associated with severe itching. The elevated areas are called **wheals** (WEELs) or hives (Figure 18–22). Scratching or rubbing the hypersensitive area can lead to formation of larger or additional wheals.

■ **DIAGNOSIS.** Diagnosis is made on the basis of physical examination of the characteristic wheal.

■ **TREATMENT.** Treatment includes antihistamines and avoidance of the allergen. (See Chapter 5, "Immune System Diseases and Disorders," for more information.)

■ **PREVENTION.** Avoiding exposure to the allergen and avoiding hot baths, showers, or exposure to the sun after a recent episode are preventive measures. Exposure to heat can cause the hives to return.

CONTACT DERMATITIS

■ **DESCRIPTION.** Contact dermatitis is an acute or chronic allergic reaction affecting the skin.

■ **ETIOLOGY.** Often, the allergen is some type of cosmetic, laundry product, plant, jewelry, paint, drug, plastic, or a variety of other agents. Frequently, it is difficult to determine the causative agent and, when found, it is sometimes impossible to avoid the causative agent completely (Figure 18–23).

■ **SYMPTOMS.** Allergic lesions can range from small, red, localized lesions to vesicular lesions that cover the entire body. A common example of a

contact dermatitis is poison ivy. (See Chapter 5 for more information.)

■ **DIAGNOSIS.** Diagnosis is not always easy. The location of the rash can help determine diagnosis if the rash appears under an item of clothing, jewelry, or an area exposed to sunlight. A use test is performed by placing a small spot of a suspected substance such as shampoo, laundry detergent, perfume, or cosmetic in another area away from the rash and watching for a reaction. Another helpful test is a patch test in which a patch containing common allergens is placed on the skin and observed for a reaction.

■ **TREATMENT.** Itching can be relieved with a number of over-the-counter topical medications containing camphor or menthol. Antihistamines such as diphenhydramine (Benadryl®) also relieve itching but cause drowsiness. Cool tub baths can also help. Treatment will not be beneficial until there is no further contact with the allergen.

■ **PREVENTION.** Avoiding the allergen is the best preventive measure. If contact with a known allergen occurs, immediately washing with soap and water might prevent the rash from developing. Application of barrier creams and wearing protective clothing are also helpful.

SCLERODERMA

Scleroderma (SKLEHR-oh-DER-mah; sclero = hardening, derma = skin) is a chronic autoimmune disorder characterized by hardening, thickening, and shrinking of the connective tissues of the body, including the skin (Figure 18–24). It is thought that this autoimmune reaction begins with the skin and

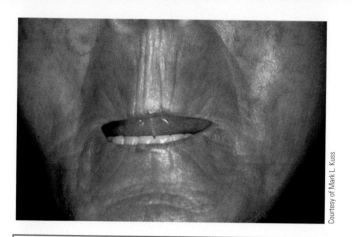

FIGURE 18–24   Scleroderma.

connective tissues, attracting lymph cells that stimulate the production of collagen, leading to the disorder. More information can be found in Chapter 5.

Idiopathic Diseases

Idiopathic diseases of the skin have no known cause but often tend to be familial. They can range from mild to severe and are generally treated symptomatically. They tend to be chronic with periods of remission and exacerbation of the disease process.

PSORIASIS

■ **DESCRIPTION.** Psoriasis (soh-RYE-uh-sis) is a very common, chronic skin disease that often affects individuals between the ages of 15 and 35. It can appear slowly or quite suddenly and usually has periods of remission (no symptoms) and exacerbation (flare-up). Psoriasis is not contagious.

A classic characteristic of the condition is the rapid replacement of epidermal cells. Normally, in a square centimeter of skin, some 25,000 cells produce 1,250 new cells with a life of 300 hours. Epidermal cells in a square centimeter of skin affected by psoriasis will number around 52,000 (twice the normal) and will produce 35,000 new cells (28 times more) with a life of only 36 hours (approximately one-eighth as long as normal).

■ **ETIOLOGY.** The cause is unknown, but some hereditary basis does exist. Stress, infection, skin trauma, and sunlight tend to cause an exacerbation of the condition.

■ **SYMPTOMS.** Psoriasis is characterized by red, raised lesions with distinct borders and silvery scales

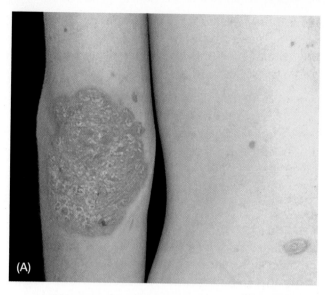

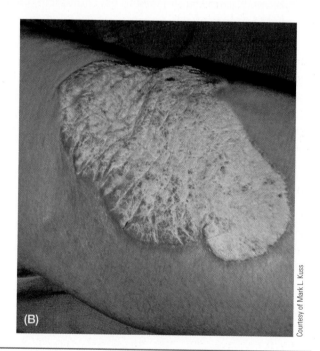

FIGURE 18–25   Psoriasis. (A) Psoriasis—mild. (B) Psoriasis—severe.

(Figure 18–25). These lesions generally occur on the elbows, knees, and scalp.

■ **DIAGNOSIS.** Diagnosis is usually made by physical examination of the skin condition. A skin biopsy might be performed to determine the exact type of psoriasis.

■ **TREATMENT.** Treatment includes medications to control itching, creams containing coal tar, creams to remove the scaling (salicylic acid), ultraviolet (UV) light treatments, steroids, and prescription medications for vitamin D or vitamin A. Several prescription medications specifically for psoriasis are also available. Oatmeal baths can also be helpful to loosen the scales.

■ **PREVENTION.** There is no way to prevent psoriasis, but certain activities can reduce flare-up of symptoms. These activities include keeping the skin moist and avoiding cold climates, skin scratches, stress, infection, and smoking.

ROSACEA

■ **DESCRIPTION.** Rosacea is a chronic skin condition characterized by inflammation and redness of the forehead, nose, cheeks, and chin but is not dangerous or life-threatening (Figure 18–26). The individual's facial skin appearance can lead to psychological damage related to loss of self-esteem.

■ **ETIOLOGY.** The cause of rosacea is unknown, but individuals affected blush easily and tend to be fair-skinned, female, and between the ages of 30 and 50. Rosacea involves enlargement of the blood vessels just under the skin and might be associated with other skin conditions such as seborrhea and acne vulgaris.

■ **SYMPTOMS.** The facial skin appears red with swelling or skin eruptions similar to acne. Other symptoms include:

- A red, bulbous nose.
- Spider-like blood vessels called telangiectasia of the face.

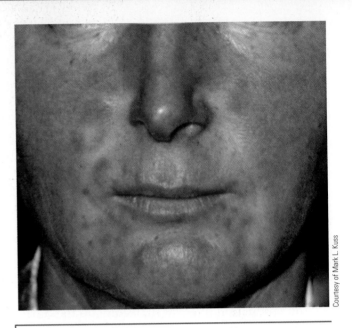

FIGURE 18–26 Rosacea.

Courtesy of Mark L. Kuss

- A burning or stinging sensation of the face.
- Bloodshot, irritated, watery eyes.

■ **DIAGNOSIS.** Diagnosis is commonly made by physical examination of the skin condition.

■ **TREATMENT.** There is no known cure. Symptoms might be controlled by identifying triggers that cause the condition to become worse. Avoiding sun exposure, prolonged exertion in hot weather, stress, spicy foods, alcohol, and hot beverages might reduce symptoms.

COMPLEMENTARY AND ALTERNATIVE THERAPY

Botanicals for Skin Conditions

Botanical extracts are often used to treat skin conditions such as acne, inflammations, infections, psoriasis, and vitiligo. Research conducted on botanicals revealed that some did have a positive effect on skin conditions. *Mahonia* (from the family Berberidaceae) is an evergreen shrub that has helped clear acne. Tea tree oil and *Saccharomyces* (fungi) have shown great potential for healing too. Some plant-based medicines like dithranol are now being used on a regular basis for treatment of psoriasis. Other plant extracts are used for topical administration to protect the skin from harmful sun rays and early aging. Extracts from tea, coffee, and some fruits and vegetables have proved promising for this application. Safety issues for some extracts have not been determined, so caution is suggested when using these botanicals.

Source: Reuter et al. (2010).

Antibiotic ointments applied to the face might control skin eruptions, and laser surgery might reduce the redness. Surgical reduction of the enlargement of the nose might be preferred to improve appearance.

■ **PREVENTION.** There is no known prevention.

Benign Tumors

Benign tumors of the skin are relatively common. They tend to be familial and often are more common in older adults.

SEBORRHEIC KERATOSIS

■ **DESCRIPTION.** Seborrheic keratosis (SEB-oh-REE-ic KERR-ah-TOH-sis) is a benign overgrowth of epithelial cells. It is one of the most common types of benign skin growth in older adults. This keratosis is synonymous with senile keratosis and does increase with age, but has also been found to appear on individuals as young as 15. Most people as they age will have at least one of these lesions (Figure 18–27).

■ **ETIOLOGY.** The cause is unknown, although it does appear to be age related.

■ **SYMPTOMS.** The lesions usually appear as a tan, brown, or black growth with a well-defined border. The surface of the lesion is covered with a warty scale that is soft on the trunk but harsh, dry, and rough on the hands, arms, and face. These lesions are rather loose and appear to be tacked onto the skin.

■ **DIAGNOSIS.** This condition is easily diagnosed by physical examination of the lesion. Seborrheic keratosis does not become cancerous, but can appear that way at times. If this is the case, a skin biopsy might be ordered.

■ **TREATMENT.** They are often easily scraped off by curettage, the treatment of choice. These skin growths are normally painless and require no treatment. They are often removed for cosmetic reasons.

■ **PREVENTION.** There is no prevention for this condition.

KELOID

■ **DESCRIPTION.** A keloid (KEE-loid) is a raised, firm, irregularly shaped mass of scar tissue that develops following trauma or surgical incision. (See Chapter 4, "Inflammation and Infection," for more information.)

■ **ETIOLOGY.** Keloids are an overgrowth of collagen during connective tissue repair; they are more common in the black population (Figure 18–28).

■ **SYMPTOMS.** Keloids can be unsightly but are generally considered harmless.

■ **DIAGNOSIS.** Diagnosis is easy and consists of a physical examination of the keloid.

■ **TREATMENT.** Surgical removal of keloids is usually not effective because it often results in the formation of another keloid. Radiation, injecting the lesion

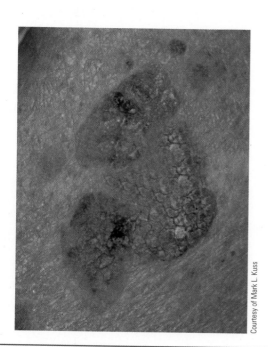

FIGURE 18–27 Seborrheic keratosis.

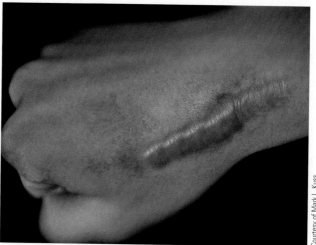

FIGURE 18–28 Keloid.

with steroids, and cryotherapy might be helpful in reducing the size of a keloid.

■ **PREVENTION.** There are no known preventive measures.

HEMANGIOMA

■ **DESCRIPTION.** Hemangioma (heh-MAN-jee-OH-mah; hem = blood, angio = vessel, oma = tumor) is the most common childhood tumor. In most cases, hemangiomas will disappear over time, with as many as 50% disappearing by age 5 and the majority disappearing by puberty. Most hemangiomas appear on the face and neck and affect females more often than males. They are also more likely to appear in twin births. Hemangiomas are congenital and do not grow on adults.

■ **ETIOLOGY.** The cause of hemangioma is unknown.

■ **SYMPTOMS.** Hemangiomas are made up of small blood vessels forming a reddish or purplish birthmark. Sometimes they present as a flat red or pink area. Common types of hemangioma include port wine stain, strawberry, and cherry hemangioma (Figure 18–29).

- **Port wine stain** A dark red to purple birthmark usually appearing on the face.
- **Strawberry hemangioma** A strawberry red, rough, protruding lesion commonly appearing on the face, neck, or trunk.
- **Cherry hemangioma** A small, red, dome-shaped lesion.

■ **DIAGNOSIS.** Diagnosis is easy and consists of a physical examination of the hemangioma.

■ **TREATMENT.** Treatment is usually not necessary because most hemangiomas will disappear with time. Surgical removal of lesions on the face is common for cosmetic reasons.

■ **PREVENTION.** There are no preventive measures.

Premalignant and Malignant Tumors

Skin cancer is the most common type of cancer in humans and, in most cases, is due to exposure to sun. Skin cancers generally occur in multiples and appear on the face, arms, and hands of middle-aged and older individuals. The most common skin cancer is basal cell carcinoma, but the most deadly is malignant melanoma. Diagnosis is made on the basis of clinical examination and positively confirmed by biopsy. Prevention for all forms of skin cancer consists of avoiding overexposure to the sun and lifelong use of sunscreen with a high sun protection factor (SPF).

ACTINIC KERATOSIS

■ **DESCRIPTION.** Actinic keratosis (ack-TIN-ick KERR-ah-TOH-sis; actinic = sun-related) is a premalignant skin condition more common in those with fair complexions, sun bathers, and individuals who have occupations in the sun such as fishermen, farmers, and construction workers (Figure 18–30).

■ **ETIOLOGY.** Actinic keratosis, also known as solar keratosis, is caused by excessive exposure to UV rays typically from the sun. These actinic lesions are slow growing, taking years to develop, and often appear first in older adults.

■ **SYMPTOMS.** Actinic keratosis is characterized by the growth of multiple wart-like lesions on sun-exposed areas of the body such as the face, backs of the hands, forearms, ears, and legs.

■ **DIAGNOSIS.** Diagnosis is made on the basis of clinical examination of the lesions.

■ **TREATMENT.** Left untreated, about 2% to 5% of actinic keratoses develop into a serious form of skin cancer called squamous cell carcinoma. Treatment is with topical medication such as Retin-A® or removal by curettage or cryotherapy.

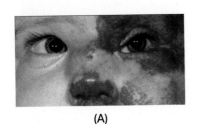 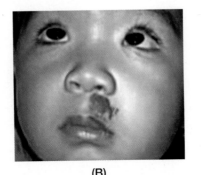 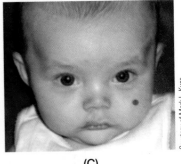

(A)   (B)   (C)

Courtesy of Mark L. Kuss

FIGURE 18–29   Hemangiomas. (A) Port wine hemangioma. (B) Strawberry hemangioma. (C) Cherry hemangioma.

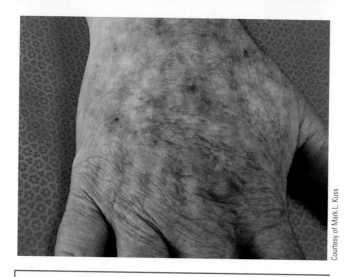

FIGURE 18–30   Actinic keratosis.

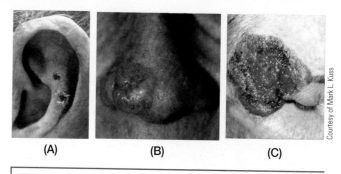

(A)   (B)   (C)

FIGURE 18–31   Basal cell carcinoma: (A) Ear. (B) Nose. (C) Near eye.

■ **PREVENTION.** Reducing sun exposure reduces or eliminates this condition.

BASAL CELL CARCINOMA

■ **DESCRIPTION.** Basal cell carcinoma is the most common type of skin cancer. It is most common in fair-skinned, blonde, and blue- or gray-eyed individuals. Basal cell carcinoma is a slow-growing, locally invading tumor that does not metastasize. This is not to say that left untreated it is not dangerous. Tumors near the eyes and mouth can invade these spaces and cause much concern. Tumors on the nose, lip, and ear can lead to the loss of these tissues.

■ **ETIOLOGY.** As with most cancers, the cause of basal cell carcinoma is unclear but does seem to be the result of a mixture of genetic and environmental factors. The most common identified environmental factor is excessive exposure to the sun.

■ **SYMPTOMS.** The appearance of this tumor varies, appearing as a raised nodule with a depressed or dented center; a smooth, shiny bump that is pink to pearly white in color; or a nonhealing lesion that bleeds easily (Figure 18–31).

■ **DIAGNOSIS.** Diagnosis is confirmed by biopsy.

■ **TREATMENT.** Treatment of basal cell carcinoma is surgical removal.

■ **PREVENTION.** Basal cell carcinomas that are related to sun exposure can be prevented by avoiding the strong midday sun, using sunscreen year round, and covering up with protective clothing if exposure is necessary.

SQUAMOUS CELL CARCINOMA

■ **DESCRIPTION.** Squamous cell carcinoma is less common than basal cell carcinoma, but it tends to grow more rapidly and become metastatic.

■ **ETIOLOGY.** This tumor, like basal cell carcinoma, tends to occur on the sun-exposed skin of those with fair complexion. It most commonly appears on people over age 50. As a general rule, basal cell carcinoma occurs on the face above the lip line, and squamous cell carcinoma occurs below the lip line. This tumor is often preceded by another skin lesion such as actinic keratosis, chronic ulcers, sinus tracts, or scars.

■ **SYMPTOMS.** Squamous cell carcinoma can appear as a firm, red nodule with crusts or a slightly elevated plaque (Figure 18–32). The nodule is usually located on the face, arm, neck, or hands but can appear in other areas. A sore that does not heal or bleeds easily might be a symptom of this cancer.

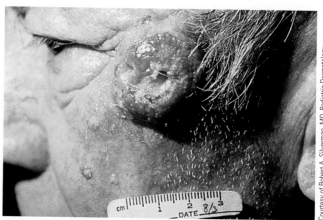

FIGURE 18–32   Squamous cell carcinoma.

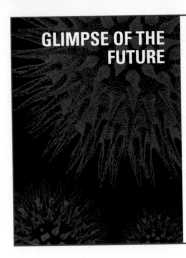

GLIMPSE OF THE FUTURE

Malignant Melanoma: New Hope in Treatments

There are some promising new treatments being used that slow the tumor growth in malignant melanoma. The drug ipilimumab (Yervoy™) works by blocking a molecule that inhibits the immune system so the immune system can be enhanced. The Food and Drug Administration (FDA) has approved the drug for late-stage melanoma. Interleukin-2 is also being used for patients with melanoma to increase longevity. The FDA also recently approved vemurafenib (Zelboraf®) for malignant melanoma. This drug causes tumor cells with a certain mutation (common in most melanomas) to die. These new treatments might significantly improve the survival rates in the future.

Source: Rice (2012).

■ **DIAGNOSIS.** Diagnosis is confirmed by skin biopsy.

■ **TREATMENT.** Squamous cell skin cancer has a high rate of cure if caught early. Treatment depends on location and size of the tumor and if there is metastasis. Wide surgical excision with radiation treatments and follow-up for at least 5 years for signs of recurrence is often the recommended treatment.

■ **PREVENTION.** Reducing sun exposure, examining the skin frequently for suspicious growths or changes in existing skin lesions, and seeking immediate treatment for these are preventive measures.

MALIGNANT MELANOMA

■ **DESCRIPTION.** Malignant melanoma (melan = black, oma = tumor) is the most serious type of skin cancer. It occurs more commonly in men and is responsible for the majority of skin cancer deaths.

■ **ETIOLOGY.** Malignant melanoma is due to an uncontrolled growth of pigment, or skin-coloring cells, called melanocytes. Growth of this tumor is caused by genetic and environmental factors, primarily sun exposure. Malignant melanoma rarely occurs before the age of 20 and can be related to a severe childhood sunburn.

■ **SYMPTOMS.** This tumor is usually tan, brown, or dark brown in color (Figure 18–33). Often, it arises in a mole and causes a change in size and color of the mole. Malignant melanoma metastasizes quickly and is highly malignant. It spreads into the lymph nodes and can metastasize to all organs of the body.

■ **TREATMENT.** Treatment depends on the degree of spread and might include wide surgical excision, radiation, and chemotherapy. Prognosis depends on the degree of spread when discovered, but approximately 20% of those diagnosed with this tumor die from effects of metastasis.

■ **PREVENTION.** Preventive measures include reducing sun exposure, examining the skin frequently for suspicious growths or changes in existing skin lesions, and seeking immediate treatment.

KAPOSI'S SARCOMA

■ **DESCRIPTION.** Prior to the discovery of AIDS, Kaposi's sarcoma (KAP-oh-seez sar-KOH-mah) was

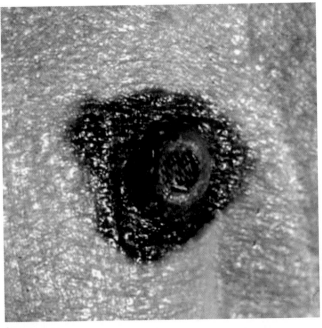

Courtesy of Mark L. Kuss

| **FIGURE 18–33**   Malignant melanoma.

HEALTHY HIGHLIGHT

Sunburn Prevention

Fair-skinned persons and those working in the sun—sailors, farmers, ranchers, road crew workers, and construction personnel—are at the greatest risk for development of sunburn and, ultimately, skin cancer. Prevention of sunburn includes:

- Avoiding sun exposure between the hours of 10:00 A.M. and 3:00 P.M., when the sun's rays are the strongest.
- Using sunscreen with SPF of 30 or higher on all exposed skin.
- Wearing a large, brimmed hat to reduce sun exposure to the face, ears, and head.
- Avoiding tanning beds.

relatively rare, but with the recent epidemic of AIDS, the development of this neoplasm has increased drastically.

■ **ETIOLOGY.** The relationship between Kaposi's sarcoma and AIDS is not fully understood. Usually, this tumor is not highly malignant except in the case of AIDS, in which it tends to be widespread and is often the cause of death in these individuals.

■ **SYMPTOMS.** This sarcoma is a malignant vascular skin tumor characterized by bluish-red cutaneous patches that grow under the skin most often on the face and legs. About one-third of the time, they show up in the lining of the nose, mouth, and throat

and can lead to pain and difficulty with eating and swallowing. The patches are usually composed of blood and cancer cells and often cause no symptoms. Tumors developing on the toes, feet, and legs often increase in number and size and spread upward. If the cancer spreads to the digestive tract or lungs, bleeding can result (Figure 18–34).

■ **DIAGNOSIS.** Diagnosis is made on the basis of a physical examination of the skin revealing painless, flat, bluish-red lesions that do not itch or drain. A skin biopsy is definitive.

■ **TREATMENT.** The most important treatment is treating AIDS. Specific Kaposi's treatments include

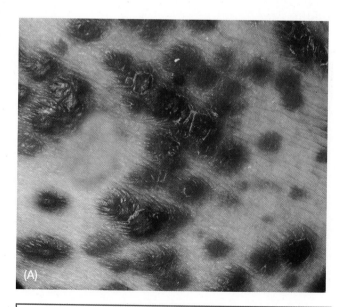

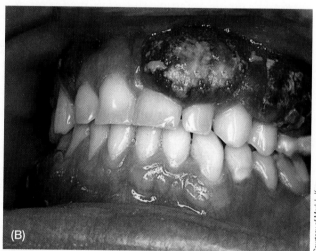

FIGURE 18–34 Kaposi's sarcoma. (A) Kaposi's sarcoma—skin. (B) Kaposi's sarcoma—mouth.

liquid nitrogen, chemotherapy, and radiation. As with AIDS, there is no cure for Kaposi's.

■ **PREVENTION.** Because most cases of Kaposi's are related to HIV infection, taking preventive measures to avoid HIV infection will usually prevent Kaposi's.

Abnormal Pigmented Lesions

The epidermis of normal skin contains melanocytes that produce melanin, the coloring pigment of skin. Skin color varies from light to dark, depending on the number of melanocytes present and protects the skin from burning. This explains why individuals with a fair or pale complexion burn more easily than individuals with a darker complexion. An individual's skin can contain several variations of abnormal lesions associated with pigment. These abnormal, pigmented lesions include ephelis, lentigo, nevus, albinism, vitiligo, and melasma. These conditions can be unsightly but are usually harmless and easily diagnosed by a physician. Moles can cause increased concern if they undergo a change in size and shape, possible indicators of cancer. Lesions can be biopsied if cancer is suspected. A brief description of abnormal pigmented lesions follows.

■ **Ephelis** Commonly called a freckle and is indicative of skin damage due to sunburn. The melanocytes in a freckle area are hyperreactive to sunlight, causing the darkened lesion. Freckles commonly occur in children and tend to fade in adults.

■ **Lentigo** A small brown spot occurring on the face, neck, and back of the hands of older adults. Commonly called liver spots, these lesions are not due to aging but to years of overexposure to the sun.

■ **Nevus** Commonly called a mole. Nevi can be brown, black, or pink-colored and are often due to a collection of melanocytes, which can appear on any area of the body, vary in size and shape, and occur singly or in multiples. Suspicious or unsightly nevi are often removed surgically.

■ **Albinism** A hereditary disorder characterized by a decrease or total absence of pigment in the skin, hair, and eyes. Individuals affected with albinism have pale skin, white hair, and pale blue or pink eyes. These individuals suffer from extreme sunburn if adequate protection is not provided.

■ **Vitiligo** (VIT-ih-LYE-go) Characterized by destruction of melanocytes in small or large patches

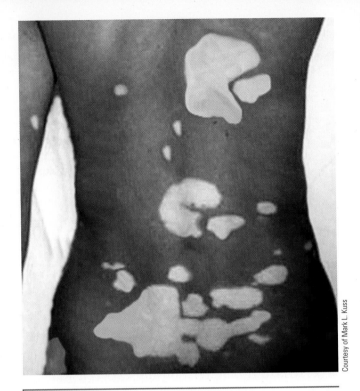

FIGURE 18–35 Vitiligo.

of skin (Figure 18–35). This condition can be due to an immune disorder.

■ **Melasma** Characterized by dark patches of skin on the face, especially the cheeks (Figure 18–36) and common in pregnant females and those taking birth control pills. It is commonly called the mask of pregnancy. Melasma usually disappears after delivery or discontinuation of birth control pills.

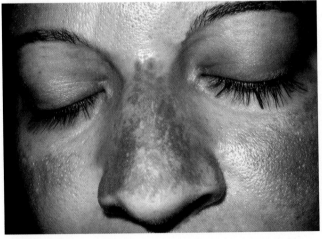

FIGURE 18–36 Melasma.

Diseases of the Nails

Nails act as coverings for the toes and fingers and can be considered extensions of the skin. Diseases of the nail can cause abnormal shape, thickening, and color changes. Fungal and bacterial infections are the most common cause of nail disease.

Bacterial infection of the nails is **paronychia** (PAR-oh-NICK-ee-ah), an infection of the skin around the nail. This condition is commonly seen in individuals whose hands are in water for long periods of time, such as dishwashers, for example. This infection can cause the nail to lift away from the bed, causing acute pain. Antibiotics are usually an effective treatment.

Fungal infections frequently affect the feet, are often chronic in nature, and commonly cause permanent nail deformity. Tinea pedis (athlete's foot) is a common cause of fungal nail infections of the feet. Fungal infections, as discussed previously in the chapter, are difficult to treat, and recurrence is common.

Diseases of the Hair

Hair color, texture, and distribution are genetically determined and influenced by hormones.

HIRSUTISM

■ **DESCRIPTION.** Hirsutism (HER-soot-izm; Latin, meaning shaggy) is excessive growth of hair. Men typically have facial and chest hair due to stimulation by male sex hormones. Hair growth in these areas in females is quite distressing, however, and is usually caused by hormone abnormalities due to such disorders as adrenal tumors, ovarian tumors, and polycystic ovaries.

ALOPECIA

■ **DESCRIPTION.** Alopecia (AL-oh-PEE-shee-ah; Greek, meaning fox mange, which causes hair loss) is partial or complete hair loss, usually from the head (Figure 18–37A).

■ **ETIOLOGY.** Alopecia can be caused by a number of factors, including aging, heredity, thyroid disease, iron deficiency, chemotherapy, radiation, and dermatitis. Alopecia can occur suddenly or over a period of time and can be temporary or permanent.

■ **TREATMENT.** Treatment of alopecia varies according to cause and usually restores hair growth.

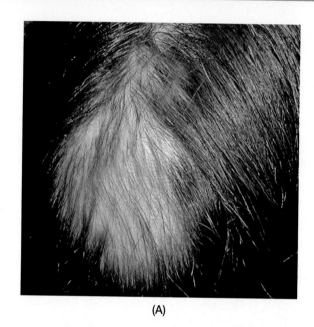

(A)

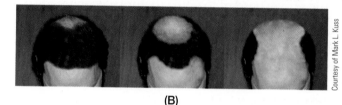

(B)

FIGURE 18–37   (A) Alopecia. (B) Male-patterned baldness.

One of the most common causes of sudden, temporary alopecia is related to chemotherapy and radiation treatment. Hair growth normally returns when treatments are stopped.

MALE-PATTERNED BALDNESS

■ **DESCRIPTION.** Male-patterned baldness is a common cause of hair loss in men and is an inherited trait passed to males by their mothers. The mother does not have this type of hair loss because it is influenced by male sex hormones, but the pattern can easily be recognized in the mother's brothers or the affected individual's maternal uncles.

■ **SYMPTOMS.** Male-patterned baldness often begins around age 30 with a receding front hairline and loss of hair on the top and back portion of the head (Figure 18–37B). In some men, these areas of alopecia eventually meet, leaving hair on only the sides of the head. Alopecia in females is usually due to a hormonal or nutritional disorder.

■ **TREATMENT.** In the case of male-patterned baldness, hair growth can be restored to some degree by

Courtesy of Mark L. Kuss

certain special medications. These medications are quite expensive, and loss of hair returns if treatment is discontinued. Other options include use of a wig, toupee, and hair transplantation.

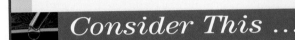

Consider This ...

A human naturally loses 40 to 100 strands of hair a day.

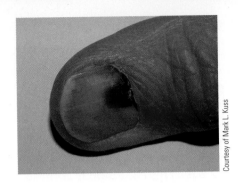

FIGURE 18–38   Bruise of the finger due to blunt trauma.

■ TRAUMA

The skin is the outermost organ of the human body and the body's first line of defense. The position of the skin exposes it to high risk for receiving frequent trauma, which might be the result of mechanical, thermal, or electrical injury or radiation or pressure injury and insect or spider bites.

Mechanical Skin Injury

Skin is exposed to mechanical trauma in a variety of ways. Mechanical trauma can be due to blunt or sharp objects and range from mild and insignificant to major and life-threatening. Types of mechanical skin injury include the following.

ABRASION

■ **DESCRIPTION.** A common mechanical trauma is caused by scraping away the skin surface. Abrasions are also called friction burns or rug burns.

■ **SYMPTOMS.** An **abrasion** is red, raw, and painful, but bleeding is usually minimal. A skinned knee is a typical example of an abrasion.

■ **TREATMENT.** Treatment generally consists of cleaning the area with soap and water, removing any embedded particles such as grass or rock, applying antibiotic ointment, and covering the area with a light sterile dressing.

BLUNT TRAUMA

■ **DESCRIPTION. Blunt trauma** can be caused when an individual is struck by items such as hammers and clubs or is thrown into objects such as steering wheels and walls. Falls also can cause blunt trauma.

■ **SYMPTOMS.** Blunt trauma often causes a large bruise called a **contusion** (kon-TOO-zhun), an accumulation of blood from injured or disrupted blood vessels in the tissue without breaking the skin (Figure 18–38).

AVULSION

■ **DESCRIPTION. Avulsion** occurs when a portion of skin or appendage is pulled or torn away. Avulsion injuries usually occur when tissue is caught up in some type of machinery (Figure 18–39). If an appendage is completely torn away, it is termed an amputation.

CRUSH TRAUMA

■ **DESCRIPTION.** Crush trauma occurs when tissue is caught between two hard surfaces. Crush injuries commonly involve fingers, hands, feet, and toes such as when hands and fingers are caught in doors or between objects or when heavy items are dropped on the fingers, hands, feet, and toes.

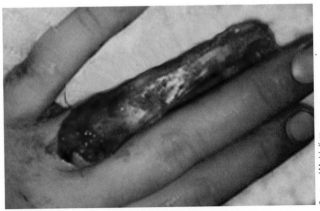

FIGURE 18–39   Avulsion of finger.

PUNCTURE INJURY

■ **DESCRIPTION.** Puncture injury occurs when a sharp object such as a knife, nail, or splinter of glass or metal is forced into the tissue. Bleeding is usually minimal. A feared complication of puncture injury is tetanus because puncture injuries set up an anaerobic condition favorable to tetanus bacteria.

LACERATION

■ **DESCRIPTION.** A **laceration** is a cut in the skin caused by a sharp object such as a knife, razor, glass, or metal. The edges of the laceration can be smooth, making repair easy, or the edges can be jagged, leading to a more difficult repair. A laceration with smooth, even edges is commonly called an **incision**.

Thermal Skin Injury

Thermal skin injury can be due to excessive heat or cold or to short- or long-term exposure to varying temperatures. Skin injury can range from mild to severe. Untreated severe skin injuries can become life-threatening.

HYPERTHERMIA

■ **DESCRIPTION.** Hyperthermia (hyper = excessive, thermia = temperature) occurs when the body is overheated from excessive exposure to the sun or a hot environment or to excessive exercise in a hot environment. There are two types of hyperthermia: heat exhaustion and heat stroke. The cause and treatment of these types of hyperthermia vary considerably.

HEAT EXHAUSTION

■ **DESCRIPTION.** Heat exhaustion is sometimes called heat prostration; it commonly occurs from excessive exercise or activity in a warm environment.

■ **SYMPTOMS.** The individual has profuse perspiration and loss of salt and water, leading to dehydration. The skin is cool and moist. The individual might feel weak and nauseated and might have muscle cramps. Body temperature is usually normal.

■ **TREATMENT.** The affected individual should lie quietly in a cool place. Fluid and salt replacement can include drinking tomato juice or other high-sodium drinks along with water. In extreme cases, the affected individual should be transported to the hospital.

HEAT STROKE

■ **DESCRIPTION.** Heat stroke is more serious than heat exhaustion. It occurs when the body's temperature-regulating mechanisms are no longer able to cope with the excessive exposure to heat.

■ **SYMPTOMS.** The body's core temperature rises above 105°F, and the skin is red and hot. The skin is dry with a noted absence of perspiration. The affected individual might feel nauseated and weak and can become mentally confused. In extreme cases, the confusion can progress to loss of consciousness with convulsions. Without rapid and effective treatment, brain damage and death can result.

■ **TREATMENT.** Treatment is aimed at immediate and aggressive cooling of the body by removing clothing and pouring cool water over the body or placing the body in a cool tub or pool. The affected individual should be immediately transported to a hospital.

BURNS

■ **DESCRIPTION.** Burns can be caused by fire, steam, exposure to hot liquids or items, chemicals, and electricity. The degree of tissue injury is related to the intensity of the heat and duration of exposure. Burns are classified by depth of skin injury and include first-, second-, and third-degree burns.

■ **ETIOLOGY.** The main complications of burns are fluid loss and infection. Open tissue affected by second- and third-degree burns can leak pints to quarts of serous fluid per day, leading to dehydration and shock. *Pseudomonas*, the bacterium often causing infection, is noted for its ability to spread to the blood, leading to septicemia and death.

■ **TREATMENT.** Treatment of burns depends on the degree and type of burn. Generally, treatment will include cooling the tissue with cool water to prevent further burning. Pain is treated with analgesics ranging from over-the-counter products to narcotic analgesics, depending on the severity of pain. Antibiotics are given orally and intravenously to prevent or treat infection. Antibiotic ointments also can be applied directly to the burned area.

Surgical débridement might be needed to remove charred and necrotic tissue. In some cases, this can be accomplished by whirlpool treatments. Surgery is often necessary to graft skin, remove excessive scar tissue, and reshape deformities. Surgical treatment might be necessary multiple times over a period of months or years to obtain the desired results.

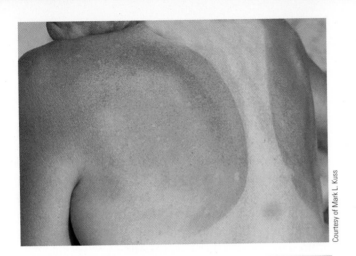

FIGURE 18–40   First-degree burn.

FIRST-DEGREE BURNS

■ **DESCRIPTION.** First-degree burns are fairly common and are characterized by pain, skin redness, and swelling. First-degree burns involve only the epidermis and are often the result of sunburn (Figure 18–40). Healing generally occurs within a week, followed by peeling of the damaged epidermis.

SECOND-DEGREE BURNS

■ **DESCRIPTION.** Second-degree burns are also called partial-thickness burns; they involve the epidermis and dermis and are characterized by extreme pain, redness, blisters, and open wounds (Figure 18–41).

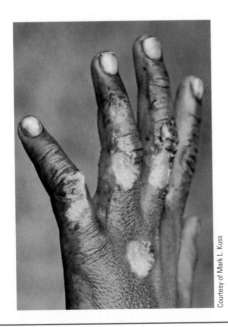

FIGURE 18–41   Second-degree burn.

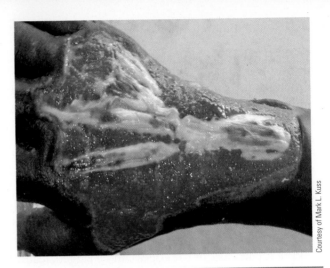

FIGURE 18–42   Third-degree burn.

Second-degree burns usually heal in 2 to 3 weeks. If the burned area becomes infected, a second-degree burn can progress into a third-degree wound.

THIRD-DEGREE BURNS

■ **DESCRIPTION.** Third-degree burns are also called full-thickness burns; they involve the epidermis and entire dermis, exposing layers of fat, muscle, and bone. Tissue burned to the third degree is painless because the nerves in the dermis have been destroyed (Figure 18–42). This is not to say that individuals with third-degree burns do not have pain; there is extreme pain, but the pain is due to a layering of degrees of burn, with first- and second-degree areas surrounding the third-degree areas.

■ **SYMPTOMS.** This burn is characterized by charred and broken tissue layers. The affected individual can exhibit signs and symptoms of shock.

■ **TREATMENT.** Third-degree burns often need tissue grafting to heal. Scarring and deformity are common with third-degree tissue damage.

The amount of body surface burned generally correlates with the chance of survival for the affected individual. Body surface may be determined by applying the rule of nines (Figure 18–43). Burns exceeding 9% of the body are serious and should be treated in large medical centers with special burn units. Generally speaking, body burns of 25% to 30% of the body are extremely serious, and 60% body burns are usually fatal.

Other factors affecting the chance of survival include age, health, quality of care, and complications. Those who are older and the very young do not survive serious burns as well as other age groups.

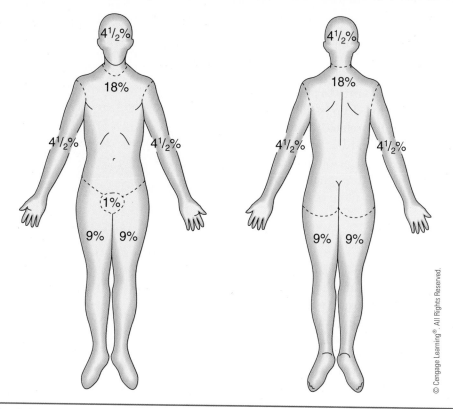

FIGURE 18–43 Rule of nines: used to calculate percentage of body surface burned.

Media Link

View an animation on bites, burns, and dislocation injuries on CourseMate.

COLD INJURIES

■ **DESCRIPTION.** Cold thermal injury is usually not as severe or life-threatening as heat or burn injuries. Hypothermia (hypo = low, therm = temperature) occurs when the body's core temperature falls below 95°F, which can occur when the body is cold for a long period of time or is exposed to extreme cold for even short periods of time. Exposure to wind and water increases the chilling effect and can lead to hypothermia in shorter amounts of time.

■ **SYMPTOMS.** Symptoms of hypothermia include extreme shivering, mental confusion, blue or cyanotic extremities, and weak pulse.

■ **TREATMENT.** Treatment includes removing wet clothing and warming the body with warm blankets, warm packs, or another person's body. Warm liquids can be given if the individual is conscious. The affected individual should be immediately transported to an emergency medical facility. Hypothermia can be fatal.

FROSTBITE

■ **DESCRIPTION.** Frostbite is the freezing of tissue, usually on the face, fingers, toes, and ears, and might or might not occur with hypothermia. Tissue affected by severe frostbite can become necrotic and need surgical débridement or amputation.

■ **SYMPTOMS.** The tissue affected by frostbite usually is painless and white in color. With warming, the skin becomes painful and turns red.

■ **TREATMENT.** Treatment includes rapid warming in warm (not hot) water baths, not rubbing the affected tissue, and emergency treatment at a medical facility.

Electrical Injury

Electrical tissue injury is the result of contacting unprotected or inadequately insulated electrical wiring or coming in contact with lightning. Whatever the cause of injury, electrical tissue damage has a point of entry and an exit point. The point of entry is the area coming in contact with the electrical source and the exit point is the grounded area. Electricity travels through the body from point of entry to point of exit, causing burns and often causing deep tissue injury.

A common cause of death related to electrical injury is from respiratory and cardiac arrest. These conditions are caused by the physical jolt of electricity and the electrical current passing through the body and interfering with the conduction system of the heart.

Radiation Injury

Radiation injury can be caused by ionizing radiation such as X-rays and by sunlight. Of the two, sunlight injury is the most common. Exposure to sunlight for short amounts of time leads to skin redness, but prolonged exposure can cause first- and second-degree burns to the skin. Fair-skinned persons are the most easily burned due to a lower number of pigment cells in the skin. Tanning of the skin occurs as a protective mechanism. Tanned skin returns to normal color when pigmented keratocytes in the epidermis are shed. Pigmented skin cells shed approximately every 30 days.

Radiation injury also can occur from exposure to tanning beds, which tan skin in the same manner as sun exposure. Tanning of the skin is a popular activity because of the cosmetically pleasant color produced, but the long-term effects of tanning are not so pleasant. Prolonged exposure to sun or tanning beds causes the skin to become prematurely dry, brittle, and wrinkled and to lose elasticity. These effects cause the skin to appear much older than its natural age. Another unpleasant effect of sun exposure is the development of skin cancers as discussed previously in this chapter.

Pressure Injury

Pressure injury is caused when placing pressure against tissue leads to a decrease in blood flow to this area. The most common type of pressure injury is a decubitus ulcer. Corns and calluses are also the result of pressure injury.

DECUBITUS (PRESSURE) ULCER

■ **DESCRIPTION.** Decubitus (dee-KYOU-bih-tus) ulcer is a pressure injury commonly called a bedsore or pressure sore (Figure 18–44). The term *decubitus* actually means the act of lying down or the position of lying down.

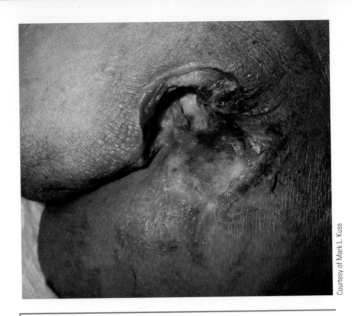

Courtesy of Mark L. Kuss

FIGURE 18–44 Decubitus ulcer.

■ **ETIOLOGY.** Decubitus ulcers commonly affect the bony areas of the body such as the heels, sacrum, elbows, and head of individuals who spend prolonged amounts of time in bed. Increased pressure in these areas slows blood flow, thus leading to tissue ischemia and necrosis.

■ **PREVENTION.** Pressure sores can be avoided by frequent turning and repositioning to decrease tissue pressure and allow blood flow to the tissues. Massaging the affected area also can improve circulation.

CORNS AND CALLUSES

■ **DESCRIPTION.** Corns and calluses are protective hyperplasias of tissue as a result of pressure. The main difference between a corn and a callus is the location. Corns are commonly found on the feet and are due to ill-fitting shoes. Corns are usually painful, and the affected individual might seek to have them surgically removed.

Calluses are found in the palms of the hands and are related to pressure injury to the hands, generally due to working with hand tools or performing labor. Calluses are usually not painful and, in fact, protect the hands from repeated abrasions and blisters.

Insect and Spider Bites and Stings

There are thousands of varieties of insects and spiders. Most bites and stings are mild and cause only itching at the site, but in a few people, these can bring about a serious reaction. Most bites and stings can be treated with home remedies.

INSECT BITES AND STINGS

■ **DESCRIPTION.** Insect bites and stings vary from bloodsucking mosquitoes, flies, and fleas, to the stings of bees, wasps, hornets, yellow jackets, and fire ants. Most of these bites and stings feel unpleasant and might cause swelling and itching at the site; however, insect bites also can transmit diseases such as malaria and yellow fever.

■ **SYMPTOMS.** Signs and symptoms of insect bites or stings often result from the injection of venom or poison into the skin. This venom incites an allergic reaction, the severity of which depends on the individual's sensitivity. Most symptoms are mild and disappear within a few days. An allergic reaction might cause intense itching, fever, and joint pain. A small percent of people develop a severe reaction called anaphylaxis, as discussed in Chapter 5.

■ **TREATMENT.** Treatment for mild reactions includes moving to an area to avoid more insects; if a stinger is involved, scraping or brushing it off with a knife or credit card; washing the affected area with soap and water; applying ice; applying hydrocortisone cream; and taking an antihistamine such as diphenhydramine (Benadryl®). Pain can usually be controlled by a mild analgesic such as Tylenol.

If a severe reaction occurs with symptoms of difficulty breathing, swelling of the face or lips, hives, tachycardia, nausea, and vomiting, call 911 for immediate assistance.

Other emergency responses include laying the victim down on his or her back with feet higher than head, loosening tight clothing, covering with a blanket, and checking for special medications the individual might have for allergic reaction, such as an EpiPen. If vomiting occurs, turn the individual on his or her side to prevent aspiration. If breathing stops, begin cardiopulmonary resuscitation.

■ **PREVENTION.** To prevent bites and stings, use insect repellent, wear protective clothing, and watch for and avoid insect nests. If you have allergies to insects, always carry an emergency epinephrine kit.

SPIDER BITES

More than 20,000 species of spiders exist in the Americas, yet only 60 are capable of biting humans and, of these, only a few have a serious bite. Most spiders are not poisonous and are helpful to have around because they eat insects that can be annoying. However, two commonly poisonous spiders are the black widow and brown recluse.

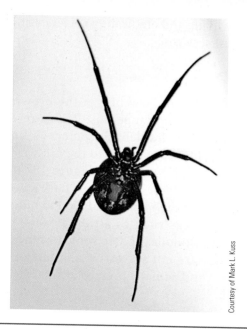

Courtesy of Mark L. Kuss

FIGURE 18–45   Black widow spider.

BLACK WIDOW BITE

■ **DESCRIPTION.** The black widow is by far the most commonly known poisonous spider due to its famous red markings in the shape of an hourglass (Figure 18–45). The name comes from a mistaken belief that the female spider kills the male after mating. They are found mostly in the southern United States but appear in all states except Alaska. They try to avoid humans and tend to live in garages and attics. Only the female bites, and this happens usually when she is disturbed or trying to protect her eggs.

■ **ETIOLOGY.** The venom of the black widow is a protein that affects the victim's nervous system. Even though this venom is one of the most potent produced by spiders, it causes severe response in only a few individuals.

■ **SYMPTOMS.** The first symptom is acute pain at the site. Other, more severe, symptoms include abdominal pain that mimics appendicitis, muscle cramps, nausea, fainting, dizziness, and chest pain.

The severity of the reaction to the bite depends on the age of the victim: the elderly and children are the most seriously affected. The bite is seldom fatal.

■ **TREATMENT.** Treatment includes cold compresses and pain relievers. Children, pregnant women, hypertensive individuals, and the elderly, if bitten, should be taken to the hospital for treatment.

■ **PREVENTION.** Prevention of bites includes taking care when reaching into dark areas where spiders might be living and eradicating spiders using professional pest services.

BROWN RECLUSE BITE

■ **DESCRIPTION.** The bite of the brown recluse spider can be very dangerous. Brown recluse spiders, also called fiddleback spider, violin spider, or brown fiddler, are native to the midwestern and southeastern United States (Figure 18–46). They live up to their name in that they have a distinctive violin shape on their backs and tend to hide in dark, warm, dry areas such as attics, closets, porches, barns, and woodpiles and, in some instances, inside shoes. They are not aggressive and bite only when threatened and actually pressed against an individual's skin.

■ **ETIOLOGY.** The bite venom is a collection of enzymes that is extremely poisonous to a level that some say is more potent than a rattlesnake's. Even so, most bite sites become firm and heal within a few days with little scarring. On occasion, however, the

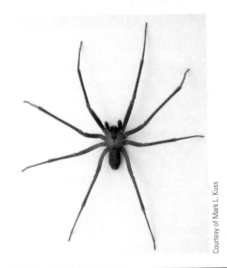

Courtesy of Mark L. Kuss

FIGURE 18–46   Brown recluse spider.

reaction in the bite area will be more severe, with redness, blistering, and blue discoloration. The venom can cause destruction to tissues, often leading to necrosis of skin, fat, and blood vessels in areas immediately surrounding the bite site (Figure 18–47).

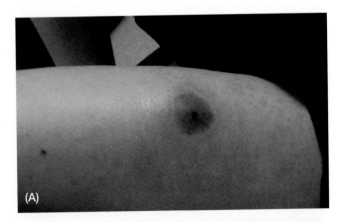

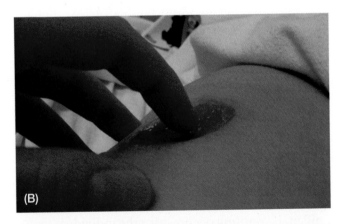

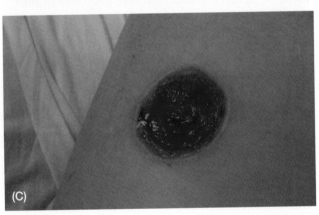

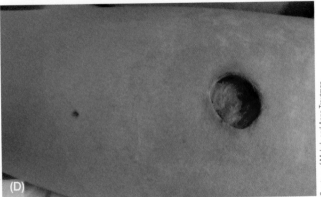

Courtesy of Melody and Anna Troutman

FIGURE 18–47   Stages of a recluse spider bite. (A) Wound—a few hours after bite. (B) Wound—1 day after bite. (C) Wound—2 days after the bite. (D) Wound—after debridement of necrotic tissue.

Bites are rarely fatal, but deaths have been reported in children younger than 7 years of age.

■ **SYMPTOMS.** Symptoms of brown recluse spider bite include severe pain, severe itching, fever, nausea, and muscle pain.

■ **DIAGNOSIS.** Diagnosis is based on a careful history and examination of the bite site, but no specific lab studies can confirm a brown recluse bite. Diagnosis can be confirmed only if the spider is available for identification.

■ **TREATMENT.** First aid consists of the application of an ice pack, administration of analgesic medications, and acquisition of prompt medical care. Further treatment includes pain medication, antihistamines, and antibiotics if infection occurs. No antivenin medication is available. A follow-up visit to the doctor might be necessary to monitor the wound, débride necrotic tissue if needed, and treat any secondary infection.

If possible, the spider should be caught in a clear, tightly closed container for future identification. It is important to seek medical treatment if a brown recluse bite is suspected because, in rare cases, necrosis can spread quickly, particularly when the venom reaches a blood vessel. When venom travels along a vein or artery, the resulting necrosis of tissue can be as large as several inches and might require extensive excising of tissue around the wound.

■ **PREVENTION.** Prevention of brown recluse spider bite includes activities to eliminate the spider by thorough house cleaning, installing tight-fitting windows and doors, and professional pest elimination services.

RARE DISEASES

Elephantiasis

Elephantiasis is characterized by hypertrophy of the skin and subcutaneous tissue, giving it an elephant-like appearance. Inflammation of the lymphatic system also leads to fluid accumulation in the legs, causing them to become enlarged. Elephantiasis is caused by a parasitic worm that enters the lymphatic system and causes obstruction of drainage and accumulation of fluids. This disease is most commonly seen in tropical areas, such as central Africa, and is spread by mosquitoes and bloodsucking flies.

EFFECTS OF AGING ON THE SYSTEM

Numerous changes develop in the integumentary system during the aging process. The epidermal layer becomes thinner and retains less water, which accounts for the easy tearing and dryness of the skin common in older adults.

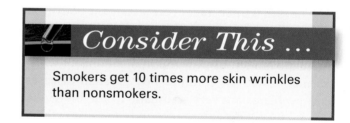
Consider This ...

Smokers get 10 times more skin wrinkles than nonsmokers.

Xerosis (zee-ROE-sis; dry skin) is a major problem in older adults, who might have flaky, scaly skin and pruritus. The sweat and sebaceous glands do not function as well, further contributing to the dry skin problem. The youthful elasticity of the skin is lost,

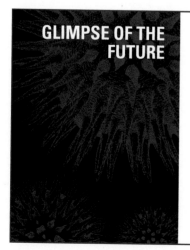
GLIMPSE OF THE FUTURE

Skin Conditions and Psychosomatic Disorders

Many skin conditions have a psychosomatic origin. The skin and the brain interact in a variety of ways. Some behaviors can cause or aggravate skin conditions. Psychotropic drugs can be beneficial in treating some of these disorders. Treatment of the underlying psychiatric condition often results in improvement of the skin condition. The difficult issue is diagnosing the problem in the first place. At times, it is hard to determine whether a skin disease is caused by or is being enhanced by an underlying psychiatric problem. Further research to find better ways to diagnose the cause of the skin problem is needed. In the future, better tests might result in finding the psychological cause for a variety of skin conditions.

Source: Shenefelt (2011).

causing wrinkles and an aged appearance. If the individual has spent a great deal of time in the sun over the years, these problems will be exaggerated. The nails become thicker and might be difficult to trim. The hair becomes thinner and brittle. There might be extensive hair loss and graying.

Skin lesions are common in older people. Keratoses and skin cancers are the most common problems, especially in individuals who have been exposed to sunlight for many years without using protection (Figure 18–48). Seborrheic dermatitis (also called senile keratosis), rosacea, and psoriasis are frequently seen disorders. Older adults with chronic disorders such as diabetes or peripheral vascular diseases are particularly prone to develop skin problems, especially pressure injuries. Older adults are also more likely to experience burn or cold injuries because they have decreased touch sensation.

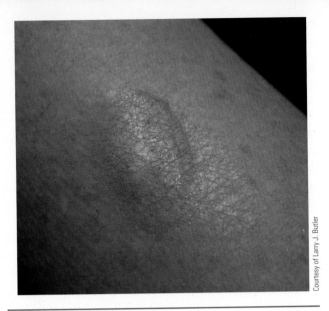

Courtesy of Larry J. Butler

FIGURE 18–48   Senile keratosis.

SUMMARY

The skin is important in protecting the body from pathogens; in providing sensations of touch, heat, and cold; and in regulating body temperature. There are numerous skin conditions, some of which are manifestations of other body system diseases. Skin problems are very traumatic to the individual because they affect appearance and can cause extreme discomfort. Skin diseases range from mild to severe and from acute to chronic. Treatment for many of the skin conditions is symptomatic. Changes in the integumentary system in the older adult cause dry skin; thick, brittle nails; and gray, thinning hair. Older people are at increased risk for secondary skin disorders related to other system diseases.

REVIEW QUESTIONS

Short Answer

1. What is the main function of the integumentary system?

2. What are the most common symptoms of integumentary system disorders?

3. Which diagnostic tests are used to diagnose integumentary system disorders?

Matching

4. Match the skin condition in the left column with its description in the right column.

_____ Herpes

_____ Verruca

_____ Folliculitis

_____ Erysipelas

_____ Tinea

_____ Scabies

_____ Eczema

_____ Psoriasis

_____ Scleroderma

a. A form of cellulitis commonly involving the face

b. A chronic autoimmune disorder characterized by hardening and thickening of the skin and connective tissue

c. A condition caused by a tiny mite that burrows into the skin

d. An inflammation and infection of the hair follicle

e. A viral disease characterized by inflammation and fluid-filled blisters

f. A chronic skin condition characterized by red, raised lesions with distinct borders and silvery scales

g. A condition caused by papillomavirus that affects the keratin cells, causing hypertrophy

h. An inflammation of the skin also known as atopic dermatitis

i. A group of contagious fungal diseases of the skin

True or False

5. T F Genital warts are a sexually transmitted disease.

6. T F Carbuncles are most commonly caused by *Staphylococcus* bacteria.

7. T F Pediculosis is an infestation of lice.

8. T F Tinea capitis is also known as jock itch because it is located in the groin area.

9. T F Comedones are plugged skin pores found in cases of acne.

10. T F A port wine stain is a type of erythema found on the neck or trunk of the body.

11. T F An avulsion is a traumatic crushing injury, often caused by heavy objects dropped on parts of the body such as the fingers.

12. T F Skin cancer is the most common type of cancer diagnosed in individuals.

13. T F Radiation injury can be caused by ionizing radiation such as X-rays and by sunlight.

14. T F In burn injuries, the amount of body surface burned generally correlates with the chance of survival of the affected individual.

15. T F Third-degree burns, also called partial-thickness burns, involve the epidermis and dermis.

16. T F Cold thermal injury is usually more severe or life-threatening than heat or burn injuries.

17. T F In the aging process, the elasticity of the skin is lost, causing wrinkles and an aged appearance only if the individual has had constant exposure to sunlight over the years.

CASE STUDIES

■ Jenny Johnson is a 21-year-old college student who has vitiligo. She has some patchy areas on her legs and just a few on her arms. She visits the health clinic on campus where you work to talk about treatment for the disorder. What options are available for her? Is vitiligo detrimental to her overall health? What can you tell her about the progression of the problem? Where might she find out more information about her disorder?

■ Mrs. Moore is a 54-year-old school teacher who has been diagnosed with psoriasis. At the present time, she has a few patches on her arms and legs but not an extensive amount. She asks you to give her more information about the disorder. She wants to know whether it will get worse, if it will eventually heal, what she can do to relieve the symptoms, whether it is contagious, whether it is genetic, and what might cause it to get worse. How would you answer her questions? How much information should you give Mrs. Moore? Where might you refer her for more information? What is her long-term prognosis?

Study Tools

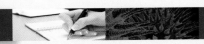

Workbook

Complete Chapter 18

Online Resources

PowerPoint® presentations

Animation

BIBLIOGRAPHY

Andersen, R. J., Campoli, J., Johar, S. K., Schumacher, K. A., & Allison, E. (2011). Suspected brown recluse envenomation: A case report and review of different treatment modalities. *Journal of Emergency Medicine 41*(2), e31–e37.

Auwaerter, P. G., Bakken, J. S., Dattwyler, R., Dumler, J., Halperin, J. J., McSweegan, E., & Wormser, G. P. (2011). Scientific evidence and best patient care practices should guide the ethics of Lyme disease activism. *Journal of Medical Ethics 37*(2), 68–73.

Bilotti, E., Gleason, C. L., & McNeill, A. (2011). Routine health maintenance in patients living with multiple myeloma. *Clinical Journal of Oncology Nursing Supplement 15*(5), S25–S40.

Centers for Disease Control and Prevention. (2009). Outline for health care associated infection surveillance. *www.cdc.gov/ncidod/* (accessed September 2012).

Coping with cold sores. (2011). *Consumer Reports on Health 23*(4), 10.

Dummer, R., Goldinger, S., Cozzio, A., French, L., & Karpova, M. (2012). Cutaneous lymphomas: Molecular pathways leading to new drugs. *Journal of Investigative Dermatology 132*(3 part 1), 517–525.

Earl, T. J. (2010). Cardiac manifestations of Lyme disease. *Medicine & Health Rhode Island 93*(11), 339–341.

Fuschiotti, P. (2011). Role of IL-13 in systemic sclerosis. *Cytokine 56*(3), 544–549.

Gannon, M., Underhill, M., Wellik, K. E., & Strickland, C. G. (2011). Which oral antibiotics are best for acne? *Journal of Family Practice 60*(5), 290–292.

Goldberg, J. L., Dabade, T. S., Davis, S. A., Feldman, S. R., Krowchuk, D. P., & Fleischer, A. B. (2011). Changing age of acne vulgaris visits: Another sign of earlier puberty? *Pediatric Dermatology 8*(6), 645–648.

Herbal medicines. (2011). *Reactions Weekly* June 11(1355), 20.

How to get rid of warts. (2011). *Harvard Women's Health Watch 19*(2), 2–4.

Isbister, G. K., & Hui Wen, F. (2011). Spider bite. *Lancet 378*(9808), 2039–2047.

It's time to really get the ticks off. (2010). *Harvard Health Letter 35*(6), 4–5.

Krishna, S., & Miller, L. (2012). Innate and adaptive immune responses against *Staphylococcus aureus* skin infections. *Seminars in Immunopathology 34*(2), 261–280.

Liu, Z., Sun, J., Smith, M., Smith, L., & Warr, R. (2012). Unsupervised sub-segmentation for pigmented skin lesions. *Skin Research & Technology 18*(1), 77–87.

Mashta, O. (2010). Beneath the surface. *Nursing Standard 25*(9), 24–25.

Monroe, J. R. (2011). Derma diagnosis. *Clinician Reviews 21*(4), 33.

Ning, S., Li, F., Qian, L., Xu, D., Huang, Y., Xiao, M., & Li, Y. (2012). The successful treatment of flat warts with auricular acupuncture. *International Journal of Dermatology 51*(2), 211–215.

Pareek, A., Suthar, M., Rathore, G. S., & Bansal, V. (2011). Feverfew (*Tanacetum parthenium* L.): A systematic review. *Pharmacognosy Reviews 5*(9), 103–110.

Reed, K. B., Cook-Norris, R. H., & Brewer, J. D. (2012). The cutaneous manifestations of metastatic malignant melanoma. *International Journal of Dermatology 51*(3), 243–249.

Reich, K. K. (2012). The concept of psoriasis as a systemic inflammation: Implications for disease management. *Journal of the European Academy of Dermatology & Venereology Supplement 26*, S3–S11.

Reuter, J., Merfort, I., & Schempp, C. M. (2010). Botanicals in dermatology. *American Journal of Clinical Dermatology 11*(4), 247–267.

Rice, J. (2012). New treatments slow deadly skin cancer. *Discover 33*(1), 68.

Roman, R. A. (2011). Immunotherapy for advanced melanoma. *Clinical Journal of Oncology Nursing, 15*(5), E58–E65.

Scalone, L., Watson, V., Ryan, M., Kotsopoulos, N., & Patel, R. (2011). Evaluation of patients' preferences for genital herpes treatment. *Sexually Transmitted Diseases 38*(9), 802–807.

Shenefelt, P. D. (2011). Psychodermatological disorders: Recognition and treatment. *International Journal of Dermatology 50*(11), 1309–1322.

Simpler cold-sore relief. (2003). *Consumer Reports on Health 15*(8), 7.

Uitto, J., Christiano, A., McLean, W., & McGrath, J. (2012). Novel molecular therapies for heritable skin disorders. *Journal of Investigative Dermatology 132*(3 part 2), 820–828.

Worried about warts? (2012). *Harvard Men's Health Watch 16*(6), 7.

Yarnell, E., Abascal, K., & Rountree R. (2009). Herbs for herpes simplex infections. *Alternative & Complementary Therapies 15*(2), 69–74.

Yellow card report indicates risk of serious side effects with TCM. (2011). *Reactions Weekly August 20*(1365), 4.

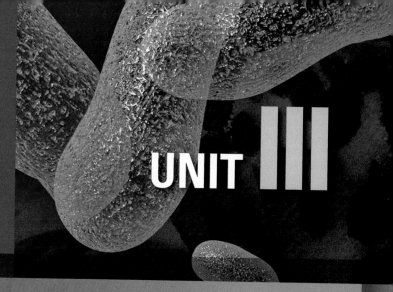

UNIT **III**

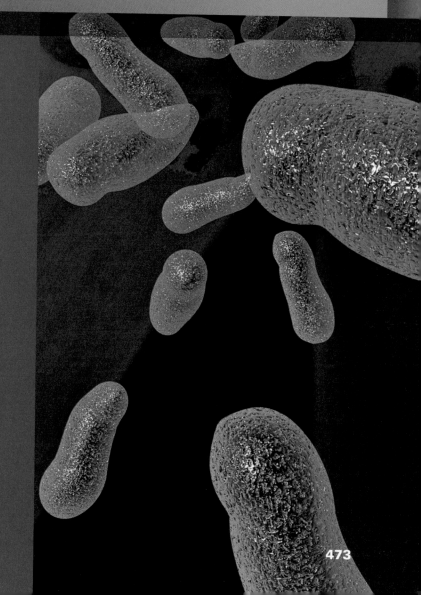

Genetic and Developmental, Childhood, and Mental Health Diseases and Disorders

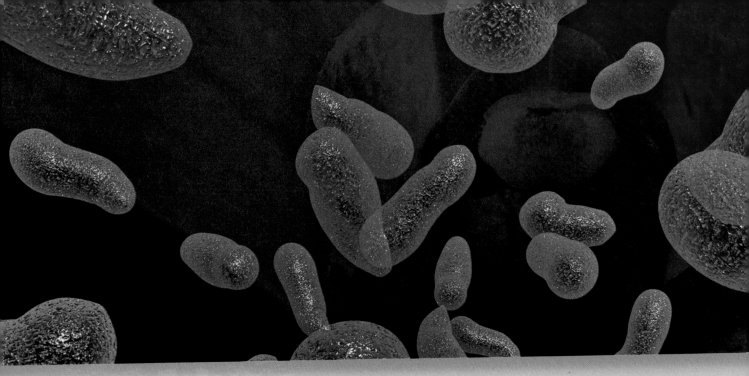

OUTLINE

KEY TERMS

Alleles (p. 477)
Atresia (p. 488)
Auscultation (p. 485)
Autosomes (p. 476)
Buccal smear (p. 476)
Congenital anomaly (p. 480)
Dominant (p. 477)
Epicanthus (p. 495)
Exocrine (p. 494)
Gene (p. 476)
Genotypes (p. 477)
Germ cells (p. 476)
Heterozygous (p. 477)
Homozygous (p. 477)
Karyotyping (p. 476)
Meiosis (p. 476)
Microcephaly (p. 495)
Mitosis (p. 476)
Murmurs (p. 485)
Phenotype (p. 477)
Pyloromyotomy (p. 490)
Recessive (p. 477)
Somatic (p. 476)
Stricture (p. 487)
Viscous (p. 494)

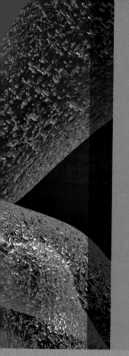

19

Genetic and Developmental Diseases and Disorders

LEARNING OBJECTIVES

Upon completion of the chapter, the learner should be able to:

1. Define the terminology common to genetic and developmental disorders.
2. Identify the important signs and symptoms associated with genetic and developmental disorders.
3. Describe the common diagnostics used to determine the type and cause of genetic or developmental disorders.
4. Identify the common genetic and developmental disorders.
5. Describe the typical course and management of the common genetic and developmental disorders.

OVERVIEW

Genetic and developmental disorders can first appear or be diagnosed at any age throughout the life span. Some are readily diagnosed at birth; others do not display symptoms until childhood, adolescence, or adulthood. Although some disorders have relatively few symptoms, others are profoundly disabling and can even result in early death. In disorders such as cystic fibrosis or Tay–Sachs disease, genetic testing can inform an individual of whether he or she is a carrier of the disease. There are many other disorders, however, for which testing is not yet available. ■

ANATOMY AND PHYSIOLOGY

The nucleus of each cell of the normal body has 46 chromosomes or 23 pairs of chromosomes. Most **somatic** (body) cells can reproduce in a process called **mitosis** (mi-TOE-sis), during which the 46 chromosomes duplicate and divide into two identical daughter cells, each containing 46 chromosomes (Figure 19–1).

Germ cells become haploid cells through a process called **meiosis** (my-OH-sis) that results in each cell carrying only half the number of chromosomes: 23 chromosomes (see Figure 19–1). The most common haploid cells are the ova and sperm cells.

Meiosis is necessary to maintain the normal 46 chromosomes in a newly formed individual. When an ovum (carrying 23 chromosomes) is fertilized with a sperm (carrying 23 chromosomes), the newly formed individual will have a combined total of the normal 46 chromosomes. Half of these, or 23 chromosomes, will have come from each parent.

Of the 46 chromosomes each individual cell possesses, 44 chromosomes, or 22 pairs, determine somatic or body function and are called **autosomes** (auto = self, somes = body). One pair (or two chromosomes) are sex chromosomes and determine the sex of the individual.

Normal females have XX chromosomes as the sex chromosome, and males have XY chromosomes. A female germ cell, or ovum, undergoes meiosis and divides into two separate X chromosomes; thus, the only chromosome a female can give is an X, or female, chromosome. Male germ cells, or sperm, undergo meiosis and divide into two separate chromosomes, one X and one Y, so the male can give an X (female) or Y (male) chromosome. This explains why the male partner, or sperm, determines the sex of the fetus.

If an X sperm combines with the ova, the result is XX, and the fetus is female. If a Y sperm combines with the ova, the result is XY, and the fetus is male. Because each male germ cell division results in one X and one Y, there is a 50/50 chance of the fetus being male or female. These two chromosomes, the sex chromosomes, are in every cell of the body and are responsible for directing the activity of the cell specifically for a female or for a male.

Chromosomes can be visualized by a process known as **karyotyping** (CARE-ee-oh-TYPE-ing), which involves taking a picture of a cell during mitosis, arranging the chromosome pairs in order of largest to smallest, and numbering them 1 through 23.

Sex chromosomes can be evaluated by a simple **buccal smear**, performed by obtaining squamous epithelial cells from the buccal cavity of the mouth, staining the cell, and microscopically observing for X chromosomes called Barr bodies. Barr bodies can be visualized when two X chromosomes are present (female). If there is no Barr body, the individual is male.

X chromosomes are much larger than Y chromosomes and carry more genetic information. The X chromosome not only carries genes for female characteristics but also for other genes essential to life, such as those for blood formation, various activities of metabolism, and immunity. The Y chromosome carries only the genes related to maleness and masculinity.

Chromosomes are made of ultramicroscopic units of deoxyribonucleic acid (DNA) arranged in a specific order, each of which is called a **gene**. Each chromosome is composed of thousands of genes located at specific positions in the chromosome.

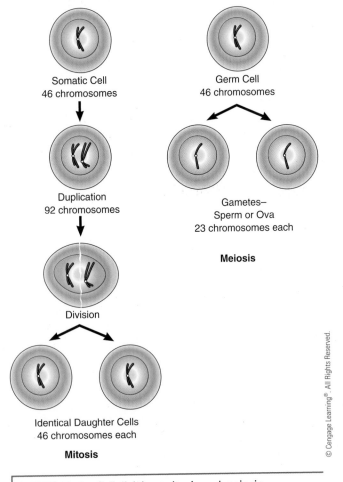

Somatic Cell
46 chromosomes

Duplication
92 chromosomes

Division

Identical Daughter Cells
46 chromosomes each

Mitosis

Germ Cell
46 chromosomes

Gametes—
Sperm or Ova
23 chromosomes each

Meiosis

FIGURE 19–1 Cell division: mitosis and meiosis.

When the chromosomes (one from each parent) pair up during fertilization of the egg, the genes on the chromosomes align and are called **alleles** (ah-LEELS). This matched gene pair determines heredity or, in other words, expresses those characteristics inherited from parents. When one thinks of genes and heredity, we usually think of facial features such as hair and eye color, but genes also determine the entire physical makeup of the individual from the length of toes to the color and texture of skin.

As discussed in previous chapters, heredity is thought to play a part in many other processes such as the development of plaque in arteries and the occurrence of rheumatic fever, obesity, and alcoholism in families, to name only a few.

To understand basic heredity, one must look at individual **genotypes**—the genetic pattern of the individual. Each gene in an allele or matched pair of genes can be **dominant** (in control) or **recessive** (lacking control). Dominant genotypes are expressed with a capital letter (B, for example), whereas recessive genotypes are expressed with a small letter (b, for example).

If the alleles, or genes in a pair, match, such as BB or bb, they are said to be **homozygous** (homo = one,

zygo = yoked or paired). If the alleles do not match, such as Bb, they are **heterozygous** (hetero = different, zygo = yoked or paired).

Expression of a trait such as brown hair or blue eyes is called **phenotype**. Generally speaking, homozygous alleles, whether dominant or recessive, will always express the trait. Heterozygous pairs will express the phenotype of the dominant gene only. Heterozygous pairs are often said to be carriers of recessive disorders because the recessive trait will not be expressed unless paired with another recessive gene (Figure 19–2).

Abnormalities can be due to chromosomal, genetic, or environmental factors or a combination of these. Chromosomal disorders are usually related to the number or placement of the chromosome. Chromosomes can fail to separate properly during cell division, causing one daughter cell to have an extra chromosome and the other daughter cell to have none.

Abnormal number or structure of autosomal (or body) chromosomes is usually incompatible with life. These chromosomes carry a large number of essential genes, and such major chromosomal abnormalities usually lead to spontaneous abortion of the fetus.

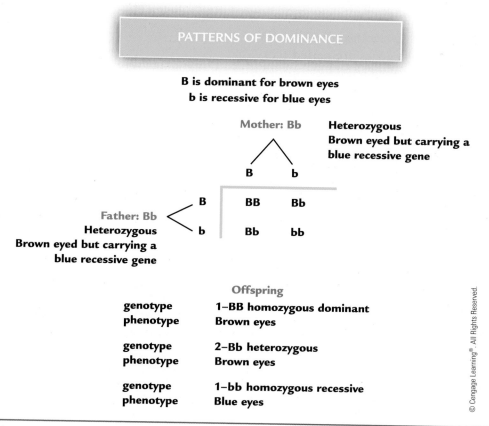

PATTERNS OF DOMINANCE

B is dominant for brown eyes
b is recessive for blue eyes

Mother: Bb   Heterozygous
Brown eyed but carrying a
blue recessive gene

	B	b
B	BB	Bb
b	Bb	bb

Father: Bb
Heterozygous
Brown eyed but carrying a
blue recessive gene

Offspring

| genotype | 1–BB homozygous dominant |
| phenotype | Brown eyes |

| genotype | 2–Bb heterozygous |
| phenotype | Brown eyes |

| genotype | 1–bb homozygous recessive |
| phenotype | Blue eyes |

FIGURE 19–2   Patterns of dominance.

The most common autosomal chromosomal disorder is Down syndrome.

An abnormal number of chromosomes in the sex chromosomes is less serious but does lead to a number of abnormalities, disorders that are not usually apparent until puberty, when sexual characteristics are found to be abnormal.

An individual can acquire an abnormal gene in two ways: (1) by mutation of the gene during meiosis, affecting the newly formed fetus, or (2) by passage of the abnormal gene from the parents (heredity).

Genetic disorders are passed to offspring in four ways: autosomal dominant, autosomal recessive, sex-linked dominant, and sex-linked recessive.

1. **Autosomal dominant** Dominant disorders are easily recognized because presence of the disorder identifies those individuals with the dominant gene. The line of inheritance is easily followed from one generation to another.

   Dominant genes will always be expressed, whether homozygous (PP) or heterozygous (Pp). An example of an autosomal dominant disorder is polydactyly, evidenced by an excessive number of fingers or toes. Refer to Figure 19–3 to see how individuals carrying a dominant gene (P) would have polydactyly.

2. **Autosomal recessive** Recessive disorders are seen only when two recessive genes are paired (cc). Cystic fibrosis is an autosomal recessive disorder.

Each parent might be phenotypically normal or without sign of the disorder but be a heterozygous carrier (Cc) of the disorder. If each parent is heterozygous, the chance of the offspring having the disorder is one in four (Figure 19–4A). If one parent has the disorder (cc), the chances increase to one in two (Figure 19–4B). If one parent is homozygous dominant (CC), none of the offspring will be affected (Figure 19–4C).

The occurrence of recessive disorders is often quite surprising to a family because this disorder can skip generations and hundreds of years before it is paired with another recessive gene and expressed.

3. **Sex-linked dominant** Like autosomal dominant disorders, these are rarer than the recessive disorders and are easily recognized.

4. **Sex-linked recessive** These disorders are typically carried by females and passed to males. The

---

AUTOSOMAL RECESSIVE PATTERN

Genotype	Phenotype
cc (affected)	cystic fibrosis
CC	normal
Cc (carrier)	normal

Mother
Normal (carrier)

		C	c
Father **C**		**CC**	**Cc**
Normal (carrier) **c**		**Cc**	cc

Offspring

| genotype | 1–CC homozygous dominant |
| phenotype | **Normal** |

| genotype | 2–Cc heterozygous (carrier) |
| phenotype | **Normal** |

| genotype | 1–cc homozygous recessive |
| phenotype | **Cystic fibrosis** |

If both parents are heterozygous, there is a 1 in 4 chance of having a child with cystic fibrosis.

(A)

AUTOSOMAL DOMINANT PATTERN

Polydactyly is dominant (P)
Normal finger number is recessive (p)

Normal mother

		p	p
Polydactyly father **P**		**Pp**	**Pp**
	P	**Pp**	**Pp**

Offspring

| genotype (all 4) | **heterozygous** |
| phenotype | **polydactyly** |

FIGURE 19–3 Autosomal dominant pattern.

FIGURE 19–4 Autosomal recessive pattern.

AUTOSOMAL RECESSIVE PATTERN

Genotype	Phenotype
cc (affected)	cystic fibrosis
CC	normal
Cc (carrier)	normal

Mother
Normal (carrier)

		C	**c**
Father	**c**	**Cc**	**cc**
Has			
cystic fibrosis	**c**	**Cc**	**cc**

Offspring

genotype	2–Cc heterozygous (carrier)
phenotype	**Normal**

genotype	2–cc homozygous recessive
phenotype	**Cystic fibrosis**

If one parent has the disorder, the chances of having a child with cystic fibrosis increase to 1 in 2.

(B)

AUTOSOMAL RECESSIVE PATTERN

Genotype	Phenotype
cc (affected)	cystic fibrosis
CC	normal
Cc (carrier)	normal

Mother
Normal (carrier)

		C	**c**
Father	**C**	**CC**	**Cc**
Normal			
(homozygous	**C**	**CC**	**Cc**
dominant)			

Offspring

genotype	2–CC homozygous dominant
phenotype	**Normal**

genotype	2–Cc heterozygous (carrier)
phenotype	**Normal**

If one parent is homozygous dominant, none of the offspring will be affected.

(C)

FIGURE 19–4 Autosomal recessive pattern (continued).

reason for this is that recessive gene disorders on the X chromosome of the female are overridden by the dominance of the normal gene on the other X chromosome.

In males, the X disorder is expressed because there is no corresponding gene on the Y chromosome. X-linked disorders usually appear every other generation because they are passed from mother to son (Figure 19–5). The affected male (son) will pass this disorder to all of his daughters, who then become carriers.

The affected male is unable to pass this disorder to his sons because the male gives a Y chromosome to sons, not an X. All the carrier daughters can then pass the disorder to their sons. If the mother is a carrier (XX Hh), there is a possibility that some of her sons will not be affected. If the mother has the disorder (XX hh), which is very rare with X-linked disorders, all her sons will have the disorder. Hemophilia and muscular dystrophy are both sex-linked recessive disorders.

SEX-LINKED RECESSIVE PATTERN

Hemophilia is recessive X linked

X and Y are chromosomes

H and h are dominant and recessive genes
found only on the X chromosome

Mother
Normal (carrier)

		XH	**Xh**
	Yo	**XHYo**	**XhYo**
Father		boy	boy
Normal		normal	hemophiliac
	XH	**XHXH**	**XHXh**
		girl	girl
		normal	normal (carrier)

FIGURE 19–5 Sex-linked recessive pattern.

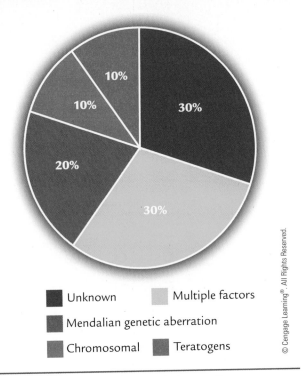

Legend:
- Unknown
- Multiple factors
- Mendalian genetic aberration
- Chromosomal
- Teratogens

FIGURE 19–6 Causes of congenital anomalies.

Approximately 2% of all newborns have a significant birth defect, or **congenital** (kon-JEN-ih-tahl; present at birth) **anomaly** (ah-NOM-ah-lee; abnormality). A high percentage of defects (60%) are due to an unknown cause.

Other causes are genetic (20%), chromosomal (10%), and teratogens (ter-AT-oh-gens) or environmental (10%) (Figure 19–6). Chromosomal and genetic causes have been discussed. Teratogens include any chemical, substance, or exposure that can cause a physical defect in a fetus during pregnancy. Teratogens are commonly thought of as environmental causes and include maternal radiation, infection, metabolic disorders, smoking, alcohol, drugs, and medications, to name only a few.

■ COMMON SIGNS AND SYMPTOMS

Signs and symptoms of the various genetic and developmental disorders vary, depending on the disorder, and are discussed individually with each disorder.

■ DIAGNOSTIC TESTS

Diagnosis of many of the genetic and developmental disorders begins with a physical examination of the affected individual. Diagnostic tests for these disorders

vary, depending on the disorder, and are discussed individually with each disorder. Prenatal diagnosis of genetic and developmental disorders is beneficial for genetic and family counseling. Tests to diagnose prenatal disorders include:

- Ultrasonography of the fetus to detect malformations of the head, internal organs, and extremities.
- Amniotic fluid analysis to determine genetic and chromosomal disorders.
- Maternal blood analysis to observe for abnormal fetal substances.

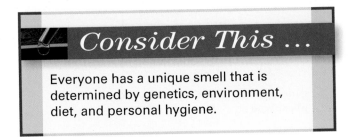

Consider This ...

Everyone has a unique smell that is determined by genetics, environment, diet, and personal hygiene.

■ COMMON GENETIC AND DEVELOPMENTAL DISORDERS

There are hundreds of genetic and developmental disorders among populations; however, most of them occur very rarely.

Genetic or developmental disorders might affect only one body system or involve several systems. Muscular dystrophy, for example, which affects the musculoskeletal system, can also be considered a neurologic system disease because it affects the neurons, thereby affecting muscle movement.

Some of the more familiar genetic and developmental disorders are covered in this chapter.

Musculoskeletal

Genetic and developmental musculoskeletal disorders are some of the more familiar severe disorders. The severity of the disease varies with the particular disorder and other problems the individual has.

MUSCULAR DYSTROPHY

■ **DESCRIPTION.** Muscular dystrophy (MD) (dys = abnormal, trophic = nourishment, growth) is a group of genetically inherited diseases characterized by progressive degeneration, or weakening, of the muscles. The affected muscles are unable to store needed protein. Malnourished muscle fibers die and are replaced with fat and connective tissue. These fibers are unable to contract and function like muscle fibers. Over a period of time, the muscle digresses from weak to useless.

■ **DESCRIPTION.** The most common type of MD is Duchenne's MD, also called pseudohypertrophic (pseudo = false, hyper = excessive, trophic = nourishment, growth) MD. The affected muscles appear healthy and bulging when, in reality, they are bulking up in size from fat deposits. This bulking of muscle mass is especially noticeable in the calf muscle.

■ **ETIOLOGY.** Duchenne's MD is a sex-linked disorder generally passed from mother to son.

■ **SYMPTOMS.** Onset is usually between the ages of 2 and 5 years. The pelvic and leg muscles are usually affected first, leading to a characteristic waddling gait, toe walking, lordosis, and Gower's maneuver (a characteristic way of getting up from a squatting position that demonstrates the weakness of the pelvic muscles) (Figure 19–7).

Affected children are usually confined to a wheelchair by age 9. Life expectancy is usually in the late teens or early 20s, with death due to respiratory or cardiac complications.

■ **DIAGNOSIS.** Diagnosis is made on the basis of physical examination, muscle biopsy, and electromyography.

■ **TREATMENT.** Although there is no cure for MD, physical therapy, orthopedic appliances such as leg braces, and exercise are quite effective in maintaining mobility and quality of life.

■ **PREVENTION.** There are no preventive measures other than genetic counseling.

CONGENITAL HIP DISLOCATION (CHD)

■ **DESCRIPTION.** CHD is an abnormality of the hip joint, or acetabulum, resulting in the femoral head, or ball, slipping out of the normal position. CHD is more common in girls and is usually obvious during the first few months of life.

■ **ETIOLOGY.** It is thought that this disorder occurs as a result of (1) improper positioning of the fetus in the uterus prior to or during birth or (2) the maternal hormones, which relax the mother's pelvic ligaments during labor, also relaxing the joint ligaments in the infant.

■ **SYMPTOMS.** The affected infant might exhibit asymmetrical folds of the affected thigh, a difference in leg length, and limited abduction, called a positive Ortolani's sign (Figure 19–8).

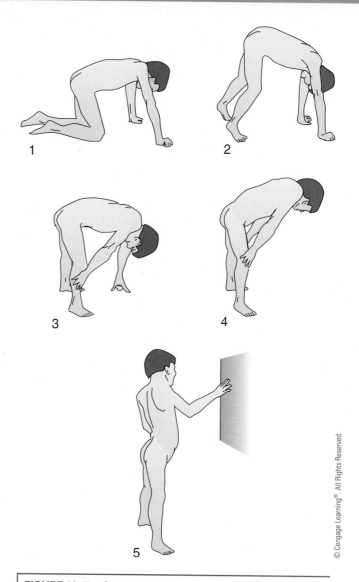

FIGURE 19–7 Gower's maneuver.

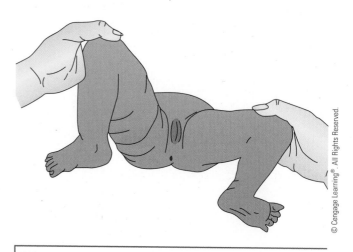

FIGURE 19–8 Asymmetrical thigh folds and Ortolani's sign in congenital hip dislocation.

■ **DIAGNOSIS.** Diagnosis is confirmed by physical examination and hip joint X-ray studies.

■ **TREATMENT.** Treatment involves closed reduction (placing the femoral head in proper position) and maintaining the normal position with a splint or cast for approximately 2 to 3 months. Treatment might require surgery in older children. The earlier the treatment is begun, the better the prognosis.

■ **PREVENTION.** Prevention is aimed at prenatal care to determine the position of the baby in the womb to assess and treat for possible CHD. The practice of swaddling, or wrapping the baby's body tightly in a blanket with legs forced into a closed, straight-together position, can lead to CHD. This position places undue stress on the hip joints.

CLUBFOOT (TALIPES EQUINOVARUS)

■ **DESCRIPTION.** Clubfoot, or talipes (talus = ankle, pes = foot) equinovarus (TAL-eh-peas ee-KWI-no-VAY-rus; equine = horse or toe walking, similar to a horse, varus = bent inward), is a frequently occurring congenital deformity of the foot.

■ **ETIOLOGY.** The cause of clubfoot is unknown, but it is thought to be due to genetic factors or fetal position in the uterus. Some positional deformities can be straightened with manipulation, but a true clubfoot deformity will not straighten with manipulation.

■ **SYMPTOMS.** The affected foot or feet turn inward with the toes pointed downward and the heel drawn upward (Figure 19–9).

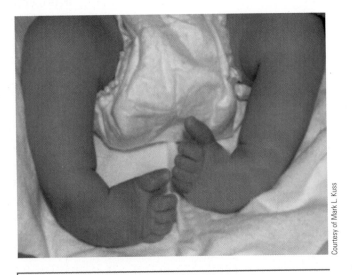

FIGURE 19–9   Talipes equinovarus (clubfoot).

Courtesy of Mark L. Kuss

■ **DIAGNOSIS.** Clubfoot is easily diagnosed with physical examination. X-rays help determine the severity of the disorder.

■ **TREATMENT.** Treatment, quite successful if begun during infancy, can involve application of a cast or splints to straighten the foot gradually. The cast or splints are changed frequently until the desired position is achieved. If casting and splinting do not achieve the desired results, surgery might be indicated. Attention must be given to the position of the child's feet throughout childhood to ensure that normal position is maintained.

■ **PREVENTION.** There are no known preventive measures.

OSTEOGENESIS IMPERFECTA

■ **DESCRIPTION.** Osteogenesis (osteo = bone, genesis = beginning) imperfecta (not perfect or normal) is characterized by abnormally brittle bones, often leading to frequent fractures.

■ **ETIOLOGY.** Osteogenesis imperfecta is an inherited condition caused by gene mutation.

■ **SYMPTOMS.** Undiagnosed children affected with osteogenesis imperfecta might be suspected as victims of child abuse due to the frequency of bone fractures. Other significant signs are an abnormally blue coloration of the sclera of the eyes, otosclerotic deafness, translucent skin, and thin dental enamel of the teeth.

■ **DIAGNOSIS.** Diagnosis is made primarily with history and physical examination. X-rays of the bones can be helpful.

■ **TREATMENT.** There is no cure for osteogenesis imperfecta, but the tendency of bones to fracture decreases with age and often disappears by adulthood.

■ **PREVENTION.** There are no preventive measures for osteogenesis imperfecta.

Neurologic

Genetic and developmental neurologic disorders are some of the most severe because of their long-term debilitating effects. Two of the most common severe disorders in this category are hydrocephalus and cerebral palsy.

HYDROCEPHALUS

■ **DESCRIPTION.** Hydrocephalus (high-droh-SEF-ah-lus; hydro = water, cephal = brain) is an abnormal accumulation of cerebrospinal fluid in the brain.

■ **ETIOLOGY.** Hydrocephalus is generally caused by obstruction of the flow of cerebrospinal fluid out of the brain, which can be from a congenital defect, an infection, or a tumor.

■ **SYMPTOMS.** The head of the affected child might be normal at birth but will rapidly enlarge over the first few months of life as the fluid accumulates. The brain tissue becomes compressed, and the skull begins to bulge. Other signs include bulging eyes, a tight scalp, prominent head veins, and a shrill, high-pitched cry. The infant is unable to lift its head, fails to develop normally, and is mentally challenged.

■ **DIAGNOSIS.** Diagnosis is confirmed with skull X-rays and angiography.

■ **TREATMENT.** Treatment of choice is surgical correction by placing a shunt from the brain to the peritoneal cavity or right atrium of the heart to drain the excess fluid (Figure 19–10). Even with early surgical intervention, the prognosis is guarded. Mortality rate is high without surgical correction.

■ **PREVENTION.** There are no preventive measures.

CEREBRAL PALSY

■ **DESCRIPTION.** Cerebral palsy (CP) (SER-ehbral PAWL-zee) is a congenital bilateral paralysis that results from inadequate blood or oxygen supply to the brain during fetal development, during the birthing process, or in infancy. CP is the most common crippler of children and more often affects premature infants and males.

■ **ETIOLOGY.** Causes of CP include maternal rubella, toxemia, birthing difficulties such as prolonged labor, anoxia, hypoxemia, asphyxia from the umbilical cord being wrapped around the infant's neck, head trauma, and meningitis. Often, the cause of CP is unknown.

■ **SYMPTOMS.** This disorder usually affects motor or muscle performance and can be noticed if the infant has difficulty sucking or swallowing. Other complications include visual and hearing deficits, seizure activity, and mental challenges. CP is characterized by hyperactive reflexes, rapid muscle contraction, and muscle weakness. The affected child commonly has a scissors gait, exhibited by toe walking and crossing one foot over the other with each step.

■ **DIAGNOSIS.** Diagnosis is based on clinical symptoms including posture, oral motor patterns, strabismus, muscle tone, postural reaction, and tendon reflexes.

■ **TREATMENT.** There is no cure for CP. Treatment involves physical therapy, speech therapy, orthopedic casting, braces, and, often, surgery to help the child reach full potential. Anticonvulsant and muscle relaxant medications also can be beneficial.

■ **PREVENTION.** There are no preventive measures.

SPINA BIFIDA

■ **DESCRIPTION.** Spina bifida (SPY-nah BIF-ih-dah), a neural tube defect (NTD), is a congenital disorder in which one or more of the vertebrae of the bony spinal column fails to close over the spinal cord, leaving an opening in the column. *Bifid* means split in two parts, which describes the vertebra in this condition. Development of the spinal cord and column occurs during the first trimester of pregnancy.

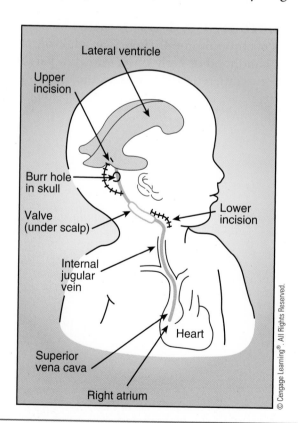

Lateral ventricle

Upper incision

Burr hole in skull

Valve (under scalp)

Internal jugular vein

Heart

Superior vena cava

Right atrium

Lower incision

FIGURE 19–10   A ventricle shunt drains spinal fluid in an infant with hydrocephalus.

■ **ETIOLOGY.** The cause of this malformation is unknown, but risk factors include maternal radiation, virus, and genetic factors. Children born with spina bifida are more often born to mothers who have other children with this defect. There are several other conditions that tend to accompany spina bifida, including hydrocephalus, cleft palate, and clubfoot. The several forms of spina bifida are illustrated in Figure 19–11 and described as follows:

- **Spina bifida occulta** The most common form of spina bifida. A spina bifida is present, but it is asymptomatic and hidden (occulta). Signs of the malformation often include a dimpling of the skin and a tuft of hair or port wine nevus on the skin surface above the defect.

- **Meningocele** Occurs when the meninges of the spinal cord protrude through the opening in the vertebral column, forming a fluid-filled sac on the skin surface. Because nerve tissue is not involved, the infant usually does not have neurologic problems.

- **Myelomeningocele** The most serious spina bifida because the meninges and a portion of the spinal cord protrude through the opening in the vertebral column, causing neurologic symptoms.

■ **SYMPTOMS.** Depending on the type and cause, common symptoms include skeletal malformation, deformed joints, paralysis of the legs, and bowel and bladder incontinence.

■ **DIAGNOSIS.** The condition is suspected in the presence of a skin defect over the spinal area along with muscular abnormalities in the legs and deformities of the feet. The diagnosis is confirmed by X-ray examination or myelography.

■ **TREATMENT.** Surgical intervention to correct the condition is usually performed in the first 24 hours of life. Additional procedures might be needed as the child grows. Some of these children are unable to walk and might die before the age of 2 or 3 years.

■ **PREVENTION.** There are no preventive methods, although there is a link between folic acid (a B vitamin) levels in pregnant women and major birth defects in the baby's brain and spine from NTDs. For this reason, women need to take folic acid every day, starting before they become pregnant, to help prevent NTDs.

HUNTINGTON'S DISEASE

■ **DESCRIPTION.** A progressive chorea (disorder characterized by involuntary muscle jerking) accompanied by increasing mental deterioration. Also known as Huntington's chorea.

■ **ETIOLOGY.** This disease is caused by a genetic defect of chromosome 4. There is an adult-onset type and a childhood or early-onset type. If a parent has the disease, there is a 50% chance the offspring will also have the defective gene and develop the disease at some time.

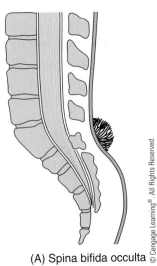 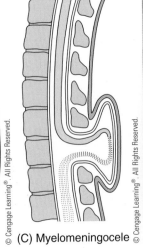 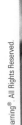 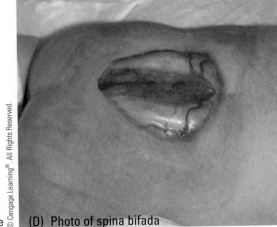

(A) Spina bifida occulta (B) Meningocele (C) Myelomeningocele (D) Photo of spina bifada

FIGURE 19–11 Types of spina bifida.

■ **SYMPTOMS.** Behavior changes are the most common symptoms. The person displays irritability, moodiness, restlessness, abnormal movements, unsteady gait, and an increasing dementia. Speech difficulties and tremors are also common.

■ **DIAGNOSIS.** The diagnosis is made based on scans, history, genetic testing, and symptoms.

■ **TREATMENT.** There is no cure for the disease, but some medications are prescribed to lessen the symptoms.

■ **PREVENTION.** There are no preventive measures other than known disease carriers not reproducing. (Huntington's disease is also discussed in Chapter 15, "Nervous System Diseases and Disorders.")

Cardiovascular

The heart and its related great vessels are the most common sites of congenital defects. The defects can be small or quite large, and consequences of these deformities can range from asymptomatic to life-threatening. Collectively, these malformations of heart structure are called congenital heart defects.

CONGENITAL HEART DEFECTS

■ **ETIOLOGY.** The cause of these defects is unknown, but a genetic tendency is strongly suspected. Certain risk factors include maternal rubella, poor maternal nutrition, smoking, and alcoholism.

■ **SYMPTOMS.** Symptoms of congenital heart defects can vary from mild cases that are asymptomatic to extreme conditions with symptoms of extreme cyanosis, breathing difficulties, and very audible heart murmurs.

■ **DIAGNOSIS.** Diagnosis is made by electrocardiogram and physical examination, including **auscultation** (listening to the chest with a stethoscope), which usually reveals heart **murmurs** (abnormal heart sounds) if present.

■ **TREATMENT.** Early diagnosis and surgical correction of these defects have improved drastically in recent years and have significantly reduced the mortality rate of infants born with heart defects.

■ **PREVENTION.** Controlling risk factors is the only preventive measure.

ATRIAL SEPTAL DEFECT

■ **DESCRIPTION.** Atrial septal defect is an opening between the right and left atria (Figure 19–12A), commonly due to the foramen ovale not closing at birth. The foramen ovale is a natural opening between the atria that allows blood to bypass the nonfunctional lungs during fetal life. After the infant is born, the act of breathing causes a change in chest cavity pressure that normally closes the foramen ovale. Atrial septal defects allow oxygenated blood to be pumped from the left atria to the right atria, which is again pumped to the right ventricle and to the lungs without ever

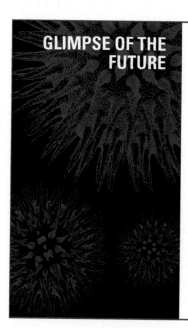

GLIMPSE OF THE FUTURE

New Treatment for Huntington's Disease

There are various cannabinoid-based medicines on the market today, and many more are being researched for potential treatment of different disorders or symptoms of diseases. Cannabinoids are the chemical components of cannabis or marijuana, such as THC. Some cannabinoid-based drugs were approved many years ago for treatment of nausea and vomiting occurring with chemotherapy treatments and eating disorders associated with acquired immunodeficiency syndrome (AIDS) patients. Recently, a new cannabinoid-based drug has been approved in some countries for the treatment of multiple sclerosis (not in the United States however). New research is looking at these preparations for other neurologic conditions like Huntington's disease. The cannabinoid-based drugs have analgesic and neurologic protective properties that show potential for helping patients with Huntington's disease. They also tend to lower some of the hyperkinetic (excessive movement) symptoms seen in the disease.

Source: Sagredo et al. (2012).

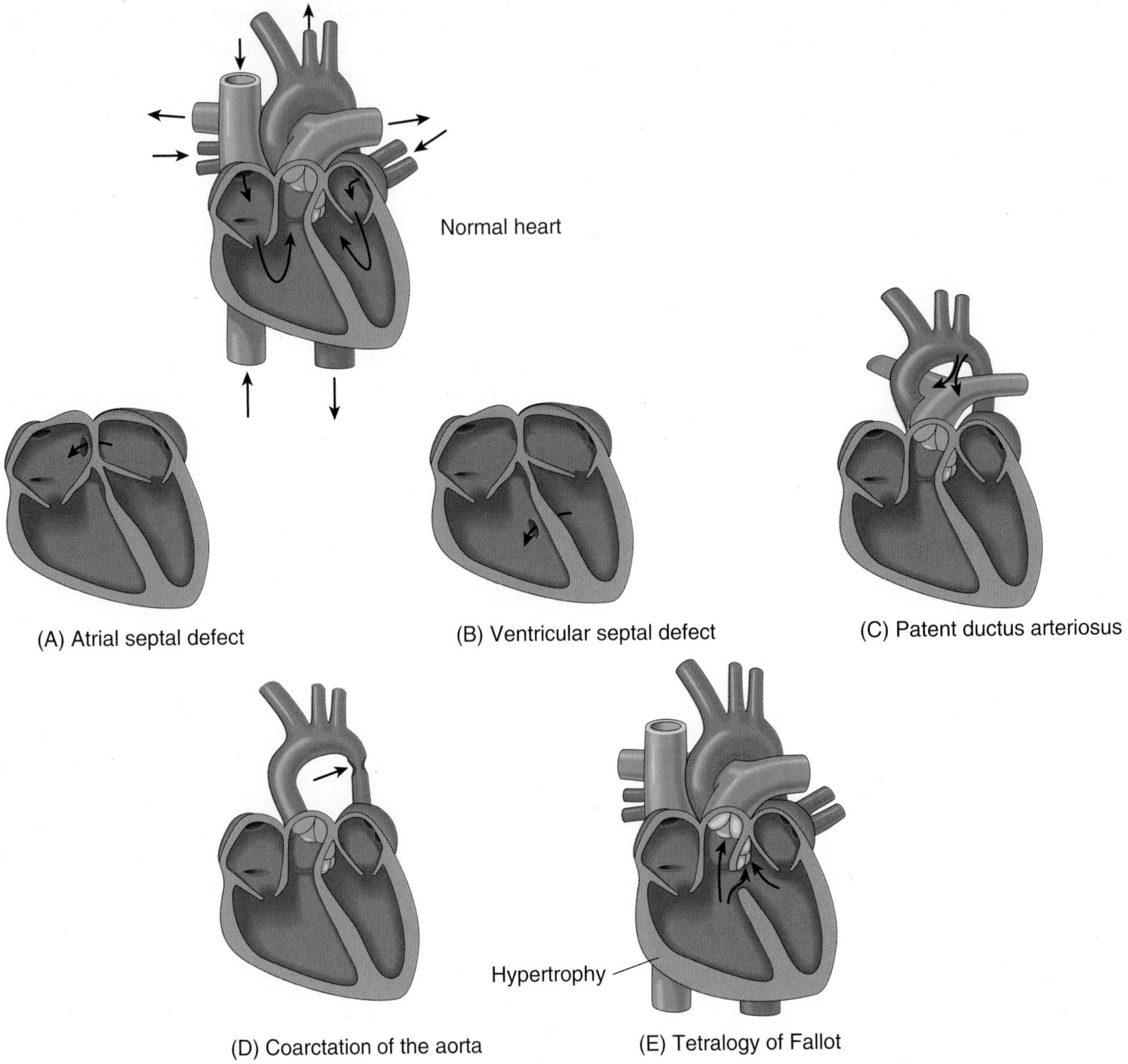

FIGURE 19-12   A normal heart and congenital heart defects (A–E).

circulating through the body. This repumping causes an increased workload on the right side of the heart. This defect occurs more commonly in girls than in boys.

VENTRICULAR SEPTAL DEFECT

■ **DESCRIPTION.** Ventricular septal defects are the most common heart defects, accounting for approximately 25% of all heart defects. As the name suggests, this defect is a hole between the right and left ventricle (Figure 19–12B) that allows blood from the left ventricle to flow into the right ventricle. Like the atrial septal defect, this oxygenated blood has to

be repumped, causing an increased workload on the right side of the heart.

PATENT DUCTUS ARTERIOSUS

■ **DESCRIPTION.** A ductus arteriosus is a connection between the pulmonary artery and the aorta of the normal fetal heart (Figure 19–12C) that allows blood to flow from the pulmonary artery to the aorta, thus bypassing the nonfunctional lungs. The ductus arteriosus, like the foramen ovale, normally closes off shortly after birth. If the structure does not close, or remains patent, the condition is called patent ductus arteriosus. With this condition, oxygenated blood shunts abnormally from the higher-pressured aorta back to the pulmonary artery. Once in the pulmonary artery, the blood is recirculated to the lungs. This condition causes an increased workload on the heart and pulmonary system and occurs twice as frequently in girls as in boys.

COARCTATION OF THE AORTA

■ **DESCRIPTION.** Coarctation is a **stricture** or narrowing. A coarctation of the aorta is a narrowing of the descending or thoracic aorta (Figure 19–12D), a condition that causes a high blood pressure proximal to the stricture and lower blood pressure distal to the stricture. Infants or children affected with coarctation of the aorta can have a high blood pressure in the arms but a lower blood pressure in the legs. Coarctation increases the workload on the heart because the heart attempts to pump blood through the narrowed vessels.

TETRALOGY OF FALLOT

■ **DESCRIPTION.** Tetralogy of Fallot (TET-traw-law-gee of fall-OH) is a combination of four (tetra) defects (Figure 19–12E) and is one of the most serious of congenital heart defects. The four defects are as follows.

1. **Pulmonary valve stenosis** The opening into the pulmonary artery is too small, restricting the amount of blood flow to the lungs.
2. **Right ventricle hypertrophy** This is due to the increased workload on the right ventricle as it attempts to pump blood through the stenotic valve.
3. **Ventricle septal defect** Allowing oxygenated blood to flow from the left ventricle to the right.
4. **Abnormal placement of the aorta** The aorta opens over the ventricle septal defect, allowing blood from both ventricles to be pumped into the aorta. The unoxygenated blood from the right ventricle enters the general circulation without passing through the lungs to become oxygenated. This unoxygenated blood from the right ventricle causes the tissues to become cyanotic (blue).

■ **SYMPTOMS.** Infants and children with tetralogy of Fallot are truly blue babies. Cyanosis increases with age, and clubbing of fingers and toes becomes evident. Older children will rest in a squatting position to breathe easier. This position also increases venous return. Other symptoms are growth retardation, severe dyspnea with exercise, and frequent respiratory infections.

Blood

Genetic and developmental disorders of the blood are more common in certain population groups. For example, some anemias are most commonly found in black populations, whereas other anemias are more common in European populations. Sickle cell anemia and hemophilia are both discussed in more detail in Chapter 7, "Blood and Blood-Forming Organs Diseases and Disorders."

SICKLE CELL ANEMIA

Sickle cell anemia is a chronic hereditary form of anemia found predominately in African American individuals.

COMPLEMENTARY AND ALTERNATIVE THERAPY

Herb Mixture for Bleeding Disorder

A mixture from several plants called Ankaferd Blood Stopper (ABS) has been used in Turkey for hundreds of years as a treatment for bleeding disorders. The mixture has a hemostatic (stopping bleeding) effect on blood cells and the vascular system. It is now becoming a well-known treatment in Turkey for bleeding problems in patients who have not reacted positively to conventional treatment measures. ABS has had therapeutic effects on wound healing and has also shown some anti-infective and antineoplastic properties. Perhaps, after further research is completed, ABS will also be the official alternative treatment for bleeding problems in the United States.

Source: Beyazit et al. (2010).

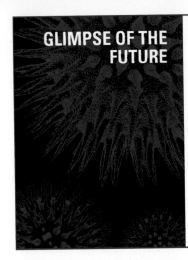

GLIMPSE OF THE FUTURE

Gene Therapy for Hemophilia

A new gene therapy that causes the liver to develop more of clotting factor IX is being tested and shows promising results. In the hereditary disease, hemophilia B, the blood does not clot properly due to a lack of clotting factor IX. These patients have to receive the clotting factor by injection to prevent excessive bleeding when cut or bruised. If this gene therapy is proven effective, the patients would just need a single infusion of the gene therapy (a harmless virus) that causes the liver to produce the necessary factor IX. It might eliminate their weekly or biweekly injections. The side effects were mild, and the therapy could last about 10 years. Further testing is planned.

Source: Seppa (2012).

HEMOPHILIA

Hemophilia is an X-linked hereditary bleeding disorder passed from a carrier mother to a son.

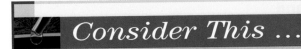

Consider This ...

In one study, 90% of breast-fed children had higher IQ scores than those who were formula fed.

Digestive

Digestive system disorders, both genetic and developmental, range from mild to severe. Many are diagnosed at birth, especially if the disorder interferes with ingestion, digestion, or elimination. Some of them are incompatible with life and must be corrected immediately or the infant will not survive.

■ **DESCRIPTION.** Several developmental malformations occur in the digestive system.

■ **ETIOLOGY.** The cause of these disorders is unknown but might be related to genetic tendencies or to maternal risk factors, including maternal rubella, poor maternal nutrition, smoking, and alcoholism.

A few of the more common malformations are briefly discussed here.

MECKEL'S DIVERTICULUM

■ **DESCRIPTION.** This is an outpouching, or diverticulum, of the ileum (Figure 19–13A). During fetal life, the intestine is connected to the yolk sac by a

duct. Failure of the duct to disappear leads to formation of this diverticulum. Meckel's diverticulum is the most common malformation of the gastrointestinal (GI) system, occurring in approximately 2% of the population. The diverticulum might be asymptomatic the entire life of the individual and found only on autopsy.

■ **SYMPTOMS.** If symptoms do occur, it is usually during infancy. The most common symptom is painless, bloody stools.

ESOPHAGEAL ATRESIA

■ **DESCRIPTION.** This is the absence of part of, or abnormal closure of, the esophagus. An **atresia** (ah-TREE-ze-ah) is the congenital absence or closure of a normal opening or lumen in the body and can occur in a variety of areas. Esophageal atresia is often accompanied by a fistula, called a tracheoesophageal fistula, connecting the trachea to the esophagus (Figure 19–13B). This is an emergency condition that allows food to pass directly into the lung.

■ **SYMPTOMS.** Reflux regurgitation of food occurs with both atresias. If a fistula is present, extreme coughing, cyanosis, and respiratory difficulties will appear.

CONGENITAL DIAPHRAGMATIC HERNIA

■ **DESCRIPTION.** This is a congenital hole in the diaphragm. Abdominal organs might herniate through this opening and into the chest cavity (Figure 19–13C).

■ **SYMPTOMS.** Difficulty breathing and chest pain are common symptoms.

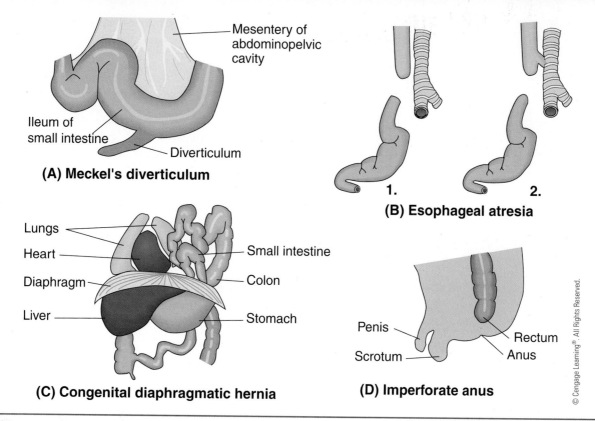

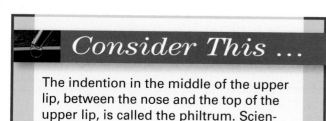

(A) Meckel's diverticulum

- Mesentery of abdominopelvic cavity
- Ileum of small intestine
- Diverticulum

(B) Esophageal atresia

1. 2.

(C) Congenital diaphragmatic hernia

- Lungs
- Heart
- Diaphragm
- Liver
- Small intestine
- Colon
- Stomach

(D) Imperforate anus

- Penis
- Scrotum
- Rectum
- Anus

FIGURE 19–13 Digestive developmental malformations.

IMPERFORATE ANUS

■ **DESCRIPTION.** This is a failure of the anus to connect to the rectum (Figure 19–13D). Infants with imperforate anus commonly have other developmental anomalies such as those affecting the heart, kidneys, esophagus, and spine.

■ **SYMPTOMS.** The primary symptom is not passing stool. Other symptoms are abdominal cramping and vomiting.

■ **DIAGNOSIS.** Diagnosis is commonly made on the basis of X-ray examination and ultrasound.

■ **TREATMENT.** Surgical correction is the treatment of choice for these malformations.

> ## Consider This ...
>
> The indention in the middle of the upper lip, between the nose and the top of the upper lip, is called the philtrum. Scientists have been unable to determine its purpose.

■ **PREVENTION.** There are no preventive measures other than controlling maternal risk factors.

CLEFT LIP AND PALATE

■ **DESCRIPTION.** Cleft (a split) lip consists of one or more abnormal splits in the upper lip (Figure 19–14A). This is a common anomaly, occurring in approximately 1 in 1,000 births. The defect occurs more frequently in boys and can vary from slight to severe.

A cleft palate involves the palate or roof of the mouth (Figure 19–14B) and is more serious than a cleft lip because it forms an opening between the nasopharynx and the nose. Cleft palate is more common in girls.

Both conditions can occur separately or in combination and can range from mild to severe.

■ **ETIOLOGY.** The cause of clefts appears to be related to a hereditary factor coupled with an alteration in intrauterine environment.

■ **SYMPTOMS.** Symptoms of cleft lip are related to difficulty feeding and speaking and, if not corrected during infancy, a struggle with positive self-image.

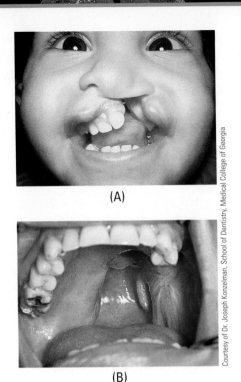

(A)

(B)

Courtesy of Dr. Joseph Konzelman, School of Dentistry, Medical College of Georgia

FIGURE 19–14   (A) Cleft lip. (B) Cleft palate.

Cleft palate includes these symptoms plus an increased risk of respiratory and middle ear infections.

■ *DIAGNOSIS.* Physical examination easily reveals this disorder. X-ray and computerized tomography (CT) may be utilized to determine the extent of the malformation.

■ *TREATMENT.* Surgical repair for cleft deformities is usually performed as soon as possible after birth. Several surgeries might be necessary to achieve the desired results. Special feeding devices and speech therapy are common needs.

■ *PREVENTION.* The only prevention is controlling maternal risk factors.

PYLORIC STENOSIS

■ *DESCRIPTION.* Pyloric stenosis is a narrowing (stenosis) of the outlet of the lower end of the stomach, the pylorus (Figure 19–15). This condition is one of the most common developmental abnormalities of the digestive tract.

■ *ETIOLOGY.* Pyloric stenosis is caused by a hypertrophy, or thickening, of the pyloric sphincter, which controls the flow of contents out of the stomach or

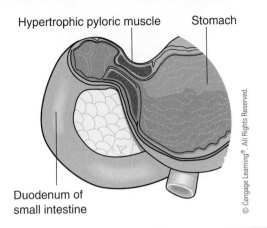

Hypertrophic pyloric muscle   Stomach

Duodenum of small intestine

© Cengage Learning®. All Rights Reserved.

FIGURE 19–15   Pyloric stenosis.

pyloric area. The hypertrophy of the pyloric sphincter slows the flow of stomach contents, resulting in a backup.

■ *SYMPTOMS.* The most common symptom of pyloric stenosis is projectile, or forceful, vomiting. Symptoms of pyloric stenosis usually begin at 2 to 4 weeks of age. This condition occurs almost exclusively in boys.

■ *DIAGNOSIS.* Diagnosis is made from history and X-ray examination (upper GI).

■ *TREATMENT.* A simple operation called a **pyloromyotomy** (pyloro = pyloric, myo = muscle, otomy = cut into), which involves incising and suturing the pyloric sphincter muscle, can be performed to correct the problem. This surgery is the standard treatment and is usually very effective.

■ *PREVENTION.* There are no known preventive measures.

HIRSCHSPRUNG'S DISEASE

■ *DESCRIPTION.* Hirschsprung's disease is due to an absence of nerves (ganglion) in a segment of the colon, usually the sigmoid colon. Without normal ganglion, the affected segment of colon lacks peristalsis, causing massive distention of the colon with feces (Figure 19–16).

■ *ETIOLOGY.* Hirschsprung's disease is seen more often in boys and those affected with Down syndrome. It has a familial tendency and occurs in approximately 1 in 5,000 births.

■ *SYMPTOMS.* Common symptoms include chronic constipation and abdominal distention.

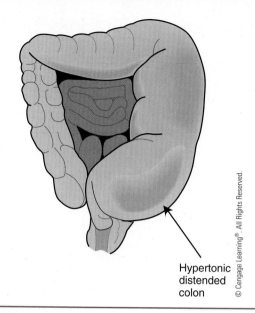

Hypertonic distended colon

© Cengage Learning®. All Rights Reserved.

FIGURE 19–16 Hirschsprung's disease.

■ **DIAGNOSIS.** Diagnosis is made on the basis of a biopsy to determine the absence of ganglion cells.

■ **TREATMENT.** Treatment is surgical removal of the affected segment. A temporary colostomy might be necessary to allow adequate healing of the colon.

■ **PREVENTION.** There is no known prevention. Genetic counseling can be offered to discuss risk and treatment options with a couple with a previous child with the condition and with those with the condition who are considering pregnancy.

PHENYLKETONURIA (PKU)

■ **DESCRIPTION.** PKU is an abnormal or faulty metabolism of the phenylalanine protein.

■ **ETIOLOGY.** PKU is a recessive genetic disorder.

■ **SYMPTOMS.** Affected individuals do not produce the enzyme necessary to break down the phenylalanine protein, which then builds up in the blood and becomes present in the urine. Phenylalanine is toxic to brain cells and causes mental disability if the condition is not corrected.

■ **DIAGNOSIS.** Diagnosis is made by PKU blood testing 72 hours after birth or after the infant has ingested proteins. This testing is mandatory in the United States.

■ **TREATMENT.** Affected infants are placed on a protein-restrictive diet. If the disease is discovered

and treated early, prognosis for normal intelligence is good. If the condition is not discovered until after age 2 or 3 years, mental challenges are inevitable and irreversible.

■ **PREVENTION.** There are no preventive measures. Genetic counseling can be offered to discuss risk and treatment options with a couple with a previous child with the condition and to those with the condition who are considering pregnancy.

Urinary

Some genetic and developmental disorders of the urinary system, such as hypospadias or epispadias, can be obvious at birth. Other disorders, such as Wilms' tumor, might not present symptoms for many years. If the condition interferes with elimination of urine, it is incompatible with life.

HYPOSPADIAS AND EPISPADIAS

■ **DESCRIPTION.** Hypospadias is an abnormal congenital opening of the male urinary meatus on the undersurface of the penis (Figure 19–17A). This abnormality can be mild, with the opening located just under the tip of the penis, or it can be more severe, with locations midshaft or near the scrotum. Hypospadias is fairly common, occurring in 1 in 250 boys.

Hypospadias can be accompanied by an abnormally downward curvature of the penis called chordee (COR-dee) (Figure 19–17B). The cause of chordee is an abnormal fibrous band of tissue.

Another similar but less common condition is epispadias, characterized by the urinary meatus located on the upper surface of the penis (Figure 19–17C).

■ **ETIOLOGY.** The cause of these conditions is unknown.

■ **SYMPTOMS.** Abnormal position of urethra is the only symptom. Chordee becomes worse with erection and can lead to difficulty with sexual intercourse.

■ **DIAGNOSIS.** Diagnosis is easily made with physical examination.

■ **TREATMENT.** Mild cases of all these conditions can be left untreated. Surgical repair is the treatment of choice for severe cases.

■ **PREVENTION.** There are no known preventive measures.

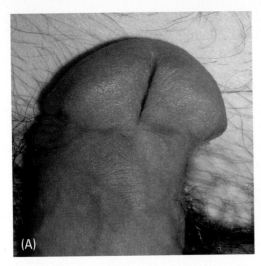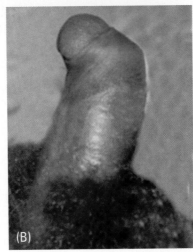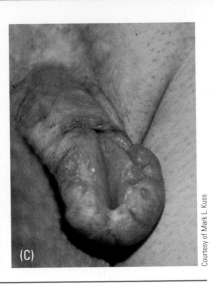

Courtesy of Mark L. Kuss

FIGURE 19–17   (A) Hypospadias. (B) Chordee. (C) Epispadias.

WILMS' TUMOR

■ **DESCRIPTION.** Wilms' tumor is the most common solid tumor affecting children and infants. Most tumors are thought to be present at birth, usually appearing between the ages of 2 and 4 years.

■ **ETIOLOGY.** The cause is thought to be genetic. It is highly malignant and usually replaces one entire normal kidney but rarely affects both kidneys.

■ **SYMPTOMS.** The tumor is usually asymptomatic until it becomes large enough to feel in the child's abdomen.

■ **DIAGNOSIS.** Most tumors are discovered by palpation of the abdomen during a routine examination by a pediatrician or by a parent.

■ **TREATMENT.** Current treatment involving chemotherapy and surgery has improved a previously dismal prognosis to a survival rate of approximately 85%.

■ **PREVENTION.** There are no preventive measures. Genetic counseling might be helpful for those who have a history of a family member affected with this condition.

Reproductive

Genetic and developmental disorders of the reproductive system are very rare disorders. Although they are not usually incompatible with life, they can have serious psychological effects on the individual because of the changes they can cause in the appearance of the person and the gender differences expected in our population.

CRYPTORCHIDISM

This developmental condition of undescended testes (crypt = hidden) is discussed in detail in Chapter 17, "Reproductive System Diseases and Disorders."

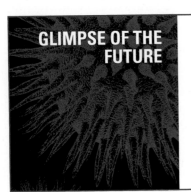

GLIMPSE OF THE FUTURE

New Information about Wilms' Tumor

There is some new genetic research occurring that may help find a cure or at least some better treatments for Wilms' tumor. The researchers have found two genes that help them understand how the tumor develops. Wilms' tumor is the most common type of kidney cancer in children. Although treatment for the disease is fairly effective, this new research should be helpful in finding the children who are at most risk of developing the cancer in the future.

Source: "Gene Research Raises Hope of New Kidney Cancer Therapies" (2010).

TURNER'S SYNDROME

■ **DESCRIPTION.** Turner's syndrome is a condition affecting females. At birth, the ovaries are abnormal or absent. Turner's syndrome is less common than Klinefelter's syndrome, a similar condition that affects males.

■ **ETIOLOGY.** Turner's syndrome is caused by a chromosomal disorder and affects approximately 1 in 3,000 females. Affected females have only one X chromosome rather than the normal XX.

■ **SYMPTOMS.** This individual fails to develop normal female secondary sex characteristics at puberty. General physical features of affected females include a short stature, broad neck, wide chest, amenorrhea, sterility, dwarfism, and impaired intelligence.

■ **DIAGNOSIS.** Physical examination and blood hormone testing aid in diagnosis.

■ **TREATMENT.** Symptoms can be reduced with growth hormone and estrogen therapy. Counseling and emotional support are often needed for the affected individual and family members to help cope with altered body image and self-esteem issues.

■ **PREVENTION.** There is no prevention for Turner's syndrome.

KLINEFELTER'S SYNDROME

■ **DESCRIPTION.** Klinefelter's syndrome is a congenital disorder that affects approximately 1 in 1,000 males.

■ **ETIOLOGY.** Klinefelter's is caused by a chromosomal disorder. Affected males have an extra X chromosome (XXY) in addition to the normal XY.

■ **SYMPTOMS.** This disorder is usually not diagnosed until puberty, when the affected individual fails to exhibit normal male sexual development. General physical features of affected males include sterility, abnormally small penis and testes, enlarged breasts, absent or scant body hair, decreased muscle development, and impaired intelligence. The affected individual has a general appearance of a eunuch with a tall, slender body and long legs.

■ **DIAGNOSIS.** Physical examination and blood hormone testing aid in diagnosis.

■ **TREATMENT.** Symptoms can be improved with testosterone therapy. Emotional and psychological counseling are often needed for the affected individual and family members to help cope with altered body image and self-esteem issues.

■ **PREVENTION.** There is no known prevention for this condition.

Other Developmental Disorders

Developmental disorders that do not fit into the previous categories of musculoskeletal, neurologic, cardiovascular, blood, digestive, urinary, or reproductive disorders are autism and stuttering.

AUTISM

■ **DESCRIPTION.** Autism, also called autistic disorder, is a developmental disorder that first presents itself in infancy or early childhood and is characterized by difficult communicating and in forming relationships.

■ **ETIOLOGY.** The cause of autism is unknown, although there might be a genetic or physical cause.

■ **SYMPTOMS.** Symptoms of autism are usually apparent in infancy when the infant exhibits an eye-to-eye gaze and blank facial expression. Affected children are so involved with themselves that they become inaccessible to others, including parents. These children might play alone happily for hours and become angry if interrupted. Approximately 10% of autistic children possess an outstanding skill such as rote memory or musical ability. An example is a child who can play a very difficult piano piece after hearing it only one time. Such children are often called autistic savants.

■ **DIAGNOSIS.** Diagnosis is confirmed on the basis of observation of behavior.

■ **TREATMENT.** Behavioral therapy to teach the child how to adapt to situations is beneficial. Prognosis is still relatively poor, and affected children rarely recover.

■ **PREVENTION.** There is no recognized prevention, although some cases can be linked to chemical exposure during pregnancy. Abstaining from alcohol and checking with a physician before taking any medications during pregnancy might aid in prevention.

STUTTERING

■ **DESCRIPTION.** Stuttering, also called stammering, is a developmental speech disorder, a common condition in young children that most of them will outgrow. If the problem persists, speech therapy might be necessary.

■ **ETIOLOGY.** Stuttering often occurs when children address an impatient or angry parent or someone who is in authority. The child's anxiety often leads to stuttering. The listener's reaction often enforces the child's anxiety, leading to more difficulties.

■ **SYMPTOMS.** Stuttering is characterized by hesitancy of starting and finishing a sound or word and prolonged pauses between words or sounds.

■ **DIAGNOSIS.** Diagnosis is usually confirmed upon physical examination, which includes talking with the child.

■ **TREATMENT.** Treatment is often based on some type of behavior modification and positive reinforcement of proper speech.

■ **PREVENTION.** There are no preventive methods, although speech therapy might help overcome the condition.

Multisystem Diseases and Disorders

Multisystem disorders are complex diseases that affect several body systems. Because of this effect, treatment is complicated and usually long term.

CYSTIC FIBROSIS

■ **DEFINITION.** Cystic fibrosis is a life-threatening hereditary disorder characterized by the production of thick secretions that block body passageways.

■ **ETIOLOGY.** Cystic fibrosis is a genetic recessive disorder affecting young children. It is passed to the child by a recessive gene from each parent.

■ **SYMPTOMS.** Cystic fibrosis affects all the **exocrine** glands (glands that excrete through a duct) of the body, causing **viscous** (thick) secretions. These viscous secretions cause obstruction in body passageways. The most serious complication of cystic fibrosis is in the lungs. The thick secretions block bronchi, causing difficulty with breathing. These thick secretions also trap bacteria and increase the

risk of respiratory infections, including pneumonia. The most common cause of death from this disease is respiratory failure.

The pancreas is also affected because blockage of these ducts decreases the amount of pancreatic enzymes delivered to the intestine, resulting in poor digestion and weight loss.

The sweat glands are also affected. Affected children perspire excessively and lose large amounts of salt (sodium). This loss of sodium causes an increase in the risk for heat exhaustion and electrolyte imbalances. This abnormal excretion of salt is usually the first sign that parents recognize as abnormal. Parents might take the child to the physician and complain that the child, when kissed, tastes salty or has sweaty baby kisses.

■ **DIAGNOSIS.** This excessive salt excretion is the basis for the sweat test that confirms the diagnosis of cystic fibrosis.

■ **TREATMENT.** Major improvements in treatment of cystic fibrosis have been made in the past few decades, but it is still considered a fatal disease. Life expectancy can reach into the late 20s or early 30s. Treatment is directed toward reducing complications and improving quality of life. Aggressive respiratory treatments include postural drainage, chest-clapping, antibiotics, bronchodilators, expectorants, and oxygen therapy. A high-calorie, high-sodium diet is provided with pancreatic enzyme supplementation. Emotional support and extensive education are needed for the affected individual and family members.

■ **PREVENTION.** There are no preventive measures. Genetic counseling can be offered to a couple with a previous child with the condition.

DOWN SYNDROME

■ **DESCRIPTION.** Down syndrome is also called trisomy 21 because it is a condition resulting in three (tri) chromosomes instead of the normal two in the 21st position of the chromosome chain. Down syndrome occurs in approximately 1 of every 700 births. It is the most common cause of genetic mental disability.

■ **ETIOLOGY.** The cause of Down syndrome is not known, but it is known that during germ cell division (usually affecting the ovum), the 21st chromosome pair fails to separate. This failure to separate results in a pair of chromosomes in position 21; if fertilized, this ovum—carrying two chromosomes—combines with the sperm—carrying one chromosome—resulting in three chromosomes in position 21. This condition is more common in children born to women age 35 years or older, suggesting that chromosomal division is affected by maternal age.

■ **SYMPTOMS.** Signs of Down syndrome include:

- Mild to severe mental disability.

- Facial features that include a flat nasal bridge, low-set ears, slanted eyes with **epicanthus** (a vertical fold of skin across the medial canthus of the eyes, giving them an Asian appearance), and a thick, protruding tongue.

- Abnormal extremities, including short arms and legs. The hands are short and wide with a crease across the entire width of the palm called a simian crease. The little finger is short and often crooked. There is an abnormally wide gap between the first (big) and second toes.

- Organ defects, especially congenital heart defects. Infertility is common in males but might not affect females.

- Other diseases are common, including anemia, leukemia, immune deficiencies, and respiratory infections.

■ **DIAGNOSIS.** Prenatal tests used to diagnose Down syndrome include ultrasound, amniocentesis, and maternal blood testing showing abnormal levels of pregnancy hormones, including human chorionic gonadotropin (HCG), and are indicative of the condition.

Diagnosis of newborns includes physical examination for symptoms along with a chromosomal karyotype that looks for the extra chromosome 21.

■ **TREATMENT.** There is no cure, but amniocentesis is an effective tool for discovery. The treatment plan is highly individual and is directed toward maximizing mental and physical abilities. Improved surgical techniques and antibiotic therapies have increased the life expectancy of affected individuals to an average of 55 years. Individuals affected with Down syndrome are known for their loving, affectionate personalities.

■ **PREVENTION.** There are no preventive measures. Genetic counseling might be beneficial.

■ TRAUMA

Failure to Thrive

Failure to thrive is a lack of physical growth and development in an infant or child. This condition was first noticed by a European psychiatrist who studied the development of infants institutionalized during their early years and who were deprived of emotional warmth and security. The condition of failure to thrive is usually reserved for infants and children who are not growing and developing due to emotional or psychological causes.

The cause of failure to thrive appears to be a disturbance in the mother–child relationship or a failure to bond. This condition tends to be associated with alcohol and drug abuse, economic stress, parental immaturity, and single parenthood. Involved mothers are often found to be victims of maternal deprivation themselves.

Symptoms of failure to thrive include weight loss or failure to gain weight and grow, irritability, anorexia or lack of appetite, vomiting, and diarrhea. Affected infants often are weak and exhibit rag-doll limpness. They can be unresponsive to affection or wary of parents or caregivers and might avoid eye contact and stiffen when cuddled.

Treatment includes teaching nurturing and mothering behaviors for the mother, promoting her self-esteem, and providing for the physical and emotional needs of the child. The prognosis for infants and children with this condition is often unknown. Decreased intelligence and social and language disabilities have been noted in children with failure to thrive. A significant number of these children die early in life.

Fetal Alcohol Syndrome

Fetal alcohol syndrome (FAS) is a group of symptoms and birth defects in an infant born to a mother who consumed alcohol during pregnancy. Infants born to mothers who chronically abuse alcohol can go through physical alcohol withdrawal shortly after birth.

Signs and symptoms of FAS include varying degrees of mental challenges, decreased physical development, irritability in infants and hyperactivity in children, **microcephaly** (micro = small, cephal = brain), and an increased occurrence of ventricular septal heart defects.

The exact amount of alcohol consumption needed to cause defects is unknown, so alcohol consumption during pregnancy should be avoided. The greatest risks for defects occur when alcohol is consumed during and after the third month of pregnancy.

Congenital Rubella Syndrome

Transmission of the rubella virus across the placenta to the unborn fetus can result in spontaneous abortion or birth of an infant with major birth defects. The most common defects are microcephaly, learning disorders, deafness, abnormal growth, heart defects, and ocular lesions such as cataracts, glaucoma, nystagmus, and strabismus.

Prevention includes immunization of all children and women of childbearing age. Women should avoid becoming pregnant for 3 months after immunization and should not be immunized during pregnancy.

▬ RARE DISEASES

Anencephaly

Anencephaly is a severe congenital malformation resulting in the absence of the brain or cranial vault. This condition is not compatible with life. Infants born with anencephaly are stillborn or die shortly after birth if they are not kept alive by artificial means.

Achondroplasia

Achondroplasia is a rare genetic disorder characterized by abnormal development of the epiphyseal cartilage, resulting in decreased long bone growth and a type of dwarfism. Interestingly, a similar condition affects basset hounds. Affected individuals might die at birth or shortly thereafter or live to a normal life expectancy.

Tay–Sachs Disease

Tay–Sachs disease is an autosomal recessive disorder primarily affecting families of Eastern Jewish origin. This condition is due to a genetic error in lipid metabolism and results in an accumulation of toxins in the brain. As a result, the brain tissue degenerates, causing mental and physical disabilities.

Symptoms usually occur by 6 months of age and include lack of developmental skills, convulsions, and blindness. A cherry-red spot on the retina of the eye is one indicative diagnostic test. Affected children usually die before age 4 years. There is no cure and no specific treatment other than symptomatic treatment.

SUMMARY

Although there are literally hundreds of genetic and developmental disorders, overall, most are relatively rare. Some are obvious at birth and can be incompatible with life; others might not be diagnosed until later in the individual's life. Because some disorders have no distinct diagnostic tests, a variety of testing might be necessary to obtain a definitive diagnosis. Other disorders can be diagnosed by genetic testing.

Many of the genetic and developmental disorders have lifelong effects on the individual and can be progressively disabling. Because of new research and extended health care services, most individuals with these disorders have longer life expectancy than in past years.

REVIEW QUESTIONS

Short Answer

1. How many chromosomes are in the nucleus of each body cell?

2. Which body cells can reproduce in a process called mitosis?

3. What is a germ cell?

4. Describe the process called meiosis.

5. What is karyotyping?

6. Why is DNA considered to be so important?

7. Name an autosomal dominant disorder.

8. Name an autosomal recessive disorder.

9. Define genotype.

10. Define phenotype.

Multiple Choice

11. Which of the following statements is the best description of MD?

   a. MD is a degenerative disorder of the nervous system.

   b. MD is a group of genetically inherited diseases characterized by degeneration or weakening of the muscles.

   c. MD is a genetic disorder most common in male children.

   d. MD is a neuromuscular disorder affecting children.

12. Which of the following statements is the best description of CP?

   a. CP is a congenital bilateral paralysis that results from inadequate blood or oxygen supply to the brain during fetal development.

   b. CP is a crippling disease caused by a genetic inherited disorder.

   c. CP is an abnormal accumulation of cerebrospinal fluid in the brain.

   d. CP is a condition of spastic movements and inability to walk caused by a genetic anomaly.

13. Coarctation of the aorta is _____.

   a. a combination of four tetra defects of the heart.

   b. a constriction or stricture of the major artery of the heart.

   c. an abnormal connection of the pulmonary artery and the aorta.

   d. a small hole in the artery at birth.

14. Some of the problems for the infant with a cleft lip and palate might include _____.

    a. a fistula connecting the trachea to the esophagus.

    b. increased risk for elimination problems.

    c. increased risk for difficulty with feedings, respiratory distress, and middle ear infections.

    d. projectile or forceful vomiting.

15. PKU is best described as _____.

    a. an absence of nerves in a particular segment of the colon, causing constipation and distention of the colon.

    b. a recessive genetic disorder of metabolism of protein.

    c. an autosomal dominant genetic disorder of digestion and absorption.

    d. a constriction of the valve in the stomach, causing a backup of food and fluid.

16. Which of the following is the most common solid tumor affecting children and infants?

    a. Osteoma

    b. Sarcoma

    c. Ewing's tumor

    d. Wilms' tumor

17. Which of the following factors are usually present in Down syndrome?

    a. Dwarf-like body, mental disability, spastic movements

    b. Organ defects, small stature, epicanthal folds, and epispadias

    c. Mental disability, immune deficiencies, and abnormal brain size

    d. Epicanthal folds, small stature, mild to severe mental disability

18. When is FAS most likely to occur?

    a. If the mother drinks alcohol during and after the third month of pregnancy

    b. If the mother drinks more than one glass of alcohol per day during the last trimester

    c. If the mother drinks alcohol during the first 2 months of pregnancy

    d. Only if the mother drinks more than two glasses of alcohol per day during the pregnancy

19. Tay–Sachs disease is an _____.

    a. autosomal dominant disease affecting the brain.

    b. autosomal dominant disease affecting metabolism, causing mental disability.

    c. autosomal recessive disease affecting metabolism, causing mental disability.

    d. autosomal recessive disease affecting the brain.

20. Failure to thrive is defined as which of the following?

    a. It is a lack of growth and development due to a genetic disease.

    b. It is a lack of physical growth and development in an infant or a child.

    c. It is an inborn error of metabolism, causing delayed growth and development.

    d. It is an inherited disease affecting growth in the infant.

CASE STUDIES

■ Heather Lee is an 8-month-old infant who is brought to the clinic because of chronic respiratory infections. Heather is weak, inactive, and underweight; she has poor skin turgor and seems very quiet except for spells of coughing. She is subsequently diagnosed with CF. Heather's mother is very upset with this diagnosis, thinking it is her fault the baby is not doing well. Is she correct in thinking this? What can you tell her about this disorder? What is the cause of CF? What is the usual treatment prescribed? What is the prognosis for Heather?

■ Abnormalities in children might be due to genetic factors. Because individuals have dominant and recessive genes, some predictions can be made about such things as color of eyes or genetic disease probabilities. If the mother has brown eyes but has a recessive gene for blue eyes and the father has blue eyes (homozygous recessive), what is the likelihood of them having a blue-eyed child? What is the likelihood of them having a brown-eyed child?

Study Tools

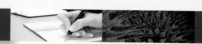

Workbook
Complete Chapter 19

Online Resources
PowerPoint® presentations

BIBLIOGRAPHY

Aschman, D. J., Abshire, T. C., Shapiro, A. D., Lusher, J. M., Forsberg, A. D., & Kulkarni, R. (2011). A community-based partnership to promote information infrastructure for bleeding disorders. *American Journal of Preventive Medicine 41*(6), S332–S337.

Baker, J. R., Riske, B., Voutsis, M., Cutter, S., & Presley, R. (2011). Insurance, home therapy, and prophylaxis in U.S. youth with severe hemophilia. *American Journal of Preventive Medicine 41*(6), S338–S345.

Barak, Y., & Achiron, A. (2011). Happiness and personal growth are attainable in interferon-beta-1a treated multiple sclerosis patients. *Journal of Happiness Studies 12*(5), 887–895.

Beyazit, Y., Kurt, M., Kekilli, M., Goker, H., & Haznedaroglu, I. (2010). Evaluation of hemostatic effects of Ankaferd as an alternative medicine. *Alternative Medicine Review 15*(4), 329–336.

Dreyer, P., Steffensen, B. F., & Pedersen, B. D. (2010). Life with home mechanical ventilation for young men with Duchenne muscular dystrophy. *Journal of Advanced Nursing 66*(4), 753–762.

Elliott, M. (2010). Injection of hope. *Nursing Standard 25*(10), 23.

Farrugia, A. A., O'Mahony, B. B., & Cassar, J. J. (2012). Health technology assessment and haemophilia. *Haemophilia 18*(2), 152–157.

Ganesh, S. S., Vennila, J. J., & Scholz, H. H. (2011). An overview and perspectives of Wilm's tumor. *International Journal of Cancer Research 7*(1), 1–7.

Gene research raises hope of new kidney cancer therapies. (2010). *Paediatric Nursing 22*(4), 4.

Genetic Disease Foundation. (2012). *www.geneticdisease-foundation.org* (accessed March 2012).

Greenop, D., Glenn, S., Ledson, M., & Walshaw, M. (2010). Self-care and cystic fibrosis: A review of research with adults. *Health & Social Care in the Community 18*(6), 653–661.

Heavey, E., & Peterson-Sweeney, K. (2010). Caring for an adult with Down syndrome. *Nursing 40*(6), 53–56.

Livingston, G., & Strydom, A. (2012). Improving Alzheimer's disease outcomes in Down's syndrome. *Lancet 379*(9815), 498–500.

Lomas, P., & Fowler, S. B. (2010). Parents and children with cystic fibrosis: A family affair. *American Journal of Nursing 110*(8), 30–39.

Markowitz, J. A., Singh, P., & Darras, B. T. (2012). Spinal muscular atrophy: A clinical and research update. *Pediatric Neurology, 46*(1), 1–12.

Murray, J., & Ryan-Krause, P. (2010). Obesity in children with Down syndrome: Background and recommendations for management. *Pediatric Nursing 36*(6), 314–319.

Muscular Dystrophy Association. (2012). *www.mda.org* (accessed March 2012).

National Hemophilia Foundation. (2012). *www.hemophilia.org* (accessed March 2012).

National Multiple Sclerosis Society. (2012). *www.nationalmssociety.org* (accessed March 2012).

Pichavant, C., Aartsma-Rus, A., Clemens, P., Davies, K., Dickson, G., Takeda, S., & Tremblay, J. (2011). Current status of pharmaceutical and genetic therapeutic approaches to treat DMD. *Molecular Therapy 19*(5), 830–840.

Pitt, V. (2011). Using human rights to fight cuts. *Community Care 1853*, 24.

Sagredo, O., Pazos, M., Valdeolivas, S., & Fernández-Ruiz, J. (2012). Cannabinoids: Novel medicines for the treatment of Huntington's disease. *Recent Patents on CNS Drug Discovery 7*(1), 41–48.

Scherer, S. S. (2011). The debut of a rational treatment for an inherited neuropathy? *Journal of Clinical Investigation 121*(12), 4624–4627.

Sekarski, L. A., & Spangenberg L. A. (2011). Hereditary hemorrhagic telangiectasia: Children need screening too. *Pediatric Nursing 37*(4), 163–168.

Seppa, N. (2012). Gene therapy helps hemophiliacs. *Science News 181*(1), 9.

Sickle Cell Disease Association of America (SCDAA). (2012). *www.sicklecelldisease.org* (accessed March 2012).

Souza, J. C., Simoes, H. G., Campbell, C. G., Pontes, F. L., Boullosa, D. A., & Prestes, J. J. (2012). Haemophilia and exercise. *International Journal of Sports Medicine 33*(2), 83–88.

Starr, S. (2012). Genetic blood disorders: Questions you need to ask. *Journal of Family Practice 61*(1), 30–37.

Susan, L., & Mueller, R. (2011). Is cystic fibrosis genetic medicine's canary? *Perspectives in Biology & Medicine 54*(3), 316–331.

Swanson, M. E., Grosse, S. D., & Kulkarni, R. (2011). Disability among individuals with sickle cell disease: Literature review from a public health perspective. *American Journal of Preventive Medicine 41*(6), S390–S397.

Wexler, N. S. (2012). Huntington's disease: Advocacy driving science. *Annual Review of Medicine 63*, 1–22.

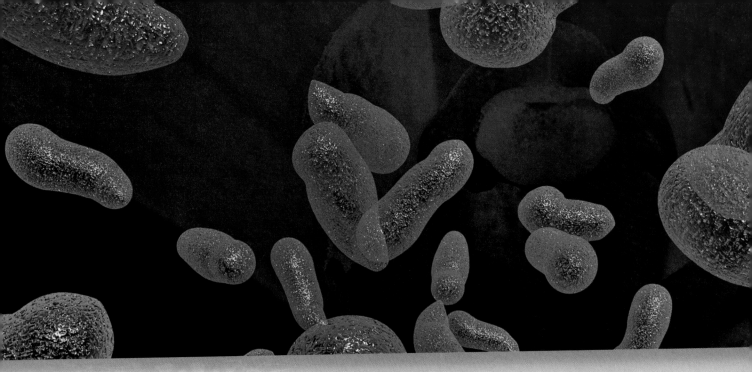

OUTLINE

KEY TERMS

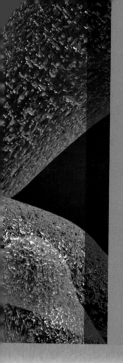

20

Childhood Diseases and Disorders

LEARNING OBJECTIVES

Upon completion of the chapter, the learner should be able to:

1. Define the terminology common to childhood diseases.

2. Identify the important signs and symptoms associated with childhood diseases.

3. Describe the common diagnostics used to determine the type and cause of childhood diseases.

4. Describe the typical course and management of the common childhood diseases.

5. State the common drugs abused by children, the effects of the drugs, and the potential health hazards of drug use.

6. List the immunizations available to prevent childhood diseases.

7. Identify the safety precautions for preventing poisonings in children.

OVERVIEW

Childhood diseases range from common infections such as tonsillitis and colds to more chronic and debilitating diseases such as Ewing's sarcoma and leukemia. In addition, traumatic events such as abuse and poisonings are very common in the young population. Childhood diseases can affect any body system, but the most commonly known ones affect the respiratory system, producing signs and symptoms of a cold or flu. Even though immunizations against many of the common childhood diseases are available, many children in this country have not been immunized at all or do not have adequate immunizations. Lack of immunization increases their likelihood of developing an acute infectious childhood disease. ■

INFECTIOUS DISEASES

More children are seen yearly by physicians for infectious disease diagnosis and treatment than for any other problem. Infectious diseases of childhood fall into four categories: viral, bacterial, fungal, and parasitic diseases. Disorders in these categories include some of the most familiar diseases such as colds, influenza, measles, pertussis, and tonsillitis, several of which can be prevented by maintenance of a regular immunization schedule (see the Healthy Highlight titled "Immunization Schedule for Children"). Many of these diseases have an **incubation period**, the time between exposure to the disease and the presence of symptoms, which lasts several days.

In general, signs and symptoms of the common infectious diseases include fever, **malaise** (a feeling of general discomfort), coughing, anorexia, nausea or vomiting, rashes, or any combination of these. Treatment varies with the specific disease. In many cases, treatment consists of symptom relief, good nutrition, and rest. Nonaspirin antipyretics are given to children with fever because aspirin has been linked to Reye's syndrome. Good hand washing is always important to prevent the spread of infectious diseases.

Viral Diseases

Viral diseases in children are usually treated symptomatically. Most children have mild cases of the disease and recuperate quickly. However, for some children, especially those who have other medical disorders, even a mild viral infection can become a critical health problem. Some viruses invade the host and remain dormant for long periods of time and activate when triggered by something. Although this concept is not well understood, it is known that stress is a common trigger for initiating the replication of a dormant virus.

MEASLES

■ **DESCRIPTION.** Measles, also called rubeola, is one of the most serious childhood diseases due to major complications such as encephalitis and meningitis. Less extreme complications include croup, ear infection, and conjunctivitis.

Since the development of immunization in 1963, measles has become rare in the United States. Outbreaks that do occur are usually a result of infected children and teens who are immigrants to this country.

■ **ETIOLOGY.** Measles is an acute viral disease commonly spread by contaminated airborne droplets.

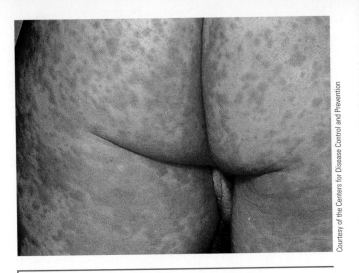

FIGURE 20–1   Maculopapular rash in rubeola.

It is highly contagious with an incubation period of 7 to 14 days.

■ **SYMPTOMS.** Symptoms include fever, inflammation of the respiratory mucous membranes, runny nose, and a generalized, dusky red maculopapular rash over the body trunk and extremities (Figure 20–1). Unique spots called **Koplik's spots** (Figure 20–2) appear in the mouth early in the disease.

■ **DIAGNOSIS.** Koplik's spots are rather unique to measles and are often the definitive symptom that confirms the diagnosis.

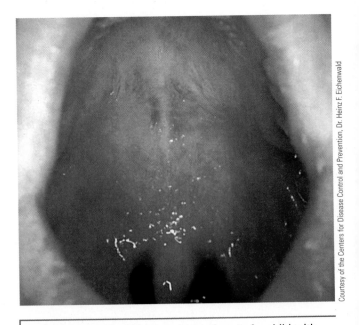

FIGURE 20–2   Koplik's spots in the throat of a child with rubeola.

■ **TREATMENT.** Treatment is usually directed at relief of symptoms and prevention of such complications as dehydration, pneumonia, or high fever. Having had one episode of the disease should provide lifetime immunity, but all children should be immunized to prevent measles (see the Healthy Highlight titled "Immunization Schedule for Children").

■ **PREVENTION.** This illness is effectively prevented with measles immunization. This immunization is often given in a combination vaccine called measles, mumps, and rubella (MMR).

RUBELLA

■ **DESCRIPTION.** Rubella is a type of measles also known as German measles or 3-day measles. It is usually a very mild disease in children but can be quite serious in pregnant women. If it occurs during the first 3 months of pregnancy, there is an 80% chance of fetal problems or congenital anomalies (birth defects) occurring. Birth defects of the eyes, heart, and brain are common.

■ **ETIOLOGY.** Rubella, like measles, is spread by contaminated airborne droplets. It is less contagious than rubeola, with an incubation period of 14 to 21 days.

■ **SYMPTOMS.** Symptoms of rubella include a classic rash similar to measles but lighter in color (Figure 20–3), lymph node enlargement, nasal discharge, joint pain, chills, and fever.

■ **DIAGNOSIS.** A blood test showing a significant rise in rubella antibodies is helpful in diagnosis. These antibodies can show whether there has been a recent or past infection with rubella.

■ **TREATMENT.** Treatment is usually symptomatic with rest, good nutrition, and prevention of spread of the infection.

■ **PREVENTION.** All children and women of childbearing age should be immunized to prevent rubella (see the Healthy Highlight titled "Immunization Schedule for Children").

MUMPS

■ **DESCRIPTION.** Mumps is an infection affecting the **parotid glands**, one of three pairs of salivary glands. These glands are located below and in front of the ears. This illness was quite common until 1906 when the vaccine was developed.

■ **ETIOLOGY.** Mumps is a contagious viral infection that is spread by saliva. The infection can be spread by breathing infected airborne droplets from coughs and sneezes or by sharing eating or drinking utensils. The incubation period is usually 16 to 18 days but can be as long as 25 days.

■ **SYMPTOMS.** Symptoms include chills, fever, ear pain, and swelling of the parotid glands (one or both) (Figure 20–4).

■ **DIAGNOSIS.** Blood test showing the presence of mumps antibodies confirms diagnosis.

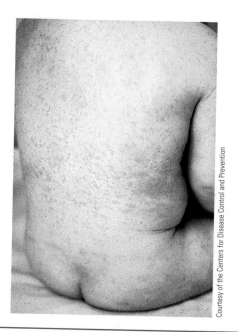

Courtesy of the Centers for Disease Control and Prevention

| **FIGURE 20–3** Rubella rash.

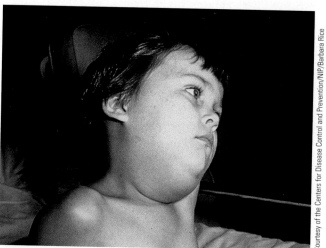

Courtesy of the Centers for Disease Control and Prevention/NIP/Barbara Rice

| **FIGURE 20–4** Parotitis (mumps).

■ **TREATMENT.** Treatment varies with the severity of the symptoms but is usually palliative (soothing or relieving symptoms). Complications of mumps include **orchitis** (or-KYE-tis; inflammation of a testis) in males and nerve conduction deafness. Although neither is common, they are a concern when mumps is diagnosed. Orchitis can result in sterility.

■ **PREVENTION.** All children should be immunized to prevent mumps (see the Healthy Highlight titled "Immunization Schedule for Children").

VARICELLA

■ **DESCRIPTION.** Varicella, more commonly known as chicken pox, is one of the most common childhood infectious diseases and a highly contagious one. After an infection, the individual usually develops lifelong protective immunity from further bouts.

■ **ETIOLOGY.** Chicken pox is the result of an infection with the herpes varicella-zoster virus. As discussed in Chapter 18, this virus causes both chicken pox (called varicella) and shingles (called herpes zoster). Varicella has an incubation period of 10 to 21 days, making it highly contagious. A person with chicken pox can be contagious up to 5 days before a rash appears. Varicella can be transmitted by airborne particles or direct contact. A common complication of chicken pox is shingles, a reactivation of the virus in an adult.

■ **SYMPTOMS.** Symptoms of varicella include a classic dew drop on a rose petal macular rash. The rose petal is the development of an irregular red macular rash with the shape of a rose petal. The dew drops are thin-walled blisters or **vesicles** (VES-ih-kuls; blister-like eruptions on the skin) that form on the rash, appearing like a drop of dew on a rose petal. This rash develops over the face, trunk, and extremities (Figure 20–5).

The rash usually develops over a period of several days with new lesions appearing every day for several days. This rash can be quite limited or very widespread and usually causes intense itching. The vesicles break, dry, and become crusty, often leaving a crater-like scar.

■ **DIAGNOSIS.** Diagnosis is by physical examination of symptoms including the classic rash.

■ **TREATMENT.** Treatment is usually symptomatic with care taken to prevent a secondary skin infection at the sites of the lesions.

■ **PREVENTION.** A vaccine has been available since 1995. Vaccine protection is recommended for children under age 13 and for adolescents and adults who have not been vaccinated and have not had chicken pox.

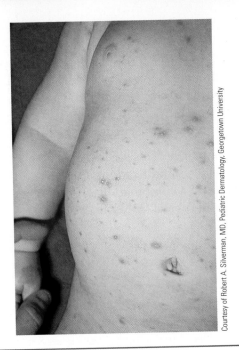

Courtesy of Robert A. Silverman, MD, Pediatric Dermatology, Georgetown University

FIGURE 20–5 Macular rash in varicella.

POLIOMYELITIS

■ **DESCRIPTION.** Poliomyelitis, also called polio, occurred in pandemics and crippled thousands of children and adults prior to the discovery of a vaccine by Jonas Salk in 1952 (Figure 20–6). Since the development of the vaccine, the number of polio cases

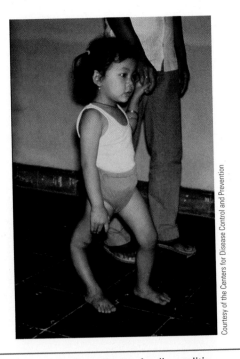

Courtesy of the Centers for Disease Control and Prevention

FIGURE 20–6 Crippling effects of poliomyelitis.

has dropped dramatically. Beginning in 1988, a global effort to eradicate polio has been led by the World Health Organization (WHO). If worldwide eradication of polio is accomplished, it will represent only the second time in history that man was able to eliminate a disease completely; the first was small pox in 1979 (Disease Eradication, 2010).

■ *ETIOLOGY.* Polio is caused by the poliovirus (PV) and is spread through an oral route or fecal–oral route from an infected individual. Abortive poliomyelitis is a mild form of the disease that does not affect the central nervous system.

The incubation period is 3 to 6 days for abortive poliomyelitis and 7 to 21 for the more severe form of poliomyelitis.

■ *SYMPTOMS.* In the more severe form of polio, early symptoms include fever, headache, sore throat, and abdominal pain. This can progress to stiffness of the neck, trunk, and extremities. Although the disease might subside at this point, it can also progress to paralysis. If the respiratory center of the brain is affected, the disease is life-threatening.

■ *DIAGNOSIS.* The disease can be suspected in an individual with symptoms of weakness or paralysis in an arm or leg that has no other reason for such symptoms. Diagnosis is confirmed by a stool sample or throat swab showing poliovirus.

■ *TREATMENT.* Treatment of polio is based on the symptoms and severity but is usually only supportive. Physical therapy is important to prevent wasting of muscles. Ventilator support is necessary if the respiratory center is affected.

■ *PREVENTION.* Forty years of an aggressive immunization program in the United States has reduced the threat of polio. However, it could still recur as a major health problem, so all children should be vaccinated against polio (see the Healthy Highlight titled "Immunization Schedule for Children").

INFLUENZA

■ *DESCRIPTION.* Influenza, or the flu, is an acute infectious respiratory disease that occurs every year in the late fall through early spring.

■ *ETIOLOGY.* Influenza is caused by viruses in the Orthomyxovirus family.

■ *SYMPTOMS.* The first symptom is commonly a sudden high fever of 100°–104°F and a dry, hacking cough. These symptoms are immediately followed by chills, headache, joint or muscle aches, and runny nose. The flu often develops very quickly and in epidemic proportions in some communities. Very young children or children with other debilitating illnesses are at risk for severe illness.

■ *DIAGNOSIS.* Physical examination with evidence of symptoms during late fall and winter can lead to diagnosis of flu, confirmed by rapid assay blood testing.

■ *TREATMENT.* Generally, treatment in children is symptomatic with rest, hydration, and antipyretics if needed. Antiviral drugs can be given for some types of influenza. A newly developed nasal spray flu vaccine is available for children 5 years of age or older.

■ *PREVENTION.* Vaccination is the primary measure for preventing influenza.

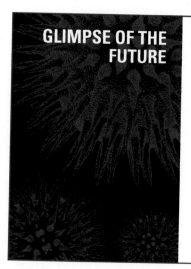

GLIMPSE OF THE FUTURE

Suppressing the Immune System May Interfere with Immunizations

Many children are taking immunosuppressive medications after organ transplantation or for other diseases. This may be required therapy, but new research is finding that it might also cause decreased responses to the routine immunizations the child receives. The immunosuppressant drugs might affect vaccines such as influenza, pneumococcal, meningococcal, hepatitis, pertussis, varicella, and herpes zoster and render them not as effective as they should be. The recommendation is to administer the immunizations prior to taking the immunosuppressive medications whenever possible. Further research still needs to be done to see which vaccines are most affected.

Source: Agarwal et al. (2012).

COMMON COLD

■ **DESCRIPTION.** The common cold is appropriately named because it is the most frequently occurring disease.

■ **ETIOLOGY.** Numerous strains of viruses can cause the common cold, but the rhinoviruses are usually the causative agent. It is transmitted by direct contact and droplet contact.

■ **SYMPTOMS.** Symptoms of the common cold include **rhinitis** (RYE-NIGH-tis; inflammation of the nasal mucous membrane), runny nose, coughing, sneezing, fever, and watery eyes.

■ **DIAGNOSIS.** There are no tests for the common cold. Diagnosis is made by physical examination of the individual's symptoms. Blood tests and throat cultures can be completed to rule out any other disease.

■ **TREATMENT.** Treatment is directed at symptom relief and getting adequate rest, hydration, and good nutrition.

■ **PREVENTION.** Good hand washing is the best preventive strategy for transmission of the cold virus.

MONONUCLEOSIS

■ **DESCRIPTION.** Infectious mononucleosis, sometimes called kissing disease (colloquially) or mono, is often joked about, but the disease can be quite serious. This infection primarily affects children and young adults. It is somewhat contagious and often will cause illness for several weeks.

■ **ETIOLOGY.** This infection is caused by the Epstein–Barr virus (EBV), which is very common. Many people have been exposed and are lifetime carriers of the virus but might never develop the illness.

The most common way to become infected with mononucleosis is by kissing someone who has been infected. Any activity involving direct contact with the saliva, such as sharing eating utensils or drinking straws, can spread the virus.

■ **SYMPTOMS.** Symptoms usually begin 4 to 7 days after infection and include fatigue, sore throat, fever, swollen lymph glands, and splenomegaly (spleen enlargement).

■ **DIAGNOSIS.** Diagnosis is confirmed by history and physical examination and a WBC count showing a marked elevation in lymphocytes.

■ **TREATMENT.** Treatment is symptomatic and includes rest, analgesics, and throat gargles. If there are no complications, symptoms of mononucleosis are usually resolved in 3 to 4 weeks. To prevent potential injury to the spleen, sports activities should be avoided for 1 month following the illness.

■ **PREVENTION.** Slowing the spread of the virus can be accomplished by frequent hand washing, covering mouth and nose when sneezing or coughing, and not sharing drinks or eating utensils.

ACQUIRED IMMUNODEFICIENCY SYNDROME

This disease is described in detail in Chapter 5, "Immune System Diseases and Disorders," but is addressed here in relation to its effect in children.

■ **DESCRIPTION.** Acquired immunodeficiency syndrome, commonly known as AIDS, has now affected thousands of children in the United States.

■ **ETIOLOGY.** AIDS is caused by the human immunodeficiency virus (HIV). During the 1980s, most children diagnosed with an HIV infection probably acquired it through a blood transfusion. Most children infected with HIV were hemophiliacs who had received transfusions or other blood products. Today, virtually all HIV infections in children are as a result of maternal–fetal transfer through blood, also called perinatal transmission.

Children not only suffer the effects of infection with the disease but also are often orphaned as a result of both parents dying with the disease. As of 2009, more than 17 million children under 18 had lost one or both parents to AIDS (Child Info, 2012). Increasing numbers of sexually active teens also are being diagnosed with HIV/AIDS. In 2009, it was estimated that 2.3 million children under age 15 were living with HIV (Africa Faith and Justice Network, 2012).

The period of time between the HIV infection and development of AIDS is much shorter in infants and toddlers than in infected older children or adults.

■ **SYMPTOMS.** Many children do not experience symptoms of the disease and live a normal life for years. However, in those with severely compromised immune systems, opportunistic infections can be overwhelming, necessitating repeated hospitalizations to sustain life.

■ **DIAGNOSIS.** As in adults, when T-cell count drops below 200 cells per microliter, the child has met the criteria set by the Centers for Disease Control and Prevention for a diagnosis of AIDS.

■ **TREATMENT.** Treatment of pediatric HIV infection and AIDS varies with the child and the severity of the symptoms. Therapy focuses on prevention and treatment of opportunistic diseases, good nutrition, antiviral drugs, and other support therapies as needed.

■ **PREVENTION.** In 2012, the United Nations Children's Fund (UNICEF) assisted in development of a Call to Action program to focus on ending preventable child deaths. The first step in the call to action is to increase efforts in the 24 countries that account for 80% of deaths in children under age 5 years.

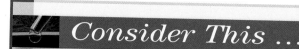

Consider This ...

Every minute of every day, a child under age 15 is infected with HIV (Africa Faith and Justice Network, 2012).

Bacterial Diseases

Bacterial diseases of childhood are caused by pathogens. There are millions of bacteria in the world, but not all bacteria are pathogenic. (See Chapter 4, "Inflammation and Infection," for more information.) Some of the common infection-causing bacteria include *Staphylococcus*, *Clostridium*, *Haemophilus*, *Escherichia coli*, and *Streptococcus*. Symptoms of bacterial infections can include coughing, fever, headache, difficulty breathing, and sore throat. Treatment is based on the causative agent along with relief of symptoms. Some bacterial diseases can be prevented by immunizations.

PERTUSSIS

■ **DESCRIPTION.** Pertussis is also known as whooping cough.

■ **ETIOLOGY.** Pertussis is an acute respiratory infection caused by *Bordetella pertussis*. The incubation period is 6 to 10 days but can be as long as 21 days. Pertussis is transmitted by direct contact with respiratory droplets.

■ **SYMPTOMS.** It is characterized by (1) a **catarrhal** (ka-TAR-al; inflammation of mucous membranes of the head and mouth with increased mucous flow) stage including cough, runny nose, and low-grade fever; (2) a

paroxysmal (PAR-ock-SIZ-mal; spasm or convulsion) stage including violent whooping coughing, cyanosis, distended neck veins, and some vomiting; and (3) a convalescent stage including some periods of the whooping coughing but with gradually less frequent episodes.

■ **DIAGNOSIS.** Diagnosis is made on the basis of symptoms. Testing is available, but because of the length of time it takes to get results, it is not considered a good diagnostic tool.

■ **TREATMENT.** Pertussis is treated with antibiotics and supportive therapy. Pneumonia is the most common complication of pertussis and can be life-threatening.

■ **PREVENTION.** All children should be immunized to prevent pertussis (see the Healthy Highlight titled "Immunization Schedule for Children"). Infants, prior to receiving vaccinations, are not immune to pertussis, so it is a serious threat to them.

DIPHTHERIA

■ **DESCRIPTION.** In 1920, there were an estimated 200,000 cases of diphtheria in the United States. With a fatality rate as high as 20% in young children, it was one of the leading causes of death among children. Since the development of a vaccine, diphtheria has almost been eradicated. There were no cases worldwide in year 2012 (WHO, 2012).

■ **ETIOLOGY.** Diphtheria is an infectious disease caused by *Corynebacterium diphtheriae* and characterized by severe inflammation of the respiratory system. It is transmitted by direct contact with droplets from an infected person. The incubation period is 2 to 5 days.

■ **SYMPTOMS.** It produces a membranous coating of the pharynx, nose, and sometimes the tracheobronchial tree. This membrane becomes a thick fibrinous **exudate** (ECKS-you-dayt; fluid composed of protein and white blood cells that seeps from tissue), causing extreme difficulty in breathing. The toxin also can produce degeneration in peripheral nerves, heart muscle, and other tissues.

■ **DIAGNOSIS.** Physical examination revealing a thick gray membrane covering the throat and tonsils, along with a positive culture of the membrane revealing diphtheria, confirms diagnosis.

■ **TREATMENT.** Treatment includes antibiotic therapy and diphtheria antitoxin.

■ **PREVENTION.** Immunization of children with the diphtheria/tetanus/pertussis (DTP) combination vaccine prevents this disease.

TUBERCULOSIS (TB)

■ **DESCRIPTION.** TB is an infectious disease primarily affecting the respiratory system. For many years, the incidence of TB was decreasing, but unfortunately, the incidence of TB in children has been increasing in recent years.

■ **ETIOLOGY.** TB is an infectious disease caused by the tubercle bacillus, *Mycobacterium tuberculosis*. Although the disease typically affects the respiratory system, it can also be found in the gastrointestinal system and the bones, brain, and lymph nodes. TB is transmitted by contaminated droplets. When the child is infected with the tubercle bacillus and the incubation period of 4 to 12 weeks is past, the skin test will test positive.

■ **SYMPTOMS.** Signs and symptoms of TB include a persistent cough, bloody sputum, lymph node enlargement, fever, and malaise. (See Chapter 9, "Respiratory System Diseases and Disorders," for more information about TB.)

Most children infected by the bacillus will not develop the symptomatic disease. The greatest percentage of cases of TB infection in children stays **dormant** (state of being inactive) and does not develop into the clinical disease.

■ **DIAGNOSIS.** Diagnosis is made by a positive skin test and sputum culture and clinical manifestations as well as a chest X-ray.

■ **TREATMENT.** For those children who develop active TB, treatment consists of drug therapy, rest, good nutrition, and prevention of spread of the disease to other family members. Children at higher risk for developing TB are those who have other chronic diseases, are HIV positive or have AIDS, are malnourished, live in poor hygienic conditions, live with adults with TB, or are otherwise immunosuppressed.

■ **PREVENTION.** The TB vaccine, bacille Calmette–Guérin (BCG), can be used for prevention and is recommended in communities where the rate of infection is greater than 1% per year.

TULAREMIA

■ **DESCRIPTION.** Tularemia is an infectious disease of rodents transmitted to humans usually through an insect bite. It may also be called rabbit fever or deer fly fever.

■ **ETIOLOGY.** Tularemia is caused by the bacterium *Francisella tularensis* and transmitted by the bite of an infected tick, deer fly, or other bloodsucking insect or by direct contact with an infected animal.

■ **SYMPTOMS.** Symptoms include headache, fever, generalized or localized pain, swelling of lymph nodes, chills, and vomiting.

■ **DIAGNOSIS.** Diagnosis is made by blood testing to identify antibodies to the bacteria. A chest X-ray can rule out pneumonia.

■ **TREATMENT.** Treatment with antibiotics given by muscle injection or intravenously is usually effective.

■ **PREVENTION.** Preventive methods include:

- Wearing long-sleeved shirt and long pants to protect the extremities from insects.
- Using insecticide containing DEET.
- Handling animals carefully. If hunting wild rabbit or deer, wearing gloves and using care in skinning and dressing the animal.
- Protecting pets by applying systemic preventives.
- Keeping away from wild or dead animals.

IMPETIGO

Impetigo is a contagious superficial **pyoderma** (PYE-oh-DER-mah; inflammatory, purulent dermatitis) commonly found on the face and hands of children (Figure 20–7). It is caused by *Staphylococcus aureus* or group A streptococci. Good hand washing is the best preventive strategy. For more information, see Chapter 18, "Integumentary System Diseases and Disorders."

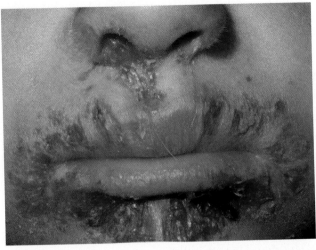

FIGURE 20–7   Impetigo.

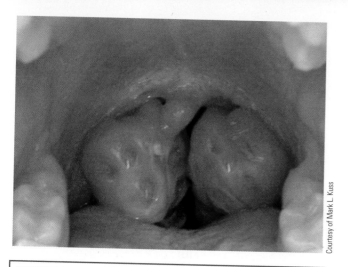

Courtesy of Mark L. Kuss

FIGURE 20–8 Acute tonsillitis.

ACUTE TONSILLITIS

■ **DESCRIPTION.** Tonsillitis is an infection of the palatine tonsils, tissue located on the posterior wall of the nasopharynx (Figure 20–8). The purpose of the tonsils is to help protect the respiratory tract from pathogens; thus, they tend to be a common site for inflammation and infection.

■ **ETIOLOGY.** Most tonsillar infections are caused by group A β-hemolytic streptococci.

■ **SYMPTOMS.** Symptoms include a sore throat, enlarged tonsils, cough, fever, and pain with swallowing.

■ **DIAGNOSIS.** Diagnosis is made by visual exam and throat culture.

■ **TREATMENT.** Antibiotics are given as supportive treatment. A **tonsillectomy** (TON-sih-LECT-toh-me; ectomy = removal; removal of the tonsils) is not recommended for children under 3 years of age but can be performed on older children who incur repeated infections.

■ **PREVENTION.** Preventive methods include avoiding contact with infected individuals, never sharing drinking glasses, and washing hands frequently with antibacterial soap. After a bout of tonsillitis, throw away the old toothbrush and begin using a new one to prevent reinfection.

OTITIS MEDIA

■ **DESCRIPTION.** Otitis media is an acute bacterial infection of the middle ear and one of the most common diseases of children.

■ **SYMPTOMS.** Symptoms include pain (in the infant, this symptom might be indicated by the child pulling on the ear); fever; drainage; and, on otoscopic examination, a bulging, reddish tympanic membrane. Treatment includes antibiotic therapy and acetaminophen for fever and pain. If the condition persists, a myringotomy with tympanoplasty tubes might be the treatment of choice. (See Chapter 16, "Eye and Ear Diseases and Disorders," for more information.)

Consider This ...

Children grow faster in the spring than in any other season.

Fungal Diseases

Fungal diseases are usually seen on the skin or mucous membranes in children. They can afflict any age, but some, such as candidiasis, are more common in infants than in older children. Most fungal infections are not severe but can be very irritating to the child and need medical intervention to halt the spread of the infection.

CANDIDIASIS

■ **DESCRIPTION.** Candidiasis, also known as a yeast infection, is a common disease in all ages as previously discussed in Chapter 18. Candidiasis in infants is commonly found in the mouth (thrush) and on the buttocks (diaper rash) (Figure 20–9).

■ **ETIOLOGY.** Candidiasis is caused by an excessive growth of *Candida albicans*. If the organism passes through the intestine, it can cause diaper rash because the continually wet diaper area is a good medium for growth. The infant can acquire the infection during delivery, or it can develop later from antibiotic therapy or unclean nipples on bottles.

■ **SYMPTOMS.** White plaques are present on the mucous membranes of the tongue and on the buttocks area.

■ **DIAGNOSIS.** Diagnosis is made by visual examination of the affected area and microscopic examination of white patch scraping or a culture of the same.

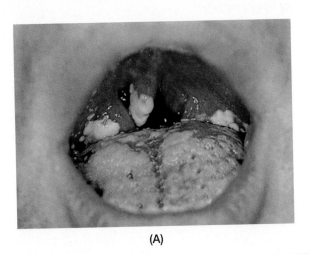

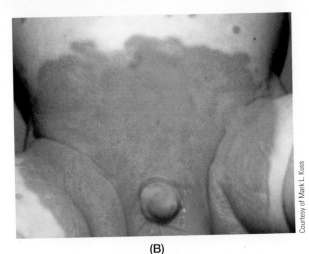

(A)   (B)

FIGURE 20–9   Candidiasis. (A) Mouth—thrush. (B) Perineal area—diaper rash.

■ **TREATMENT.** The treatment of choice is nystatin oral suspension or ointment.

■ **PREVENTION.** Thrush in infants can be prevented by breastfeeding rather than bottle feeding. If the babies are bottle fed, do not put them to bed while still feeding and avoid using pacifiers for long periods of time.

Prevention methods for young children include having them rinse their mouths after eating candy, regularly replacing their toothbrushes, and serving them yogurt on a regular basis.

To prevent diaper rash, keep the baby's diaper area clean and dry. Check the diaper soon after the infant goes to sleep because this is often a time they might wet. Allow time for the skin to dry thoroughly between changes before applying another diaper. Let the baby's skin dry by allowing them to go without a diaper as often as possible.

TINEA

■ **DESCRIPTION.** Tinea infections encompass a group of diseases commonly known as ringworm. They usually affect the scalp and area between the toes in children. Teens, primarily young males, commonly have the infection in their toes (athlete's foot) and groin area (jock itch) (Figure 20–10). For more information, see Chapter 18.

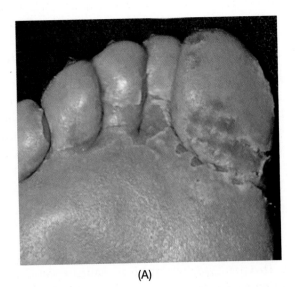

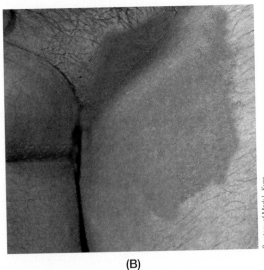

(A)   (B)

FIGURE 20–10   Tinea. (A) Foot and toes—athlete's foot. (B) Groin area—jock itch.

Parasitic Diseases

Parasitic diseases include all disorders that are caused by an organism that feeds on another organism, such as a worm that lives in the intestine of an individual. Parasites are common in areas where poor nutrition, contaminated water, and low socioeconomic conditions are widespread. The parasitic diseases common to children in the United States include giardiasis, pediculosis, and some helminth (worm) infestations.

GIARDIASIS

■ **DESCRIPTION.** Giardiasis is infection with a parasite called *Giardia*. Young children are affected three times more often than adults, leading some to believe that as we age, we develop some immunity to the parasite. An entire family can be affected with symptoms varying from mild to severe. As many as two-thirds of infected individuals are asymptomatic.

■ **ETIOLOGY.** Giardiasis is caused by the *Giardia lamblia* protozoan, which affects the digestive system. These protozoa lodge in the lining of the small intestines and absorb nutrients from the host.

■ **SYMPTOMS.** Symptoms of giardiasis include watery diarrhea, nausea, cramping, **flatulence** (excessive gas), fever, and anorexia (loss of appetite). This condition affects the body's ability to absorb fat, so the stool will float and be shiny and quite foul-smelling. Chronic giardiasis often leads to weight loss and signs of poor nutrition in children.

■ **DIAGNOSIS.** Diagnosis is by laboratory stool examination. It might take as many as three samples to detect the presence of the protozoan.

■ **TREATMENT.** Treatment usually includes furazolidone or similar drugs and symptom relief as needed. Clear liquids are given to prevent dehydration, a dangerous complication of the disease.

■ **PREVENTION.** Guidelines for prevention include:

- Drinking only clean water approved by the local health authorities.
- Drinking bottled water if the quality of the local water is questionable.
- Washing hands before preparing meals.
- Encouraging children to wash their hands after they use the bathroom and especially before eating.
- Washing raw fruits and vegetables thoroughly before eating them.

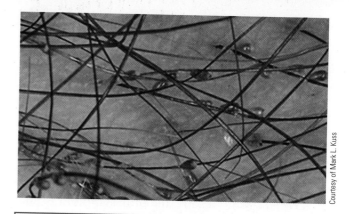

Courtesy of Mark L. Kuss

FIGURE 20–11   Pediculosis—hair nits.

PEDICULOSIS

Pediculosis is infestation with lice. Lice infestations reach epidemic levels in many school systems throughout the United States. Lice are transmitted from human to human by direct contact and reproduce rapidly with the adult female parasite producing about six eggs every 24 hours. Lice on the head and lice eggs (**nits**) attached to hair are easy to see (Figure 20–11). The most effective treatment is permethrin 1% crème rinse. In addition, vinegar and water can loosen the nits prior to combing with a delousing comb. This treatment should be performed every day until all nits are removed. For more information, see Chapter 18.

PINWORMS

■ **DESCRIPTION.** Pinworms, also known as seatworms or threadworms, are parasitic nematodes (specific type of helminthes or worms) that infect the intestines and rectum. They do not cause physical harm, other than itching, and never infect the blood. Pinworms can infect anyone because they live on objects and are easily transmitted.

■ **ETIOLOGY.** The causative organism is *Enterobius vermicularis*. Pinworms are transmitted by ingestion or inhalation of the eggs, usually by hand-to-mouth contact. These eggs can survive on most surfaces for 2 to 3 weeks. Individuals become infected by touching any infected surface, such as towels, door knobs, toilet seats, toys, or drinking glasses, to name a few. Pets do not give humans pinworms, but these eggs can be picked up off the fur if an infected individual recently touched the animal. When the eggs are on the hands, touching the mouth or food that is placed in the mouth moves these eggs to the digestive system.

The ingested eggs pass through the digestive system and attach to the inside wall of the large intestine. A few weeks later, the female pinworm leaves the intestine to move to the rectum. They often come out of the rectum at night and lay 10,000 to 20,000 eggs around the anus, causing intense itching. Scratching around the anus during sleep is common and moves the eggs to the fingers and fingernails. Contaminated fingers then move the eggs to any surface the infected individual touches, and the cycle starts over.

■ **SYMPTOMS.** Usually, the only symptom is anal itching. Pinworms can be seen as tiny white threads about the size of a staple, noticeable in the commode after a bowel movement or in the child's underwear in the morning.

■ **DIAGNOSIS.** Diagnosis is by microscopic examination of stool revealing pinworms. Pinworm eggs can be obtained for microscopic examination by pressing a piece of clear scotch tape to the child's anus early in the morning. The eggs stick to the tape and can be easily viewed under a microscope (Figure 20–12).

■ **TREATMENT.** Treatment includes over-the-counter or prescription drug therapy and instructions in good hand washing. Treatment might have to be repeated in approximately 2 weeks, and the entire family might need treating. Cleaning bed linens, clothing, and surfaces helps reduce surface infection.

■ **PREVENTION.** Good hand washing, good toileting habits, not placing fingers in or around the mouth, and not biting fingernails are all preventive measures.

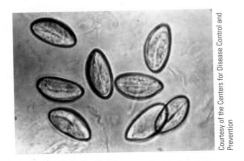

Consider This …

Only humans sleep on their backs.

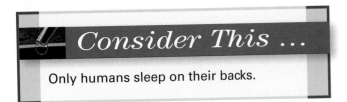

FIGURE 20–12   Microscopic view of pinworm eggs.

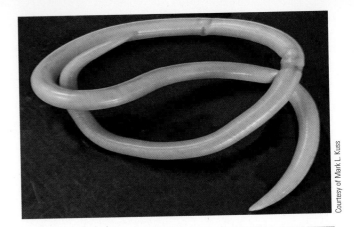

Courtesy of Mark L. Kuss

FIGURE 20–13   Roundworm.

ROUNDWORMS

■ **DESCRIPTION.** Roundworms (*Ascaris lumbricoides*) are commonly found in soil. A handful of dirt can easily contain thousands of roundworms (Figure 20–13).

■ **ETIOLOGY.** These parasites are easily ingested by infected hand-to-mouth activity. In the digestive system, these parasites lodge in the intestine, absorbing nutrients from the host. Roundworms, like pinworms, are transmitted by transfer of the eggs to the mouth or nose.

■ **SYMPTOMS.** Symptoms can be more severe than in pinworm infestations, depending on how long they reside in the intestine before treatment. The child might complain of abdominal pain, excessive gas, loss of appetite, or weight loss. Vomiting also can occur. If the helminthes are inhaled, symptoms of pneumonia might be present.

■ **DIAGNOSIS.** Diagnosis is usually made by identification of the parasites in a stool specimen.

■ **TREATMENT.** Treatment is the same as for pinworms.

■ **PREVENTION.** Good hand washing and keeping the fingers away from the mouth are preventive measures.

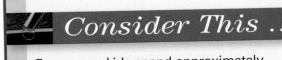

Consider This …

Every year, kids spend approximately one-half billion dollars on chewing gum.

RESPIRATORY DISEASES

Respiratory illnesses are the most common childhood diseases seen by physicians. Infants are extremely susceptible to upper respiratory problems because their immune systems are not fully developed, and they have very small air passages, so even a minor amount of mucus can obstruct a passage and cause respiratory distress. Preschool and school-aged children are very vulnerable to the contagious respiratory diseases because they have a great deal of person-to-person and hand-to-mouth contacts. Several of the viral and bacterial respiratory diseases were covered previously in this chapter.

Sudden Infant Death Syndrome (SIDS)

■ **DESCRIPTION.** Sudden infant death syndrome, or SIDS, is the abrupt unexplainable death of an infant under age 1. It is also known as crib death because the infant is found dead after being put in bed to sleep.

■ **ETIOLOGY.** There are several theories about the cause of SIDS, but none have been proven at this time. It is now recommended that infants be placed in bed in the **supine** (SUE-pine; on the back) position rather than **prone** (on the stomach side) because more cases of SIDS have occurred in children lying in the prone position. Children at higher risk for SIDS include premature infants and siblings of SIDS infants and those with sleep apnea and respiratory problems.

■ **SYMPTOMS.** The only sign is a death of unknown cause in an infant.

■ **DIAGNOSIS.** Diagnosis might be suspected when the child is taken to the emergency department, but SIDS can be confirmed only by autopsy and investigation. A diagnosis of SIDS is very traumatic to parents and families, who experience not only loss and grief but also guilt.

■ **TREATMENT.** SIDS often elicits a 911 emergency call.

■ **PREVENTION.** Counseling, along with further education, should be available for these families so SIDS might be prevented in future children.

Croup

■ **DESCRIPTION.** Croup, also known as laryngotracheobronchitis, is an upper respiratory infection.

■ **ETIOLOGY.** Croup is caused by parainfluenza viruses 1 and 2 and affects children from 3 months to 3 years of age.

■ **SYMPTOMS.** It is characterized by a harsh barking cough, fever, **inspiratory stridor** (STRYE-dor; high-pitched sound during inspiration through blocked airways), laryngeal spasms, and increased difficulty in breathing at night.

■ **DIAGNOSIS.** Diagnosis is made by physical examination.

■ **TREATMENT.** Treatment usually includes high humidity, fluids, rest, racemic epinephrine (racemic epinephrine provides bronchodilatation with only a minimal increase in heart rate and blood pressure), and antipyretics if needed. Complications can be serious if a **patent** (open) airway is not maintained.

■ **PREVENTION.** Preventive activities include:

- Good and frequent hand washing.
- Avoiding sick children.
- Teaching children to sneeze or cough into a tissue or into their elbow.
- Keeping immunizations current, especially *Haemophilus influenzae* type b (Hib).

Media Link

View an animation on croup on the Online Resources.

Adenoid Hyperplasia

■ **DESCRIPTION.** Adenoid hyperplasia is the enlargement of the pharyngeal tonsils, lymphoid tissues located on the posterior wall of the nasopharynx above the palatine tonsils. Hyperplasia of the adenoids is a very common occurrence in children.

■ **ETIOLOGY.** Adenoid hyperplasia can be caused by infection or a congenital defect.

■ **SYMPTOMS.** The enlarged adenoids can block the Eustachian tubes, causing ear problems such as otitis media. Because of the location of the adenoids, enlargement also can cause some obstruction of the airway, resulting in breathing difficulty.

COMPLEMENTARY AND ALTERNATIVE THERAPY

Massage Therapy to Improve Lung Function

Researchers studied the effect of massage therapy on the lung function of children with asthma and found that it was beneficial in improving their breathing. The participants in the experimental group received 20 minutes of massage therapy every night for 5 weeks before going to bed. In addition, they continued to receive their usual therapy and medications. The control group just used the traditional therapy regimen. The results showed that the group receiving the massage therapy had improvement in their pulmonary function tests. Thus, massage therapy might be an adjunct or alternative therapy for children with asthma. The researchers cautioned that continued research needs to be done before this becomes a recommended treatment for children with asthma.

Source: Fattah & Hamdy (2011).

■ **DIAGNOSIS.** Physical examination revealing enlarged, infected tonsils that might have deep pockets or crypts is indicative of the condition. Children with recurring middle ear infections may well have adenoid hyperplasia. A throat culture also can be performed.

■ **TREATMENT.** Treatment focuses on correcting the cause of the hyperplasia. If repeated infections are the cause, antibiotic therapy is instituted. If the enlargement cannot be corrected, an **adenoidectomy** (AD-eh-noy-DECK-toh-me; ectomy = removal; removal of the adenoids) might be necessary.

■ **PREVENTION.** Prompt and effective diagnosis and treatment of sore throats usually prevent the condition. Avoiding children with respiratory infections will help reduce the spread of these illnesses.

Asthma

■ **DESCRIPTION.** Asthma is a serious, chronic respiratory system disease. More than 5 million children under the age of 18 have been diagnosed with asthma. It is the most common chronic childhood disease and the number one cause of school absence for illness in children today. Approximately one of every four children is affected by asthma. The cost of asthma in the United States is estimated to be $56 billion a year (Centers for Disease Control and Prevention, 2011).

■ **ETIOLOGY.** The cause of asthma is unknown.

■ **SYMPTOMS.** Asthma is characterized by acute episodes of coughing, wheezing, and shortness of breath. Stimuli (called triggers) of an asthmatic episode vary and include cigarette smoke, dust mites, chemicals, pollen, animal hair and feathers, molds, cold air, and excessive exercise. Regardless of the trigger, the result is airway swelling and blockage causing the symptoms of respiratory distress.

■ **DIAGNOSIS.** Diagnosis is made by physical examination, chest X-rays (although they usually show normal results except in severe cases), pulmonary function studies, and allergy tests.

■ **TREATMENT.** Treatment of asthma in the child includes avoidance of the triggers, medications such as bronchodilators and anti-inflammatory agents, and careful monitoring of the disease. A peak flow meter is used to monitor the breathing capacity of the child. This device measures the flow of air in a forced exhalation and reports it in liters per minute. The value of peak expiratory flow indicates the degree of airway obstruction. The data obtained can help identify the onset of an asthmatic episode. The physician might use the information from the chart of measurements kept by the child to prescribe the appropriate medication regimen.

■ **PREVENTION.** There is no known prevention for asthma, but asthma management is helpful in preventing episodes. Educating the child and family is very important in effective asthma management programs. This allows the child to live a normal life with appropriate activity levels, prevents acute asthmatic attacks, and helps the child avoid hospitalization for severe episodes. (See Chapters 5 and 9 for more information on asthma.)

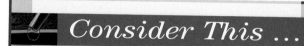

Consider This ...

In children age 5 to 17 years, asthma is the leading cause of school absences from chronic illness.

Media Link

View an animation about asthma in a child on the Online Resources.

Pneumonia

■ *DESCRIPTION.* Pneumonia is an infection marked by acute inflammation of the lung parenchyma.

■ *ETIOLOGY.* Pneumonia can be of viral or bacterial origin. It is characterized by the alveolar air spaces in the lungs becoming filled with exudate, inflammatory cells, and fibrin.

■ *SYMPTOMS.* The symptoms include cough, fever, wheezing, and malaise.

■ *DIAGNOSIS.* Diagnosis is made by chest X-ray and auscultation of the chest.

■ *TREATMENT.* Treatment is supportive in viral pneumonia, but antibiotics can be used in bacterial pneumonia. Viral pneumonia usually runs its course in children in about 5 to 7 days, but bacterial pneumonia can be more severe. (See Chapter 9 for more information.)

■ *PREVENTION.* Avoiding causative agents, promptly treating other respiratory illnesses, and good hand washing are preventive activities.

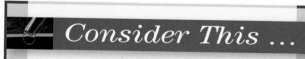

Consider This ...

Boys get hiccups more often than girls.

DIGESTIVE DISEASES

Ingestion, digestion, absorption, and elimination are essential body functions. Children with digestive diseases can experience serious growth and development problems from a lack of these. Fluid and electrolyte imbalances are frequently more severe in children, especially in infants, than in adults. The imbalances can be caused by vomiting, diarrhea, or other digestive diseases that inhibit the child's ability to ingest or digest and absorb food and fluids.

Colic is a common symptom of digestive problems or disease in children. It is particularly common in young infants. Symptoms of colic include paroxysms of gastrointestinal pain with crying and irritability. It can be due to a variety of causes such as emotional upset, overfeeding, or swallowing air.

Fluid Imbalances

Children have a higher metabolic rate than adults and thus have a higher exchange of fluids. This fact puts them at risk for serious complications if they experience bouts of vomiting or diarrhea. Children can become dehydrated and develop severe electrolyte imbalances in a very short period of time. Dehydration is life-threatening in very young children and infants. Diagnosis is made by reported history of continued vomiting, diarrhea, or both; physical examination; and laboratory data.

Treatment focuses on replacement of the fluids and electrolytes. If the child cannot retain fluids because of vomiting, intravenous therapy is necessary. If fluids continue to be lost because of diarrhea, treatment focuses on correcting the cause of the diarrhea, administering medications to prevent the hyperactive bowel problems, and giving replacement fluids and electrolytes either orally or intravenously.

Nonprescription oral electrolyte solutions are available for infants and young children and for older children. Children who are active in sports in very warm weather should drink electrolyte replacement fluids frequently to prevent dehydration.

Food Allergies

A food allergy is an overreaction of the immune system to a particular food or ingredient in the food. The reaction can occur rapidly within seconds or take several hours after ingestion of the food. Symptoms of food allergies include nausea, diarrhea, abdominal

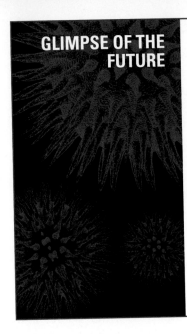

Preventing Food Allergy Reactions

The numbers of children with allergies/allergic reactions to various foods is increasing at an incredibly high rate. It seems that the immune system is quite vulnerable to the environmental changes in recent decades. Historically, the treatment was often just to avoid the allergen. However, this has been ineffective in many cases, especially when the allergen is unknown. The new strategy to reduce or eliminate allergy problems includes restoring the body's internal balance and the use of probiotic supplements. Other nutrients being studied include antioxidants and vitamin D. Some tips on how to prevent allergic reactions/allergies in children still include avoiding cigarette smoke and promoting breastfeeding. Avoiding the allergen is still a good practice, but it is now usually left off the recommendations list since it is often very difficult to do. More research on the use of probiotics, specific dietary guidelines, and what nutrients are most beneficial to reduce the effects of allergens is still needed.

Source: Prescott & Nowak-Węgrzyn (2011).

pain, coughing, wheezing, itching, rash, headache, and swelling of hands, face, and lips.

Food allergies are more common in children than in adults but still affect only a small number of children. The greatest incidence of food allergy occurs in children under age 1, and the most common allergies are to cow's milk and eggs. Most of these allergies disappear by age 3 to 5. Allergies to peanuts and fish seem to last much longer but usually disappear by the time the child is in school.

If the food allergy develops after age 3, it usually continues into adult life. Children at higher risk of developing food allergies are those who have parents with food allergies or those who were high-risk infants prenatally and at birth. Children with food allergies as infants are at greater risk for developing respiratory allergies as they get older.

The best method for preventing allergies is to avoid giving children, especially high-risk children, the common allergenic foods. Children can be tested for allergic antibodies if necessary. Medications are not given for food allergies, but some might be necessary to relieve the symptoms of the allergic reaction. (For more information, see Chapter 5.)

Eating Disorders

Eating disorders have become a major problem among children, especially adolescent females. The two most common types of eating disorders are anorexia nervosa and bulimia. Anorexia is characterized by the inability to eat over long periods of time, which results in extreme weight loss, fluid and electrolyte imbalances, and a life-threatening state. Bulimia is characterized by binge eating followed by purging the food. Both of these conditions are discussed in detail in Chapter 21, "Mental Health Diseases and Disorders."

CARDIOVASCULAR DISEASES

Most cardiovascular diseases in children are related to genetic or developmental disorders, which are discussed in Chapter 19, "Genetic and Developmental Diseases and Disorders."

MUSCULOSKELETAL DISEASES

Musculoskeletal disorders in children are common because of their high activity levels and rapid growth patterns. Such problems range from soft-tissue injuries and fractures to joint and bone deformities and degenerative muscle disorders. Some of these have already been discussed in Chapter 6, "Musculoskeletal System Diseases and Disorders," and Chapter 19.

Legg–Calvé–Perthes

■ **DESCRIPTION.** Legg–Calvé–Perthes (LCP) disease is an avascular necrosis of the upper end of the femur. The blood supply to the femoral head is reduced, causing changes in bone growth. The disease is known as a disorder of growth that is most common in boys aged 4 to 8 years.

■ **ETIOLOGY.** The cause is unknown.

■ **SYMPTOMS.** In most cases, the only symptom is pain that increases with walking or running.

■ **DIAGNOSIS.** Diagnosis is made by examination and X-ray.

■ **TREATMENT.** The treatment objective is to maintain the correct position of the femoral head in the acetabulum of the hip until healing occurs. This is accomplished by bed rest for a week to 10 days along with range-of-motion exercises. Traction, casts, or braces also can be used to maintain the correct position of the femoral head. If this does not correct the condition, surgical intervention might be necessary. An osteotomy may be performed to place the femoral head in the correct position. If left uncorrected, permanent deformity can result.

■ **PREVENTION.** There is no known preventive measure.

Ewing's Sarcoma

■ **DESCRIPTION.** Ewing's sarcoma, also known as Ewing's tumor, is a malignant neoplasm that occurs before age 20. It is more common in males than in females and is usually located in a long bone such as the femur.

■ **ETIOLOGY.** The cause of the tumor is unknown.

■ **SYMPTOMS.** Symptoms include swelling and pain.

■ **DIAGNOSIS.** Diagnosis is made by X-ray, computerized tomography (CT) or magnetic resonance imaging (MRI), and bone scan. A biopsy is necessary to differentiate the exact type of tumor from other kinds of bone tumors.

■ **TREATMENT.** Treatment usually includes chemotherapy and, in some cases, radiation therapy. Surgery might be performed but is not usually the first choice of treatment, especially if the tumor is in the leg or arm, because that would necessitate amputation of the extremity. Ewing's sarcoma is quickly metastatic and highly malignant, but if no metastasis has occurred, the prognosis is very good.

■ **PREVENTION.** There is no known way to prevent this disease.

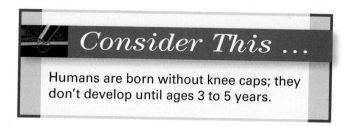

Consider This ...

Humans are born without knee caps; they don't develop until ages 3 to 5 years.

■ BLOOD DISEASES

One of the most common disorders of the blood and blood-forming organs in children is leukemia, a type of cancer. Many of the other blood disorders diagnosed in children are chronic diseases such as hemophilia and sickle cell disease. These, as well as acute disorders of the blood such as iron deficiency anemia and some cancers such as Hodgkin's disease, are discussed in Chapter 7 "Blood and Blood-Forming Organs Diseases and Disorders" and are not repeated in this chapter.

Leukemia

■ **DESCRIPTION.** Leukemia (leuk = white, emia = blood) is a malignancy of the blood-forming cells located in the bone marrow. Leukemia is the most common form of cancer in children. Approximately 3,800 children are diagnosed each year with leukemia (Leukemia and Lymphoma Society, 2012). Leukemia is diagnosed more frequently in boys than in girls.

■ **ETIOLOGY.** The cause of the disease is unknown, but factors that increase the risk for developing leukemia include exposure to radiation and the presence of genetic or immunologic disorders.

The most common type of leukemia in children is acute lymphoblastic leukemia (ALL), characterized by a proliferation of immature white blood cells. As the marrow becomes filled with the diseased white cells, platelets, red cells, and healthy white-cell production decrease, causing symptoms to appear.

■ **SYMPTOMS.** Symptoms include pallor (pale skin); easy bleeding or bruising; fatigue; joint, bone, or abdominal pain; and fever.

■ **DIAGNOSIS.** Leukemia is diagnosed by medical history, complete blood count, and bone marrow biopsy.

■ **TREATMENT.** Childhood leukemias are now among the most curable diseases of all types of childhood cancers. Treatment for ALL in children is directed at killing all cancer cells.

Chemotherapy is the treatment of choice. **Intrathecal** (IN-trah-THEE-kal; intra = within, thecal = spinal cord; injected into the spinal fluid) medications are used to destroy any cancer cells in the central nervous system. Then, other combinations of the chemotherapeutic agents are given to prevent reappearance of the cancer cells.

Radiation also can be used in some cases. One of the complications of this therapy is the reduced ability to fight off infections.

■ **PREVENTION.** There is no way to prevent most types of leukemia.

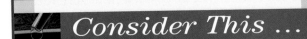

Consider This ...

What children learn in the first 8 years of their lives has lifelong influence in shaping their personality and career.

NEUROLOGIC DISEASES

There are many neurologic disorders in children. Some of them, such as meningitis and encephalitis, are covered in Chapter 15, "Nervous System Diseases and Disorders." The genetic and developmental ones, including cerebral palsy, are discussed in Chapter 19.

Reye's Syndrome

■ **DESCRIPTION.** Reye's syndrome is an acute **encephalopathy** (en-SEF-ah-LOP-ah-thee; encephalo = brain, opathy = disease; disorder of the brain) seen in children under age 15 who have had a viral infection.

■ **ETIOLOGY.** The cause is unknown, but a relationship has been found between the disease and the use of aspirin for febrile illnesses in children. Thus, it is recommended that aspirin not be given to children and acetaminophen used instead.

■ **SYMPTOMS.** Reye's syndrome is characterized by nausea, vomiting, liver enlargement, lethargy, seizures, coma, and in many cases, death.

■ **DIAGNOSIS.** This should be suspected in a child who has had a recent viral illness and begins vomiting and having episodes of unconsciousness. Blood testing of liver enzymes that are abnormally high, along with lumbar puncture to rule out encephalitis and meningitis, might be necessary.

■ **TREATMENT.** This is a life-threatening illness that requires prompt diagnosis and treatment. Most cases are managed in an intensive care unit.

■ **PREVENTION.** Avoiding aspirin and products containing aspirin for children and young people is the best prevention.

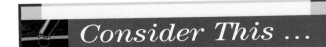

Consider This ...

Children burn more calories sleeping than they do watching TV.

EYE AND EAR DISEASES

Children are curious and use their senses even more than adults during the learning and growing process, so problems with the eyes and ears can have profound effects on the child's ability to learn and develop. Some of the common eye and ear problems have been covered in previous chapters and in other sections of this chapter.

Strabismus

Strabismus, also known as lazy eye or crossed eyes, is a condition of lack of parallelism of the eyes. This can be normal in the very young infant but should not be present after about 4 months of age. For more information, see Chapter 16, "Eye and Ear Diseases and Disorders."

Deafness

■ **DESCRIPTION.** Hearing losses in children range from mild to complete.

■ **ETIOLOGY.** The cause of deafness can be unknown or genetic or from trauma, infections, or exposure to ototoxic drugs.

■ **SYMPTOMS.** The primary symptom is a loss of hearing.

■ **DIAGNOSIS.** Audiometric testing is needed for an accurate diagnosis of the extent of hearing loss.

■ **TREATMENT.** Treatment depends on the cause and severity of the loss. If the hearing loss is the nonconductive type, some medications or surgical interventions can be helpful in restoring all or part of the lost hearing. Several types of hearing aids are designed especially for children for use in the ear, over the ear, and attached to the eyepieces of glasses, which can be fitted by professional hearing specialists. Cochlear implants are now being inserted surgically. They stimulate the eighth cranial nerve (vestibulocochlear nerve) and send out electrical impulses to the inner ear.

■ **PREVENTION.** Reduction in noise levels and avoiding ototoxic medications are preventive measures.

TRAUMA

Trauma in children is a major cause of debility and death. Child abuse is found at all ages, but some types of trauma such as drug abuse and suicide are much more common in adolescents. Poisonings are at peak levels in toddlers.

Child Abuse

Child abuse is a serious problem in the United States. It is more common than most other pediatric illnesses and is frequently fatal. It has been difficult to define because limits of punishment such as spanking are hard to set. However, it is generally defined as purposeful (not accidental), significant, or demonstrable harm to a child, whether in the form of physical, sexual, or emotional harm. It also can be in the form of neglect, which accounts for a major portion of the child abuse diagnosed. Neglect is defined as failing to provide basic needs such as food, clothes, and schooling for the child.

Physical child abuse, and sometimes neglect, is usually diagnosed by physical examination, review of verbal explanations from the child and parents, and investigation by authorities. It can be difficult to diagnose or prove at times because of conflicting stories reported by those involved. Many children try to cover up the abuse due to fear of retaliation by the abuser or because of shame.

The most frequent instrument to inflict physical abuse is the hand, although belts, clubs, and other items are also used. Burns by cigarettes are also common, especially in very young children. Fractures in children under age 3 are suggestive of physical abuse. One of the most common injuries in infants is the shaken baby syndrome. This is a serious injury to the brain caused by vigorous shaking of the child and can result in death.

Sexual abuse has become an epidemic problem. It is defined by specific acts and might or might not include intercourse. Unfortunately, sexual abuse of children frequently occurs for years before being reported, and the emotional effects are often more serious than the physical effects. The easiest way to identify sexual abuse is to listen to the child, ask open-ended questions, and report suspected abuse to appropriate persons.

Emotional abuse is the most difficult form of child abuse to recognize and diagnose. Constant stigmatizing, berating, or ignoring a child is considered emotional abuse. The effects of this abuse are manifested in symptoms such as failure to thrive, learning disabilities, eating disorders, social isolation, acting-out behaviors, depression, and other behavior and personality disorders.

Recognizing child abuse early can save the life of the child, and most states have mandatory reporting laws. Usually, these laws protect the person reporting the suspected abuse from any litigation due to the report. Teachers, clergy, health professionals, and law enforcement personnel are usually listed as the persons mandated to report suspected cases, but all individuals should be aware of the problem and report any suspicions of abuse to authorities.

Suicide

The overall suicide rate among youth has declined in the past decade, but it is still the third leading cause of death among young people (15–24 years of age). Firearms were used in 57% of male suicides (Traylor et al., 2010). The incidence is much less for females than for males of the same ages but is still significant.

The suicide rate for males has increased significantly in the past two decades. It is thought that most teens who commit suicide do so during or immediately after a period of depression. The depression can be due to a variety of factors such as low self-esteem, chemical abuse, sociological makeup, family problems, abuse, or any combination of these. Alcohol abuse has also been found to be a contributing factor, as are other risky behaviors such as drug abuse and gang membership.

Suicide attempts are highest in incarcerated youths. Females have a higher rate of suicide ideation and attempts than males but a much lower incidence of death. Sexual abuse also contributes to suicide ideation and suicide attempts. Some children have been involved in suicide pacts with others, but this is not common. Gay and bisexual youths have a higher suicide rate than heterosexual youths of the same age.

Early intervention is the key to preventing suicides in children. Recognition of problems in adolescents and involvement in treatment programs is imperative, and even casual statements about death or killing oneself need to be taken seriously by parents, counselors, teachers, and friends. These youths need to be referred to special counseling programs as soon as possible. In addition, early intervention in dysfunctional families and prevention of sexual abuse and alcohol and drug abuse is extremely important.

Drug Abuse

Illicit drug, alcohol, and tobacco use among children, especially adolescents, is occurring in epidemic proportions in the United States. The most common drugs used by children and adolescents include marijuana, cocaine, methamphetamine, alcohol, cigarettes, LSD, inhalants, and anabolic steroids. Children continually use and abuse many other drugs, stimulants, and depressants on a daily basis.

Almost any product that gives the individual an altered sense of reality has been used improperly by children and teens. Products such as glue, cough syrup, correction fluid, mouthwash, and a variety of other products have been used to obtain a high. Unfortunately, many of these can be deadly, especially when mixed with alcohol or other drugs. More detailed information about drug abuse is discussed in Chapter 21 in the section titled "Substance-Related Mental Disorders."

Poisoning

Accidental poisoning can occur when a child ingests medications, cleaning products, alcohol, cosmetics, or other toxins. Parents and other adults frequently fail to recognize how toxic certain substances can be

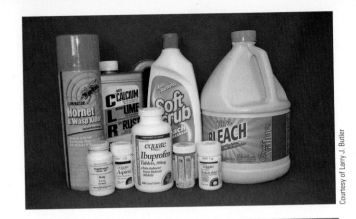

FIGURE 20–14 Various common household poisons and medicines that can be dangerous for children.

or do not realize the consequences of leaving them in places accessible to children (Figure 20–14).

Accidental poisoning is among the top five causes of death in children under 10 years of age. About 75% of all poisonings occur in children under 6 years of age. Children are inquisitive and tend to put things in their mouths, with a devastating consequence when the substance is toxic.

Most poisonings are due to common substances found in the home such as cleaning products, medicines, and plants. Generally, the poisoning is an acute event, and treatment is provided at a physician's office or emergency room. Symptoms and treatment depend on the substance ingested.

Lead poisoning, however, is a chronic event. Children suffering neurologic symptoms, chronic anemia, or difficulty with coordination should be evaluated for lead poisoning. The diagnosis is made by checking the blood for lead levels. Chelation therapy treatment is instituted to remove the lead from the blood.

Every state has poison control centers, most with an 800 number to call for emergency information in case of an accidental poisoning. Generally, local hospitals also have an emergency poison control information number.

Although over-the-counter medications to induce vomiting are available, it is wise to check with one of the poison control services prior to instituting treatment in the home. Many products should not be vomited up by the child because they are caustic and can do further damage if treated in that manner. All individuals should be aware of the problem of poisoning and prevent poisonings in the home by following a few guidelines as stated in the following Healthy Highlight.

HEALTHY HIGHLIGHT

Preventing Poisonings in Children

Medication Safety

- Store all medications—prescription and nonprescription—in a locked cabinet, far from children's reach.
- Never leave vitamin bottles, aspirin bottles, or other medications on the kitchen table, countertops, bedside tables, or dresser tops. Small children might decide to emulate adults and help themselves.
- Do not ever tell a child that medicine is candy.
- Take special precautions when you have houseguests. Be sure their medications are far from reach, preferably locked in one of their bags.
- Do not keep aspirin or other medicines in a purse; children can find them when searching for gum or a toy.
- Child-resistant packaging does not mean childproof packaging. Do not rely on packaging to protect your children.
- Never administer medication to a child in the dark; you might give the wrong dosage or even the wrong medication.
- After taking or administering medication, be sure to reattach the safety cap and store the medication away safely.

Chemical Safety

- Store household cleaning products and aerosol sprays in a high cabinet far from reach. Do not keep any cleaning supplies under the sink, including dishwasher detergent and dishwashing liquids.
- Never put cleaning products in old soda bottles or containers that were once used for food.
- When cleaning or using household chemicals, never leave the bottles unattended if a small child is present.
- Never put roach powders or rat poison on the floors of your home.
- Keep hazardous automotive and gardening products in a securely locked area in your garage.
- Do not leave alcoholic drinks where children can reach them. Take special care during parties; guests might not be conscious of where they have left their drinks. Clean up promptly after the party.
- Keep bottles of alcohol in a locked cabinet far from children's reach.
- Keep mouthwash out of the reach of children. Many brands of mouthwash contain substantial amounts of alcohol.

Lead Paint

- If you have an older home, have the paint tested for lead.
- Do not use cribs, bassinets, high chairs, painted toys, or toy chests made before 1978. These can have a finish that contains dangerously high levels of lead.

Other Toxic Items

- Never leave cosmetics and toiletries within easy reach of children. Be especially cautious with perfume, hair dye, hair spray, nail and shoe polish, and nail polish remover.
- Learn the names of all the plants in your house and remove any that could be toxic.
- Discard used button-cell batteries safely and store any unused ones far from children's reach. (Alkaline substances are poisonous.)

HEALTHY HIGHLIGHT

Immunization Schedule for Children

- Birth to 4 months:
  Hepatitis B—doses 1 and 2 of 3
- 2 months:
  Diphtheria, tetanus, and acellular pertussis (DTaP)—dose 1 of 5
  Haemophilus influenzae type b (Hib)—dose 1 of 4
  Inactivated poliovirus (IPV)—dose 1 of 4
  Pneumococcal conjugate (PCV13)—dose 1 of 4
  Rotavirus (RV)
- 4 months:
  DTaP—dose 2 of 5
  Hib—dose 2 of 4
  IPV—dose 2 of 4
  PCV13—dose 2 of 4
  RV
- 6 months:
  DTaP—dose 3 of 5
  Hib—dose 3 of 4
  PCV13—dose 3 of 4
  RV
  Hepatitis B—dose 3 of 3
  IPV—dose 3 of 4
  Influenza—annual dose
- 12 months:
  Hib—dose 4 of 4
  PCV13—dose 4 of 4
  Measles, mumps, rubella (MMR)—dose 1 of 2
  Chicken pox (varicella)—dose 1 of 1
  Hepatitis A—2 doses (6 months apart)
- 15 months:
  DTaP—dose 4 of 5
- 2 years:
  PCV13
  Influenza
  Pneumococcal polysaccharide vaccine (PPSV)
  Meningococcal conjugate vaccine (MCV4)
  Hepatitis A
  Between ages 2 and 6 years, children who haven't had the hepatitis A vaccine can receive the series.
- 4 to 5 years:
  DTaP—dose 5 of 5
  IPV—dose 4 of 4
  MMR—dose 2 of 2
  Chicken pox (varicella)
  Influenza

(Continued)

HEALTHY HIGHLIGHT (continued)

- 7 years:
  Tetanus toxoid, reduced diphtheria toxoid, and acellular pertussis (Tdap) vaccine
  MCV4
  PCV13
  PPSV
  Hepatitis A
  Influenza
- 11 years:
  Influenza
  Tdap vaccine
  It is recommended to have a tetanus-diphtheria (Td) booster every 10 years.
  MCV4
  Human papillomavirus (HPV) vaccine (HPV vaccination is recommended for both boys and girls at age 11 or 12, but it can be given as early as age 9; it is a series of three injections over a 6-month period).

SUMMARY

Childhood is a time for rapid physical, emotional, and intellectual growth and development. Some childhood diseases can interfere with normal growth and development, but most are acute illnesses that are common among young people. The most common diseases in children are infectious respiratory illnesses. Following a regularly scheduled immunization program can prevent many of the infectious diseases of children. Individuals with congenital disorders, premature infants, and children in low socioeconomic households are at highest risk for contracting one of the common childhood diseases. Trauma affects children of all ages, races, and socioeconomic status and is one of the leading causes of disability and death in children.

REVIEW QUESTIONS

Short Answer

1. What are the most common diseases affecting children?

2. What are the common signs and symptoms of these diseases?

3. What immunization is available to prevent each of the following diseases?
   a. Mumps
   b. Measles
   c. Pertussis

     d. Polio

     e. Diphtheria

     f. Influenza

     g. Rubella

     h. Tetanus

     i. Hepatitis

4. TB is found in which body system?

5. What are the four types of child abuse?

6. How do children contract HIV?

7. What is the most common type of cancer diagnosed in children?

8. At what age are children at greatest risk for ingesting a poisonous substance?

9. What fungal diseases are common in children?

CASE STUDIES

■ Jason is a 14-year-old who has a severe case of itching in the groin area. He comes to you, the school nurse, for help with this problem. Although he is rather embarrassed about it, he explains to you that he thinks he has jock itch. What do you say to him? How can you be sure that is his problem? What is the medical name for this condition? What should you do for him? Is there a treatment for his problem?

■ Janette Brenner is a nurse who also runs a day care center in a local community. She plans to offer an educational session on preventing poisonings in children with the parents of her day care attendees. What are the most important points she should cover? What other safety issues are important besides talking about medication safety? What should she tell them about inducing vomiting if a child ingests a poisonous material?

Study Tools

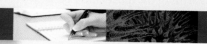

Workbook

Complete Chapter 20

Online Resources

PowerPoint® presentations

Animation

BIBLIOGRAPHY

Africa Faith and Justice Network. (2012). Forgotten victims: Children infected with HIV/AIDS: Report 2-3m. *http://www.afjn.org/* (accessed October 2012).

Agarwal, N., Ollington, K., Kaneshiro, M., Frenck, R., & Melmed, G. Y. (2012). Are immunosuppressive medications associated with decreased responses to routine immunizations? A systematic review. *Vaccine 30*(8), 1413–1424.

Andrade, A., Toscano, C. M., Minamisava, R., Costa, P., & Andrade, J. (2011). Pneumococcal disease manifestation in children before and after vaccination: What's new? *Vaccine 29*, C2–C14.

Baguley, D., Lim, E., Bevan, A., Pallet, A., & Faust, S. N. (2012). Prescribing for children: Taste and palatability affect adherence to antibiotics: A review. *Archives of Disease in Childhood 97*(3), 293–297.

Beltrão, B., da Silva, V., de Araujo, T., & Lopes, M. (2011). Clinical indicators of ineffective breathing pattern in children with congenital heart diseases. *International Journal of Nursing Terminologies & Classifications 22*(1), 4–12.

Centers for Disease Control and Prevention. (2011). Asthma in the United States. *www.cdc.gov* (accessed October 2012).

Chiapponi, C. C., Stocker, U. U., Mussack, T. H., Gallwas, J. J., Hallfeldt, K. K., & Ladurner, R. R. (2011). The surgical treatment of Graves' disease in children and adolescents. *World Journal of Surgery 35*(11), 2428–2431.

Child health: Key questions—Childhood skin conditions. (2012). *Pulse 72*(3), 23–24.

Child Info. (2012). Open estimates: Statistics by area: HIV/AIDS. *www.childinfo.org* (accessed September 2012).

Clinical digest. Infant respiratory disorders unaffected by corticosteroids. (2011). *Nursing Standard 25*(39), 16.

Cooper Robbins, S., Ward, K., & Skinner, S. (2011). School-based vaccination: A systematic review of process evaluations. *Vaccine 29*(52), 9588–9599.

Cortes, J. E., Curns, A., Tate, J. E., Cortese, M. M., Patel, M. M., Parashar, U. D., & Zhou, F. (2011). Rotavirus vaccine and health care utilization for diarrhea in U.S. children. *New England Journal of Medicine 365*(12), 1108–1117.

Crawford, D. (2011). Understanding childhood asthma and the development of the respiratory tract. *Nursing Children & Young People 23*(7), 25–36.

Disease eradication—history of vaccine. (2010). *www.historyofvaccines.com* (accessed September 2012).

Fattah, A. M., & Hamdy, B. (2011). Pulmonary functions of children with asthma improve following massage therapy. *Journal of Alternative & Complementary Medicine 17*(11), 1065–1068.

Gawthrop, M. (2012). Travelling with babies and toddlers. *Practice Nurse 42*(2), 26–30.

Gene research raises hope of new kidney cancer therapies. (2010). *Paediatric Nursing 22*(4), 4.

Goldberg, J. L., Dabade, T. S., Davis, S. A., Feldman, S. R., Krowchuk, D. P., & Fleischer, A. B. (2011). Changing age of acne vulgaris visits: Another sign of earlier puberty? *Pediatric Dermatology 28*(6), 645–648.

Hepp, N. (2011). Protecting children from toxicants. *ASHA Leader 16*(14), 12–15.

Kulik, T. J., Harris, J. E., & McElhinney, D. B. (2011). The impact of pulmonary venous hypertension on the pulmonary circulation in the young. *Congenital Heart Disease 6*(6), 603–607.

Lawton, K., & Kasari, C. (2012). Brief report: Longitudinal improvements in the quality of joint attention in preschool children with autism. *Journal of Autism & Developmental Disorders 42*(2), 307–312.

Leukemia and Lymphoma Society. (2012). Facts. *www.lls.org* (accessed September 2012).

Lo, S. (2012). Diagnosis, treatment and prevention of autism via meridian theory. *American Journal of Chinese Medicine 40*(1), 39–56.

McDowell, D., Noone, D., Tareen, F., Waldron, M., & Quinn, F. (2012). Urinary incontinence in children: Botulinum toxin is a safe and effective treatment option. *Pediatric Surgery International 28*(3), 315–320.

Nelson, R. (2011). Childhood vaccinations. *American Journal of Nursing 111*(11), 19–20.

Niederhauser, V., & Baker, D. (2011). What's new in child and adolescent immunizations? *Nurse Practitioner 36*(10), 39–44.

Oz, M. (2012). Charms of the quiet child. *Time, 179*(5), 46.

Paul, S., Wellesley, A., & O'Callaghan, C. (2011). Meningococcal disease in children: Case studies and discussion. *Emergency Nurse 19*(4), 24–29.

Pozzi-Monzo, M. (2012). Ritalin for whom? Revisited: Further thinking on ADHD. *Journal of Child Psychotherapy 38*(1), 49–60.

Prescott, S., & Nowak-Węgrzyn, A. (2011). Strategies to prevent or reduce allergic disease. *Annals of Nutrition & Metabolism 59*(Suppl), 28–42.

Rise in tuberculosis prompts plans for blanket vaccination. (2011). *Nursing Children & Young People 23*(6), 4.

Rollins, J. A. (2011). Protecting children from HPV: Challenges and opportunities. *Pediatric Nursing 37*(6), 292–301.

Round, J., Fitzgerald, A., Hulme, C., Lakhanpaul, M., & Tullus, K. (2012). Urinary tract infections in children and the risk of ESRF. *Acta Paediatrica 101*(3), 278–282.

Scarfe, G., Redshaw, S., Wilson, V., & Dengler, L. (2012). Heart to heart: A program for children on a cardiac ward. *British Journal of Nursing (BJN) 21*(2), 108–114.

Spence, K., Swinsburg, D., Griggs, J., & Johnston, L. (2011). Infant well-being following neonatal cardiac surgery. *Journal of Clinical Nursing 20*(17/18), 2623–2632.

Traylor, A., Price, J. H., Tulljohann, S. K., King, K., & Thorpon, A. (2010). Clinical psychologists' firearm risk management and perception. *Journal of Community Health 35*(1), 60–67.

Tullus, K. (2012). What do the latest guidelines tell us about UTIs in children under 2 years of age. *Pediatric Nephrology 27*(4), 509–511.

UNICEF. (2012). Child survival call to action. *www.unicef.org* (accessed October 2012).

Wick, J. Y. (2011). Pediatric skin conditions: Prevention and treatment. *Pharmacy Times* 16–18.

World Health Organization. (2012). Vaccine preventable diseases: monitoring system 2012. Global summary. *www.who.int* (accessed September 2012).

Yarnell, E., & Abascal, K. (2011). Undervalued herbs: Use in clinical practice and need for validating research. *Alternative & Complementary Therapies 17*(4), 220–224.

Young-Ju, K. (2011). A systematic review of factors contributing to outcomes in patients with traumatic brain injury. *Journal of Clinical Nursing 20*(11/12), 1518–1532.

Zastrow, R. L. (2011). Pertussis on the rise: A troubling picture of waning immunity, with unvaccinated children especially vulnerable. *American Journal of Nursing 111*(6), 51–56.

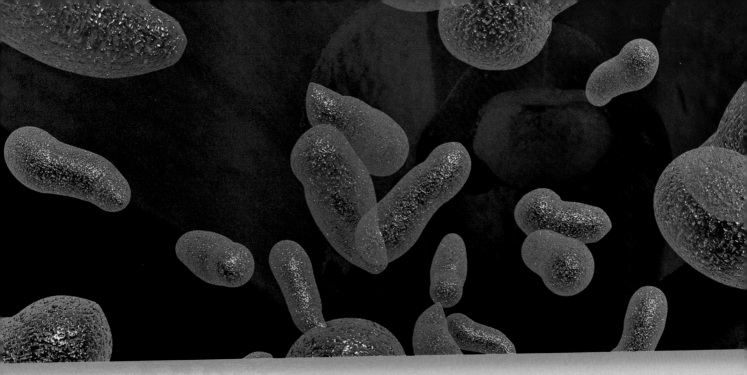

OUTLINE

- Common Signs and Symptoms
- Diagnostic Tests
- Common Mental Health Diseases and Disorders
  Developmental Mental Health Disorders
  Substance-Related Mental Disorders
  Organic Mental Disorders
  Psychosis
  Mood or Affective Disorders
  Dissociative Disorders
  Anxiety Disorders
  Somatoform Disorders
  Personality Disorders
  Gender Identity Disorder
  Sexual Disorders
  Sleep Disorders

- Trauma
  Grief
  Suicide

- Rare Diseases
- Mental Health Disorders in the Older Adult
- Summary
- Review Questions
- Case Studies
- Bibliography

KEY TERMS

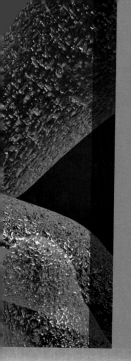

21

Mental Health Diseases and Disorders

LEARNING OBJECTIVES

Upon completion of the chapter, the learner should be able to:

1. Define the terminology common to mental health disorders.

2. Identify the important signs and symptoms associated with mental health disorders.

3. Describe the common diagnostic tests used to determine the type and/or cause of mental health disorders.

4. Identify common mental health disorders.

5. Describe the typical course and management of the common mental health disorders.

6. State the mental health disorders found in the older population and the effects of these disorders.

OVERVIEW

Mental health disorders are some of the most difficult diseases to diagnose and understand. Symptoms can range from mild behavior changes to severe personality disturbances. Because of the variety of symptoms, the difficulty in diagnosing some disorders, and the lack of understanding of the physiologic cause, many mental health disorders are misdiagnosed and can go untreated for years. Although some mental health problems are not yet well understood, many more are relatively easy to diagnose and treat. ■

COMMON SIGNS AND SYMPTOMS

For mental health disorders, there are only a few common signs and symptoms. Typically, symptoms of mental health problems begin with behavioral changes. These are often slow developing and very subtle, so symptoms might not be noticed early in the development of a disorder, and many of the symptoms, such as forgetfulness, anxiety, or temper tantrums, are attributed to age, stress, or other illnesses. Typical symptoms of each mental health problem are discussed with the specific disorder.

DIAGNOSTIC TESTS

A variety of diagnostic tests is used to determine the specific mental health problem. When symptoms first appear, the physician usually orders physiologic assessments such as laboratory tests, brain scans, electroencephalograms (EEGs), and magnetic resonance imaging (MRI) scans to determine whether the cause is an organic problem; then the individual might be referred to a psychiatrist for psychological testing to determine a diagnosis. These tests can include an aptitude test, personality test, and several others, depending on the symptoms presented and the severity of the symptoms.

COMMON MENTAL HEALTH DISEASES AND DISORDERS

Mental health disorders range from mild to severe. A few disorders have a genetic base, others are due to behavior choices, and some are of unknown cause. Early diagnosis and treatment are essential to assist the individual either to overcome the disorder or to improve the quality of life.

Developmental Mental Health Disorders

Developmental mental health disorders are those usually discovered during infancy, childhood, or adolescence. These disorders might diminish or worsen as the child matures. Developmental disorders that are carried into adulthood can be mild, allowing the involved individual to function in an adult role, or be so severe that institutionalization is necessary.

INTELLECTUAL DISABILITY

■ **DESCRIPTION.** Intellectual disability is a condition of decreased intelligence leading to a decrease in the ability to learn, socialize, and mature. Intellectual disability varies in degrees from mild and moderate to severe and profound.

PHARMACOLOGY HIGHLIGHT

Common Drugs for Mental Health Disorders

CATEGORY	EXAMPLES OF MEDICATIONS
Antidepressants Drugs used to treat depression	fluoxetine, citalopram, paroxetine, imipramine, isocarboxazid, or sertraline
Antipsychotics Drugs used to treat psychotic disorders	risperidone, aripiprazole, haloperidol, loxapine, or clozapine
Antianxiety Drugs used to treat anxiety disorders	buspirone, lorazepam, diazepam, or clonazepam
Mood Stabilizers Drugs used to treat mood disorders	carbamazepine, lithium carbonate, or gabapentin
Stimulants Drugs used to treat attention-deficit hyperactivity disorder	amphetamine, dextroamphetamine, or methylphenidate

TABLE 21–1   Genetic and Acquired Causes of Intellectual Disability

Genetic	Acquired
Down syndrome Phenylketonuria (PKU) Hypothyroidism (cretinism)	Prenatal maternal rubella Prenatal maternal syphilis Blood type incompatibility Prematurity Anoxia Birth injury Poor nutrition Head trauma

■ **ETIOLOGY.** The cause of intellectual disability is often unknown. Known causes fall into two categories: genetic and acquired (Table 21–1). Some types of intellectual disability can be avoided by providing prenatal care.

■ **SYMPTOMS.** Affected children might not show signs of intellectual disability until entry into school. Difficulty learning and keeping up with other children of the same age can be indicative of this disorder.

■ **DIAGNOSIS.** Diagnosis is confirmed on the basis of observation and IQ testing. IQ testing is a controversial issue today because many feel this testing is culturally biased. If testing is used, the most common types are the Wechsler and Stanford–Binet systems. IQ scores of 90 to 109 are considered normal intelligence. Scores of 71 to 89 are considered borderline in intellectual functioning. Scores below 70 indicate profound disability with an inability to perform the simplest tasks of daily living.

■ **TREATMENT.** Treatment of intellectually disabled individuals varies with the amount of disability. Many mildly disabled individuals grow up and find employment in a suitable occupation and lead fairly normal lives. Others might need special, dependent-living facilities, but very few are disabled to the level of needing institutionalization.

■ **PREVENTION.** Many cases are not preventable, but one common cause that can be prevented is fetal alcohol syndrome. Prenatal care, education, and encouragement to avoid alcohol when pregnant are helpful measures to prevent intellectual disability due to this cause.

Another preventable cause is kernicterus, a brain damage that occurs when a baby has too much bilirubin in the blood, causing excessive jaundice. Treatment of kernicterus can prevent intellectual disability.

ATTENTION-DEFICIT HYPERACTIVITY DISORDER (ADHD)

■ **DESCRIPTION.** ADHD is a mental health disorder characterized by an inability to concentrate, hyperactivity, and impulsiveness.

■ **ETIOLOGY.** The cause of ADHD is unknown, but there does appear to be a familial pattern. This behavior can be apparent at any age but is usually observed before the age of 7, becoming more obvious in school situations.

■ **SYMPTOMS.** Examples of ADHD behavior include forgetfulness, not appearing to listen, difficulty in remaining seated or waiting one's turn, squirming, excessive running, climbing, talking, inability to complete detailed work, messy work, and an inability to organize. These behaviors tend to become more exaggerated in a group situation.

■ **DIAGNOSIS.** Diagnosis is made on the basis of observation of the age-inappropriate behavior. It is now recognized that in many youngsters with this condition, the hyperactivity component might not be a major factor (especially in girls), and the term *attention-deficit disorder (ADD)* would serve better, but ADHD has become the accepted diagnosis.

■ **TREATMENT.** Treatment of ADHD with amphetamines has shown varying degrees of effectiveness. Behavior modification by rewarding appropriate behavior also has been successful.

■ **PREVENTION.** Preventive measures to reduce the incidence of ADHD are not known at this time. Early detection and treatment can reduce the symptoms.

EATING DISORDERS

■ **DESCRIPTION.** An eating disorder is a compulsion to eat, or avoid eating, that affects the mental and physical condition of the individual. Eating disorders have a negative impact on all aspects of the individual's life, including school, work, and personal relationships. These disorders affect approximately 5 in 100 females in the United States. Two common eating disorders are **anorexia nervosa** and **bulimia**.

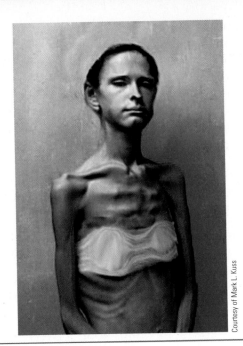

Courtesy of Mark L. Kuss

FIGURE 21–1   Anorexia nervosa.

- **Anorexia** (AN-oh-RECK-see-ah; an = without, orexia = appetite) **nervosa** is a disorder of self-imposed starvation resulting from a distorted body image (Figure 21–1).

- **Bulimia** (boo-LIM-ee-ah) is a disorder characterized by episodes of binge eating (an intake of approximately 5,000 calories in 1 to 2 hours) followed by activities to negate the calorie intake by purging.

■ **ETIOLOGY.** The exact cause of these eating disorders is not known. It is thought that one factor relates to the great emphasis Americans place on the thin, perfect, female body. To obtain this ideal figure, many females go to dieting extremes.

■ **SYMPTOMS.** The effects of these disorders can range from decreased energy levels, growth retardation, and menstrual dysfunction to more severe effects such as cardiac disturbances, delayed puberty, personality changes, inability to perform activities of daily living, and death. The affected female's excessively thin body often appears prepubescent in shape, which can help reduce stress by decreasing the fears of growing up, sexuality, and developing a sexual identity.

The term *anorexia* is a misnomer because the appetite is not diminished, but the affected individual simply refuses to eat from fear of becoming fat. The

typical characteristics of an individual with anorexia nervosa include:

- Adolescent female
- Meticulous, high achiever
- Distorted body image (feels fat no matter how thin)
- Intense fear of becoming fat
- Performs excessive exercise

Affected individuals often come from families exhibiting conspicuous togetherness characterized by over-protectiveness and conflict avoidance. The mother is often controlling and domineering, whereas the father is distant and uninvolved. The family unit often fails to support the idea that the adolescent female is competent and able to function in an independent way.

Bulimic individuals exhibit purging behaviors including self-induced vomiting or excessive laxative use. Excessive vomiting often leads to electrolyte imbalances and erosion of the teeth.

Individuals affected with bulimia are usually older than anorexics, more obese, and experience a wide fluctuation in weight. Bulimic individuals, like anorexics, tend to have perfectionist personalities and a dread of becoming fat.

■ **DIAGNOSIS.** Eating disorders are diagnosed by physical examination, diet history, and reports from the affected individual, family, and close friends.

■ **TREATMENT.** Anorexia and bulimia are both classified as psychiatric disorders. Treatment of either is often difficult and lengthy, involving both restoring normal nutrition and resolving psychological problems.

Early intervention is critical to prevent severe complications, and the entire family must be involved in the individual's recuperation plan. Usually, this can be accomplished on an outpatient basis, but in severe cases, the individual might need hospitalization for treatment or forced feedings until stable.

Several clinics in the United States specialize in treating eating disorders. The use of antidepressant medications can be beneficial. Death from starvation is often due to compromised cardiac function.

■ **PREVENTION.** There is no known prevention for eating disorders. Educational programs that promote health and early identification of these disorders are helpful, and early treatment is the best course to prevent progression of the disorder and potential complications.

TIC DISORDERS

■ **DESCRIPTION.** Tic disorders include a variety of conditions characterized by sudden, rapid muscle movement or vocalization.

■ **ETIOLOGY.** The cause of tics is unknown, but there is some evidence that maternal emotional stress during pregnancy might play a part in development. Tic tends to develop in children ages 5 to 10 years. Tics are irresistible but tend to increase with stress and decrease with sleep or preoccupation with another activity.

■ **SYMPTOMS.** Examples of tics include eye blinking, facial grimacing, neck or shoulder jerking, throat clearing, snorting, and grunting, to name just a few.

■ **DIAGNOSIS.** Physical examination is typically all that is needed for diagnosis.

■ **TREATMENT.** Treatment depends on how this condition is affecting the individual's life. Medication and psychotherapy are used only if the condition is having a major impact on school, job, and other life activities. Dopamine blocker medications such as risperidone and pimozide are used to treat tics, but these are not always successful.

■ **PREVENTION.** There are few preventive measures for tic disorders, but avoiding emotional stress during pregnancy might be helpful. Because tic disorders appear more often when individuals are stressed, avoiding or minimizing stress can also aid in prevention of symptoms.

ENURESIS

■ **DESCRIPTION.** Enuresis (EN-you-REE-sis), commonly called bedwetting, is a condition of urinary incontinence after the age of bladder training (usually considered as 5 years of age). Enuresis is more common in males than in females and commonly affects firstborn children.

■ **ETIOLOGY.** The cause of enuresis is unknown, but it does have familial tendencies and is thought by some to be due to inadequate or poor attempts at toilet training.

■ **SYMPTOMS.** The only symptom is involuntary bedwetting that occurs at least twice a month.

■ **DIAGNOSIS.** A physical examination is usually completed to rule out any physical conditions. A bedwetting diary outlining dates of wetting episodes along with time of meals, fluid intake, and sleep time can be helpful.

■ **TREATMENT.** Treatment involves encouraging the child to participate in planning and carrying out a program to reduce and finally eliminate the episodes. Planning might include restriction of fluids after the evening meal, bladder training to help enlarge the capacity of the bladder, urinating before bedtime, and awakening the child during the night to void. Reprimanding, ridiculing, and shaming the child should be avoided because these activities tend to make the condition worse.

■ **PREVENTION.** Getting plenty of sleep and developing a habit of using the bathroom at scheduled times during the day and evening hours might prevent some episodes of bedwetting.

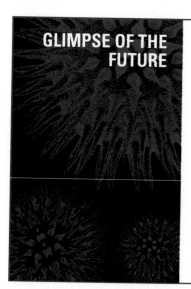

GLIMPSE OF THE FUTURE

Alcohol and the Teenage Brain

Alcohol affects the teenage brain differently than the adult brain. Many teens are the size of adults and thus might be expected to react to alcohol in the same way, but their brains are different, so they react to alcohol differently. The Centers for Disease Control and Prevention (CDC) has reported that 25% of teens use alcohol and participate in binge drinking. This is dangerous behavior. A researcher noted that the teen brain has less white matter, and thus, the teen cannot make judgments and decisions as the adult can. Teens have a greater tendency to make quick decisions and engage in impulse-driven behaviors. This might be why there are many more fatal car accidents and dangerous sexual encounters in the teen population. Ongoing research is looking at all aspects of teen behavior, and new recommendations for caution might be forthcoming soon.

Source: Paturel (2011).

Substance-Related Mental Disorders

Substance-related mental disorder is now the diagnosis used in place of the term *drug addiction*. The annual cost of substance abuse in the United States has been estimated at more than $193 billion a year (Substance Abuse and Mental Health Services Administration, 2011). It is a national problem that needs continued investigation, education, and monitoring.

Common terms used in substance-related mental disorders include *addiction*, *dependency*, *tolerance*, and *withdrawal*. **Addiction** means a physical and or psychological dependence on a substance. **Dependency** is a psychological craving for a substance that might or might not be accompanied by a physical need. **Tolerance** is the ability to endure a larger amount of a substance without an adverse effect or the need for a larger amount or dose of the drug to attain the same effect. **Withdrawal** is the unpleasant physical and psychological effects that result from stopping the use of the substance after an individual is addicted.

ALCOHOLISM

■ **DESCRIPTION.** Alcoholism, a physical and mental dependence on a regular intake of alcohol, is one of the most common mental disorders, with approximately 10% of the population affected. It is a chronic, progressive, and often fatal disease. Onset of alcoholism is often insidious, beginning in the teen years. Excessive use can be related to stress, depression, or some other stressful life event.

Alcoholism is a major drug problem that causes approximately 100,000 deaths per year and adversely affects the physical, mental, social, and spiritual health of the affected individual. Chronic alcoholism causes physical damage to nearly every organ system. Some of the common problems include heart disease, hypertension, cirrhosis, pancreatitis, peripheral neuropathy, and gastrointestinal problems (including an increased risk of stomach and esophageal cancer).

Mental disorders include anxiety, depression, insomnia, impotence, and amnesia. These physical and mental problems, along with the associated accidents, injuries, and violence associated with alcoholism, can be psychologically, socially, and economically devastating to affected individuals and their families.

■ **ETIOLOGY.** The cause of alcoholism is unknown. There is no universally accepted explanation for alcoholism, although recent research points toward a biological explanation or at least a genetic predisposition. Other causal factors can include depression, poverty, peer pressure, and condoning of substance abuse by peers and family members. Individuals raised in homes in which both parents are alcoholics are at very high risk for also becoming alcoholics.

Alcohol is absorbed in the mouth and small intestine and is broken down by the liver. A normal-sized individual can metabolize or break down approximately 30 milliliters of alcohol, or 1 ounce of whiskey, every 90 minutes. If taken in higher amounts or consumed more frequently, alcohol causes a sedative effect and can depress breathing and lead to death.

■ **SYMPTOMS.** An individual is **intoxicated** when the blood alcohol level reaches 0.10% or more. Four to 6 hours after intoxication occurs, the individual experiences a hangover with symptoms of nausea, vomiting, fatigue, sweating, and thirst. The primary cause of a hangover is the accumulation of alcohol in the blood and hypoglycemia.

COMPLEMENTARY AND ALTERNATIVE THERAPY

Family Therapy for Drug Abuse

Family therapy may be an effective alternative treatment for drug abuse in adolescents and adults. Researchers have found that family-based therapy programs show the best effects with both the families and young drug abusers. Drug abuse affects the entire family and causes distress and disruptions to all members. The family-based treatment regimen is recommended as an alternative modality for drug abuse. These programs have proven to be an effective approach to treating drug abusers and helping families of abusers.

Source: Rowe (2012).

Alcoholics become physically dependent on alcohol and can experience symptoms of withdrawal if alcohol is withheld for 24 to 48 hours. Symptoms of withdrawal include **hallucinations** (a false sensation of sight, touch, sound, or feel), tremors of the hands, mild seizures, and **delirium tremens (DTs)**.

Symptoms of delirium tremens can include agitation, memory loss, anorexia, seizures, and hallucinations. DTs usually last 1 to 5 days and can be fatal if not properly treated. Treatment for withdrawal includes tranquilizers, anticonvulsive medication, adequate nutrition, and antiemetic (anti = against, emetic = nausea or vomiting) medications.

The National Institute on Alcohol Abuse and Alcoholism (NIAAA) defines problem drinking as more than 7 drinks per week for women and more than 14 drinks per week for men. Diagnosis is frequently difficult because affected individuals are often embarrassed and not forthcoming with information. A history of alcohol abuse is often obtained from family members. Blood tests including blood alcohol and liver enzymes can be helpful.

■ **TREATMENT.** Treatment of chronic alcoholism includes rehabilitation designed to meet the alcoholic's physical and psychological needs and supports total abstinence from alcohol. Many alcoholics have found success with self-help groups.

MARIJUANA ABUSE

■ **DESCRIPTION.** Marijuana is a mixture of the dried leaves and flowers of an Indian hemp plant, *Cannabis sativa* (Figure 21–2). This mixture is crushed and rolled into cigarettes or joints. It can also be smoked in a pipe.

Hashish, a resin from the flowering top of the hemp plant, is thought to be four to eight times stronger than marijuana. Both marijuana and hashish usually produce a euphoric effect or sense of well-being. This effect is immediate and lasts approximately 2 to 3 hours.

■ **ETIOLOGY.** All forms of marijuana are mind-altering because they contain delta-9-tetrahydrocannabinol (THC), the active chemical in the plant. THC disrupts the nerve cells in the brain, making it difficult to problem-solve, remember events, and participate in activities with normal skill and coordination. THC is absorbed by fatty tissue in the body and can be detected in urine samples for weeks after use.

■ **SYMPTOMS.** The short-term effects of marijuana use include memory loss, slowed ability to learn, distorted perception, loss of coordination, and increased heart rate. Long-term effects of use include the short-term effects as well as problems in the respiratory, immune, and reproductive systems.

True tolerance does not develop with marijuana use, but chronic use can lead to a psychological dependence. Marijuana use has not been proven to lead to the use of hard drugs, but users often experiment with other drugs.

Beneficial uses of marijuana include a lowering of intraocular pressure in glaucoma patients and relief of nausea and vomiting in individuals on chemotherapy.

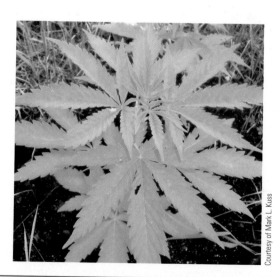

Courtesy of Mark L. Kuss

FIGURE 21–2   Marijuana (*Cannabis sativa*) plant.

SYNTHETIC CANNABIS ABUSE

■ **DESCRIPTION.** Synthetic cannabis, or "fake weed," also known as "K2" and "Spice," is a psychoactive designer drug made from a mixture of herbal and spice plants sprayed with chemicals that mimic the effects of marijuana. This designer drug began selling in 2000. It was originally thought that these blends achieved an effect through a mixture of legal herbs, but chemical analysis of the ingredients showed that these blends actually contained synthetic cannabinoids that acted on the body in a similar way as marijuana.

In an effort to continue legal sales in the United States, a large variety of synthetic cannabinoids were sold under various brand names and marketed as herbal incense online and in head shops. The Synthetic Drug Abuse Prevention Act of 2012 banned synthetic compounds commonly found in synthetic marijuana, making them a controlled substance and therefore illegal to possess or use in the United States.

■ *SYMPTOMS.* Symptoms and side effects mimic those of marijuana.

COCAINE ABUSE

■ *DESCRIPTION.* Cocaine is one of the most addictive drugs abused by individuals. It is estimated that one in two Americans between the ages of 25 and 35 has tried cocaine, and 3.6 million Americans are regular cocaine users (National Institute on Drug Abuse, 2009).

Cocaine is a powerful stimulant that accelerates the central nervous system and an anesthetic that numbs whatever part of the body it touches. The anesthetic properties of powdered cocaine make it an ideal legal medication for patients undergoing nasal surgery.

Effects of the drug include increased blood pressure, dilated pupils, increased heart rate, hyperstimulation, reduced fatigue, and a high associated with pleasure. The length of the effect depends on the route of administration and amount used.

Cocaine is obtained from either the leaves of the coca plant found in South America or synthetic production. Cocaine is a pure white powder referred to as coke. It is quite expensive at $100 per gram.

The powder form of cocaine is commonly cut into lines, or doses, with a razor blade and snorted (drawn up) through the nose with a straw or tightly rolled dollar bill (Figure 21–3). Drug paraphernalia include a piece of glass or mirror and a razor blade. Snorting produces a slower response than injecting, with effects lasting approximately 20 minutes. Complications of snorting cocaine include disintegration of the mucous membrane of the nose and ulceration through the nasal septum.

Cocaine powder can also be mixed with water, heated to help with the dissolving process, and injected. Drug paraphernalia, in this case, includes syringes, spoons, and straws. Injecting cocaine and sharing needles increase the risk of human immunodeficiency virus (HIV).

Another form of cocaine is called crack or freebase. Crack cocaine is currently made by heating a mixture of powder cocaine, water, and ammonia or baking soda, causing the material to precipitate into a hardened form of small chips or chunks. Historically,

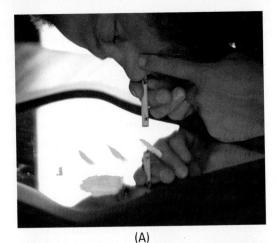

(A)

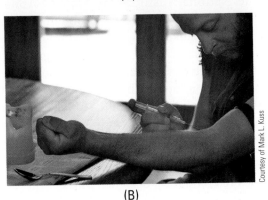

(B)

Courtesy of Mark L. Kuss

FIGURE 21–3   Cocaine paraphernalia and use. (A) Snorting lines of cocaine. (B) Injecting cocaine.

this process involved the use of ether and other flammable bases rather than ammonia and baking soda. Processing with the ether method is very dangerous due to the flammability of this product.

Crack cocaine is four to five times stronger, and much more addictive, than powder cocaine. Crack is smoked rather than snorted or injected. Manufacturing and smoking crack cocaine is called freebasing. When smoked, crack reaches the brain within seconds, giving an intense high, or rush, to the body. The high lasts approximately 5 to 15 minutes and then fades into a restless desire for more of the drug.

Crack is sold by the size of the rock and ranges from $5 to $40. This cost is initially less expensive than powdered cocaine, but the intense addiction this drug causes leads to increased use and cost. Addiction often leads to theft, prostitution, and dealing to obtain the money needed to purchase more cocaine.

Crack cocaine is usually smoked with marijuana, tobacco cigarettes, or in a glass pipe. Overdosing with crack is more common than with powder cocaine.

In some instances, death has occurred with the first dose taken. However, most deaths associated with the drug are related to overdosing, mixing the drug with other drugs or alcohol, or both.

When mixed with alcohol, the liver combines the drugs, creating a third substance called cocaethylene, which intensifies the **euphoric** (sense of well-being) effects of cocaine but increases the risk of sudden death.

■ **TREATMENT.** Treatment for cocaine addiction includes behavior modification along with some pharmacologic agents. Recent research in antiaddiction medications is aimed at development of opioid receptor blocking. Infants born to cocaine-using mothers are often addicted and exhibit low birth weight, hyperactivity, tremors, and frantic sucking activities.

METHAMPHETAMINE ABUSE

Methamphetamine is a white, odorless powder that acts as an addictive, potent stimulant that affects the central nervous system. It is one of the most abused drugs. It is popular among the young because it is relatively cheap to purchase and is easily produced in home laboratories. It can be taken by mouth, injected, smoked, or sniffed.

The effects of the drug include decreased appetite, decreased fatigue, anxiety, and a general euphoric state. After the initial rush, the effects can last up to 8 hours. Long-term use has many negative consequences including severe dental problems called "meth mouth," extreme weight loss, anxiety, confusion, insomnia, mood disturbances, and violent behavior.

Repeated abuse of methamphetamine can lead to addiction accompanied by chemical and molecular changes in the brain. Chronic users can develop psychotic features including visual and auditory hallucinations, paranoia, and delusions. A common delusion involves insects crawling under the skin.

ECSTASY (MDMA) ABUSE

■ **DESCRIPTION.** Ecstasy (MDMA, 3,4-methylenedioxymethamphetamine) is a synthetic, psychoactive drug similar to the methamphetamine. Street names are Ecstasy, Adam, beans, and love drug. Ecstasy is an illegal psychedelic stimulant that produces an energizing effect and distortions in time and perception.

■ **SYMPTOMS.** Ecstasy primarily affects the brain and may cause persistent memory problems. It also can affect the body's ability to regulate temperature,

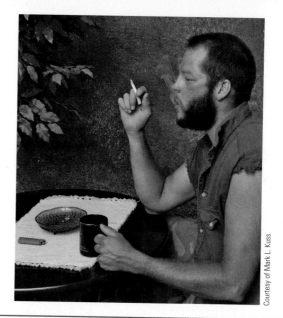

FIGURE 21–4 Nicotine and caffeine—two of the most common addictive substances.

leading to hyperthermia. Other symptoms may include increased heart rate and blood pressure, muscle tension, involuntary teeth clenching, nausea, confusion, depression, sleep problems, drug craving, and severe anxiety.

CAFFEINE AND NICOTINE ABUSE

Two of the most common addicting substances in our society are caffeine and nicotine (Figure 21–4). Caffeine is a stimulant found in coffee, chocolate, tea, cola drinks, and some over-the-counter medications. Caffeine causes vasoconstriction and, over a long period of time, can lead to circulatory problems.

Individuals addicted to caffeine often experience severe withdrawal headaches, anxiety, drowsiness, fatigue, and nausea. Caffeine tends to cause breast tenderness in females and intensify the symptoms of premenstrual syndrome (PMS). Caffeine is the cheapest and most abused drug in the United States.

Tobacco use in this country is on the rise, especially among the teen population. Cigarettes are the most widely used drug by adolescents, despite widespread knowledge of the devastating effects of nicotine on the cardiovascular and respiratory systems. Nicotine is a stimulant that narrows blood vessels and raises the heart rate and blood pressure. It has been theorized that nicotine is as addictive as cocaine. Symptoms of withdrawal include depression, irritability, anger, anxiety, and an increase in appetite and weight gain.

Smoking during pregnancy can result in spontaneous abortion and premature birth. Nicotine patches that reduce nicotine intake gradually have been successful in helping millions of affected individuals quit smoking.

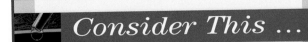

Consider This ...

Antidepressants decrease brain levels of dopamine, a brain chemical of pleasure that plays an important role in creativity and love/romance.

SEDATIVES OR DEPRESSANTS ABUSE

Drugs in this category are commonly antianxiety medications (Librium or Valium), barbiturates (Nembutal and Seconal), and hypnotics (Dalmane and Placidyl). Individuals addicted to these medications can use as much as 65 milligrams of Valium or 600 milligrams of Seconal a day.

The most severely abused group of sedatives or depressants is the barbiturates. Street names for these drugs include downers or barbs, or they might be known by the color of the capsules (reds, yellow jackets, or rainbows). These medications are often prescribed to treat insomnia, hypertension, and seizure disorders. Barbiturates distort mood, leading to euphoria; slow down reaction times, causing an increase in automobile and home accidents; and, in some cases, cause hallucinations.

Taking barbiturates with alcohol potentiates, or enhances, the effect of alcohol. Addiction and tolerance to barbiturates develop quickly and commonly lead to overdosing of barbiturates, causing a slowing of the heart and breathing that often results in death. Barbiturate use is one of the main causes of accidental death and is the most common method of suicide. Sudden withdrawal from barbiturates also can be life-threatening. It is recommended that withdrawal be conducted under the guidance of a physician. Affected individuals are usually hospitalized and the drug is withdrawn slowly to prevent nausea, delirium, and seizures.

A nonbarbiturate sedative, methaqualone (Quaalude), was introduced in the United States in the mid-1960s and was marketed as having no effect on sleep patterns and little potential for abuse. Since that time, it has been discovered that Quaalude,

commonly called ludes, does interfere with rapid eye movement (REM) sleep and does cause psychological and physical dependence. Withdrawal symptoms can last 2 to 3 days and can include insomnia, anxiety, nausea, hallucinations, and nightmares.

AMPHETAMINE ABUSE

Amphetamines are stimulant drugs that cause a release of the body's natural epinephrine, leading to an increase in heart rate, respiration, and digestion. Commonly, amphetamines are called speed, uppers, bennies, and pep pills. These drugs are often used by obese individuals to lose weight, by truck drivers to stay awake, and by college students to stay alert for studying. Amphetamines are addictive and do lead to tolerance. Chronic use often leads to an opposite effect, that is, to drowsiness. Depression and suicide can result from sudden withdrawal.

HALLUCINOGEN ABUSE

Hallucinogens, also called psychedelic drugs, commonly produce hallucinations. These drugs cause a heightened and distorted response to visual, auditory, and tactile stimuli and induce the affected individual to see flat objects take on shape, stationary objects to move, and colors to become more vivid. Hallucinogenic drugs include lysergic acid diethylamide (LSD), mescaline, and phencyclidine (PCP).

LSD

LSD is the most commonly abused drug in the **hallucinogenic** (producing psychedelic or bizarre alterations in mental functioning) class. It is a colorless, tasteless, and odorless synthetic substance primarily produced in illegal laboratories. It can be added to the food or drink of an unsuspecting victim or to chewing gum, hard candy, postage stamps, or stickers. LSD is a very potent drug; an amount of drug visible to the eye is enough to cause an 8-hour hallucination.

With LSD, the heart rate increases, pupils dilate, blood pressure increases, and appetite diminishes. **Delusions**, hallucinations, and abnormal thought processes can cause temporary or permanent mental changes. Controversy exists over whether LSD might also cause chromosomal damage. Surprisingly, LSD is not addictive. It appears that this drug is abused to escape reality rather than to help cope with reality. Abusers of LSD do have a high tendency to abuse marijuana, barbiturates, and amphetamines.

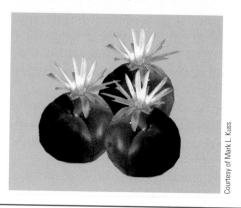

Courtesy of Mark L. Kuss

FIGURE 21–5 Peyote cactus.

The danger of this drug lies in the fact that the activities of an individual under the influence of LSD are totally unpredictable. The person might attempt to fly or exhibit episodes of violence and self-destruction. Flashbacks (recurrence of a trip) can occur months after the drug was taken because it is stored in fat tissue and might be released at a later time.

Mescaline

Mescaline is similar to LSD but much weaker. It is an active chemical found in the Mexican peyote cactus that also can be produced synthetically (Figure 21–5). Native Americans use this cactus as part of their traditional religious ceremonies.

PCP

PCP, also known as angel dust, peace pill, and peace weed, is a depressant that was introduced in the 1950s as an animal tranquilizer. Its use has since been abandoned because of unpredictable side effects. PCP is easily produced in illegal laboratories and can be taken as pills or injections or by snorting or smoking. Danger lies in the poor and varied quality of the product sold on the street. PCP can cause memory lapses lasting for several days. Other symptoms are coma, convulsions, and respiratory arrest.

NARCOTIC ABUSE

Narcotics are depressants that are primarily prescribed as analgesics or painkillers. Demerol, methadone, morphine, heroin, and opium are classified as narcotics and are commonly abused. Narcotics lower blood pressure and slow nerve and muscle action and the rate of the heart and breathing. Physical and psychological dependence and tolerance rapidly develop with the use of narcotics. Overdose symptoms include slurred speech, confusion, staggering, coma, and respiratory arrest.

Opium

Opium is an air-dried, milky residue obtained from the unripe opium poppy. References to opium smoking are common in Oriental history, and some people in Asian countries still smoke opium. Users in the Western countries, including the United States, prefer opium derivatives such as morphine and heroin. Opium contains approximately 10% morphine. Heroin is a derivative of morphine but is approximately eight times stronger. Heroin is very addictive and is commonly called smack and horse. Heroin is the narcotic most widely used by narcotic addicts today.

Heroin

Heroin is a fine white powder that is usually mixed with water and injected intravenously in a process

COMPLEMENTARY AND ALTERNATIVE THERAPY

Herbs for Addictions Abuse of opium-based drugs is increasing, and researchers are continuing to search for effective treatment measures. Chinese medicines such as WeiniCom (also known as Xuan Xia) have been used as an alternative treatment for opium addictions for centuries and also in conjunction with traditional treatments. Another herbal product used for opium addiction is kratom, which comes from a leaf of a tree found in Southeast Asia. The problem is that most of these herbs have not been well-researched to determine their effectiveness, toxicity, and therapeutic dosages.

Source: Ward et al. (2011).

called mainlining. It also can be snorted or smoked. Heroin use usually gives a rush, or intense feeling of well-being, followed by a sleepy, drowsy state. Withdrawal from heroin without medical treatment is called going cold turkey. Withdrawal is often uncomfortable but not usually life-threatening. Symptoms of withdrawal include sweating, shaking, diarrhea, vomiting, and sharp pain and cramps in the stomach and legs.

INHALANT ABUSE

Inhalants are chemicals that produce a vapor that can be inhaled and that produce a mind-altering effect. Young people are more likely to abuse inhalants than adults and often treat the use of inhalants as a game or a way to get a cheap high. This is a very dangerous activity and has caused death in many adolescents.

Inhalants include over 1,000 legal substances, including glue, spray paint, hair spray, nail polish, lighter fluid, and gasoline. These substances commonly contain harmful hydrocarbons and an oily base that, when inhaled, coats the inner lining of the lungs. Inhalant abuse refers to intentionally breathing the vapors of a substance to get high. This intentional breathing in is commonly called huffing, snuffing, or bagging. The effect is similar to alcohol intoxication.

Bagging is the most dangerous because it entails placing a plastic bag over the head to get a longer effect. Using inhalants over a period of time can result in permanent brain, heart, kidney, and liver damage. Some products, such as paint and gasoline, contain lead and can lead to death from lead poisoning.

Inhalant abuse is the third most common substance abused by individuals aged 12 to 14 years, surpassed only by alcohol and tobacco. Symptoms of inhalant abuse include spots or sores around the mouth, a glassy-eyed look, fumes on the breath or clothing, anxiety, and loss of appetite.

ANABOLIC STEROID ABUSE

Anabolic steroids are the synthetic derivatives of testosterone, the male hormone. They are widely abused by athletes and others trying to promote growth of skeletal muscle and increase lean body mass. From the fitness craze of the 1980s, the use of anabolic steroids has increased significantly in young males and even in females who want to develop athletic, lean bodies.

Steroids are taken orally or injected. They do produce increases in muscle strength, lean body mass, and improved performance over periods of time, but the long-term effects are dangerous. The side effects include shrinking of the testes, reduced sperm count, infertility, and baldness in males; and growth of facial hair, changes in menstruation, enlargement of the clitoris, and a deepened voice in females.

A spectrum of behaviors is exhibited by people on anabolic steroids that range from being somewhat more assertive, to being frankly aggressive, to displaying what is described as "roid rage." Roid rage is commonly thought to account for some instances of road rage because this activity is not uncommon for those on steroids. A variety of extreme behaviors is exhibited by those on anabolic steroids.

Adolescents or preteen children can experience accelerated puberty changes and growth cessation from premature skeletal maturation. Other effects reported include mood swings, depression, and irritability.

Organic Mental Disorders

Organic mental disorders are those associated with some type of known physical cause. These disorders affect the cognitive abilities—the abilities to think, remember, and make judgments by the affected individual. These disorders can be temporary or permanent.

DEMENTIA

■ **DESCRIPTION.** Dementia is common in the elderly; it was called senility in the past and thought to be caused by aging. Dementia is a progressive deterioration of mental abilities due to physical changes in the brain. The most common form of dementia is Alzheimer's disease. It accounts for 50%–75% of all cases of dementia.

■ **ETIOLOGY.** We now know that dementia is not part of the normal aging process but, rather, is caused by a variety of medical conditions. Factors important in determining whether dementia will occur in an individual include nutritional status, family history, chronic diseases, and general state of health. Causes of dementia are listed in Table 21–2. Dementia might or might not be reversible, depending on cause.

■ **SYMPTOMS.** Symptoms often develop gradually and show a progressive deterioration of cognitive or mental abilities, including severe memory loss, disorientation, impaired judgment, and the inability to learn new information. An affected individual might lose items, get lost when driving even in familiar areas,

TABLE 21–2   Physical Causes of Dementia and Delirium

Drugs

Prescribed medications
Alcohol
Abused substances

Metabolic Disorders

Endocrine gland disorders

Nutritional Disease

Vitamin deficiencies
Malnutrition

Infection

Meningitis
Encephalitis
Brain abscess
AIDS

Trauma

Head injury

Vascular Disorders

Cerebrovascular accidents (CVA)
Arteriosclerosis

Neoplastic

Brain tumors

Neurologic

Epilepsy

get confused in conversations, and lose the ability to perform common tasks such as balancing a checkbook. As the disease progresses, symptoms become more noticeable. Symptoms of dementia can become severe enough to interfere with the individual's ability to care for himself or herself.

■ **DIAGNOSIS.** The diagnosis of dementia requires a thorough medical, physical, and neurologic examination. The American Psychiatric Association has established two criteria to support the diagnosis of dementia. The first is loss of memory. The second is the loss of one of the following functions: language,

motor activity, recognition, and executive function (unable to plan, organize, or think abstractly).

■ **TREATMENT.** Treatment focuses on correction of all reversible factors. These include correcting drug doses, ensuring that prescribed medications are being taken correctly, withdrawing misused drugs, treating depression and other medical conditions, and ensuring proper nutrition and hydration.

■ **PREVENTION.** Researchers have found that activity in the elderly reduces the risk of dementia. Activities such as reading, playing musical instruments, dancing, playing board games, and doing puzzles are beneficial.

DELIRIUM

■ **DESCRIPTION.** Delirium is not a disease but a clinical syndrome, or set of symptoms, that might result from a disease. Thorough assessment is necessary to distinguish it from other psychiatric disorders. Deliriums commonly affect 1 in 10 hospitalized patients and as many as 80% of those in intensive care units. Delirium is more common in the elderly and, although it is not a disease in and of itself, those who have it usually do not do as well as those with the same illness who do not have delirium.

■ **ETIOLOGY.** Delirium is an acute condition that can develop suddenly or over a period of days. There are a variety of causes of delirium, including medications, alcohol, fever, dehydration, or physical illness. Causes of delirium are also listed in Table 21-2.

■ **SYMPTOMS.** The classic symptom of delirium is a fluctuating level of consciousness with periods of calmness and extreme anxiety. The affected individual is often frightened and disoriented in place and time and has illusions, hallucinations, and incoherent speech. Individuals with delirium expend great amounts of energy, continually wandering and performing aimless activities.

■ **DIAGNOSIS.** Diagnosis is made after a thorough medical history and physical and mental status examinations. The most important activity is determining the cause of the delirium. Tests can include blood and urine test, computerized tomography (CT), MRI, EEG, electrocardiogram (ECG), and lumbar puncture.

■ **TREATMENT.** A calm, quiet atmosphere along with simple, clear communication, especially from family members, might help with symptoms. Physical restraints might be needed to keep the individual safe. Prompt and effective treatment of the cause often reverses the symptoms of delirium.

■ *PREVENTION.* Prevention is focused on avoiding or treating the causes.

ALZHEIMER'S DISEASE

■ *DESCRIPTION.* Alzheimer's disease is a progressive and irreversible form of dementia. Alzheimer's accounts for 50% of all dementias and commonly occurs after age 65 but can occur as early as age 40.

■ *ETIOLOGY.* The cause of Alzheimer's is unknown, but theories include an inherited chromosomal defect, viral infection, a deficiency in neurochemicals in the brain, and an immunologic defect. Interestingly, postmortem studies have revealed a high level of aluminum in the brain and a higher incidence of a serious head injury. Physical changes noted during autopsy include brain plaques and neuronal tangles.

■ *SYMPTOMS.* Symptoms begin with mild memory loss and progress to impaired mental function, personality changes, and speech and language problems. In the final stage, the affected individual is often depressed and paranoid and might have hallucinations. At this stage, the individual with Alzheimer's depends on another individual for total care and might need institutionalization. Death usually occurs in 10 to 15 years from onset and is usually due to complications of immobility.

■ *DIAGNOSIS.* A thorough medical history involving family members and physical examination of the individual are needed along with testing to rule out other conditions. Test can include hearing exam, blood sugar levels, thyroid level, screening for depression, cognitive testing, and brain scanning with MRI or positron emission tomography (PET). Alzheimer's can usually be diagnosed with 80%–90% accuracy. The only definitive diagnosis is postmortem brain tissue examination.

■ *TREATMENT.* Treatment is aimed at relieving symptoms and managing behavior problems. (See Chapter 15, "Nervous System Diseases and Disorders," for more information.)

■ *PREVENTION.* Research suggests that preventing or slowing the symptoms of Alzheimer's can be accomplished by lifestyle changes including:

■ Wearing helmets and seatbelts and preventing falls to protect the brain from jarring or injury.

■ Staying active with family and friends.

■ Exercising your body and your brain.

■ Eating a healthy diet.

Psychosis

Psychosis is a term describing conditions characterized by a disintegration of one's personality and a loss of contact with reality. Psychotic individuals have delusions, hallucinations, impaired communication skills, and an inability to deal with life's demands. These mental disturbances might or might not have a physical or structural change in the brain. One of the most common psychotic disorders is schizophrenia.

SCHIZOPHRENIA

■ *DESCRIPTION.* Schizophrenia, meaning split mind, is a serious type of psychosis. It is not a split-personality disorder.

■ *ETIOLOGY.* Various theories exist as to the cause of schizophrenia, including genetics, brain biochemical disorders, and structural alterations. It is generally agreed that schizophrenics have a genetic vulnerability because an individual with a schizophrenic parent, sibling, or other close relative has an increased possibility of becoming schizophrenic. Another theory suggests that schizophrenic individuals were deprived of meaningful relationships with family members during childhood years. This theory is supported by the fact that most schizophrenics felt that as children, they were unloved, unwanted, and unimportant.

■ *SYMPTOMS.* This disorder often appears in individuals aged 16 to 25 and is more common in females than in males. Schizophrenics lose touch with reality and act on imagined or fantasized reality. Specific symptoms include delusions, hallucinations, flat tone of voice, incoherent speech, bizarrely disorganized behavior such as lack of speech, unresponsiveness, and muscular rigidity.

■ *DIAGNOSIS.* Verbal screening tests are used to help determine the diagnosis. If one or more of the symptoms persist for 6 or more months, the diagnosis may be confirmed.

■ *TREATMENT.* Drug treatment is the primary therapy. Studies indicate, however, that an integrated approach, using a variety of therapies, prevents relapses better than routine care (medication, monitoring, and access to rehabilitation programs).

■ **PREVENTION.** There is no known way to prevent schizophrenia. Activities that reduce or prevent relapses include recognizing the first signs of relapse so early intervention is possible, reducing stress, avoiding alcohol and illegal drugs, and taking medications as prescribed.

DELUSIONAL DISORDERS

■ **DESCRIPTION.** Delusional disorders are characterized by a firm belief in a delusion in an otherwise normally adjusted and balanced personality. The delusions often center on feelings of persecution and grandiosity and often involve romance, religion, and politics. These delusions often develop slowly and involve a false interpretation of an actual occurrence. Delusional individuals become firmly convinced that something is true no matter how convincing evidence is to the contrary. Types of delusional disorders affecting the thinking of affected individuals include the following:

- Grandiose—an inflated sense of self-worth, power, and knowledge.

- Jealous—belief that their sexual partner is unfaithful.

- Erotomanic—belief that someone of higher status is in love with them.

- Persecutory—seeing suspicious actions and having feelings that people are spying on them with harmful intentions.

- Somatic—belief that they have a physical disease or disorder.

   People with delusional disorder can often continue to socialize and function normally apart from their delusion. This ability to function in society is unlike other psychotic disorders. This disorder is more common in women and tends to occur in middle to late life.

■ **ETIOLOGY.** The exact cause is not known, although genetic, biological, environmental, and psychological factors are thought to be involved.

■ **SYMPTOMS.** Nonbizarre delusion is the most common symptom. Other symptoms include an irritable, angry, or low mood and hallucinations of sight, hearing, or things that are not really there.

■ **DIAGNOSIS.** After a thorough medical and physical examination, if there is no physical reason for the condition, referral to a psychiatrist or psychologist is needed. A diagnosis is made if the individual has non-bizarre delusions for at least 1 month.

■ **TREATMENT.** The most common medications used to treat delusional disorders are antipsychotics. These disorders are usually chronic, but if properly treated, many get relief from symptoms. Unfortunately, many will not seek help because they do not recognize that they are ill. Without treatment, these disorders can last a lifetime.

■ **PREVENTION.** There is no known way to prevent delusional disorders, although treatment can improve the individual's life.

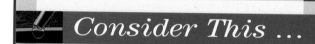

Consider This ...

A study found that individuals who believe they are always treated unfairly are 55% more likely to have a heart attack. The authors recommended that these individuals focus on getting over the idea that life isn't fair.

Mood or Affective Disorders

Mood or affective disorders are those that involve the emotions (**mood**) and the outward expression of those emotions (**affect**). Mood ranges on a spectrum with extreme depression at one end and extreme elation or happiness at the other.

   Individuals normally experience times of sadness and moments of joy. When these emotions are not appropriate to the events of life, last for an inappropriate length of time, or are extreme in nature, mood disorders might be suspected. Some individuals with mood disorders can have extreme depression, whereas others will exhibit both extreme depression and extreme elation at alternating times (bipolar disorder).

DEPRESSION

■ **DESCRIPTION.** Depression is a prolonged feeling of extreme sadness or unhappiness, despair, and discouragement. It is different from grief, which is a realistic sadness related to a personal loss. Prolonged grief might become depression because depression is often associated with loss of a loved one, possessions, self-esteem, and youth.

■ **ETIOLOGY.** The cause of depression can include genetic, biological, and environmental factors. In some cases, the cause can be singular, whereas in others, it might be multifactorial. In some cases, the cause is never known.

For some, the cause appears to be due to a decrease in chemicals in the brain known as neurotransmitters. These chemicals typically affect mood and appear to play a part in depression. Causes of depression include:

■ Heredity—Certain types of depression run in families.

■ Personality—People who are negative thinkers, are pessimistic, have low self-esteem, or are ineffective stress managers.

■ Situations—Difficult life events, including death of family members or a friend, loss of job, or loss of financial status.

■ Medical conditions—Heart disease, stroke, diabetes, cancer, menopause, or Parkinson's and Alzheimer's diseases.

■ Medication—Birth control pills, prednisone, and medications for hypertension.

■ Substance abuse—Although depression can lead to substance abuse, it is now realized that substance abuse can also lead to depression.

■ Diet—Deficits in folic acid, B12, and some vitamins.

■ Gender—Females are more at risk.

■ Age—The elderly are more often affected.

■ Status—Lower socioeconomic status.

■ Weight—Obesity.

■ Social isolation—Living alone, recently widowed.

■ **SYMPTOMS.** A depressed individual often exhibits the following characteristics:

■ Feels rejected, helpless, and worthless

■ Is indecisive and disinterested in surroundings

■ Does not enjoy pleasurable events

■ Has a low energy level; always feels fatigued

■ Is unable to sleep or sleeps excessively

■ Might cry easily and often

■ Might have thoughts of suicide

Depression more commonly occurs during critical periods along the life cycle, including adolescence, menopause, and old age.

■ **DIAGNOSIS.** A thorough history and physical examination are completed to rule out other conditions. Tests might include blood test, X-rays, MRI, or CT scan. A psychological questionnaire can also be helpful in diagnosis.

■ **TREATMENT.** Treatment of depression can include psychotherapy and antidepressant medications. The majority of individuals with serious depression will show improvement in only a few weeks. Depression is often untreated, with only one in every three affected individuals seeking assistance.

■ **PREVENTION.** Prevention might not be possible, but activities that reduce risk of developing depression and help prevent recurrence include eating a balanced diet, exercising regularly, getting adequate sleep, avoiding drugs and alcohol, seeking help with the first symptoms of depression, and taking medications as prescribed.

SEASONAL AFFECTIVE DISORDER (SAD)

■ **DESCRIPTION.** SAD, also called winter depression, is a depressive condition that occurs more commonly during the winter months. Onset of depression typically begins in the fall, becomes progressively worse through the winter months, and clears or improves in the spring. SAD tends to recur each year with the change of seasons.

■ **ETIOLOGY.** The cause of SAD is thought to be related to an increase in the melatonin hormone, which is released by the pineal gland during dark hours and is suppressed by light. Increased amounts of melatonin cause drowsiness and fatigue, so individuals with SAD are thought to be affected by high levels of melatonin.

Another theory suggests that SAD is caused by a delay in the individual's **circadian rhythm** (a normal 24-hour cycle of biological rhythms including sleep, metabolism, and glandular secretions), causing a type of hibernation.

■ **SYMPTOMS.** Symptoms include chronic fatigue, excessive sleep, and excessive eating with weight gain. SAD occurs more commonly in women and those living at higher latitudes with shorter daylight hours.

■ **DIAGNOSIS.** Diagnosing SAD is difficult because many other types of depression and mental health conditions have similar symptoms. Diagnosis depends on the individual having bouts of depression for at least 2 consecutive years during the same season, the symptoms resolving for a period of time, and the absence of other explanations for the mood change.

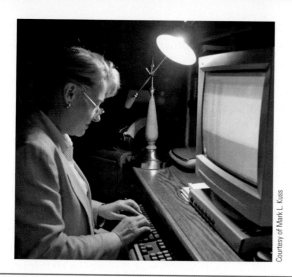

Courtesy of Mark L. Kuss

FIGURE 21–6   Seasonal affective disorder: many individuals with seasonal affective disorder will experience less depression when using light therapy.

■ **TREATMENT.** Medications to treat SAD may include some serotonin reuptake inhibitors. Daily exposure to bright light during the winter months has also improved depression in individuals affected by SAD (Figure 21–6).

■ **PREVENTION.** There is no way to prevent SAD, although steps to manage symptoms include starting treatment before symptoms would normally appear and continuing treatment past the time the symptoms usually disappear.

BIPOLAR DISORDER (MANIC DEPRESSIVE)

■ **DESCRIPTION.** Bipolar disorder is a type of depression in which extreme depression and mania (extreme elation or agitation) occur. The mania is not truly a state of happiness but rather a state of elated depression. Affected individuals experience a normal state of depression but also exhibit dramatic swings between extreme depression and extreme mania.

■ **ETIOLOGY.** The cause of bipolar disorder is unknown. Current theories suggest genetics and a biochemical deficiency in the brain.

■ **SYMPTOMS.** Symptoms of extreme depression have already been discussed. Symptoms of mania include:

- Feelings of euphoria
- Increased energy, activity, and restlessness

- Rapid thoughts and racing speech
- Unrealistic beliefs in one's abilities
- Extreme irritability
- Unusual behavior and denial that anything is wrong

■ **DIAGNOSIS.** Bipolar disorder is difficult to diagnose because individuals do not seek medical treatment in the manic phase, only in the depressed stage. A history of the condition often reveals only symptoms of depression, not of mania. There is no blood test to help with diagnosis. A mood disorder questionnaire (MDQ) is a checklist that aids the physician in identifying symptoms and thus diagnosis.

■ **TREATMENT.** Current treatment includes psychotherapy and lithium medication to control mood swings.

■ **PREVENTION.** Bipolar disorder cannot be prevented. Taking prescribed medications can control mood swings.

Dissociative Disorders

■ **DESCRIPTION.** Dissociative disorders are characterized by escape of reality in involuntary and unhealthy ways ranging from suppressing memories to assuming alternate identities. These disorders commonly develop in reaction to a trauma and include psychogenic amnesia, psychogenic fugue, depersonalization disorder, and multiple personality.

- **Psychogenic amnesia** is characterized by a sudden loss of memory that is more than simple forgetfulness. This disorder tends to occur after a major stress event and is considered to be a way of escape.

- **Psychogenic fugue** is characterized by suddenly leaving home, traveling some distance, forgetting one's identity and past, and often changing one's name. Fugue usually occurs after a major natural disaster such as an earthquake or during wartime. This disorder often lasts only a few days but can last for several months.

- **Depersonalization disorders** often occur following severe depression, stress, fatigue, or recovery from drug addiction. The affected individuals feel disconnected from mind and body and can feel like they are viewing life from a distance. Often, individuals feel that they are losing their minds.

- **Multiple personality** is a rare disorder characterized by exhibition of two or more distinct personalities. The dominant personality determines the actions and activities of the affected individual. The dominant personality is usually not aware of the secondary personality(ies), but the secondary personality(ies) are aware of the dominant personality. Change from one personality to another usually occurs quite suddenly and usually follows a stressful event.

■ *ETIOLOGY.* These disorders commonly develop during childhood as a mechanism for coping with trauma that includes physical, sexual, or emotional abuse and a frightening home environment. Adults rarely develop these disorders.

■ *SYMPTOMS.* Symptoms include memory loss (amnesia), depression, anxiety, blurred sense of identity, and a sense of being detached from self (depersonalization).

■ *DIAGNOSIS.* Physical exam to rule out conditions such as head trauma, brain diseases, and sleep disorders is needed. A mental health professional might use medication and hypnosis to identify alternate personalities to confirm diagnosis.

■ *TREATMENT.* Psychotherapy, also known as talk therapy, is the primary treatment for this disorder. This course of therapy is often long and difficult but frequently very effective.

■ *PREVENTION.* Protecting children from physical, sexual, and emotional trauma is the best prevention. If children are traumatized, seeking professional help immediately is a preventive measure.

Anxiety Disorders

■ *DESCRIPTION.* Normally, anxiety is a temporary response to stress, but for some individuals, anxiety becomes a chronic problem. Affected individuals often experience anxiety that is exaggerated or of inappropriate proportion to the situation. Anxiety disorders, previously known as neuroses, represent the largest group of mental health disorders in the United States.

■ *ETIOLOGY.* The cause of anxiety disorders might be related to genetic factors, severe stress, biochemical alterations, and, in some cases, physical causes such as hyperthyroidism.

■ *SYMPTOMS.* Symptoms of each type of anxiety disorder, including generalized anxiety, panic, phobia, obsessive-compulsive, and post-traumatic stress, are covered in the following list.

- **Generalized anxiety disorder**, also called excessive worry, is a continuous state of mild to intense anxiety. The anxiety is not related to a specific event and, for this reason, is often called free-floating anxiety. This state of constant anxiety often leads to physical symptoms including dry mouth, nausea and vomiting, diarrhea, and muscle aches.

- **Panic disorder** is a state of extreme, uncontrollable fear commonly called a panic attack. Onset of an attack is usually sudden and peaks in 10 minutes or less and can include a feeling of impending doom and a need to escape. Other symptoms include diaphoresis, chest pain, increased pulse, nausea, and dissociation (the feeling that the incident is happening to someone else).

- **Phobia disorder** is the most common anxiety disorder. A phobia is an intense and irrational fear of an object, situation, or thing, resulting in a strong desire to avoid the feared stimulus. The affected individual usually realizes that the phobia is irrational but is still unable to control the fear. There are over 700 known phobias (see Table 21–3 for a partial listing of these). Fears of spiders, snakes, and enclosed areas are some of the more common phobias.

- **Obsessive-compulsive disorder** (OCD) is an anxiety disorder with two distinct parts. **Obsession** is repetition of a thought or emotion. **Compulsion** is a repetitive act the affected individual is unable to resist performing. With OCD, the individual is unable to stop the thought or the action. Behavior becomes ritualistic, and thoughts or attempts to stop the thought or action bring about extreme anxiety. This behavior becomes very time-consuming, usually taking more than an hour a day, and can become so disruptive that the individual is unable to perform daily activities or hold a job. Examples of compulsive activities include hand washing, cleaning objects, checking an object, and locking and unlocking locks.

- **Post-traumatic stress disorder** (PTSD) develops as a response to a psychologically distressing event the individual could not control and is outside the normal range of human experience. This disorder is a new addition to anxiety disorders and was observed frequently in Vietnam veterans.

TABLE 21–3 Phobias

Phobia	Fear
Acrophobia	High places
Algophobia	Pain
Androphobia	Men
Arachnophobia	Spiders
Astrophobia	Thunder, lightning, storms
Avioidphobia	Flying
Claustrophobia	Closed, tight, or narrow spaces
Hematophobia	Blood
Hydrophobia	Water
Iatrophobia	Physicians
Kakorrhaphiophobia	Failure
Lalophobia	Public speaking
Monophobia	Being alone
Ochlophobia	Crowds
Olfactophobia	Odor
Ophidophobia	Snakes
Pathophobia	Disease
Phasmophobia	Ghosts
Phobophobia	Fear
Ponophobia	Work
Pyrophobia	Fire
Sitophobia	Food
Thanatophobia	Death
Toxophobia	Being poisoned
Traumaphobia	Injury
Triskaidekaphobia	The number 13
Xenophobia	Strangers
Zoophobia	Animals

In addition to war, individuals who are victims of rape, child incest, or abuse or survive natural disasters or acts of violence are often affected. Police and firemen are at great risk for PTSD. The feelings and fears associated with the trauma do not normally diminish with the passing of time. Affected individuals often relive this trauma for weeks, months, or years in painful recollections or dreams and frequently go to extremes to avoid any reminder of the trauma.

Symptoms can occur immediately or not arise for months after the trauma. Symptoms include:

- Flashbacks with the individual reliving the traumatic event
- Difficulty developing and maintaining relationships
- Irritability and agitation
- Depression
- Social withdrawal
- Drug dependency

■ **DIAGNOSIS.** A thorough medical and physical exam is necessary to rule out other conditions. Diagnosis is made by confirming a history of symptoms without other causes or conditions.

■ **TREATMENT.** Hypnosis, stress reduction, relaxation therapy, physical exercise, and biofeedback can be used to treat the condition, depending on severity and cause.

■ **PREVENTION.** Education on stress and stress reduction techniques, along with a good support system, might prevent this condition.

Somatoform Disorders

■ **DESCRIPTION.** Somatoform (somato = body) disorders are characterized by physical symptoms that lead one to believe in a physical disease, but no organic or physiologic cause can be found. Additionally, the physical symptoms appear to be associated with unconscious mental factors or conflicts.

■ **ETIOLOGY.** The cause of somatoform disorders is not clear. The problem appears to be multifactorial and might include genetic influences, environmental causes, high parental expectations that the child feels pressured to meet, sexual abuse, and a poor ability to express emotions.

■ **SYMPTOMS.** The symptoms of somatoform disorders are very real to the affected individual except in the case of factitious disorders (Munchausen and malingering). Individuals with somatoform disorders characteristically are described as frustrated, dependent, emotionally deprived, and resentful of family members and physicians. Somatoform disorders include conversion, hypochondriasis, pain disorder, malingering, Munchausen syndrome, and Munchausen by proxy. Each condition is described, along with typical symptoms, in the following list.

- **Conversion disorder,** formerly known as hysterical neurosis, is a very striking disorder characterized by dramatic physical symptoms such as paralysis of an arm or leg, blindness, numbness, and deafness. The affected individual usually exhibits a calm, indifferent attitude about the situation. These physical symptoms enable the individual to avoid a stressful or unacceptable situation and, at the same time, gain attention from others who might not usually give them attention.

- **Hypochondriasis** is a condition characterized by an abnormal anxiety about one's body and health. Affected individuals are commonly called hypochondriacs. These individuals have an astounding knowledge of medical conditions and are constantly watchful of symptoms. Hypochondriacs have an unrealistic fear that they are ill, despite medical assurance to the contrary. Affected individuals have difficulty establishing and maintaining relationships because so much of their energy and conversation revolve around their perceived illnesses.

- **Pain disorder** can occur at any age but commonly occurs in adolescent and young females. This disorder is characterized by pain that does not have a physiologic cause or, if a cause is discovered, the pain is greater than normally expected. This pain causes interference with the individual's social, occupational, and basic activities of life. Long-standing pain often leads to depression and suicide. This condition is not fictitious, as is malingering.

- **Malingering** is the fictitious display of symptoms to gain financial or personal reward. Returning to work after a work-related injury commonly leads to malingering. Symptoms are usually exaggerated and fraudulent. Diagnosis is often difficult because many of the symptoms are subjective and difficult to disprove.

- **Munchausen syndrome** is a group of disorders in which the affected individuals simulate illness for no other apparent reason than to receive treatment. Often, the individuals will go to extremes to present false tests, for example, scratching or cutting themselves to add blood to urine specimens. An affected person also might self-inject a variety of substances into the blood or tissues to cause an illness. Generally, this individual has an extensive knowledge of diseases, medical treatments, terminology, and hospital routine.

Affected individuals often present to emergency departments with reports of a variety of symptoms. Multiple tests and procedures are undergone willingly. When testing does not support the stated symptoms, the individual often reports different symptoms. There is usually a history of repeated hospitalizations with undetermined diagnosis. When the behavior is discovered, the confronted individual often becomes hostile and seeks attention at a different facility.

- **Munchausen by proxy** is the same disorder except the parent projects the disorder onto a child. The parent might inject the child or otherwise cause illness and then present the child for treatment. Illness commonly tends to be gastrointestinal or genitourinary in nature, and the parent denies any knowledge of the cause of the illness. Munchausen by proxy can be carried to the extreme and actually cause the death of the child.

■ *DIAGNOSIS.* A thorough history and physical examination are necessary to rule out other medical or neurologic disorders from somatoform disorders. A history of ongoing symptoms is often the key to diagnosis.

■ *TREATMENT.* Because somatoform disorders usually have a long medical history, it is beneficial to develop a long-term relationship with a trusted physician. This aids in diagnosis and often prevents unnecessary tests and treatments.

Antianxiety and antidepressant medications are sometimes prescribed because these conditions often coexist with somatoform disorders. Psychoanalysis is usually not used, but supportive approaches might be beneficial to reduce symptoms and secure the individual's personality. In some cases, hypnosis might also be helpful. Other therapies that are of some benefit include acupuncture, therapeutic message, homeopathic treatments, hydrotherapy, and meditation, to name a few.

■ *PREVENTION.* There is some evidence to suggest that allowing children to express emotional pain without ridicule of being weak or a sissy might be a preventive measure.

Personality Disorders

■ *DESCRIPTION.* An individual's personality is formed during the early years of life and is affected or molded by genetics and environmental factors such as early life experiences. Much of what is learned aids the individual in adapting to life situations. A person might be funny, social, quiet, or reserved, depending on these factors. The basic personality is fixed by adulthood and remains intact throughout life.

Individuals with personality disorders have traits or factors that make them feel and behave in unacceptable or unsocial ways. This behavior limits relationships and can affect home and work life. A vast number of people have maladaptive patterns of seeing, relating to, and thinking about their environment. These individuals fit on a mental health spectrum at some point between mentally healthy and mentally ill.

■ **ETIOLOGY.** The cause of personality disorder can be due to genetics and environmental factors. Although there is no clear-cut cause, it is known that those at risk are children who have:

- A family history of personality disorders.
- An alcoholic parent.
- Been raised in a chaotic or abusive family.
- Been sexually abused.
- Suffered some type of head trauma.

■ **SYMPTOMS.** Most individuals with personality disorders have disturbances in emotional development, are maladjusted socially, and often have incapacitating, acute episodes of their mental disorder; most believe that others are responsible for their condition.

Personality disorders include paranoid, schizoid, antisocial, narcissistic, and histrionic behaviors. Each condition is described, along with typical symptoms, in the following list.

- **Paranoid personalities** are characterized by traits of jealousy, suspicion, envy, and hypersensitivity. These individuals exhibit extreme mistrust of others and suspect their motives and intents as deliberately harmful to them. Paranoid individuals are often angry, hostile, cold, and unemotional.

- **Schizoid personalities** are loners. They lack warm or tender feelings for others and have few friends. The opinions of others have little effect on their feelings, and they have difficulty expressing anger.

- **Antisocial personalities** usually are identified in the teen years by troublesome behavior including fighting, stealing, running away, and cruelty. The antisocial individual is selfish, irritable, aggressive, and impulsive. These individuals do not express feelings of guilt and do not learn from mistakes.

- **Narcissistic personalities** have an exaggerated sense of self-importance and self-love. They need constant attention and admiration. If criticized, they react with rage or humiliation and lack ability to express empathy.

- **Histrionic personalities** are overly dramatic with expressions of emotion. They exhibit theatrical

mannerisms and overreact to events. This personality is vain and demanding, needs to be the center of attention, and constantly seeks approval and reassurance.

■ **DIAGNOSIS.** There are no specific tests for personality disorders. Diagnosis is usually made by a mental health professional based on evaluation of symptoms and emotional and mental history.

■ **TREATMENT.** Treatment of personality disorders includes psychotherapy and drug therapy. Common medications include antidepressants, anticonvulsants, and antipsychotics. Hospitalization might be needed during acute episodes.

■ **PREVENTION.** There is no way to prevent personality disorders. Avoiding acute symptoms might be possible by regularly attending counseling sessions and taking medications as prescribed.

Gender Identity Disorder

Gender identity disorder is a condition in which the person is uncomfortable or distressed with his or her sexual identity. Affected children might state a preference for being the opposite sex, cross-dress, choose members of the opposite sex for best friends, play games stereotypical of the opposite sex, show disgust with their genitals, and express a desire for genitals of the opposite sex.

In adults, the disorder is characterized by a stated desire to be the opposite sex and a conviction that they have feelings and attitudes of the opposite sex and that they were born the wrong sex. Adults with gender identity try to rid themselves of secondary sex characteristics and might seek hormonal and surgical intervention for a gender reassignment.

Sexual Disorders

■ **DESCRIPTION.** Sexual disorders include sexual dysfunction and paraphilias, sexual deviations. Sexual dysfunction is discussed in Chapter 17, "Reproductive System Diseases and Disorders." Paraphilia is a sexual disorder in which the person experiences repeated and intense sexual arousal from bizarre fantasies, often involving objects or nonconsenting persons. The majority of paraphiliacs are male. Many of these disorders are considered socially unacceptable at the least and criminal at worst.

■ **ETIOLOGY.** There are many theories concerning the origin of sexual disorders, but in reality, no one has a certain answer. Some think these are formed during sexual development near or during puberty. The idea is that social development, or how the individual has been treated, has somehow gone off course, leading to the inability to develop relationships. This inability, along with the lack of meaningful relationships, is expressed in the form of sexual disorders.

■ **SYMPTOMS.** Sexual disorders include exhibitionism, fetishism, transvestic fetishism, frotteurism, pedophilia, sexual sadism, sexual masochism, and voyeurism. Each condition is described, along with typical symptoms, in the following list.

- **Exhibitionism** is a very common disorder and involves a male exposing his genitals to an unsuspecting female.
- **Fetishism** involves sexual arousal with a nonliving object.
- **Transvestic fetishism** involves arousal by cross-dressing (Figure 21–7).
- **Frotteurism** involves sexual arousal from touching or rubbing against a nonconsenting person.
- **Pedophilia** is a condition of being sexually aroused by a child. This disorder occurs primarily in impotent men. Pedophiles usually do not rape the involved child but, more often, want to fondle the child and request the child to fondle them. This activity is criminally classified as child molestation. Homosexuals are usually not child molesters. The usual case is a teen or adult male with a prepubescent female.
- **Sexual sadism** involves sexual arousal of the sadist when the victim suffers physical or psychological pain.
- **Sexual masochism** involves sexual arousal of the masochist when the masochist is humiliated or made to suffer by being beaten or bound.
- **Voyeurism** is a common disorder and involves arousal by secretly watching others undress or engage in sexual activity. Voyeurs are commonly called peeping toms.
- **Other paraphilia** include arousal with animals (zoophilia), corpses (necrophilia), and obscene telephone calls (scatologia).

■ **DIAGNOSIS.** Individuals with sexual disorders are not easily diagnosed, usually due to embarrassment about the condition. Those affected are often found out and reported. After the individual is assessed by a mental health professional, the diagnosis is usually confirmed.

■ **TREATMENT.** Professional treatment that assists the affected individual with suppressing the activity is often beneficial. Treatment with androgen (hormones) can influence the frequency and intensity of the episodes.

■ **PREVENTION.** There are no clear-cut actions for prevention.

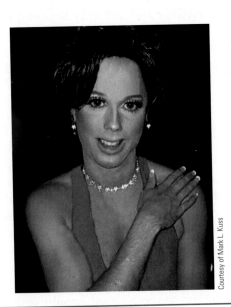

Courtesy of Mark L. Kuss

FIGURE 21–7   Cross-dresser.

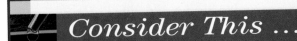

Consider This ...

The colder the room you sleep in, the greater is the risk of having bad dreams.

Sleep Disorders

■ **DESCRIPTION.** Sleep disorders (somnipathy) are medical disorders of sleep. Some disorders are serious enough to disrupt the individual's ability to function at home and work. These disorders include dyssomnias and parasomnias. Dyssomnias are disorders related to falling asleep and include insomnia, narcolepsy, and sleep apnea. Parasomnias are disorders related to staying asleep and include nightmares, sleep terror, and sleepwalking disorders.

■ *ETIOLOGY.* Some causes of sleep disorders are easy to recognize, whereas others are more difficult to determine. Common causes include shift work, anxiety, pain, incontinence, noise, and certain medications.

■ *SYMPTOMS.* Sleep disorders include insomnia, narcolepsy, apnea, nightmare, sleep terror, and sleepwalking. Each condition is described, along with typical symptoms, in the following list.

- **Insomnia** is the inability to fall or stay asleep. The affected individual might awaken early and feel mentally and physically fatigued. Insomnia commonly affects females and tends to increase in incidence with age. Intake of stimulants such as coffee or tea before bedtime often causes the condition, as do physical disorders such as thyroid conditions. Anxiety and stress also can lead to insomnia. Treatment can include treating physical disorders, removing stress and anxiety, obtaining psychotherapy, and, as a last resort, taking sleeping medications.

- **Narcolepsy** is a daily uncontrollable attack of sleep. Affected individuals might fall asleep any time they are sedentary such as driving, studying, reading, or eating. Narcolepsy usually occurs in the late teens or early 20s. Seizure disorder and sleep apnea must be ruled out prior to treatment. Scheduled naps and establishing a sleeping routine will usually resolve the disorder.

- **Sleep apnea** is a dyssomnia characterized by short periods of breathlessness during sleep, possibly due to respiratory or neurologic problems. This condition is discussed in Chapter 15.

- **Nightmare disorder** is a condition in which the involved individual is awakened by anxiety-provoking dreams. Once awakened, the individual is quickly oriented. Common subjects of nightmares include falling, death, and being attacked. Children usually outgrow this condition, but adults might need treatment with Valium.

- **Sleep terror** is an awakening due to nightmares, but individuals are so terrified that they do not become quickly oriented. The individual can be confused and cannot be comforted by family members. Night terrors can be reduced by not allowing the child or affected individual to watch disturbing movies or television programs.

- **Sleepwalking disorder** is a condition characterized by the individual getting up at night and walking without awakening. The individual can be awakened, usually with some difficulty, but does not remember the episode. The primary concern with sleepwalking is the increased potential for injury to the sleeping individual.

■ *DIAGNOSIS.* Most disorders can be diagnosed by a sleep history. Sleep studies including a polysomnogram, along with medical testing, help the physician confirm the diagnosis.

■ *TREATMENT.* When the source of the problem is identified, several treatment options exist, including bright-light therapy, continuous positive airway pressure (CPAP), medications such as melatonin, and surgery.

■ *PREVENTION.* Depending on the cause, some activities that might help prevent sleep disorders include:

- Going to bed at the same time every night.
- Avoiding caffeine, nicotine, and alcohol late in the day.
- Avoiding a large meal late in the day.
- Getting regular exercise.
- Eating a healthy diet.
- Creating a routine to wind down just before sleep, such as reading or taking a warm bath.

TRAUMA

Grief

Grief is a natural process of coping with a loss, such as the loss of a family member or friend or the prospect of one's own impending death. The loss might also be of less weight and include the loss of a body part or body function, a job, or a valued possession.

No matter the cause, grief is real and is a natural part of life. Grieving is a healthy process. Those unable to grieve and complete the grieving process often have difficulty coping with life.

People grieve differently in different cultures, and individuals within each culture might grieve differently. Some individuals are very emotional, whereas others remain solemn.

TABLE 21–4 Dr. Elisabeth Kübler-Ross's Five Stages of Grief/Death and Dying

Stage	Key Ideas	Behavior
Denial	No, not me	Refusal to believe; must be a mistake
Anger	Why me?	Envy those not dying or grieving; frustrated
Bargaining	If I could have one more chance	Becomes religious and good in an effort to bargain for time
Grief/Depression	Realizes bargaining is not working	Depressed, cries, gives up
Acceptance	OK, I give up, but I might not like it	Expects death, might call family members near, completes unfinished business, prepares to die

The normal grieving process passes through several stages that were defined by Dr. Elisabeth Kübler-Ross in the 1970s and remain true today (Table 21–4). Not everyone is able to move through all the steps. Grieving individuals might stop in one stage and need assistance to move on, or they might retreat to a lower stage before moving forward again. The speed at which a person moves through the grieving process is, again, very individual.

An important aspect of a funeral ceremony is to allow those who are grieving to say good-bye and to have closure of the situation. Individuals who were never allowed to say good-bye to a deceased or missing loved one, such as families of servicemen killed overseas or of missing children or persons, can suffer with extreme depression. Inability to grieve and complete the grieving process can lead to depression, poor coping skills, and the need for psychological counseling.

Suicide

Suicide was discussed in Chapter 20, "Childhood Diseases and Disorders," as a major concern for teenagers, but it is also a common problem among individuals with mental health disorders. Depression is a main cause of suicide. Suicidal individuals have feelings of depression, guilt, hopelessness, and helplessness. As previously stated, changes in the life cycle—including aging—can lead to depression and suicide.

It is estimated that more than one-third of people over age 65 try to commit suicide. Individuals diagnosed with a terminal illness often consider suicide as a means of living the remainder of life with dignity. Widowed, older white men; minority groups; and the unemployed are also at risk.

RARE DISEASES

Several of the disorders discussed in this chapter are considered to be rare but are included to maintain the order of the outline and assist the learner in categorizing mental illnesses. There are, however, many other very rare mental health disorders affecting individuals from children to the older adult population.

MENTAL HEALTH DISORDERS IN THE OLDER ADULT

There are many mental health disorders that can affect the older adult. Some of these might have begun early in life, whereas others occur very late in life. Some disorders of the neurologic system cause symptoms such as memory lapses, behavior changes, and confusion that mimic symptoms of mental health problems but really are a physiologic or system-specific disorder. Others, such as Alzheimer's disease, although a neurologic system problem, are also considered to be a mental health disorder.

Many other disorders found in the older adult population are like this. Because of the changes that occur in the aging process, some symptoms seen in the older population might just be normal changes and not related to mental health disorders at all. Unfortunately, older adults are often labeled as having a mental health problem when they are merely dealing with the normal process of aging.

The most common mental health problems in the older population include depression, insomnia, isolation, stress, and disorders related to or caused by other system diseases. In addition, some individual medications or medication interactions can cause symptoms of mental health problems such as confusion, forgetfulness, dizziness, and speech problems.

SUMMARY

M ental health disorders are some of the most misunderstood health problems. Although some are difficult to diagnose and treat, many more can be either controlled or cured with proper diagnosis and intervention.

Some of the symptoms of mental health problems are very slow to appear and are quite subtle, making it difficult to determine whether a real problem exists. In the older adult, many neurologic disorders and the normal changes occurring in the aging process are often incorrectly attributed to a mental health disorder. Early diagnosis and treatment of any type of mental health disorder are important to assist the affected individual to live a quality life.

REVIEW QUESTIONS

Short Answer

1. What are some of the common signs and symptoms of mental health disorders?

2. What are some common tests used to diagnose mental health problems?

3. List some of the treatments used to control or cure mental health disorders.

Matching

4. Match the mental health disorder in the left column with the appropriate category in the right column. Items in the right column may be used more than once.

_____ Conversion	a. Developmental mental disorders
_____ Alcoholism	b. Substance-related mental disorders
_____ Depression	c. Organic mental disorders
_____ Panic disorder	d. Psychoses
_____ Delusional disorder	e. Mood disorders
_____ Dementia	f. Anxiety disorders
_____ ADHD	g. Somatoform disorders
_____ PTSD	
_____ OCD	
_____ Drug abuse	
_____ Mental retardation	
_____ Munchausen	
_____ Schizophrenia	

5. Match the drugs listed in the left column with the best description in the right column.

_____ Marijuana

_____ Cocaine

_____ Methamphetamine

_____ LSD

_____ Anabolic steroids

_____ Alcohol

_____ Nicotine (cigarettes)

_____ Solvents

a. The most used hallucinogenic drug

b. An addictive stimulant also known as speed and crank

c. Chemicals with breathable vapors that produce the effect of being intoxicated

d. The most widely used drug by adolescents

e. Contains the active chemical THC

f. Drug taken to enhance muscular development

g. An intoxicating drug that is implicated in thousands of motor vehicle accidents

h. A strong central nervous system stimulant that produces a euphoric state

CASE STUDIES

■ Jenny Stanson is a 20-year-old college student who lives with her grandmother. She has noticed that her grandmother seems confused at times, forgets things she has told her, and is often rather short-tempered. This does not seem to be her usual manner and happens only infrequently, but Jenny is concerned. Someone stated her grandmother might be suffering from early Alzheimer's disease. She wants to know what she should do about this. She also wants more information about Alzheimer's disease. How can you help her? What resources might be helpful?

■ Jim Wolf is a 45-year-old auto-parts store owner who constantly washes his hands. He also continually checks and rechecks parts lists, equipment, and his employees' schedules. His wife, Mary, who works in the business with Jim, has convinced him to seek medical intervention for his problem because his anxiety level has been interfering with his work performance and his ability to sleep. After testing and referral to a psychiatrist, he has been diagnosed with an OCD. What can you tell Jim and Mary about this disorder? Jim asks you if you think he is crazy. How would you respond to that question? What type of treatment might he expect?

Study Tools

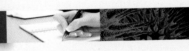

Workbook

Complete Chapter 21

Online Resources

PowerPoint® presentations

BIBLIOGRAPHY

Brennaman, L., & Lobo, M. L. (2011). Recovery from serious mental illness: A concept analysis. *Issues in Mental Health Nursing* 32(10), 654–663.

Browne, G., Cashin, A., & Graham, I. (2012). Models of case management for working with young children: Implications for mental health nurses. *International Journal of Mental Health Nursing* 21(2), 123–130.

Clinical Digest. (2011). People with schizophrenia show improved symptoms after cognitive treatment. *Nursing Standard* 26(13), 14–15.

Cooper, G. L. (2011). Untapping mental health capital. *Health Promotion International* 26(Suppl), 1–3.

Donnelly, J. R. (2011). The need for ibogaine in drug and alcohol addiction treatment. *Journal of Legal Medicine* 32(1), 93–114.

Donnelly, T., Hwang, J., Este, D., Ewashen, C., Adair, C., & Clinton, M. (2011). If I was going to kill myself, I wouldn't be calling you. I am asking for help: Challenges influencing immigrant and refugee women's mental health. *Issues in Mental Health Nursing* 32(5), 279–290.

Drug overuse in women. (2011). *Consumer Reports on Health*, 23(12), 10.

Finfgeld-Connett, D., & Johnson, E. (2011). Therapeutic substance abuse treatment for incarcerated women. *Clinical Nursing Research* 20(4), 462–481.

Flaskerud, J. H. (2012). Mental health care and health literacy. *Issues in Mental Health Nursing*, 33(3) 196–198.

French, L. (2011). Student voices. Seeing schizophrenia from the patient's viewpoint. *Nursing* 41(10), 18–19.

Harris, B. A., & Shattell, M. M. (2012). A critical nursing perspective of pharmacological interventions for schizophrenia and the marginalization of person-centered alternatives. *Issues in Mental Health Nursing* 33(2), 127–129.

Heilig, M., Goldman, D., Berrettini, W., & O'Brien, C. P. (2011). Pharmacogenetic approaches to the treatment of alcohol addiction. *Nature Reviews Neuroscience* 12(11), 670–684.

Injured employee? He or she may be at high risk for opioid addiction. (2011). *Occupational Health Management* 21(11), 121–122.

Kaufman, E., McDonell, M. G., Cristofalo, M. A., & Ries, R. K. (2012). Exploring barriers to primary care for patients with severe mental illness: Frontline patient and provider accounts. *Issues in Mental Health Nursing*, 33(3) 172–180.

Kozlak, J. B. (2011). Psychotic symptoms in home health clients. *Home Health Care Management & Practice* 23(4), 295–298.

Mcdougall, T. (2011). Mental health problems in childhood and adolescence. *Nursing Standard* 26(14), 48–56.

Monroe, T., Hamza, H., Stocks, G., Davies Scimeca, P., & Cowan, R. (2011). The misuse and abuse of propofol. *Substance Use & Misuse* 46(9), 1199–1205.

National Institute on Drug Abuse (NIDA). (2009). What is the scope of cocaine use in the United States? *www.drugabuse.gov* (accessed October 2012).

Paturel, A. (2011). Buzz kill: How does alcohol affect the teenage brain? *Neurology Now* 7(6), 23–24, 26–28.

Powell, G. (2011). Wound care for injecting drug users: Part 1. *Nursing Standard* 25(46), 51–60.

Quinn, C., Happell, B., & Browne, G. (2012). Opportunity lost? Psychiatric medications and problems with sexual function: A role for nurses in mental health. *Journal of Clinical Nursing* 21(3/4), 415–423.

Roush, K. (2012). Examining our biases about mental illnesses. *American Journal of Nursing* 112(2), 7.

Rowe, C. L. (2012). Family therapy for drug abuse: Review and updates 2003–2010. *Journal of Marital & Family Therapy* 38(1), 59–81.

Sacks, S., McKendrick, K., Vazan, P., Sacks, J. Y., & Cleland, C. M. (2011). Modified therapeutic community aftercare for clients triply diagnosed with HIV/AIDS and co-occurring mental and substance use disorders. *AIDS Care* 23(12), 1676–1686.

Scott, D., & Happell, B. (2011). The high prevalence of poor physical health and unhealthy lifestyle behaviors in individuals with severe mental illness. *Issues in Mental Health Nursing* 32(9), 589–597.

Sturgess, J. E., George, T. P., Kennedy, J. L., Heinz, A., & Müller, D. J. (2011). Pharmacogenetics of alcohol, nicotine and drug addiction treatments. *Addiction Biology* 16(3), 357–376.

Substance Abuse and Mental Health Services Administration. (2011). The economic impact of illicit drug use on American society. U.S. Department of Health and Human Services. *www.samhsa.gov* (accessed September 2012).

Torchalla, I. I., Okoli, C. C., Malchy, L. L., & Johnson, J. L. (2011). Nicotine dependence and gender differences in smokers accessing community mental health services. *Journal of Psychiatric & Mental Health Nursing* 18(4), 349–358.

Ward, J. (2010). Addiction: A search for transformation. *Healthcare Counseling & Psychotherapy Journal* 10(4), 25–29.

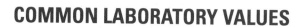

Appendix A

COMMON LABORATORY VALUES

Test	Explanation/Normal Values
Complete blood count (CBC)	Indicates oxygen-carrying capacity of blood and presence of infection.
White blood cells (WBCs)	4,300–10,000 mm^3
Red blood cells (RBCs)	4.2–5.4/mm^3
Hemoglobin (Hg)	
males	13–18 gm/dl
females	12–16 gm/dl
Hematocrit (Hct)	
males	40–62%
females	37–47%
Electrolytes	Test determines blood electrolyte levels.
Sodium (Na)	136–145 mEq/L
Potassium (K)	3.5–5.4 mEq/L
Chloride (Cl)	98–106 mEq/L
Carbon dioxide (CO$_2$)	22–30 mEq/L
Magnesium (Mg)	1.5–2.5 mEq/L
Arterial blood gases (ABGs)	Indicates respiratory and metabolic functioning.
	pH = 7.35–7.45
	PCO$_2$ = 35–45 mm Hg
	HCO$_3$ = 21–28 mEq/L
	PaO$_2$ = 80–100 mm Hg
	O$_2$ saturation = 95–100%
Culture and sensitivity (C&S)	Culture determines presence of microorganism. Sensitivity determines antibiotic that will kill or inhibit growth of microorganism. Normal value is negative for microorganism growth.
Urinalysis	Diagnoses problems in the urinary system.
Color	Clear to amber
Odor	Pleasantly aromatic
Albumin (protein)	Negative
Acetone	Negative
Red blood cells	2–3/HPF
White blood cells	4–5/HPF
Bilirubin	Negative
Glucose	Negative
Specific gravity	1.005–1.030
Bacteria	Negative
Casts	Rare
pH	4.6–8.0
Cholesterol	Less than 180 mg/dl desirable
	200–239 mg/dl borderline high
	240 mg/dl and above high
LDL	Less than 100 mg/dl
HDL	60 mg/dl and above

Author's note: Lab values/ranges may vary some depending on the laboratory running the test. Check the laboratory used for their normal ranges.

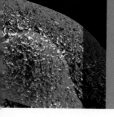

Appendix B

METRIC CONVERSION TABLES

LENGTH	Centimeters	Inches	Feet
1 centimeter	1.00	0.394	0.0328
1 inch	2.54	1.00	0.0833
1 foot	30.48	12.00	1.00
1 yard	91.4	36.00	3.00
1 meter	100.00	39.40	3.28

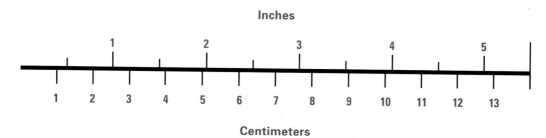

Comparison of Centimeters and Inches

VOLUMES	Cubic Centimeters	Fluid Drams	Fluid Ounces	Quarts	Liters
1 cubic centimeter	1.00	0.270	0.033	0.0010	0.0010
1 fluid dram	3.70	1.00	0.125	0.0039	0.0037
1 cubic inch	16.39	4.43	0.554	0.0173	0.0163
1 fluid ounce	29.6	8.00	1.00	0.0312	0.0296
1 quart	946.00	255.00	32.00	1.00	0.946
1 liter	1000.00	270.00	33.80	1.056	1.00

WEIGHTS	Grains	Grams	Apothecary Ounces	Pounds
1 grain (gr)	1.00	0.064	0.002	0.0001
1 gram (gm)	15.43	1.00	0.032	0.0022
1 apothecary ounce	480.00	31.1	1.00	0.0685
1 pound	7000.00	454.00	14.58	1.00
1 kilogram	15432.00	1000.00	32.15	2.205

Rules for Converting One System to Another

Volumes

Grains to grams	divide by 15
Drams to cubic centimeters	multiply by 4
Ounces to cubic centimeters	multiply by 30
Minims to cubic millimeters	multiply by 63
Minims to cubic centimeters	multiply by 0.06
Cubic millimeters to minims	divide by 63
Cubic centimeters to minims	multiply by 16
Cubic centimeters to fluid ounces	divide by 30
Liters to pints	divide by 2.1

Weights

Milligrams to grains	multiply by 0.0154
Grams to grains	multiply by 15
Grams to drams	multiply by 0.257
Grams to ounces	multiply by 0.0311

Temperature

Multiply centigrade (Celsius) degrees by $\frac{9}{5}$ and add 32 to convert Fahrenheit to Celsius

Subtract 32 from the Fahrenheit degrees and multiply by $\frac{5}{9}$ to convert Celsius to Fahrenheit

Common Household Measures and Weights

1 teaspoon	= 4–5 cc or 1 dram	1 cup	= 8 fluid ounces or ½ pint
3 teaspoons	= 1 tablespoon	1 tumbler or glass	= 8 fluid ounces or 240 cc
1 dessert spoon	= 8 cc or 2 drams	1 wine glass	= 2 fluid ounces or 60 cc
1 tablespoon	= 15 cc or 3 drams	16 fluid ounces	= 1 pound
4 tablespoons	= 1 wine glass or ½ gill	4 gills	= 1 pound
16 tablespoons (liquid)	= 1 cup	1 pint	= 1 pound
12 tablespoons (dry)	= 1 cup		

Glossary

A

abdominocentesis (ab-DOM-ih-no-sén-**TEE**-sis) pacentesis of the abdomen; a procedure in which a puncture is made into the abdominal cavity to withdraw fluid.

abortion a spontaneous or induced interruption of a pregnancy.

abrasion a scraping away of skin surface.

abscess a localized collection of pus.

achlorhydria (a-klor-**HIGH**-dree-ah) absence of hydrochloric acid.

achondroplasia a hereditary disorder of cartilage formation leading to dwarfism.

acne an inflammatory skin disease that affects the sebaceous glands and hair follicles; often seen at puberty.

acromegaly (ACK-roh-**MEG**-ah-lee; acro = extremity, megaly = enlargement) a condition of extremity enlargement as a result of excessive growth hormone in the adult.

acute (a-CUTE) a disease that is short term.

addiction a physical and/or psychological dependence on a substance.

Addison's disease hypoadrenalism; an uncommon undersecretion of hormones by the adrenal cortex.

adenocarcinoma (Ad-eh-NO-Kar-sin-oh-mah) a malignant tumor involving ductal or glandular epithelium, often found in the colon.

adenoidectomy (AD-eh-noy-**DECK**-toh-me; ectomy = removal) surgical removal of the adenoids.

adenoma (AD-eh-**NO**-ma; adeno = gland, oma = tumor) a tumor of glandular tissue.

adhesions (ad-HE-zhun) parts of tissue that cling to the surface of adjoining organs as normal fibrous scar tissue develops in an operative site, resulting in a fibrous band.

affect outward expression of emotions.

AIDS acquired immunodeficiency syndrome.

albinism absence of skin pigment.

albumin (al-BYOU-men) a blood protein distributed throughout the body; responsible for osmotic pressure of the blood.

albuminuria (al-BYOU-mih-**NEW**-ree-ah; albumin = a blood protein, uria = urine) albumin in the urine; usually albumin but may also be globulin; usually indicative of a disease process.

aldosterone (al-doh-STER-ohn) a mineralocorticoid; acts on the kidney to assist in maintaining electrolyte balance.

alleles matched pairs of genes; the term used to refer to the product when the chromosomes (one from each parent) pair up during fertilization of the egg; the genes on the chromosomes align.

allergen the environmental substance that causes a reaction.

allergy the state when the immune response is too intense or hypersensitive to an environmental substance.

alopecia (AL-oh-**PEE**-shee-ah; in Greek, meaning fox mange, which caused hair loss) a partial or complete hair loss, usually from the head.

amblyopia (AM-blee-**OH**-pee-ah) a decrease in the vision of the affected eye due to a lack of visual stimuli.

amenorrhea (ah-MEN-oh-**REE**-ah; a = without, menorrhea = menses) the absence or cessation of menses.

amnesia (am-NEE-zee-ah) loss of memory.

amylase an enzyme; often elevated in pancreatic disorders.

anaerobic (an = without, aerobic = air) living without oxygen.

analgesic (AN-al-**GEE**-sick) a medication that relieves pain.

anaphylaxis (AN-ah-fih-**LACK**-sis) an immediate allergic reaction characterized by contraction of smooth muscle and dilation of capillaries, leading to severe respiratory distress or failure.

anaplastic (AN-ah-**PLAST**-ic) abnormal tissue, the more undifferentiated tissue.

anastomosis connection of two tubular structures.

androgens hormones secreted by the adrenal cortex and responsible for male characteristics.

anemia (ah-NEE-me-ah; an = without, emia = blood) any decrease in oxygen-carrying ability of the red blood cell.

anencephaly a congenital malformation resulting in the absence of the brain or cranial vault.

aneurysm a weakening in the wall of an artery that allows the vessel to bulge or rupture.

angina (an-JIGH-nah) a severe pain, angina pectoralis is pain in the chest.

angiogenesis (AN-jee-oh-**JEN**-eh-sis; angio = vessel, genesis = formation) new growth of blood vessels.

angiography (AN-jee-**OG**-rah-fee; angio = vessel, graphy = procedure to record) a radiographic study of blood vessels after injection of fluorescein dye.

angioplasty (AN-jee-oh-**PLAS**-tee; angio = vessel, plasty = surgical repair) a procedure that involves passing a catheter into the artery and inflating a balloon on the catheter to push the plaque against the vessel wall, thus widening the lumen of the vessel.

ankle-brachial index (ABI) a comparison of the blood pressure in the lower legs to the blood pressure in the arms.

anomaly (ah-NOM-ah-lee) any abnormality.

anorexia nervosa (AN-oh-**RECK**-see-ah; an = without, orexia = appetite) a disorder of self-imposed starvation, resulting from a distorted body image.

anoxia (ah-NOCK-see-ah) no oxygen.

antibody(ies) immunoglobulins that develop in response to an antigen; also called immune bodies; proteins that the body produces to react to and render the antigen harmless.

antigen(s) (AN-tih-jens) a cell marker that induces a state of sensitivity after coming in contact with an antibody; any substance that causes the body some type of harm, thus setting off this specific reaction.

antipyretics (anti = against, pyretic = fever) a class of medications given to reduce an elevated temperature.

anuria (ah-NEW-ree-ah; an = without, uria = urine) no urine output.

apnea (ap-NEE-ah; a = without, pnea = breathing) the condition of not breathing; a term used to describe the absence of respirations for a period of time.

appendicitis inflammation of the appendix.

arrhythmia abnormal heart rhythm.

arterial blood gases (ABGs) the laboratory test that measures the amounts of oxygen and carbon dioxide in blood.

arteriosclerosis hardening of arterial walls.

arthritis inflammation of a joint.

articular relating to a joint surface.

articular fracture one that involves a joint surface.

ascites (ah-SIGH-teez) fluid in the abdomen (peritoneal cavity).

asthma a chronic allergic condition characterized by bronchospasm, wheezing, and excessive mucus formation.

asymptomatic (a = without, symptomatic = symptoms) not displaying symptoms.

atherosclerosis accumulation of lipids in the arterial walls or hardening of the arteries.

atresia the congenital absence or closure of a normal opening or lumen in the body; it may occur in a variety of areas.

atrophy (AT-tro-fee) a decrease in cell size, which leads to a decrease in the size of the tissue and organ.

audiometry (AW-dee-**OM**-eh-tree; audio = sound, metry = measure) the basic test used to measure hearing.

aura symptoms occurring at the onset of a partial epileptic seizure or migraine headache; it may include tingling of the fingers, ringing in the ears, and visual disturbances.

auscultation (AWS-kul-**TAY**-shun) using a stethoscope to listen to body cavities and organs.

autodigestion autolysis or digestion of self or one's own cells.

autoimmunity or autoimmune the state when the immune response attacks itself.

autosomes (auto = self, somes = body) a chromosome other than a sex chromosome; they determine body function.

avulsion skin pulled or torn away.

avulsion fracture one where there is a separation of a small bone fragment from the bone where a tendon or ligament is attached.

B

bacteria a one-celled microorganism that may be aerobic or anaerobic and free-living, saprophytic, parasitic, or pathogenic.

bariatrics the branch of medicine that deals with obesity.

Bence Jones protein a special protein found in the blood and urine, indicative of multiple myeloma.

benign (beh-NINE) having limited growth, noncancerous.

bimanual examination (bi = two, manual = handed) an examination in which the physician places one hand on the abdomen and inserts fingers of the other hand into the vagina to feel the female organs between the two hands.

bioethics a branch of ethics concerned with what is right and wrong within life decisions.

biopsy (BYE-op-see) removing a small piece of tissue for microscopic examination.

bleeding time a test to determine the length of bleeding time or time it takes the blood to clot.

blood urea nitrogen (BUN) a test to determine the level of urea nitrogen or waste in the blood.

blunt trauma a wound or injury (trauma) caused by an object with a flat, dull, or not sharp area (blunt).

body mass index (BMI) A measurement obtained by dividing the individual's weight in pounds by his or her height in inches. A BMI scale uses these figures to determine levels of obesity.

bone mass density (BMD) a measure of bone density or weight. A thinning bone results in a lower bone density.

bronchiectasis (BRONG-key-**ECK**-ta-sis) a chronic or long-term dilatation of a bronchus or bronchi along with an infection.

bronchoscopy (brong-KOS-koh-pee; broncho = bronchus or lung passageways, oscopy = procedure to look into) a diagnostic or surgical procedure in which a scope is passed through the mouth into the bronchus.

bronchospasm (BRONG-ko-**SPA**-zm) muscular constriction of the bronchi of the respiratory tract.

buccal smear a test for evaluating chromosomes; this test is performed by obtaining squamous epithelial cells from the buccal cavity, staining the cell, and microscopically observing for X chromosomes called Barr bodies.

bulimia (boo-LIM-ee-ah) an eating disorder characterized by episodes of binge eating (an intake of approximately 5,000 calories in 1 to 2 hours) followed by activities to negate the calorie intake by purging.

C

cachexia (ca-KACK-see-ah) a term used to describe any individual who has an ill, thin, wasted appearance.

calcaneal the heel area of the foot.

cancer a malignant tumor.

caput medusae tortuous, unsightly varicosities spreading from the umbilicus outward across the front of the abdomen.

carcinogen (kar-SIN-oh-jen) cancer-causing agent or substance.

carcinogenesis (KAR-sin-oh-**JEN**-eh-sis) cancer development.

carcinoma (KAR-sih-**NO**-mah) the most common type of malignant neoplasm arising from epithelial tissue.

carcinoma in situ atypical cells residing in the epithelial layer of tissue, not having broken through the basement membrane and invading other local tissues.

cardiac catheterization (KATH-eh-ter-eye-**ZAY**-shun) an invasive procedure used to sample the blood in the chambers of the heart to determine the amount of oxygen content and blood pressure in the chambers.

cardiac palpitations an unusually strong, rapid, or irregular heart rate that is so abnormal the individual can feel it.

cardiomyopathy a variety of diseases affecting the heart muscle.

carotid endarterectomy (END-ar-ter-**ECK**-toh-me; endo = inside, arter = artery, ectomy = excision of) surgical intervention to remove plaque in the carotid arteries to improve blood flow and reduce the risk of a thrombus.

catarrhal (ka-TAR-all) inflammation of mucous membranes of the head and mouth with increased mucus flow.

catheterization (KATH-er-ter-eye-**ZAY**-shun) a sterile procedure consisting of passing a soft catheter through the urethra and into the bladder for the purpose of (1) instilling or pouring fluids or medication into the bladder or (2) removing urine.

cauterization (KAW-ter-eye-**ZAY**-shun) the electrical burning of tissue to stop bleeding; used most frequently during surgery to stop bleeding from vessels.

cellulitis (SELL-you-**LYE**-tis) inflammation of connective tissue.

cephalalgia (SEF-ah-**LAL**-jee-ah; cephal = head, algia = pain) headache.

cerebrovascular accident (CVA) poor blood flow to the brain, commonly called a stroke.

cerumen (se-ROO-men) ear wax.

cervicitis (SER-vih-**SIGH**-tis) inflammation of the cervix.

chancre (SHANG-ker) a painless, highly contagious lesion occurring in the primary stage of syphilis.

chemotaxis the movement of cells or organisms in response to chemicals.

chemotherapy using pharmacologic therapy in the treatment of cancer.

cholecystectomy (KOH-lee-sis-**TECK**-toh-me; chole = gall or bile, cyst = bladder, ectomy = removal) surgical removal of the gallbladder.

chorea (ko-REE-ah) a constant, jerky, uncontrollable movement.

chronic a disease that persists for a long time.

circadian rhythm a normal 24-hour cycle of biological rhythms including sleep, metabolism, and glandular secretions.

clean catch a term used to describe a clean urine collection method involving cleansing the urethral area prior to urinating and catching the voided urine specimen.

closed or simple fracture a fracture that does not break through the skin.

clubbing a condition affecting the distal portion of the finger; characterized by soft tissue enlargement and an abnormal curvature of the nail.

Colle's fracture a fracture of the lower end of the radius with displacement of the fragment.

colorectal pertaining to both the colon and rectum.

colostomy (co-LOSS-toh-me) an artificial opening in the colon.

comedones (KOM-eh-dohns) plugged skin pores; the open form is a blackhead; the closed form is a whitehead.

comminuted fracture one in which there are more than two ends or fragments.

complete blood count (CBC) a laboratory test that identifies the number of red blood cells (RBCs), white blood cells (WBCs), and platelets per cubic millimeter.

complete fracture   the fracture is completely through the bone.

complication   the onset of a second disease or disorder in an individual who is already affected with a disease.

compound (open) fracture   a fracture involving the bone puncturing through the skin, or an object puncturing the skin, making an opening through the skin to the fracture site.

compression fracture   one in which the bone appears to be mashed down.

compulsion   a repetitive act the affected individual is unable to resist performing.

computerized axial tomography (CAT or CT)   imaging by a cross-sectional plane of the body; also called computed tomography.

congenital   (kon-JEN-ih-tahl) present at birth; usually concerning a congenital anomaly or an abnormality present at birth.

congenital anomaly   (kon-JEN-ih-tahl ah-NOM-ah-lee; congenital = present at birth, anomaly = abnormality) a birth defect.

contusion   (kon-TOO-zhun) a large bruise.

convulsion   an abnormal muscle contraction; a violent spasm or jerking of the face, trunk, or extremities.

corticosteroids   (KORT-ti-ko-STEHR-oyds) powerful anti-inflammatory hormones.

cortisol   hydrocortisone; a steroid hormone secreted by the adrenal cortex.

cortisone   a glucocorticoid; it affects carbohydrate metabolism and influences the nutrition and growth of connective tissues.

creatinine   (kree-AT-in-in) one of the two most common nitrogenous waste products that are normally filtered from the blood, the final product of creatine catabolism.

creatinine clearance test   a diagnostic test for kidney function that measures the rate the kidneys excrete creatinine, a waste product from muscle contraction that is carried in small amounts in the blood, filtered by the kidney, and excreted in urine. An increased blood or urine level indicates a disturbance in kidney function.

cretinism   congenital hypothyroidism.

cryptorchidism   (krip-TOR-kih-dizm; crypt = hidden, orchid = testicle, ism = condition) undescended testicle(s).

culture and sensitivity   a test to identify a pathogen and the type of treatment needed.

curative   something that corrects or cures the disease or condition.

cyanosis   (SIGH-ah-NO-sis; cyano = blue, osis = condition) a bluish condition of the skin due to lack of oxygen in the blood.

cystogram   (cysto = bladder, gram = picture) an X-ray picture of the bladder that helps determine the shape and function of the bladder.

cystoscopy   (sis-TOS-koh-pee; cysto = bladder, scopy = procedure to look) an invasive procedure to look into the urethra and bladder by using a lighted scope.

cytologic   (SIGH-toe-LAW-gic) pertaining to cytology.

cytology   (SIGH-TOL-oh-jee; cyto = cell, logy = study) the examination or study of cells.

cytotoxic   (cyto = cell, toxic = killing) something that kills cells.

D

débridement   (day-breed-MENT) a process of washing or cutting away necrotic tissue and foreign material.

decompress   a release of pressure.

defecate   to have a bowel movement.

degenerative   diseases related to aging, or destruction of tissue, functions, and use.

dehiscence   (dee-HISS-ens) separation of tissue margins.

delirium tremens (DTs)   (dee-LIR-ee-um TREE-mens) a serious form of delirium due to alcoholic withdrawal after a period of sustained intoxication.

delusions   false beliefs that are firmly adhered to although they are not shared by others.

dementia   (dee-MEN-she-ah) a loss of mental ability due to the loss of neurons or brain cells.

densitometry   measurement of bone thickness.

dental plaque   tough, sticky material that adheres to the tooth enamel; caused by bacteria.

dependency   a psychological craving for a substance that may or may not be accompanied by a physical need.

diabetic retinopathy   (DYE-ah-BET-ick RET-ih-NOP-ahthee, retino = retina, opathy = disease) disease of the retina of the eye, often resulting in blindness; caused by degeneration due to diabetes mellitus.

diagnosis   (DIE-ag-KNOW-sis) the identification or naming of a disease.

diapedesis   (DYE-ah-pe-DEE-sis) passage of blood, or its formed elements, through the intact walls of blood vessels.

diastolic   (dye-as-TOL-ick) relating to cardiac diastole; the process of the heart resting as the chambers refill with blood.

differential   a detailed white blood cell count identifying the number of each type of leukocyte.

differentiation   the process of individual specialization of cells.

digital rectal examination   a manual examination in which the physician feels the prostate for abnormal enlargement (hypertrophy or hyperplasia) and tumors.

dilatation and curettage (**KYOU**-reh-**TAHZH**) or D&C, a procedure that involves a dilation of the cervix (dilatation) and scraping (curettage) of the uterine endometrial tissue; a D&C is commonly performed for abnormal uterine bleeding and following a spontaneous abortion.

diplopia (dih-**PLOH**-pee-ah) double vision.

disease a change in structure or function within the body that is considered to be abnormal; any change from normal.

diskectomy surgery to remove a vertebral disk.

disorder a derangement or abnormality of function.

displaced fracture one in which fragments are out of position.

dominant in control.

Doppler a device that may be placed over arteries to magnify the sound of blood flow.

dormant state of being inactive.

dowager's hump abnormal curvature in the upper thoracic spine.

dual energy X-ray absorptiometry (DEXA) the most widely used technology to measure bone density. Two X-ray beams are aimed at the patient's bones and the density of the bone is determined by the absorption of each X-ray beam.

dwarfism a decrease in growth hormone (GH) that leads to impaired growth of all body tissues.

dysentery an acute inflammation of the colon; colitis.

dysmenorrhea (DIS-men-oh-**REE**-ah; dys = painful, menorrhea = menses) pain with menstrual periods.

dyspareunia (DIS-pa-**ROO**-nee-ah) painful sexual intercourse.

dysphagia (dis-**FAY**-jee-ah; dys = difficulty, phagia = swallowing) difficulty swallowing.

dysphasia (dis-**FAY**-zee-ah; dys = difficulty, phasia = speaking) difficulty speaking.

dysplasia (dis-**PLAY**-zee-ah) an alteration in size, shape, and organization of cells.

dyspnea (disp-**NEE**-ah; dys = difficult, pnea = breathing) difficulty breathing.

dysuria (dis-**YOU**-ree-ah; dys = difficult or painful, uria = urine) difficulty or pain with urination.

E

E test (epsilometer test) an antibiotic-permeated strip that identifies the kill zone of bacteria on a culture plate and also shows the concentration of antibiotic needed to kill the organism.

ecchymoses (ECH-ih-**MOH**-ses) large areas of bruising or hemorrhage.

eclampsia (eh-**KLAMP**-see-ah) a condition of pregnancy characterized by all the symptoms of toxemia or preeclampsia, plus the symptoms of convulsions.

ectopic (eck-**TOP**-ick) out of normal place.

electrocardiogram (ECG or EKG; ee-**LECK**-troh-**KAR**-dee-oh-**GRAM**; electro = electrical, cardio = heart, gram = picture) the graphic drawing produced by an electrocardiograph, a machine that receives electrical information and draws heart action.

electromyography (EMG; ee-**LEK**-troh-my-**OG**-ra-fee) a diagnostic test in which a small needle is inserted into muscle tissue and the electrical activity is recorded.

embolus (**EM**-boh-lus) material floating in the blood that may stick in a vessel and occlude or stop blood flow, leading to ischemia or death of the organs supplied by that vessel.

empyema (**EM**-pye-**EE**-mah) an accumulation of pus in a body cavity.

encapsulated enclosed in a capsule.

encephalopathy (en-**SEF**-ah-**LOP**-ah-thee; encephalo = brain, opathy = disease) any disease or disorder of the brain.

endarterectomy (**END**-ar-ter-**ECK**-toh-me; endo = inside, arter = artery, ectomy = excision) a surgical procedure involving opening an artery and cleaning out the plaque.

endometritis (**EN**-doh-me-**TRY**-tis) inflammation of the uterus lining.

enteral relating to the small intestine.

enterotoxin intestinal poison.

enucleation removal of the eyeball.

epicanthus a vertical fold of skin across the medial canthus of the eye, giving the eyes an Asian appearance.

epidural (hematoma) (**EP**-ih-**DOO**-ral; epi = above, dural = dura, outer meninges) blood collecting between the skull and the dura mater.

epistaxis (**EP**-i-**STACK**-sis) hemorrhage or bleeding from the nose; nosebleed.

erythema (**ER**-ih-**THEE**-mah) skin redness.

erythrocytopenia (erythrocyte = red cell, penia = decrease) a deficiency of red blood cells.

erythrocytosis (erythrocyte = red cell, osis = condition) a condition of increased red blood cells.

esophageal varices (eh-**SOF**-ah-**JEE**-al **VAYR**-ih-seez) varicosities (varicose veins) of the esophagus.

estrogen a term used to describe the hormones responsible for female characteristics.

etiology (**ET**-tee-**OL**-oh-jee) the study of cause or the cause of a disease.

euphoric a sense of well-being.

exacerbation   (x-AS-er-**BAY**-shun) a time when symptoms flare up or become worse.

exocrine (glands)   glands that excrete through a duct.

exophthalmos   (ECK-sof-**THAL**-mos) abnormal protrusion of the eyeballs.

exsanguination   loss of circulating blood volume.

extracapsular fracture   a fracture outside or not involving the joint capsule.

exudate   (ECKS-you-dayt) fluid that has seeped out of tissue or capillaries because of injury or inflammation.

F

familial   runs in or common to a family; for example, a disease that tends to occur in several members of the same family.

fascia   (FASH-ee-ah) a thick fibrous connective tissue.

fatal   inevitable or causing death.

feces   evacuated bowel contents; commonly called bowel movement or BM.

femoral neck fracture   a fracture involving the neck of the femur.

fibrillation   (FIH-brih-**LAY**-shun) a heart rhythm that is wild and uncoordinated; a cardiac arrhythmia.

fissure   a crack, split, or ulcer-like sore; a groove or slit.

fistula   (FIS-tyou-lah) a tract that connects two organs or cavities to each other or to the surface of the skin.

flatulence   excessive gas in the stomach or intestine.

florescent treponemal antibody absorption test (FTA-ABS)   an indirect fluorescent antibody test used to confirm a diagnosis of syphilis.

frequency   how often the individual urinates.

frostbite   the freezing of tissue, usually on the face, fingers, toes, and ears.

frozen section   a technique that enables a pathologist to make a rapid determination of a tumor condition, either malignant or benign.

fulminant   (FULL-ma-nant) occurring suddenly, rapidly, and intensely.

fungi   forms of yeast and molds; microscopic plant-like organisms.

G

gangrene   (GANG-green) a condition occurring when saprophytic (dead tissue–loving) bacteria become involved in necrotic tissue.

gene   the unit on the chromosome that carries DNA information.

genotypes   the genetic pattern of the individual.

germ cells   sex cells.

giantism   a condition of overgrowth due to hyperpituitarism occurring before puberty and during the growing years.

gingivitis   inflammation of the gums.

glucagon   a hormone secreted by the alpha cells in the islets of Langerhans in the pancreas; responsible for elevating blood glucose concentration.

glucocorticoids   a group of steroids of the adrenal cortex that affects metabolism such as causing glycogen storage and causing an anti-inflammatory effect.

glucose tolerance test   a blood test that determines how long it takes to clear glucose levels in the blood.

glycogen   (GLYE-ko-jen) the form that extra sugar is stored in, primarily in the liver.

glycosuria   (GLYE-koh-**SOO**-ree-ah; glyco = glycogen or sugar, uria = urine) the spilling of sugar into the urine; a common symptom of diabetes mellitus.

goiter   (GOI-ter) noticeable protrusion of the thyroid gland.

goitrogenic   goiter producing, as in foods or drugs such as turnips, cabbage, and lithium.

gonad   a sex organ; a testis or an ovary.

grading   determining the degree of differentiation of cells through microscopic examination.

grand mal   a term applied to seizures that are the type most often thought of as epilepsy; these seizures are characterized by convulsions, loss of consciousness, urinary and fecal incontinence, and tongue biting.

greenstick fracture   a common incomplete fracture that occurs in children; it appears to have broken partially like a sap-filled green stick.

gumma   (GUM-mah) a characteristic soft, gummy lesion caused by bacteria that invade organs throughout the body; found in the tertiary stage of syphilis.

gynecomastia   (GUY-ne-koh-**MAS**-tee-ah) abnormal breast enlargement.

H

hallucinations   (hah-LOO-sih-**NAY**-shun) false sensations of sight, touch, sound, smell, or taste.

hallucinogenic   (hah-LOO-sih-no-**JEN**-ick) producing psychedelic or bizarre alterations in mental functioning.

heat exhaustion   a reaction to heat, marked by prostration, weakness, and collapse; caused by severe dehydration.

heat stroke   a serious and possibly fatal illness caused by exposure to excessively high temperatures.

helminths   intestinal parasites; also called worms; nematodes, cestodes, and trematodes.

hemarthrosis   (hem = blood, arthro = joint, osis = condition) bleeding into joints.

hematemesis   (HEM-ah-**TEM**-eh-sis; hema = blood, emesis = vomiting) vomiting blood.

hematochezia (HEM-at-toe-**KEE**-zee-ah) bright red blood in the feces.

hematocrit (he-**MAT**-oh-krit) a measurement of the amount of red cell mass as a proportion of whole blood.

hematoma (HEM-ah-**TOH**-mah) a large tumor or swelling filled with blood; also called a bruise or contusion.

hematuria (HEM-ah-**TOO**-ree-ah; hema = blood, uria = urine) blood in the urine.

hemicolectomy surgical removal of part of the colon.

hemiparesis (HEM-ee-**PAR**-ee-sis; hemi = one half, paresis = paralysis) weakness or paralysis affecting one side of the body.

hemoglobin (Hgb) a measurement of the amount of hemoglobin, or oxygen-carrying potential, available in the blood.

hemolytic (HE-moh-**LIT**-ick) destruction of red blood cells.

hemolyzed broken-down cells.

hemoptysis (he-**MOP**-tih-sis; hemo = blood, ptysis = saliva) coughing up blood.

hemothorax (hemo = blood, thorax = chest) blood in the chest cavity.

hepatomegaly (HEP-ah-toh-**MEG**-ah-lee) enlarged liver.

heterozygous (hetero = different, zygo = yoked or paired) having different paired genes.

hirsutism (**HER**-soot-izm) abnormal hair on the face and body of the female.

histamine a substance that causes local arterioles, venules, and capillaries to dilate, resulting in an increase in blood flow to the area; released in response to injury or irritation.

holistic medicine the concept of considering the whole person rather than just the physical being.

homeostasis (HOME-ee-oh-**STAY**-sis) the state of sameness or normalcy that the body strives to maintain.

homozygous (homo = one, zygo = yoked or paired) having identical genes.

hydrocortisone a steroid hormone secreted by the adrenal cortex.

hydrophobia (hydro = water, phobia = fear) fear of the water.

hyperemia (HIGH-per-**EE**-me-ah; hyper = increased, emia = blood) increased blood flow in response to a release of histamine.

hyperglycemia (HIGH-per-glye-**SEE**-me-ah; hyper = excessive, glyc = glycogen or glucose, emia = blood) high blood sugar level.

hyperplasia (HIGH-per-**PLAY**-zee-ah) an increase in cell number; overgrowth in response to some type of stimulus.

hypersensitivity a condition in which there is an excessive response by the body to the stimulus of a foreign body.

hypertrophy (HIGH-**PER**-tro-fee) an increase in the size of the cell, leading to an increase in tissue and organ size.

hypoglycemia (HIGH-poh-gly-**SEE**-me-ah; hypo = decreased, glyc = glucose, emia = blood) a low blood sugar level.

hypothermia (hypo = low, thermia = heat or temperature) a significantly low body temperature.

hypovolemia (HIGH-poh-voh-**LEE**-me-ah) low or decreased blood volume.

hypoxemia (high-**POX**-SEE-me-ah; hypo = not enough, ox = oxygen, emia = blood) not enough oxygen in the circulating blood.

hypoxia (HIGH-**POX**-see-ah) not enough oxygen in tissues.

hysterosalpingogram (hystero = uterus, salpingo = fallopian tubes, gram = picture) an X-ray picture of the uterus and fallopian tubes.

I

iatrogenic (eye-AT-roh-**JEN**-ick; iatro = medicine, physician, genic = rising from) a problem arising due to or related to a prescribed treatment.

idiopathic (ID-ee-oh-**PATH**-ick) an unknown cause of disease.

ileus (**ILL**-ee-us) absence of peristalsis.

immunodeficiency the state when the immune response is unable to defend the body due to a decrease or absence of leukocytes, primarily lymphocytes.

impacted fracture one that has a bone end forced over the other end.

impotent (**IM**-poh-tent) inability in the male to achieve or maintain a penile erection.

in and out catheterization a catheterization procedure in which the catheter is removed as soon as the urine is drained; the catheterization is temporary.

incision a laceration or cut with smooth, even edges.

incomplete fracture the bone is fractured but not in two.

incubation period the time between exposure to the disease and the presence of symptoms, which might last several days.

induration (IN-dur-**RAY**-shun) hardened tissue.

indwelling catheter a catheter that is placed for a longer period of time than an in and out catheter as commonly occurs for urinary incontinence; a balloon on the end of the catheter is inflated to hold the catheter in the bladder.

infarct (in-**FARKT**) necrosis of cells or tissues due to ischemia.

infection (in-**FECT**-shun) invasion of microorganisms into the tissue, causing cell or tissue injury, thus leading to the inflammatory response.

inflammation   (IN-flah-**MAY**-shun) a basic pathologic process of cytologic and chemical reactions that occur in the blood vessels and tissues in response to an injury or irritation; a protective immune response that is triggered by any type of injury or irritant.

inspiratory stridor   (STRYE-dor) high-pitched sound during inspiration due to blocked airways.

insulin   a hormone secreted by the beta cells in the islets of Langerhans in the pancreas; responsible for glucose usage.

intermittent claudication   (KLAW-dih-**KAY**-shun) the condition of developing muscle cramps that are relieved with rest and increased with activity.

interphalangeal   (inter = between, phalangeal = finger bones) usually referring to joints between the finger bones.

intertrochanteric fracture   one that is in the trochanteric area of the femur.

intoxicated   when the blood alcohol level reaches 0.10% or more.

intracapsular fracture   a fracture inside the joint capsule.

intractable   difficult to stop or control.

intrathecal   (IN-trah-**THEE**-kal; intra = within, thecal = spinal cord) injected into the spinal fluid.

intravenous pyelogram (IVP)   (IN-trah-**VEE**-nus **PYE**-ehloh-GRAM) an X-ray picture taken after injecting dye into the individual's bloodstream; the dye accumulates in the urinary tract and improves the ability to identify obstructions, tumors, and deformities.

intrinsic factor   a substance secreted by the stomach lining necessary for absorption of vitamin B$_{12}$.

intussusception   (IN-tus-sus-**SEP**-shun) the telescoping of one part of the intestine over the adjoining section.

invasion   spreading into surrounding or local tissue.

ischemia   (iss-**KEE**-me-ah) hypoxia of cells or tissues caused by decreased blood flow.

islets of Langerhans   specialized cells in the pancreas that act as an endocrine gland secreting hormones, primarily insulin.

isoimmune   a high level of a specific antibody as a result of antigen stimulation from the red blood cells of another individual; isoimmunization may occur when an Rh-negative person is treated with a transfusion of Rh-positive blood.

J

jaundice   (JAWN-dis) a yellowish color in the skin and sclera due to increased bile pigments in the blood.

K

Kaposi's sarcoma   (KAP-oh-seez sar-KOH-ma) blood vessel cancer that causes reddish-purple skin lesions.

karyotyping   a method of identifying chromosomes; this process involves taking a picture of a cell during mitosis, arranging the chromosome pairs in order from largest to smallest, and numbering them 1 to 23.

keloid   (KEE-loid) excessive collagen formation, often resulting in a hard, raised scar.

keratin   a tough protein substance in nails, hair, and body tissues.

ketoacidosis   acidosis seen in diabetes mellitus caused by overproduction of ketone bodies.

ketones   waste products produced when tissue cells burn fats and proteins.

kidneys-ureter-bladder (KUB)   a common X-ray of the structures of the urinary tract to determine abnormalities.

Koplik's spots   spots seen in the mouth in the early stage of measles; these spots are rather unique to measles and are often the definitive symptom that confirms the diagnosis.

L

laceration   a cut in the skin.

laminectomy   surgery to cut away part of the vertebra to open the area around the spinal nerve.

laparoscopy   (LAP-ah-**ROS**-ko-pee; laparo = abdomen, scopy = scope procedure) looking inside the abdominal cavity with a lighted scope; commonly used to view the female organs for abnormalities, diagnose endometriosis, and perform a tubal ligation.

lesion   (LEE-zhun) any discontinuity of tissue.

lethal   something that kills.

leukemia   (loo-KEE-me-ah; leuk = white, emia = blood) a progressive overgrowth of abnormal leukocytes; a malignant disease of the bone marrow.

leukocytopenia   (leukocyte = white cell, penia = decrease) a decrease in white cell count.

leukocytosis   (leuko = white, cyto = cell, osis = condition) an increase in white cell count.

leukorrhea   (LOO-koh-**REE**-ah; leuk = white, orrhea = flow or discharge) a white, usually foul-smelling, vaginal discharge.

lipids   fats or fat-like substances.

lithotripsy   (litho = stone, tripsy = breaking) a procedure for breaking kidney or gallbladder stones.

longitudinal fracture   one that runs the length of the bone.

lumen   (LOO-men) the inner open space or width of a tubular structure or anatomical part.

lymph   a clear liquid similar to plasma containing many white cells.

lymphadenopathy   (lim-FAD-eh-**NOP**-ah-thee; lymph = lymph, adeno = gland, opathy = disease) any disease of the lymph glands.

lymphangiography (lim-FAN-jee-**OG**-rah-fee; lymph = lymph, angio = vessel, ography = procedure) a radiographic procedure consisting of injecting a contrast dye and taking X-rays of lymphatic vessels.

lymphangiopathy (lim-FAN-jee-**OP**-ah-thee; lymph = lymph, angio = vessel, opathy = disease) a general term to describe any disease of the lymph vessels.

lymphedema (lymph = lymph, edema = swelling) an abnormal collection of lymph fluid, usually observed in the extremities.

lymphocytes white blood cells formed in lymphatic tissue.

lymphocytopenia or lymphopenia a decrease in lymphocytes.

lymphocytosis increase in number of lymphocytes.

lymphoma (lim-FOH-ma) malignant neoplasms of blood-forming organs.

M

macrophage (macro = large, phage = eat) a monocyte that leaves the bloodstream and moves into the tissue and becomes phagocytic.

magnetic resonance imaging (MRI) a diagnostic radiologic test using nuclear magnetic resonance technology.

malaise general ill feeling.

malignant (mah-LIG-nant) deadly or progressing to death; cancerous.

mammography (mam-OG-rah-fee; mammo = breast, ography = procedure to take a picture) a procedure of taking an X-ray picture of breast tissue.

mammoplasty (**MAM**-oh-PLAS-tee; mammo = breast, plasty = surgical repair or restructuring) a surgical procedure that involves reconstruction of the breast with plastic surgery and prosthetic breast implants.

mania extreme elation or agitation.

mast cells also called tissue histiocytes; found in all tissues of the body; play a major role in the inflammatory process.

mastectomy (mas-TECK-toh-me; mast = breast, ectomy = excision) surgical removal of the breast.

mastoidectomy (MAS-toy-**DECK**-toh-me; ectomy = removal or excision) a procedure used to prevent complications and preserve hearing by removing the bony partitions forming the mastoid cells.

medical ethics values and decisions in medical practice including relationships to patient, patient family, peer physicians, and society.

meiosis the process of reproduction of germ cells in which they divide before duplication.

melena (meh-LEE-nah) dark tarry stool due to blood in feces.

meniscus semilunar articular cartilage found inside the knee joint.

metacarpophalangeal (meta = beyond, carpo = wrist, phalangeal = finger bones) referring to the metacarpus and the phalanges; specifically, the articulations between them.

metaplasia (MET-ah-**PLAY**-zee-ah) a cellular adaptation in which the cell changes to another type of cell.

metastasis (meh-TAS-tah-sis) spreading to distant sites.

metastasize (meh-TAS-tah-sighz) move or spread.

metastatic (MET-ah-**STAT**-ic) moves from a site of origin to a secondary site in the body.

metatarsophalangeal (meta = between, tarso = foot, phalangeal = toe bones) referring to the metatarsus and the phalanges; specifically, the articulations between them.

microcephaly (micro = small, cephal = brain) having an abnormally small head; usually associated with mental retardation.

mineralization a process that causes the characteristic hardness of bones.

mineralocorticoids one group of steroids of the adrenal cortex that influences sodium and potassium metabolism.

mitosis the process of reproduction of cells in which the 46 chromosomes duplicate and divide into two identical daughter cells, each containing 46 chromosomes.

mood emotion.

morbidity the state of being diseased.

mortality the quality of being mortal or destined to die.

mortality rate (also called death rate); it is related to the number of people who die with a disease in a certain amount of time.

motility ability to move.

multiparity (mul-TIP-ah-rah-tee) multiple births.

murmur an abnormal sound in the heart or vascular system.

MVAs motor vehicle accidents.

myelogram an X-ray picture taken after injecting dye into the spinal canal to reveal compression on the spinal cord or spinal nerves.

myringotomy (MIR-in-**GOT**-oh-me; myringo = eardrum, tomy = incision into) incision into the eardrum to remove fluid.

myxedema (MECK-seh-**DEE**-mah) advanced hypothyroidism in an adult.

N

necrosis (nee-CROW-sis) cellular death.

neoplasia (nee-oh-PLAY-zee-ah) the development of a new type of cell with an uncontrolled growth pattern.

neoplasms (new growths) an increase in cell number, leading to an increase in tissue size; commonly called tumors.

nephrectomy (neh-FREC-toh-me; nephr = kidney, ectomy = excision or removal) the surgical removal of the kidney.

neutropenia a decrease in neutrophils.

nits lice eggs.

nocturia (nock-TOO-ree-ah; noc = night, uria = urine) excessive voiding at night.

nondisplaced fracture one in which the fragments are still in correct position.

nosocomial (NOS-oh-**KOH**-me-al) a disease acquired from the hospital environment.

nuchal rigidity a stiffness in the neck that resists bending the neck forward or sideways.

O

oblique fracture a fracture that runs in a transverse pattern.

obsession repetition of a thought or emotion.

occult blood hidden blood; invisible except under microscopic examination.

oliguria (OL-ih-**GOO**-ree-ah; olig = scanty or few, uria = urine) a decrease in urine output.

oncology (ong-KOL-oh-jee) the study of tumors.

oophoritis (OH-of-oh-**RYE**-tis) inflammation of the ovary.

open (compound) fracture a fracture involving the bone puncturing through the skin, or an object puncturing the skin, making an opening through the skin to the fracture site.

ophthalmoscope (aft-THAL-moh-skope; ophthalm = eye, scope = instrument used to look) the instrument used for a basic examination of the eye.

opportunistic normal flora bacteria that take the "opportunity" to cause infection in the host.

orchiectomy (OR-kee-**ECK**-toh-me; orchi = testicle, ectomy = removal) removal of the testicle(s).

orchitis (or-KYE-tis) inflammation of a testis.

organ rejection when the body recognizes an organ (after a transplant) as foreign and attacks it, leading to organ death.

organic related to an organ or physical component.

ORIF (open reduction, internal fixation) surgical opening over a fracture site and internally fixing the fracture with plates, screws, or pins.

orthopnea (or-THOP-nee-ah; ortho = straight, pnea = breathing) the condition in which an individual has difficulty breathing in a lying position, or is able to breathe with less difficulty when standing or sitting straight up.

osteomyelitis inflammation or infection of the marrow of the bone.

ostomy (OS-toh-me) an artificial opening, which may be temporary or permanent, often involving the intestines or urinary tract.

otalgia (oh-TAL-gee-ah; oto = ear, algia = pain) ear pain.

otoscope (OH-toh-skope; oto = ear, scope = instrument to look) the instrument used to examine the ear.

ova and parasite (O&P) an examination of a stool specimen for the presence of adult parasites or their eggs (ova).

P

palliative (PAL-ee-ay-tiv) something that is directed toward relief of symptoms but does not cure.

pallor (PAL-or) lack of color; paleness.

palmar erythema (ER-ih-**THEE**-mah) unusual redness of the palms of the hands.

palpation feeling lightly or by pressing firmly on internal organs or structures.

pancytopenia (pan = all, cyto = cell, penia = decrease) severe decrease or total absence of erythrocytes, leukocytes, and thrombocytes.

panhypopituitarism (pan = all, hypo = decreased) the condition in which the secretion of all anterior pituitary hormones is inadequate or absent; caused by a variety of disorders.

panhysterectomy (pan = all, hyster = uterus, ectomy = excision) the surgical removal of the ovaries, fallopian tubes, and uterus.

Pap test also called Papanicolaou test; a screening for cancer using and examining the cells scraped from the cervical area.

paralytic obstruction a decrease or absence of peristalsis that causes intestinal blockage.

paraplegia (PAR-ah-**PLEE**-jee-ah; para = beyond or two like parts, plegia = paralysis) a loss of movement and feeling in the trunk and both legs.

parenteral (pah-REN-ter-al) a delivery route for fluid or medications that includes subcutaneous, intramuscular, or intravenous administration.

paresthesia (PAR-es-**THEE**-see-ah) abnormal sensation, burning, tingling, or numbness.

paronychia (PAR-oh-**NICK**-ee-ah) an infection of the skin around the nail.

parotid glands the salivary glands located just in front of the ears.

paroxysmal (PAR-ock-**SIZ**-mal) spasm or convulsion.

patency openness.

patent open.

pathogenesis (PATH-oh-**JEN**-ah-sis; patho = disease, genesis = arising) a description of how a particular disease progresses.

pathogens (PATH-oh-jens) microorganisms or agents that cause disease.

pathologic (path-oh-LODGE-ick) caused by a pathogen or a disease.

pathologic fracture (path-oh-LODGE-ick) a fracture caused by weakness from another disease.

pathologist   (pah-THOL-oh-jist; patho = disease, logist = one who studies) one who studies disease.

pathology   (pah-THOL-oh-jee; patho = disease, ology = study) the study of disease.

percussion   (per-KUSH-un) tapping over various body areas to produce a vibrating sound.

perforation   an abnormal opening in an organ or tissue.

perfusion   (per-FYOU-zuhn) to pour through or supply with blood.

peristalsis   the contraction of muscles along the gastrointestinal tract to move food and fluid.

peritonitis   (PER-ih-toe-**NIGH**-tis) an inflammation of the peritoneum.

petechiae   (pee-TEE-kee-ee) small hemorrhages in the skin.

petit mal   a term applied to a type of seizure; these seizures consist of a brief change in the level of consciousness without convulsions; the involved individual may show symptoms of blank staring, blinking, and/or twitching of the eyes or mouth.

phenotype   the physical expression of a genetic trait such as eye, hair, and skin color.

phimosis   (figh-MOH-sis) abnormally tight foreskin of the penis.

photophobia   (photo = light, phobia = fear) an abnormal fear of light.

pilonidal cyst   (PYE-loh-**NIGH**-dal) a particular type of sebaceous cyst found in the midline of the sacral area.

plaque   (PLACK) a patch; dental plaque is a sticky mass of microorganisms growing on teeth.

***Pneumocystis carinii* (NEW-moh-*SIS*-tis kah-RYE-neeeye) pneumonia**   a protozoan infection of the lungs, commonly occurring in immunodeficient individuals.

polydipsia   (POL-ee-**DIP**-see-ah; poly = many, dipsia = thirst or drinking) excessive thirst.

polyp   (POL-ip) an inward projection of the mucosal lining of the colon.

polyuria   (POL-ee-**YOU**-ree-ah; poly = many, uria = urine) excessive urination.

portal hypertension   increased pressure in the portal system frequently seen in cirrhosis.

Pott's fracture   fracture of the lower part of the fibula and tibia, with outward displacement of the foot.

precocious (puberty)   premature (early) sexual development.

predisposing factors   also known as risk factors; make a person more susceptible to disease.

preeclampsia   (PREE-ee-**KLAMP**-see-ah) the development of hypertension with proteinuria and/or edema due to pregnancy; also called toxemia.

prevalent   occurring more often.

preventive   something that reduces risk.

primary union   also called healing by first intention; involves approximating the edges of the wound.

primigravid   (PRE-mih-**GRAV**-id; primi = first, gravid = pregnancy) the term used to describe a female who is pregnant with her first child.

productive cough   coughing up sputum or excessive mucus.

progesterone   (pro-**JESS**-ter-ohn) a female sex hormone produced by the ovary.

prognosis   (prawg-KNOW-sis) the predicted or expected outcome of the disease.

prone   positioned face down on the stomach.

prophylactic   (pro-fil-LACK-tic) something that works to prevent.

prosthesis   (pros-THEE-sis) an artificial part.

proteinuria   protein in the urine; specific protein or albumin may be identified, resulting in albuminuria.

protozoa   a parasite of the phylum Protozoa; a single-celled microscopic member of the animal kingdom.

pruritus   (proo-RYE-tus) itching.

puerperal   (pyou-ER-pier-al) relating to childbirth.

purpura   (PER-pew-rah) a bleeding disorder characterized by bleeding into the skin and mucous membranes initially turning the affected areas purplish in color.

purulent   (PURR-you-lent) loaded with dead and dying neutrophils, tissue debris, and pyogenic (pus-forming) bacteria.

pus   white or yellow exudate due to death of numerous neutrophils mixed with exudate or blood fluid.

pustules   (PUS-tyoul) small, pus-filled lesions.

pyloromyotomy   (pyloro = pyloric, myo = muscle, otomy = cut into) a surgical procedure that involves incising and suturing the pyloric sphincter muscle.

pyoderma   (PYE-oh-**DER**-mah) inflammatory, purulent dermatitis.

pyogenic   (PIE-oh-**JEN**-ick; pyo = pus, genic = arising) pus forming.

pyuria   (pye-YOU-ree-ah; py = pus, uria = urine) pus in the urine.

Q

quadriplegia   (KWAD-rih-**PLEE**-jee-ah; quadri = four, plegia = paralysis) the loss of movement and feeling in the trunk and all four extremities with the accompanying loss of bowel, bladder, and sexual function.

R

radial keratotomy   (KER-ah-**TOT**-oh-me; kerato = cornea, otomy = incision) a surgical procedure to correct myopia; incisions are made in a radial fashion in the cornea to flatten the cornea, thus shortening the length of the eyeball and correcting the refractive error.

radiation   the process of using light, short waves, ultraviolet or X-rays, or any other rays.

radical cystectomy   (radical = a treatment that seeks to cure; aggressive, not palliative or conservative; sis-TECT-toh-me; cyst = bladder, ectomy = excision or removal) the removal of the entire bladder, usually done as treatment for cancer of the bladder.

radiologic   relating to medical imaging using X-rays, ionizing radiation, nuclear magnetic resonance, or ultrasound.

rales   (RALZ) an abnormal discontinuous breath sound caused by narrowed bronchi and heard primarily on inspiration during auscultation of the chest.

recessive   lacking control; weak.

Reed–Sternberg cell   a large connective tissue cell found in lymphatic tissue indicative of Hodgkin's disease.

remission   a time when symptoms are diminished or temporarily resolved.

rhinitis   (RYE-**NIGH**-tis) inflammation of the nasal mucous membrane.

rhinorrhea   (rhino = nose, orrhea = run through) a runny nose.

rhonchi   (RONG-kigh) abnormal wheezing breath sounds caused by partial airway blockage and heard during inspiration, expiration, or both during auscultation of the chest.

RICE   acronym for Rest, Ice, Compression, and Elevation, the activities to manage soft tissue trauma like those often associated with sports injuries.

rickettsiae   (ric-KET-see-ah) microscopic organisms that are intermediate between bacteria and viruses. They live in the host and are spread by lice, fleas, ticks, and mites.

RPR (rapid plasma reagin)   a blood test for syphilis.

S

Salmonella   (SAL-moh-**NEL**-ah) a group of gram-negative bacteria often responsible for intestinal infections.

salpingitis   (SAL-pin-**JIGH**-tis; salping = fallopian tube, itis = inflammation) inflammation of the fallopian tube.

sarcoma   (sar-KO-mah) a malignant neoplasm arising from connective tissue.

scar   skin lesion resulting from fibrous connective tissue repair.

sciatica   pain along the sciatic nerve, often radiating down the leg and caused by pressure on the spinal nerve.

sebum   oil produced by the sebaceous glands.

secondary union   also called healing by secondary intention; the same process as primary union, but involving a larger degree of tissue damage and more inflammation to resolve.

seizure   a sudden onset or attack, but the term is commonly used to indicate a convulsive seizure as occurs in epilepsy.

self-antigen   the body's own antigen.

septicemia   (SEP-tih-**SEE**-me-ah; septic = dirty, contaminated, emia = blood) a systemic disease caused by the spread of microorganisms in the blood; also called blood poisoning.

signs   observable or measurable factors used to determine a diagnosis.

simple (closed) fracture   a fracture that does not break through the skin.

sinus   a tract or opening to the surface of the body formed by a large ruptured abscess.

somatic   related to the body.

spasms   uncontrolled muscle contractions.

spider angiomas   telangiectasias or small dilated vessels in the skin; commonly seen on the face and chest of individuals with cirrhosis of the liver.

spinal stenosis   (stenosis = narrowing) the condition of narrowing of nerve root openings in the spinal column.

spiral fracture   a fracture that twists around the bone.

splenomegaly   (SPLEE-no-**MEG**-ah-lee) enlargement of the spleen.

sputum   (SPYOU-tum) fluid or secretions coughed up from the lungs.

staging   determining the degree of spread of a malignant tumor.

stapedectomy   (STAY-peh-**DECK**-toh-me; stape = stapes, ectomy = removal or excision) a procedure that removes the stapes bone in the middle ear and replaces it with a prosthesis.

status asthmaticus   (AZTH-**MAH**-ti-kus) a severe asthma attack that lasts for several days.

status epilepticus   a life-threatening event; a state of continued convulsive seizure with no recovery of consciousness; it is a medical emergency.

stellate fracture   a fracture that forms a star-like pattern.

sterility   inability to conceive. In the female, an inability to become pregnant. In the male, an inability to impregnate a female, often related to sperm quality or quantity.

stoma   (STO-mah) a mouth-like opening; the opening on the abdominal wall for an ostomy.

stool   fecal matter; feces; bowel movement (BM).

strep throat   an acute form of pharyngitis caused by *Streptococcus*.

streptococcal   (**STREHP**-toh-**KAHK**-al) relating to the organism *Streptococcus*; an anaerobic, gram-positive bacteria.

stress fracture   related to too much weight or pressure.

striae   stretch marks on the skin.

stricture   a narrowing.

subcapital fracture   a fracture below (sub) the head (caput) of the femur.

subdural (hematoma)   (SUB-**DOO**-ral) blood collecting between the outer (dura mater) layer and the middle (arachnoid) layer of the meninges.

supine   (SUE-pine) positioned on the back.

suppurative   (SUP-you-**RAY**-tive) formation of pus.

suprapubic catheter   a catheter that is inserted surgically through the pelvic wall as is often done after urinary tract surgeries.

symptoms   what patients report as their problem or problems.

syncope   (SIN-koh-pee) fainting.

syndrome   (SIN-drome) a group of symptoms that may be caused by a specific disease but also may be caused by several interrelated problems.

systemic   refers to the entire or whole body rather than to a part or region.

systolic   (sis-TALL-ick) relating to cardiac systole; the process of cardiac contraction (heartbeat) when blood is ejected into the systemic circulation.

T

tachycardia   (TACH-ee-**KAR**-dee-ah; tachy = rapid, cardia = heart rate) a rapid heart rate; usually a rate over 100 beats per minute.

tachypnea   (TACK-ihp-**NEE**-ah; tachy = rapid, pnea = breathing) a severely increased respiratory rate.

tetany   (TET-ah-nee) hyperirritability of muscles causing a spasm-like condition; usually the result of a lack of calcium.

thoracentesis   (THOR-rah-sen-**TEE**-sis; thora = chest, centesis = puncture) a procedure in which a puncture is made into the chest cavity to withdraw air (or fluid); a chest tube also may be inserted to help the lung reexpand.

thrombocytopenia   (THROM-boh-SIGH-toh-**PEE**-nee-ah; thrombocyte = platelet, penia = decrease) a decrease in platelets, leading to a coagulation problem.

thrombocytosis   (THROM-boh-sigh-**TOH**-sis; thrombocyte = platelet, osis = condition of) an increase in platelets.

thrombus   (THROM-bus) a blood clot attached to a vein or artery.

thyroid storm   a sudden life-threatening exacerbation of all symptoms of hyperthyroidism.

tinnitus   (tin-EYE-tus) ringing in the ears.

tolerance   the ability to endure a larger amount of a substance without an adverse effect, or the need for a larger amount or dose of the drug to have the same effect.

tonometry   (toh-NOM-eh-tree; tono = tone or pressure, metry = measurement) a procedure to measure the pressure inside the eye.

tonsillectomy   (TON-sih-**LECT**-toh-me; ectomy = removal) the surgical removal of the tonsils.

tophi   small, whitish nodules of uric acid.

topical   placed on the skin.

TPN   total parenteral nutrition; intravenously giving a special solution that meets the total nutritional needs of the individual.

transurethral resection (TUR)   (trans = through, urethral = uretha; resection = partial excision) a surgical procedure that may be performed to remove a tumor, visualize a structure, or take a piece of tissue for biopsy; a cystoscope is passed through the urinary meatus and the urethra for this procedure.

transverse fracture   one that runs across or at a 90-degree angle.

trauma   (TRAW-mah) a physical or mental injury.

triage   (tree-AUZH) the prioritizing of care.

Trichomonas   (TRICK-oh-**MOH**-nas) a parasitic protozoan that commonly infects the vagina and causes trichomoniasis.

tumor   "swelling" or growth, originally used in the description of the swelling related to inflammation.

tympanoplasty   (TIM-pah-no-**PLAS**-tee; tympano = eardrum, plasty = surgical correction) surgery to repair the tympanic membrane.

tympanostomy   (TIM-pan-**OSS**-toh-me; tympano = eardrum, ostomy = new opening) a procedure in which tubes, commonly called PE tubes or pediatric ear tubes, are placed through the tympanic membrane to prevent the accumulation of fluid.

U

ulcer   a crater-like lesion in the skin or mucous membranes.

undifferentiated   change in a cell that is more general or appears more malignant; not clearly or easily identified.

urea   a common nitrogenous waste product that is normally filtered from the blood.

uremia   (you-REE-me-ah; ur = urine, emia = blood) a toxic condition of the blood due to high levels of waste products.

urgency   the severe need to urinate.

urinalysis   (YOU-rih-**NAL**-ih-sis; urine analysis) a laboratory urine test for pH, specific gravity, protein, glucose or sugar, and blood; it also includes a microscopic examination to determine the presence of bacteria, crystals, and casts.

urine culture and sensitivity (C&S)   a laboratory analysis that determines the type of bacteria present and the most effective antibiotic to prescribe for treatment.

urticaria   (UR-tih-**KAR**-ree-ah) an allergic reaction resulting in a skin eruption of wheals that causes intense itching.

V

vasopressin   antidiuretic hormone (ADH) secreted by the posterior portion of the pituitary gland.

Venereal Disease Research Laboratory (VDRL)   a blood test to screen for syphilis.

vermiform   (VER-my-form) worm-like.

vertigo   (VER-tih-go) dizziness.

vesicles   (VES-ih-kuls) blister-like eruptions on the skin.

virilism   (VIR-ill-izm) masculinization; used to describe the occurrence or presence of male characteristics in a female or prepubescent male.

virulent   (VIR-u-lent; infectious) difficult to kill; able to produce disease.

viruses   a large group of infectious agents; they are much smaller than bacteria and must be viewed with an electron microscope. They can pass through fine filters that would retain most bacteria.

viscous   (VIS-cuss) thick.

volvulus   (VOL-view-lus) the bowel twisted on itself.

W

wheal(s)   round, slightly reddened, spot(s) on the skin, usually accompanied by intense itching; also called urticarial lesion(s) or hives; caused by an allergic reaction to something such as food or medication.

wheezing   a whistling, musical, or raspy sound during breathing, usually indicative of partially blocked respiratory passages.

withdrawal   the unpleasant physical and psychological effects resulting from stopping the use of a substance after an individual is addicted.

X

xerosis   (zee-ROE-sis) dry skin.

Index

A

sleep disorders, 552–553
somatoform disorders, 549–550
substance-related, 536–542
Mescaline, 541
Metabolic diseases, integumentary system, 447
Metacarpophalangeal joints, 109
Metaplasia, 22, 23, 24f, 36
Metastasis, 35–36
  bloodstream, 35–36
  cavity, 36
  defined, 30
Metastatic cancers, 18
Metatarsophalangeal joint, 111
Methamphetamine abuse, 539
Methaqualone (Quaalude), 540
Methicillin-resistant *Staphylococcus aureus* (MRSA), 61–62, 66, 441–442
Metrorrhagia, 396
Microcephaly, 495
Microthrombi, 87, 145
Middle ear, 361
Migraine headache, 340
Mineralization, osteomalacia and, 108
Mineralocorticoids, 304, 312
Miscarriage (spontaneous abortion), 409
Mitosis, 476, 476f
Mitotic cells, facultative mitotic, 57
Monocytes, 74
Mononucleosis, 141, 220, 508
Monovision, 367
Mood disorders, 545–547
Mood or affective disorders, 545–547
Mood stabilizers, 532
Morbidity, 25
Morning sickness, 409
Mortality rate, 9
Motility, 228
Motion sickness, 379
Motor vehicle accidents (MVAs), 16
Mouth
  cancer of, 232
  diseases of, 231–233
  trauma to the, 251–252
Mouth tightening, scleroderma and, 87
MRI (magnetic resonance imaging), 102
  of head, 103f

MRSA (methicillin-resistant *Staphylococcus aureus*), 61–62, 66, 441–442
Multiparity, 410
Multiple myeloma, 143–144, 143f
Multiple personality disorder, 548
Multiple sclerosis, 353
Mumps, 505–506
Munchausen by proxy, 550
Munchausen syndrome, 550
Murmur, heart, 173
Muscle relaxants, 104
Muscles. *See also* Musculoskeletal system
  diseases of, 112–114
  functions of, 101
Muscular dystrophy (MD), 112–113, 480–481
Musculoskeletal system, 99–126
  aging and, 126
  anatomy and physiology of, 100–102
  diseases and disorders of, 102–126. *See also* Trauma
    common drugs for, 104
    de Quervain's disease, 125
    diagnostic tests, 102
    diseases of the bone, 102–108
    diseases of the joints, 108–112
    diseases of the muscles and connective tissue, 112–114
    ganglion cyst, 113, 113f
    genetic and developmental, 480–482
    gout, 111
    hallux valgus, 111–112, 112f
    kyphosis, 104
    lordosis, 104, 105f
    muscular dystrophy (MD), 112–113
    myasthenia gravis, 126
    osteoarthritis (degenerative joint disease), 109–111, 109t, 110f
    osteomalacia, 108
    osteomyelitis, 107–108, 108f
    osteoporosis, 105–107, 106f, 107f, 107t
    Paget's disease, 125
    rare diseases, 125–126
    scoliosis, 105, 105f
    spinal deformities, 103–104
    temporomandibular joint syndrome (TMJ), 112
    tetanus, 113–114
    tuberculosis (TB) of the bone, 125

Myasthenia gravis, 83–85, 84f, 85f, 126
Mycobacterium tuberculosis, 199–200
Myelogram, 120
Myelomeningocele, 484
Myocardial infarction (MI), 158, 169–170, 170f
Myocarditis, 81, 173
Myofibrils, 101
Myopia, 365, 366, 366f
Myringotomy, 374
Myxedema, 310

N

Nails, 433
Narcissistic personalities, 551
Narcolepsy, 553
Narcotics abuse, 541
Nasogastric tube, 19
Natural resistance, 75
Necrosis, 24
Needle aspiration, 392f
Neoplasia, 22, 24
Neoplasms, 17–18, 30t. *See also* Cancer; Tumors
  appearance and growth pattern of, 30
  benign, 17, 30
    appearance and growth pattern of, 30
    growth of, 32–33
  cellular changes progressing to, 36, 37f
  cellular growth patterns, 32f
  classification of, 30–31, 31f
  comparison of benign and malignant, 33t
  defined, 30
  examples of, 18t
  growth of, 31–33
  hyperplasias and, 33, 34
  malignant. *See* Cancer
  origins and names for, 31t
  terminology related to, 30
  tissue of origin of, 30
Nephrectomy, 292
Nervous system, 327–354, 328f
  anatomy and physiology, 328–330
  cerebral lobes, 329f
  diseases and disorders, 331–354
    aging and, 353–354